SEX STEROIDS

Edited by **Scott M. Kahn**

Sex Steroids
Edited by Scott M. Kahn

Published by InTech
Janeza Trdine 9, 51000 Rijeka, Croatia

Publishing Process Manager Bojan Rafaj

Technical Editor Teodora Smiljanic

Cover Designer InTech Design Team

Additional hard copies can be obtained from orders@intechopen.com

Sex Steroids, Edited by Scott M. Kahn
p. cm.
ISBN 978-953-307-857-1

For EU product safety concerns:
IN TECH d.o.o., Prolaz Marije Krucifikse Kozulić 3, 51000 Rijeka, Croatia,
info@intechopen.com or visit our website at intechopen.com.

Meet the editor

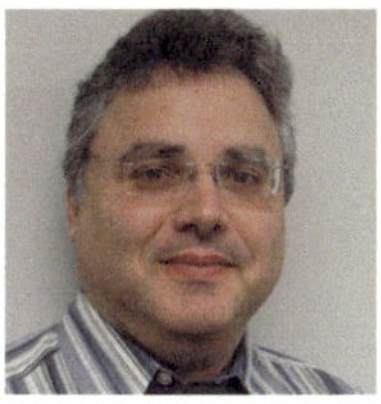

Dr Scott M. Kahn, Ph.D. is Director of Basic Urologic Research at St. Luke's-Roosevelt Institute for Health Sciences in New York City, and Member of the Herbert Irving Columbia Presbyterian Comprehensive Cancer Center, with an appointment in the Department of Urology. Additionally, Dr. Kahn serves as Biomarkers Council Chairman for the International Cancer Advocacy Network. Since receiving his Ph.D. from SUNY at Stony Brook in 1988, Dr. Kahn's research has covered a broad spectrum of cancer biology, including work on signal transduction, cell cycle control, cancer genetics, microsatellite instability, biomarker detection, and oncogene addiction. His more recent studies have focused on intracellular expression of the steroid binding protein, sex hormone-binding globulin in the prostate and breast, and its role in androgen and estrogen signaling.

Contents

Preface

In "Sex Steroids", we have compiled a collection of insightful and timely chapters meant to provide the reader with expert analyses on our current state of knowledge in select areas of sex steroid research. Sex steroids are central players in many fundamental biologic processes. In addition to their roles in reproduction, development, growth, differentiation, homeostasis, behavior, memory, etc., sex steroids are fundamentally involved in many diseases and disorders. Throughout the years, great progress have been made in our understanding of sex steroid actions at the molecular level. The classical model of sex steroid signaling involves diffusion of an androgen, estrogen, or progesterone across the cell membrane, where it binds to its cognate steroid receptor. This receptor then translocates to the cell nucleus, where it modulates the expression of steroid responsive genes. While many of the pleiotropic effects attributed to sex steroids are explained by this classical model, we know that their mechanisms of action are far more complex and intricate.

Aberrant sex steroid signaling programs are responsible for many aspects of altered sexual characteristics and development. Furthermore, the pioneering work of visionaries, such as George Beatson and Charles Huggins on hormone ablation as treatment for breast and prostate cancer, respectively, highlights the importance of sex steroids in the development and progression of these diseases. Sex steroids are implicated in cardiovascular disease, CNS diseases, memory loss, and a host of other afflictions. In this age of advancements in "–omics", platforms, computational and systems biology, and many other rapidly emerging areas, we should continue to anticipate tremendous advances in our understanding of sex steroid actions, their biologic properties, and their influence on disease prevention and progression.

The initial section of "Sex Steroids" entitled, "The Biology of Sex Steroids", features chapters on the evolutionary and functional overview of sex steroids, sex hormone-binding globulin and its effects on androgen responsiveness, estrogens and growth hormone action in the liver, hormonal feedback, and reproductive aging. Additional chapters include sex steroid receptors in teleocytes, and the influence of sex steroids on stress responsiveness. This is then followed by "Sex Steroids, Memory, and the Brain", which offers chapters on estrogen and brain protection, and estrogen influences on cognition and memory. The third section, "Sex Steroids and the Immune Response", includes chapters describing the fish immune response, the reciprocal nature of the reproductive and immune systems during ontogeny, modulation of the immune response by menopause and hormone therapy, and the role of sex steroids in the host-parasite interaction. The final section, entitled, "Therapy", presents chapters on the effect of postmenopausal therapy on adipose tissue, gonadotropin-suppressive therapy, and hormonal therapy for the treatment of malignant salivary gland tumors.

It is my hope, as editor of "Sex Steroids", that this book provides insights into the fascinating complexity of sex steroid biology that are of interest to seasoned researchers in this field. In addition, I hope it will stimulate newer investigators who are intrigued by the many exciting areas of sex steroid research that remains to be explored. I offer my sincerest appreciation to the many authors and scientists who devoted themselves to the work presented in this book.

I would like to close on a personal note. Earlier this year, the field of sex steroid research lost one of its most devoted and highly respected colleagues. Dr. Jonathan J. Li was a beloved mentor, and also a generous and dear friend who dedicated his professional life to understanding the role that estrogens play in breast cancer. For those of us who were fortunate to spend long hours with Dr. Li on the history of sex steroid research, discussing his views on the interplay between steroids and cancer, he will be greatly missed. Dr. Li, together with his wonderfully bright and talented wife, Sara, have impacted many areas of hormonal research, most recently on estrogen as an initiator of breast cancer. As one who greatly valued discourse in science and the field of sex hormones and cancer, Jonathan co-founded the International Symposium on Hormonal Oncogenesis (ISHO). As one of the more successful and highly acclaimed academic research symposia, the ISHO series has brought together renowned leaders from all over the world, as well as junior researchers in a warm and collegial manner. It is with this spirit of Jonathan's that I hope this book serves the complex and captivating field of sex steroids.

Scott M. Kahn
Director of Basic Urologic Research St. Luke's-Roosevelt Health
Science Center Adjunct Associate Research Scientist Department of Urology Member,
Herbert Irving Comprehensive Cancer Center Columbia University Chairman,
Biomarkers Council, International Cancer Advocacy Network (ICAN), New York,
USA

Part 1

Biology of Sex Steroids

1

Evolutionary Perspectives on Sex Steroids in the Vertebrates

Nigel C. Noriega
University of California at Davis,
Department of Neurobiology,
Physiology and Behavior
USA

1. Introduction

The term "sex-steroids" refers to estrogen, androgen and progestin products of vertebrate gonads. Sex steroids were so named for their influence on the sexually dimorphic development of the reproductive tract, secondary sex characters and central nervous system, which cause subsequent sexually dimorphic behavior and physiology (Phoenix et al. 1959b; Breedlove & Arnold 1983b). Receptors for sex-steroids are present in almost all tissues, and sex-steroids may be synthesized from cholesterol in the gonads, adrenals and brain. Although commonly described as endocrine components released into the bloodstream, sex-steroids may be generated through conversion from other (particularly adrenal) circulating steroids (Hinson et al. 2010) or generated de novo from cholesterol via intracrine pathways, as in the case of the brain neurosteroids (Baulieu 1997).

In this chapter we examine how sex-steroids fit into the larger themes of metazoan physiology and reproduction, and examine why these compounds may function the way they do in vertebrates. I aim to present broad concepts in a manner that is easily accessible to the non-specialized reader. It will be useful for the reader to be able to navigate modern versions of metazoan systematics. Therefore I aim to utilize the open-source nature of this publication by providing links that encourage the reader to use the Tree of Life web project (http://tolweb.org/tree/) for up-to-date "locations" of animals within the organization of living things. Navigation instructions for the Tree of Life web project are located at: (http://tolweb.org/tree/home.pages/navigating.html). In summary, clicking the leftward-pointing arrow on a given tree will navigate to the next broader category. Clicking text on the right side of the tree will navigate inside the highlighted group (the next narrower category).

2. Hormonal axes, gonadotropins and gonadotropin releasing hormones

In vertebrates, gonadal activity and steroid release are stimulated by members of a family of glycoprotein hormones known as gonadotropins. Follicle Stimulating Hormone (FSH) and Luteinizing Hormone (LH) typify the gonadotropins, which may be derived from multiple sources, but have highly conserved functionality across species. For example, chorionic gonadotropins (CG) are produced by primate fetus, placenta and pituitary gland (Cole 2009). The human chorionic gonadotropin (hCG) is an effective gonadotropin in amphibians

(Holland & Dumont 1975), fish (Targonska & Kucharczyk 2010) and reptiles (Arslan et al. 1977). This example is included to illustrate the conservative nature of gonadotropin function.

LH and FSH are released from the pituitary gland and regulated by Gonadotropin Releasing Hormone (GnRH) secreted from the hypothalamus of the brain. Several versions of GnRH also may be derived from multiple sources within the body, but the hypothalamus in the brain releases the organism-specific GnRH version that regulates gonadotropins. This control route: Hypothalamus → Pituitary → Gonad, is called the hypothalamic-pituitary-gonadal (HPG) axis, and is one of several highly conserved hypothalamic-pituitary-hormonal axes in the vertebrates.

The hypothalamus and pituitary operate under negative feedback control regulated by levels of gonadotropins and sex-steroids. These HPG axis feedback loops are in turn influenced by complex interactions between additional neurotransmitter and hormonal systems, which are themselves influenced by feedback from a vast array of additional hormones and signaling molecules (Williams & Larsen 2003; Oakley et al. 2009). Although the HPG axis is conceptually simple, it is one of several hubs in a network. This system is connected to other systems through complex interactive networks. The theme of interactive complexity is critical in modern considerations of endocrinology.

Reproduction is coordinated with growth and development, which is tied to metabolism. At the core of metabolic and developmental regulation is the Hypothalamic-Pituitary-Thyroid (HPT) axis. The pituitary gonadotropins (LH and FSH), thyroid stimulating hormone (TSH) as well as thyrostimulin (Nakabayashi et al. 2002) and chorionic gonadotropin (CG) are members of a family of heterodimeric glycoproteins (sharing a common α subunit but unique β subunits) which likely evolved from a common ancestral molecule (Kawauchi & Sower 2006). The discovery of thyrostimulin homologs in invertebrates suggests that this most ancestral heterodimeric glycoprotein hormone existed before the divergence of vertebrates and invertebrates (Sudo et al. 2005). This finding also supports hypotheses for the existence of early, overlapping yet functional HPG and HPT endocrine systems prior to extant vertebrates (Sower et al. 2009).

2.1 Separation of hormonal axes

Operating on similar principles of negative feedback inhibition, the hypothalamic-pituitary-gonadal (HPG) axis, the hypothalamic-pituitary-thyroid (HPT) axis and the hypothalamic-pituitary-adrenal (HPA) axis target organs are gonads, thyroid gland and adrenal glands respectively. Pituitary glycoproteins are used in both the HPG and HPT axes, with luteinizing hormone (LH) and follicle stimulating hormone (FSH) in the HPG axis and thyroid stimulating hormone (TSH) in the HPT axis. Although these axes appear separated in more derived vertebrates, they are less specified in evolutionarily older taxa. Agnathans (hagfishes and lampreys) are the oldest extant lineage of the vertebrates. The endocrine control of reproductive and thyroid functions in lamprey may reflect an intermediary stage on the evolutionary pathway to the highly specialized HPG and HPT axes currently observed in jawed vertebrates (gnathostoma: http://tolweb.org/Vertebrata) (Sower et al. 2009).

2.2 GnRH

Because the role of GnRH at the head of the HPG regulatory cascade is so highly conserved across vertebrates, GnRH has been referred to as the master molecule of reproduction. This master molecule acts in coordination with a host of other molecules. In order to facilitate this coordination, hypothalamic GnRH neurons are influenced by over 30 neurotransmitters, neuropeptides cytokines, hormones and growth factors in the brain (Gore 2002).

GnRH binding sites have been detected in several regions of the mammalian brain (Jennes et al. 1997), testicular Leydig cells (Bourne et al. 1980), the placenta (Bramley et al. 1992), ovarian luteal and granulosa cells (Hazum & Nimrod 1982), adrenal cortex (Eidne et al. 1985), immune tissues including thymus (Marchetti et al. 1989), spleen, blood lymphocytes (Marchetti et al. 1998), and several other tissues (Gore 2002). Although the HPG function of GnRH is highly conserved, possible alternative roles for GnRH molecules are poorly understood and rarely investigated. For example, the prevalence of GnRH-II in the midbrain of most vertebrates and its association with sensory and motor functions implies that GnRH molecules may have been important neural regulators (Tsai & Zhang 2008). However, interruption of GnRH function produces sterility in all vertebrate classes, and the pattern of GnRH expression in brains across vertebrate classes is so ubiquitous that some authors have proposed the existence of GnRH "lineages" such as a conserved GnRH-II or mesencephalic lineage, and a hypothalamic or "releasing" lineage (Somoza et al. 2002).

Such ubiquity may be indicative of more generalized roles for GnRH in ancient organisms. The presence of multiple GnRH genes in all vertebrate classes, as well as the homology of functional GnRH peptides and receptors between vertebrates, and tunicates (compare Craniata and Urochordata in http://tolweb.org/Chordata/2499) indicate that GnRH genes were present before the evolution of vertebrates (Somoza et al. 2002). It is suggested that in ancestral chordates, before the evolution of the pituitary, GnRH was released from sinuses near the gonads into the bloodstream and acted directly on the gonads (Powell et al. 1996).

Because, GnRH molecules are small (10-15 peptides), diverse, and can serve multiple functions in the same organism, it is difficult to assess the significance or evolutionary directionality of single peptide changes in GnRH structure. The short length of these peptides also makes statistically rigorous sequence comparisons difficult, and raises questions as to whether GnRH genes in distant evolutionary lineages are the result of convergent evolution or orthologous genes. Despite these difficulties, phylogenetic analyses have elucidated relationships among the vertebrate GnRH peptides and receptors (Levavi-Sivan et al. 2010). The discovery of a receptor for octopus GnRH with sequence (Kanda et al. 2006) and functional similarity to vertebrate GnRH receptor (Millar et al. 2004) suggests that a common GnRH ancestor may have been shared between chordates and protostomes (Tsai & Zhang 2008). Even in modern times, various GnRH molecules show cross functionality between the protostomes and deuterostomes (Table 1).

2.3 System complexity: Sex-steroid coordination with other hormone systems

Dynamic changes in serum sex-steroid levels are associated with sexual behavior. This is accomplished through HPG coordination with other hormonal systems where metabolic regulators such as Polypeptide YY, ghrelin, glucose, insulin and leptin influence GnRH release (Fernandez-Fernandez et al. 2006; Gamba & Pralong 2006; Tena-Sempere 2008; Roland & Moenter 2011). Progesterone acts in coordination with estradiol to regulate female sexual receptivity in reptiles (Wu et al. 1985). Opiates modulate gonadotropin secretion in mammals (Brooks et al. 1986). Adrenal steroids such as corticosterone affect courtship behavior in amphibians (Moore & Miller 1984). What often appear to be effects of testosterone are mediated through the conversion of testosterone to other androgens or estrogens (Callard 1983).

Source taxon	Molecule	Effect	Recipient	Recipient taxon	Reference
cnidarian	GnRH (HPLC purified)	LH release	Sea porgy pituitary cells	fish	(Twan et al. 2006)
vertebrate	chicken GnRH-II*	Δ in neuronal discharge from reproductive cells	California sea slug	gastropod	(Zhang et al. 2000)
gastropod	GnRH (HPLC purified)	gonadotropin release	goldfish pituitary cells	fish	(Goldberg et al. 1993)
cephalopod	GnRH (HPLC purified)	LH release	quail pituitary cells	bird	(Iwakoshi et al. 2002)
mammal, bird, fish lamprey	GnRH (5 commercial preps)	[^{3}H]thymidine incorporation	*Crassostria gigas* gonial cells	bivalve	(Pazos & Mathieu 1999)
mammal	mammal GnRH	mitosis	*Mytilus edulis* mantle cells	bivalve	(Pazos & Mathieu 1999)
yeast	α-factor	LH release	rat pituitary cells	mammal	(Ciejek et al. 1977) (Loumaye et al. 1982)

Table 1. Examples showing GnRH cross functionality between organisms whose evolutionary divergence pre-dates the split between protostomes and deuterostomes.

The steroid hormone binding globulins (SHBG) form a third class of steroid binding protein in addition to nuclear and membrane bound receptors (Section 3), and are distinguished by their rapid dissociation constants (Pardridge 1987). Increased ligand specificity in more recently derived lineages indicates that SHBGs may have been important in the evolution of complex endocrine systems. For example, circulating steroid binding proteins appear scarce in the lampreys (Hyperoartia: http://tolweb.org/Vertebrata/14829) where an α1 globulin is specific to progesterone and a β globulin is specific to estradiol, but neither is specific to testosterone or corticosteroids. Chondrichthyes (http://tolweb.org/Gnathostomata/14843) show plasma SHBGs with generalized specificities for estradiol, testosterone, progesterone and corticosterone. In the osteichthyes, plasma SHBGs are more specific to estradiol and testosterone compared to progesterone and corticosterone (Bobe et al. 2010). In mammals (http://tolweb.org/Therapsida/14973), SHBGs regulate the accessibility of sex-steroids to various organs. For example, bound estradiol is unable to pass the blood brain barrier, whereas unbound testosterone has relatively high access to the brain (Pardridge et al. 1980). SHBGs may also bind environmental compounds that influence hormonal activity (Crain et al. 1998).

Prostaglandins act as local intra and inter-cellular regulators (Stacey 1987) that modulate gonadotropin release, ovulation and sexual behavior in vertebrates ranging from fish to mammals. The neurohypophysial peptide hormones released from the neural lobe of the pituitary act in coordination with steroids such as aldosterone and cortisol, as well as prolactin to regulate osmotic and fluid pressure (Nishimura 1985).

Kisspeptins are a family of neuropeptides expressed in the hypothalamus that act as important regulators of GnRH neuron activity and the HPG axis. Sex steroids directly influence kisspeptin neurons, which in turn directly influence GnRH neurons (Han et al. 2005; Pielecka-Fortuna & Moenter 2010). Other physiologically important molecules interacting with Kisspeptin neurons include neurokinin B (NKB), and dynorphin (Lehman et al. 2010), leptin, proopiomelanocortin (POMC), neuropeptide Y (NPY) (Backholer et al. 2010), and Gonadotropin Inhibiting Hormone (GnIH) (Smith et al. 2008). Kisspeptins are key players in the integration of behavioral, maturational and metabolic feedback control of gonadotropins by sex-steroids (Norris & Lopez 2011a; Roa et al. 2011).

Using the variety of systems acting on the HPG axis, estrogen-mediated behavior, such as lordosis in sexually receptive rats, involves coordination of multiple steroid hormones, neuropeptides and prostaglandins (Sodersten et al. 1983; Sirinathsinghji 1984). Similarly, sexual behavior of the male rough-skinned newt *Taricha granulosa* is regulated by complex endocrine coordination of GnRH-regulated androgenic and estrogenic sex-steroids (Moore 1978; Moore & Miller 1983) together with GnRH, arginine vasotocin (AVT), and melanocyte stimulating hormone (MSH), as well HPA axis components; adrenocorticotropic hormone (ACTH), corticotropin releasing factor (CRF) and the adrenal steroid corticosterone (Moore et al. 1982; Moore & Miller 1984).

The evolution of complex coordination may offer finer appropriation of sex-steroid mediated behavioral responses to complex, nuanced or varied stimuli, and may allow robustness of important behaviors when uncoupled from what may once have been key regulators (Crews & Moore 1986; Moore 1987). For example, sexual behaviors of male garter snakes and white-crowned sparrows occur in the absence of plasma testosterone (Moore & Kranz 1983; Crews et al. 1984) although testicular androgens still regulate male secondary sex characters in these species (Crews et al. 1985). Such interactive complexity allows for the sex-specific evolution of environmentally and socially contingent use of sex-steroids within members of the same species. Interactive complexity may be a means by which diversity of behavioral modes involving olfactory, tactile, visual, auditory, photoperiodic, nutritional, habitat selection and conspecific display cues affecting fertility and fitness evolved in vertebrates (Crews 1987b).

3. Before the vertebrates: Sex steroids in the bilaterian animal lineages (Bilateria: http://tolweb.org/Animals/2374)

3.1 Steroids in evolution

Steroid and thyroid hormones were originally thought to bind only to receptors found in the cell nucleus, where effects were exerted via gene transcription. We now know that in addition to binding to nuclear receptors, estrogens also illicit rapid non-genomic responses via membrane bound receptors (Pietras & Szego 1977). The nuclear receptors are grouped in a superfamily of ligand-activated transcription factors (Whitfield et al. 1999; Robinson-Rechavi et al. 2003) which are specific to animals (http://tolweb.org/Animals) and bind compounds such as steroids, thyroid hormones, and retinoids (Bertrand et al. 2004). Because steroids are lipids, their structures provide little phylogenetic information. However, we can examine the evolution of steroid receptors because they are proteins encoded by genes. Construction of a truly reliable animal phylogenetic tree is currently a difficult objective because expansion of techniques across molecular, developmental and evolutionary biology, as well continued discoveries of new taxa reveal common secondary simplifications of morphology and developmental processes that repeatedly challenge the validity of assumptions that evolution proceeds from simple to more complex (Telford & Littlewood 2009). The converse, that rapid evolution is associated with simplification, may be just as well founded. When using extant species for evolutionary clues, it must be noted that groups like ascidians (urochordates: http://tolweb.org/Chordata/2499), nematodes (in Ecdyzoa: http://tolweb.org/Bilateria/2459), and acoel flatworms (in Platyhelminthes:

http://tolweb.org/Bilateria/2459) are characterized by high rates of molecular evolution that can lead to large amounts of secondary gene loss (Ruiz-Trillo et al. 1999; Hughes & Friedman 2005).

Steroid receptors evolved in two main branches from an ancestral steroid receptor (ancSR1) that was likely to be estrogen-activated (Thornton et al. 2003) (Figure 1). One branch contains the estrogen receptors (ER) and is descended from ancSR1. The other branch likely evolved from a gene duplication of the original ancSR1. This duplicate gave rise to an ancSR2 which was altered to bind 3-ketosteroids. This 3-ketosteroid receptor group derived from ancSR2 contains diversified steroid receptors for androgens (AR); progestins (PR); glucocorticoids (GR); and mineralocorticoids (MR) (Schwabe & Teichmann). Only representatives of the ER branch have been detected in fully sequenced genomes of molluscs and annelids (both in Lophotrochozoa: http://tolweb.org/Bilateria/2459) (Eick & Thornton 2011). However, the lancelets (cephalochordate: http://tolweb.org/Chordata/2499) contain two steroid receptors, one from the ER branch and one possibly derived from the 3-ketosteroid receptor (AR/GR/MR/PR) branch (Bridgham et al. 2008; Katsu et al. 2010).

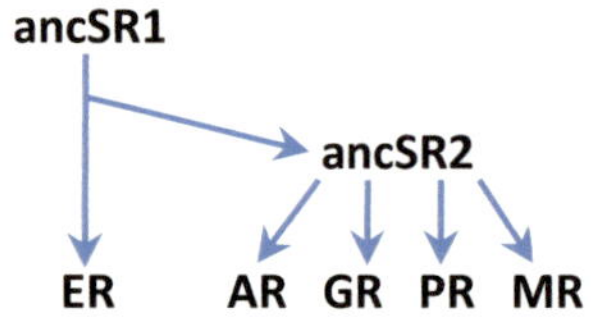

Fig. 1. Simplified schematic of proposed steroid receptor evolution (Thornton et al. 2003). ancSR = ancestral steroid receptor; AR = androgen receptor; ER = estrogen receptor; GR = glucocorticoid receptor; PR = progesterone receptor; MR = mineralocorticoid receptor.

3.2 Estrogen receptors in animal evolution

Estrogen receptor (ER) orthologs have recently been discovered in well-known molluscs: *Aplysia californica* (California sea slug) and *Octopus vulgaris* (the common octopus), as well as annelid marine polychaete worms, *Platynereis dumerilii* and *Capitella capitata* (Lophotrochozoa: http://tolweb.org/Bilateria/2459). All of these organisms are protostomes, indicating that the ancestral steroid receptor was likely present before the separation between protostomes and deuterostomes. This evidence supports the hypothesis that the ER was secondarily lost in taxa such as arthropod and nematode protostomes (Maglich et al. 2001), or the urochordate and echinoderm deuterostomes where definitive orthologs have not been detected (reviewed in Eick & Thornton (2011).

Care is suggested for interpreting the steroidogenic potential of GnRH molecules in molluscs (Tsai & Zhang 2008). This is because the estrogen receptor (ER) orthologs for molluscs like the California sea slug, common octopus, pacific oyster *Crassostrea gigas* and the marine snail *Thais clavigera* are constitutively active and unresponsive to estrogens or other vertebrate steroid hormones (Thornton et al. 2003; Kajiwara et al. 2006; Keay et al. 2006; Matsumoto et al. 2007).

3.3 Androgens and progestins

In early animals, more generalized versions of the roles we currently associate with sex-steroids may have been assigned to alternative compounds. Steroids which at one point were intermediate compounds in the synthesis of ligands for a particular receptor, may have become ligands for alternative "orphan" receptors (Thornton 2001).

Steroid receptors for androgens (AR) and progestins (PR) likely arose out of adaptations for specialized endocrine systems through such use of intermediary steroid metabolites (Eick & Thornton 2011).

For example, the agnathans (lampreys and hagfish in Craniata: http://tolweb.org/Chordata/2499) may be illustrative of the evolutionary stage before gene duplication of the original ER-like ancSR1 generated ancSR2. Remember that ancSR2 (section 3.1) is believed to be ancestral to the modern 3-ketosteroid receptor (AR/GR/MR/PR) family (Thornton 2001; Thornton et al. 2003). An example of evidence for this hypothesis is that in the European river lamprey, (*Lampetra fluviatilis*) and the arctic/Japanese lamprey (*Lampetra japonica*), testosterone concentrations range from low to non-detectable, and do not seem correlated to life stage or gender (Fukayama & Takahashi 1985; Klime & Larsen 1987). However, androstenedione (an androgen), is responsive to GnRH (see below) and acts as a hormone, increasing the development of secondary sex characteristics and accelerating maturation in sea lampreys (*Petromyzon marinus*) (Bryan et al. 2007). These findings are significant because androstenedione is an androgenic precursor in vertebrates, but in lampreys, GnRH may be eliciting release of steroids for much less specific steroid receptor binding than we see in animals with more complex endocrine systems. Additional support for this hypothesis comes from observations that progesterone and estradiol have been detected in sea lamprey plasma of both sexes, and concentrations of both of these hormones change in response to GnRH stimulation (Gazourian et al. 1997).

3.4 The noteworthy case of the octopus

The common octopus, *Octopus vulgaris,* is the first invertebrate species shown to possess representatives of three classes of sex-steroids found in vertebrates (progestins, androgens and estrogens) as well as binding proteins for these steroids (Di Cosmo et al. 2001). The octopus also possesses a progesterone receptor (Di Cosmo et al. 1998) and an estrogen receptor (Di Cosmo et al. 2002). Another vertebrate-like trait of the octopus is the expression of two peptides belonging to the oxytocin/vasopressin superfamily (Kanda et al. 2005) as well as associated receptors for one such peptide (Kanda et al. 2003). In addition, enzymatic (3beta-Hydroxysteroid dehydrogenase) activity has been detected in the ovary, indicating that the octopus reproductive system is a source of steroidogenesis (Di Cosmo et al. 2001). These findings display an astonishing level of functional parallelism with vertebrates, especially in consideration of the vast evolutionary distance between cephalopods (mollusca) and gnathostomes (deuterostomia) among the bilateria (http://tolweb.org/Bilateria/2459). These findings further support the hypothesis that secondary loss of ancestral steroid receptor function occurred in the arthropod and nematode protostomes, as well as urochordate and echinoderm deuterostomes (Maglich et al. 2001; Eick & Thornton 2011).

4. Reproductive variability among the vertebrate classes (http://tolweb.org/Gnathostomata/14843)

Sex steroids were largely characterized based on their roles in sex-determination and sex-differentiation as described for gonochoristic species. These are species with two sexes (male and female) where once the sex of an individual is determined, the individual differentiates into that sex only once during its lifetime. Mechanisms of sex determination are characterized as genetic, temperature-dependent, and behavioral (Crews 1993). Sex steroids are integral to sex-specific differentiation of the reproductive tracts and development of corresponding secondary sex characteristics and behaviors in all vertebrate groups (Norris & Lopez 2011a). In many fish species, an individual may normally undergo sex differentiation on multiple occasions during a lifetime (Thresher 1984). The spectrum of reproductive strategies utilized by vertebrates (Figure 2) is illustrative of the variety of sex-steroid mediated behavioral and physiological modifications that are feasible (Lombardi 1998; Norris & Lopez 2011a).

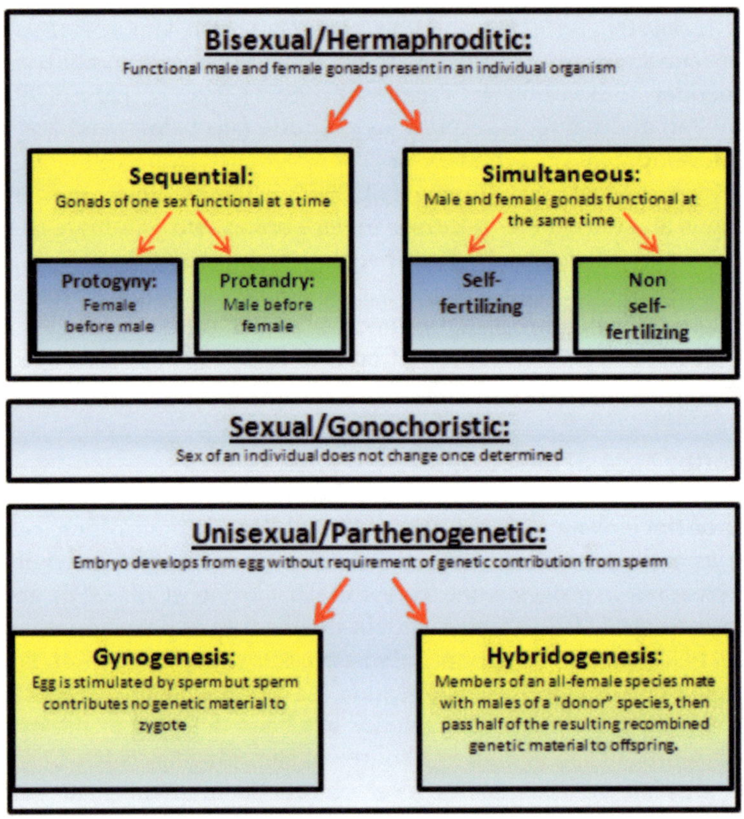

Fig. 2. Summary of vertebrate reproductive strategies (Harrington 1961; Schultz 1973) (Charnov et al. 1976; Potts et al. 1984; Crews 1987b; Paul-Prasanth et al. 2011).

4.1 Fishes

Living members of fishes include the Sarcopteriygii, Actinopterygii and Chondrichthyes of the jawed vertebrates (http://tolweb.org/Gnathostomata/14843). Fishes include groups that show a faster evolution of protein sequences and conserved noncoding elements than mammals, and some of the highest "evolvability" observed in vertebrates (Ravi & Venkatesh 2008)

Fish also exhibit the highest degree of reproductive plasticity and diversity of strategies observed in vertebrates (Potts et al. 1984; Crews 1987b; Paul-Prasanth et al. 2011). Often, combinations of sex-determining mechanisms are observed in a single species, such as the internally self-fertilizing bisexual cyprinodont *Rivulus marmoratus,* in which both temperature-dependent and genetic sex-determining mechanisms are utilized (Harrington 1961; Harrington & Crossman 1976). Sex reversal and sequential hermaphroditism is well described (Shapiro 1984) in many species of reef fishes. Sex changing fish can perform both male-typical and female-typical sexual behaviors and functions during a single lifetime. Functional sex reversal can also be induced with hormonal treatment in fish that do not normally undergo sex change.

Many fish species have multiple male phenotypes where each phenotype makes different types of investments in reproduction. Each of these types of males requires different endocrine settings as well as neuroendocrine and behavioral parameters. The theme of two types of males within a species becomes more complicated when considering sex-changing reef fishes such as wrasses and parrotfish. Here the "primary" males are small with female like coloration, and sneak in on spawning aggregations or the matings of secondary (terminal) males. Terminal males are large and brightly colored, and maintain territories. The development of terminal males varies according to species, and may occur through transformation of primary males as well as through sex change of a female (Warner 1982).

Sex change in fishes can be induced by social conditions and relative size of neighboring conspecifics (Thresher 1984; Warner 1984). Sex change may also be initiated through application of exogenous testosterone (Chan & Yeung 1983; Kramer et al. 1988). Rapid color changes observed in sex-changing fish involve integration of visual stimuli with sex-steroid and GnRH action (Demski 1987).

4.2 Amphibians (http://tolweb.org/Amphibia)

Body compartmentalization adaptations necessary for transitioning from aquatic to terrestrial life are abundant in amphibians. Both genetic and temperature-dependent mechanisms may interact to influence sex determination in this clade (Nakamura 2009; 2010). Although the naturally occurring range of observed developmental plasticity is narrower than in fishes, many amphibians can be sex-reversed with sex-steroid application. For example, estrogen effects on gonadal differentiation range from masculinization to feminization, and vary widely according to species, administration protocol, and interactions with other steroids (Hayes 1997b). Much of this variation may be related to the physiological stage of the animal at the time of exposure (reviewed in Hayes (1998). Sex steroid effects on amphibian rates of metamorphosis (Sluczewski & Roth 1950) as well as adrenal steroid effects on courtship behavior (Moore & Miller 1984) and gonadal differentiation (Hayes 1998) are reflective of high levels of cross-connectivity between HPG, HPA and HPT systems (Hayes et al. 1993). Developmental timing can vary dramatically between closely related species (Buchholz & Hayes 2000), and differences in developmental timing may affect ages or stages when animals have achieved the organizational capacity to exhibit hormone-induced effects (Hayes 1997a).

Sex-steroids exert their most potent effects on sexual differentiation only during specific stages of development (Chang & Witschi 1956; Villalpando & Merchant-Larios 1990). This theme of "critical windows" of development is common in the vertebrates. It is an important consideration in evaluations of sex-steroid effects as well as effects of non-steroidal compounds such as atrazine (Hayes et al. 2002) or o,p'DDT (Noriega & Hayes 2000) which affect sex-steroid mediated development of primary and secondary sex characters.

4.3 Reptiles (Compare testudines and diapsida in: http://tolweb.org/Amniota/14990)

Reptilian use of sex-steroids shows the greatest diversity of sexual differentiation modes observed among extant amniotes. Temperature sex determination is observed in all crocodilians (Crocodylomorpha: http://tolweb.org/Archosauria/14900) examined (Deeming & Ferguson 1989), many chelonians and some squamates (Bull 1980). It is in the reptiles that we see the beginnings of mutual exclusivity between genetically determined sex and temperature determined sex (Bull 1980). Studies in reptiles have clarified that genetic and temperature dependent sex determining mechanisms operate along much more of a continuum than was originally perceived (Norris & Lopez 2011b). Of the 80 or so vertebrate taxa displaying unisexual reproduction, squamate reptiles are the only vertebrates shown to reproduce entirely in the absence of males (Kearney et al. 2009) (Neaves & Baumann 2011). Variations in sex-steroid levels appear to underlie behavioral and morphological differences among males with differences in functional roles such as "sneaker" vs. "territorial" or males displaying one color type vs. another (Norris & Lopez 2011b).

Well studied examples include several all-female parthenogenetic species of whiptail lizards (*Cnemidophorus*) secondarily evolved from sexual species which display male courtship behavior, but no such behavior between females (Cuellar 1977). In the all-female parthenogens, females have adopted displays of courtship and copulatory behavior that are identical to those of males from the ancestral species. This pseudomale copulatory behavior is not essential for reproduction (Cuellar 1971), but does increase fecundity (Crews & Fitzgerald 1980). In addition to pseudomale copulatory behavior, there are instances in gonochoristic species where courtship behavior is required for reproduction but does not lead to fertilization. These scenarios lend credence to hypotheses that copulatory behavior may be used to facilitate sociality as well as to deliver environmental or conditional cues important for overall fitness (Crews 1982; Crews & Moore 1986).

Female red-sided garter snakes *Thamnophis sirtalis* release an estrogen-dependent pheromone that attracts male garter snakes. Typical males do not express the female pheromone, but a subset of "she-males" release a similar or identical attractant as the females. "She-males" are genetic males with typical male morphology, and are able to achieve high mating success by using their pheromone release to lure typical males away before returning to mate with the then unattended females (Mason & Crews 1985). Males receiving exogenous estrogen produce the female pheromone (Garstka & Crews 1981), and estrogen administered to neonatal males causes them to be courted by adult males (Crews 1985). "She-males" have high circulating testosterone concentrations although estrogen concentrations are comparable to typical males, and it is hypothesized that aromatic conversion of testosterone to estrogens may be important for "she-male" pheromone production (Crews 1987a).

4.4 Birds (http://tolweb.org/Aves/15721)

In birds, temperature sex determination appears to have been lost, although it is still ubiquitous in the other living archosaur group (http://tolweb.org/Archosauria/14900), the crocodilians (Deeming & Ferguson 1989). One interesting exception is the case of the Australian brush-turkey (*Alectura lathami*), a member of the megapodes, a family which builds mound nests that are ambiently incubated in a manner reminiscent of crocodilians. Sex ratios in hatchling *A. lathami* are influenced by incubation temperature (Goth & Booth 2005). Birds are functionally gonochoristic. There are occasional reports of viable male offspring from unfertilized eggs (Olsen & Marsden 1954; Sarvella 1974), but parthenogenesis does not seem to be currently used as a reproductive strategy in birds.

Compared to the reptiles, amphibians and fishes, reproductive strategies in birds are conservative. The overall chromosomal sex determination appears uniform, where females (ZW) are heterogametic and males (ZZ) are homogametic, resulting in a "default" male phenotype which occurs in the absence of endocrine influence (Mittwoch 1971; Adkins 1975; 1976; Elbrecht & Smith 1992). The ZZ/ZW female heterogametic sex determination system is opposite to the XX/XY male heterogametic scheme employed by mammals (section 4.5). In birds, conversion of testosterone to estrogen during critical windows of development (section 5) is required for demasculinization and feminization in the normal sexual differentiation of the female. Blockage of this conversion results in genetic females exhibiting male secondary sex characteristics and behavior (Elbrecht & Smith 1992).

Sex-steroids link the physiology of sexual differentiation, sexually dimorphic behavior, seasonality, parental care and brain changes related to song development (Norris & Lopez 2011c). In species where males provide significant parental care, plasma testosterone is kept at minimal levels needed to maintain the gonads, secondary sex characteristics and territorial behavior without interfering with expression of parental behavior (Wingfield & Moore 1987). In white-crowned and golden-crowned sparrows, photoperiodic cues influence levels of gonadal androgens in both sexes to affect appetite control centers of the brain in coordination with migration. Sex-steroids synchronize courtship behavior and reproductive status with seasonal environmental cues (Ramenofsky 2011).

4.5 Mammals (http://tolweb.org/Mammalia)

Mammals are a gonochoristic group using an XX/XY male heterogametic sex determination scheme where temperature sex determination appears to have been lost. In contrast to birds, the "default" sexual morphology is that of the homogametic female (XX), and androgens during critical windows of development (section 5) are required to defeminize and masculinize the default female morphology in order to generate a normal male morphology. However, deviations from the norm provide some of the most fascinating insights into the endocrinology of sex steroids. Spotted hyenas *Crocuta crocuta* represent an interesting paradox where females show a physical appearance and some behaviors that are more masculinized than males. Females have masculinized external genitalia, no external vaginal opening and give birth though a large pseudopenis. Female masculinization is evident at birth and maintained throughout life (Neaves et al. 1980; Frank et al. 1990). This masculinization of females is due to high levels of androgens originating from the adrenals and ovaries where steroidogenic pathways are altered compared to ovaries of typical placental mammals (Lindeque et al. 1986; Glickman et al. 1992). In addition, the placenta converts ovarian androstenedione to testosterone (Licht et al. 1992; Yalcinkaya et al. 1993).

Interactions between behavior, signaling molecules, HPA and HPG axes and the comparative evolution of complexity in endocrine systems across many species are well described in mammals (Park & Rissman 2011; Uphouse 2011). For example, the role of sex-steroids in parturition is peripheral to influences from prostaglandins in the marsupial tammar wallaby (*Macropus eugenii*) (http://tolweb.org/Marsupialia/15994). However, a coordinated interplay between fetal and maternal estrogens and progestins as well as the fetal HPA axis and placental hormones is observed in primates (http://tolweb.org/Primates/15963) (Young et al. 2011).

5. Applied considerations

With respect to ontogenetic development of sexual dimorphism in individuals, the effects of sex-steroids are commonly discussed using the "organizational" vs. "activational" nomenclature (Phoenix et al. 1959b; a; Arnold & Breedlove 1985). For a given structure, "organizational" typically refers to effects of sex-steroid exposure during a critical time window in early development which determines the type of response or morphology that the affected structure will have. "Activational" refers to acute effects of sex-steroids on the structure after the critical window during which the structure was organized (Whalen & Edwards 1967). The type of activation is dependent on the organizational effect that occurred during the critical window of development (Guillette et al. 1995).

5.1 Brain dimorphism

Naturally occurring dramatic sexual dimorphism in vertebrate brains are exemplified in canaries (*Serinus canaria*) and zebra finches (*Taeniopygia guttata*) where three vocal control areas in the brain are strikingly larger in males (Nottebohm & Arnold 1976). Sex steroid effects on sexually dimorphic brain development was originally investigated in mammals (Raisman & Field 1973) and have since been described in the broader central nervous system (Breedlove & Arnold 1983b; a) for all vertebrate classes (Norris & Lopez 2011a). Correspondingly, sexual dimorphisms of brain neurotransmitter systems are also now evident (De Vries et al. 1984) (Simerly et al. 1985). Note that while this classical view of sex-steroid involvement in the dimorphic brain development is very robust, the paradigm has shifted to incorporate sex differences due to gene expression which occur before gonadal differentiation and subsequent organizational effects of sex-steroids (Mccarthy & Arnold 2007; Arnold 2009).

6. The "endocrine disruptor" hypothesis

Organisms encounter many environmental compounds that approximate, diminish or enhance the activity of sex-steroids. As explained in the sections on fish and amphibians, exposure to sex-steroids can morphologically and functionally reverse the sex of many vertebrate species. Here, a brief history of subsets of key events characterizing the development and expansion of the endocrine disruptor hypothesis is outlined. Emphasis is placed on the types of compounds that have received attention due to their observed effectiveness, abundance or distribution in this regard. Arguments in this section are also described with reference to some of the hormone-treatment experiments leading to current perspectives regarding the endocrine disruption of normal reproductive behavior, development and function in wildlife and laboratory species.

Naturally-occurring compounds as well as anthropogenic compounds released into the environment due to human activity have been hypothesized to affect endocrine function in vertebrates by mimicking the action of endogenous hormones (Colborn & Clement 1992), thereby 'disrupting' normal endocrine settings. In cases of endocrine disruption, exposure levels are typically too low to have toxic or acute effects on adults (Colborn et al. 1993), but affect organisms during critical organizational periods of early life stages (Guillette et al. 1995). Tissue contaminant levels previously considered safe are sufficient to alter endogenous chemical mediation in fish (Sumpter & Jobling 1995; Jobling et al. 2006), amphibians (Hayes et al. 2002; Hayes et al. 2006; Hayes et al. 2010), reptiles (Crews et al. 1995; Guillette et al. 2000), birds (Ottinger et al. 2009), and mammals (Colborn et al. 1993).

Pasture-specific variations in plant-derived estrogens (Walker & Janney 1930) affect livestock fertility according to grazing location. Hormones and hormone analogs are routinely used to manage production of agricultural animals (Brooks et al. 1986) and byproducts of steroid analogs used in livestock production have endocrine activity and are likely to affect wildlife (Orlando et al. 2004; Soto et al. 2004; Durhan et al. 2006). Sex-steroids or their analogs are routinely applied in aquaculture and agriculture to manipulate the sex ratios, behavior and physiology of commercially reared vertebrates.

Metabolites of steroids applied to livestock have biological activity that may affect animals at sites removed from the source of application (Shelton 1990; Lone 1997; Meyer 2001). Similarly, effluent from pulp mills, paper mills and sewage treatment plants affecting the endocrinology of aquatic vertebrates are transported far from sites of entry into the environment (Jobling & Tyler 2003a; b).

A key feature in the development of the endocrine disruptor hypothesis was the concept of "environmental estrogens". The environmental estrogen was a hallmark of the hypothesis because estrogenic properties of the compounds first identified as endocrine disruptors were well described. For example, widespread use of the synthetic estrogen diethylstilbestrol (DES) in humans (Morrell 1941; Smith & Smith 1949b; a) continues to be one of the most well studied examples of endocrine disruption where effects in the exposed mothers are minimal compared to effects in their offspring who were exposed during critical windows of development (Giusti et al. 1995). Organochlorine pesticides and environmentally persistent chlorinated hydrocarbons designed to be harmless to exposed vertebrates tended to bioaccumulate and affect offspring of exposed animals. Key players in the environmental estrogen story included the synthetic estrogen DES; the organochlorine pesticides, DDT and methoxychlor; a host of polychlorinated biphenyls (PCB's); and the plasticizers bisphenol-A, nonylphenol, and octylphenol. Compounds of concern were identified based partially on their ability to bind to nuclear estrogen receptors (Blair et al. 2000), and activity observed using *in vivo* biological assessments of estrogen activity such as the rat uterotropic assay (Gray et al. 2004), and production of the egg yolk protein vitellogenin (Sumpter & Jobling 1995). *In vitro* induction of estrogen-responsive breast cancer cell lines (Klotz et al. 1996) and tests of transcription in response to estrogen receptor binding (Ernst et al. 1991) were also primary means of screening compounds for estrogenic activity. With mechanistic knowledge came distinctions between feminizing and demasculinizing effects, and the concept of anti-androgens were more carefully considered (Wilson et al. 2008) in addition to estrogens or anti-estrogens. Key anti-androgens were originally characterized by their antagonism of androgen receptor (AR). Further characterization was based on extensive batteries of *in vivo* reproductive tract and secondary sex character examinations in the laboratory rat. In these studies, androgen action *in utero*, or on pubertal development were examined (Gray et al. 2004; Owens et al. 2007). Recognized antiandrogens fell into classes including dicarboximide (Gray et al. 1994; Kelce & Wilson 1997) and imidazole fungicides (Vinggaard et al. 2002; Noriega et al. 2005), organochlorine insecticides (Kelce et al. 1995), urea-based herbicides (Gray et al. 1999; Lambright et al. 2000), phthalate esters used as plasticizers (Parks et al. 2000; Howdeshell et al. 2007), and polybrominated diphenyl ethers (PBDEs) used as flame retardants (Stoker et al. 2005).

Natural hormones (Stumm-Zollinger & Fair 1965) and birth control agents (Tabak et al. 1981) occurring in wastewater prompted concern over sewage effluents. Some compounds, such as the phthalate esters, diethylhexyl phthalate (DEHP), dibutyl phthalate (DBP) and benzylbutyl phthalate (BBP), originally considered estrogenic (Jobling et al. 1995), also exhibited anti-androgenic properties by decreasing testosterone production in fetal testes and reducing the expression of steroidogenic genes after *in utero* exposure (Parks et al. 2000; Wilson et al. 2004).

Although effects of endocrine disruptors are well documented, as explained earlier in the chapter, complex endocrine interactions with other steroids, peptides and lipids are integral to the function of sex-steroids in living vertebrates. Therefore it is critical to consider the enormous range of physiological variation that occurs in vertebrates under "normal" conditions that would be considered "uncontaminated" (Orlando & Guillette 2007). Using terms like "estrogenic" or "androgenic" may limit the scope of investigation because androgens and estrogens have well-characterized function in a very small percentage of species. In addition, phylogenetic assessments discussed earlier in this chapter may expand the scope of sex-steroid considerations outside of the vertebrates. For example, the recently characterized ER in molluscs is not responsive to steroid ligands (Thornton et al. 2003) (Keay et al. 2006; Matsumoto et al. 2007) and the cephalochordate ER acts as a constitutive repressor of estrogen response element (ERE) function (Bridgham et al. 2008; Paris et al. 2008). It is important to note that although compounds may be defined based on a given outcome or mechanism of action, almost all chemicals influence multiple physiological systems and influence the way physiological systems interact with each other. For example, compounds such as linuron (a urea-based herbicide) and prochloraz (an imidazole fungicide) act as anti-androgens via multiple mechanisms of action (Lambright et al. 2000; Wilson et al. 2004; Noriega et al. 2005).

6.1 A case study using prochloraz

Any number of compounds can be used to demonstrate endocrine disruption via an endocrine active chemical (EAC). However, prochloraz provides a highly illustrative example because it affects development of external mammalian genitalia with which readers will have prior familiarity. Much of the reason that an imidazole fungicides like prochloraz kill fungi is because they affect members of the diverse cytochrome P450 enzyme family (Mason et al. 1987; Riviere & Papich 2009), a group of enzymes catalyzing electron transfer in representatives of all classes of cellular life (Nebert et al. 1989; Lewis et al. 1998; De Mot & Parret 2002; Nelson 2011). These enzymes have been evolutionarily co-opted for vertebrate steroidogenesis, as well as the metabolism of steroids and xenobiotics (Gibson et al. 2002). In addition to affecting steroidogenic cytochrome P450 enzymes and reducing androgen production, prochloraz is an androgen receptor antagonist (Vinggaard et al. 2002; Noriega et al. 2005) and inhibits testicular expression for insulin-like hormone 3 (insl3), which affects gubernacular development (Wilson et al. 2004). An example of laboratory-administered *in utero* prochloraz exposure (Noriega et al. 2005) can be used for a discussion on effects of a non-steroidal compound on sex-steroid action as viewed throughout the historical development of the endocrine disruptor hypothesis. Namely:

1. Exposure (ingestion) over a time course (5 days) and dosage that produced no observable effects on directly exposed mothers, was sufficient to produce severe abnormalities in offspring of those mothers (figure 3) through secondary *in utero* exposure during critical windows for sex-steroid sensitive development;
2. Abnormalities such as vaginal morphology in males (figure 4), that might have initially been classified as "feminization" in the early history of the field are more accurately described as extreme cases of de-masculinization towards a default female morphology for the species in question.

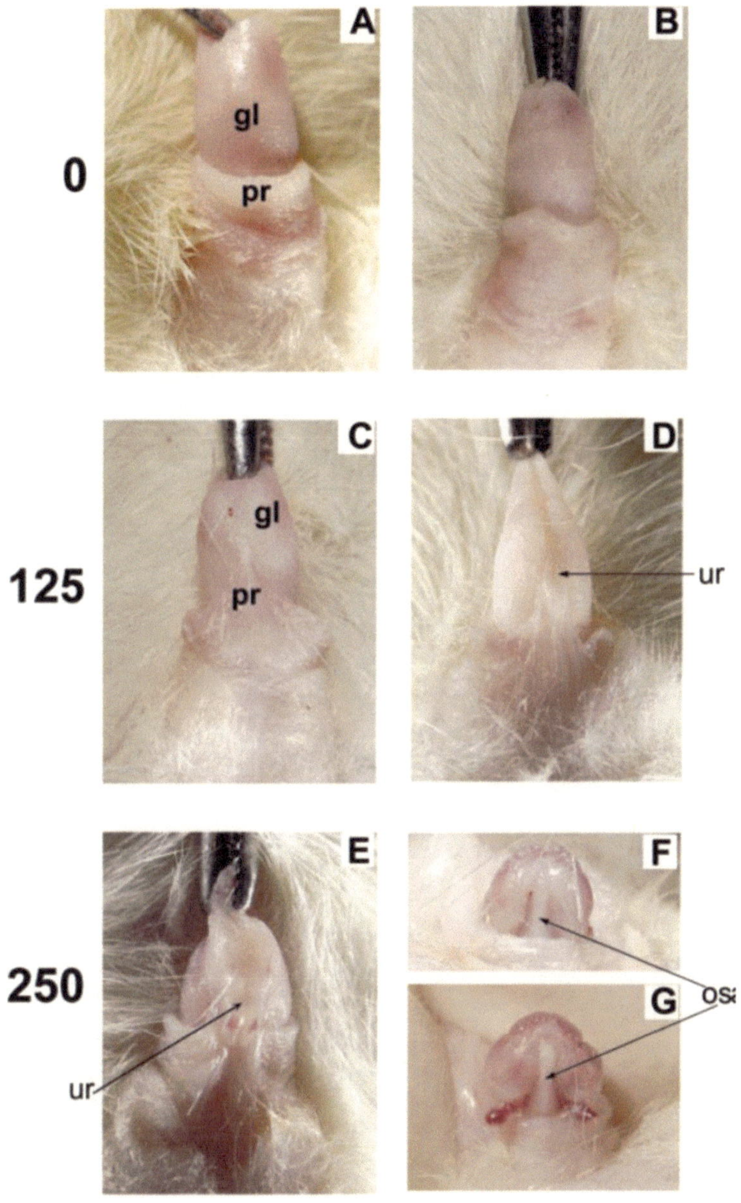

Fig. 3. Phallus abnormalities in adult male rats receiving a 5-day *in utero* exposure to prochloraz. Panels are arranged from left to right according to dosage group indicated by numbers to the left of the diagram. **A** and **B**) Variation within controls. **C** and **D**) Animals with a maternal dose of 125 mg/kg per day. **E–G**) Animals with a maternal dose of 250 mg/kg per day. gl, glans penis; pr, prepuce; ur, urethral opening; os, os penis. Hypospadias is evident in the two highest dosage groups and (**C–E**) show examples of incomplete preputial separation. Severe phallus clefting and exposure of the os penis is evident in the highest dosage group (**F** and **G**). (Noriega et al. 2005) modified with permission from the Society for the Study of Reproduction.

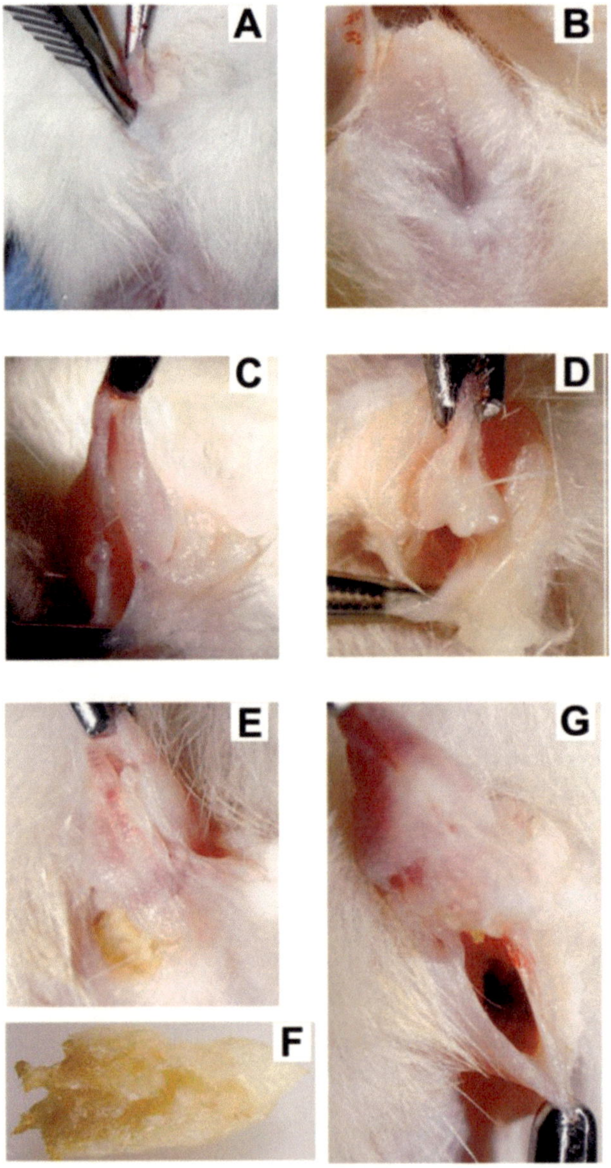

Fig. 4. Prochloraz-induced vaginal morphology in adult male rats receiving a 5-day *in utero* exposure. **A**) Panoramic view of a vaginal pouch (forceps inserted) in a male from the 250 mg/kg maternal dosage group. **B**) A close-up of a control female phallus and vaginal opening. **C** and **D**) Vaginal pouch and phallus deformity variations in males from the 250 mg/kg maternal dose group. **E–G**) The most severely affected animal from the 125 mg/kg maternal dose group. In this male, an ejaculatory plug (**F**) was found embedded (**E**) in the vaginal opening (**G**). (Noriega et al. 2005) modified with permission from the Society for the Study of Reproduction.

7. Conclusion

The terminology used in discussions of endocrinology, evolution and behavior is changing in light of the growing body of knowledge regarding the complexity of hormonal interactions. This chapter is intended to provide the reader with a panoramic snapshot of sex-steroid function compared to what is normally encountered in specialized fields of study. The summaries of concepts presented here will hopefully be catalysts for further investigation of topics in more detail than presented here. Existing paradigms regarding "disruption", "variation" and "adaptation" are increasingly seen as parts of a continuum. Thus the scope of "endocrine disruptor" assessment has already expanded beyond currently established definition parameters (Guillette 2006; Marty et al. 2011; Norris & Lopez 2011a). For example, the term "Endocrine Active Chemical" (EAC) is now used in favor of terms implying "disruption" (Norris & Lopez 2011a).

The claim has long been made that distinctions such as endocrine system vs. nervous system are arbitrary (Roth et al. 1986). Evolutionary constraints lead to reduced variation in reproductive strategies used by birds and mammals compared to evolutionarily older clades represented by fishes, reptiles and amphibians. However, the evolution of complex neuroendocrine systems may provide time and context-specific behavioral avenues for adaptive radiation in the face of external influences on peripheral hormone levels (Wingfield et al. 1997; Adkins-Regan 2008). We have only a brief window of perspective on the cycle of extinction and adaptive radiation. The ability to include expansive, as well as reductionist perspectives may facilitate new thresholds in our evaluation of environmental, social, behavioral and clinical aspects of sex-steroid biology.

8. Abbreviations

ancSR = Ancestral Steroid Hormone Receptor; AR = Androgen Receptor; CG = Chorionic Gonadotropin; ER = Estrogen Receptor; FSH = Follicle Stimulating Hormone; GR = Glucocorticoid Receptor; hCG = Human Chorionic Gonadotropin; HPA = Hypothalamic-Pituitary-Adrenal; HPG = Hypothalamic-Pituitary-Gonad; HPT = Hypothalamic-Pituitary-Thyroid; insl3 = Insulin-like hormone 3; LH = Lutenizing Hormone; MR = Mineralocorticoid Receptor; SHBG = Steroid Hormone Binding Globulin; TSH = Thyroid Stimulating Hormone;

9. References

Adkins-Regan, E. (2008). Review. Do hormonal control systems produce evolutionary inertia? *Philosophical transactions of the Royal Society of London. Series B, Biological sciences* Vol. 363, No. 1497, pp (1599-1609), 0962-8436

Adkins, E. K. (1975). Hormonal basis of sexual differentiation in the Japanese quail. *Journal of comparative and physiological psychology* Vol. 89, No. 1, pp (61-71), 0021-9940

Adkins, E. K. (1976). Embryonic exposure to an antiestrogen masculinizes behavior of female quail. *Physiology & Behavior* Vol. 17, No. 2, pp (357-359), 0031-9384

Arnold, A. P. (2009). The organizational-activational hypothesis as the foundation for a unified theory of sexual differentiation of all mammalian tissues. *Hormones and behavior* Vol. 55, No. 5, pp (570-578), 1095-6867

Arnold, A. P. & Breedlove, S. M. (1985). Organizational and activational effects of sex steroids on brain and behavior: a reanalysis. *Hormones and Behavior* Vol. 19, No. 4, pp (469-498), 0018-506X

Arslan, M., Lobo, J., Zaidi, A. A. & Qazi, M. H. (1977). Effect of mammalian gonadotropins (HCG and PMSG) on testicular androgen production in the spiny-tailed lizard, Uromastix hardwicki. *General and Comparative Endocrinology* Vol. 33, No. 1, pp (160-162), 0016-6480

Backholer, K., Smith, J. T., Rao, A., Pereira, A., Iqbal, J., Ogawa, S., Li, Q. & Clarke, I. J. (2010). Kisspeptin cells in the ewe brain respond to leptin and communicate with neuropeptide Y and proopiomelanocortin cells. *Endocrinology* Vol. 151, No. 5, pp (2233-2243), 1945-7170

Baulieu, E. E. (1997). Neurosteroids: of the nervous system, by the nervous system, for the nervous system. *Recent progress in hormone research* Vol. 52, pp (1-32), 0079-9963

Bertrand, S., Brunet, F. G., Escriva, H., Parmentier, G., Laudet, V. & Robinson-Rechavi, M. (2004). Evolutionary genomics of nuclear receptors: from twenty-five ancestral genes to derived endocrine systems. *Molecular biology and evolution* Vol. 21, No. 10, pp (1923-1937), 0737-4038

Blair, R. M., Fang, H., Branham, W. S., Hass, B. S., Dial, S. L., Moland, C. L., Tong, W., Shi, L., Perkins, R. & Sheehan, D. M. (2000). The estrogen receptor relative binding affinities of 188 natural and xenochemicals: structural diversity of ligands. *Toxicological sciences : an official journal of the Society of Toxicology* Vol. 54, No. 1, pp (138-153), 1096-6080

Bobe, J., Guiguen, Y. & Fostier, A. (2010). Diversity and biological significance of sex hormone-binding globulin in fish, an evolutionary perspective. *Molecular and cellular endocrinology* Vol. 316, No. 1, pp (66-78), 0303-7207

Bourne, G. A., Regiani, S., Payne, A. H. & Marshall, J. C. (1980). Testicular GnRH receptors--characterization and localization on interstitial tissue. *The Journal of clinical endocrinology and metabolism* Vol. 51, No. 2, pp (407-409), 0021-972X

Bramley, T. A., Mcphie, C. A. & Menzies, G. S. (1992). Human placental gonadotrophin-releasing hormone (GnRH) binding sites: I. Characterization, properties and ligand specificity. *Placenta* Vol. 13, No. 6, pp (555-581), 0143-4004

Breedlove, S. M. & Arnold, A. P. (1983a). Hormonal-Control of a Developing Neuromuscular System .2. Sensitive Periods for the Androgen-Induced Masculinization of the Rat Spinal Nucleus of the Bulbocavernosus. *Journal of Neuroscience* Vol. 3, No. 2, pp (424-432), 0270-6474

Breedlove, S. M. & Arnold, A. P. (1983b). Hormonal control of a developing neuromuscular system. I. Complete Demasculinization of the male rat spinal nucleus of the bulbocavernosus using the anti-androgen flutamide. *The Journal of neuroscience : the official journal of the Society for Neuroscience* Vol. 3, No. 2, pp (417-423), 0270-6474

Bridgham, J. T., Brown, J. E., Rodriguez-Mari, A., Catchen, J. M. & Thornton, J. W. (2008). Evolution of a new function by degenerative mutation in cephalochordate steroid receptors. *PLoS genetics* Vol. 4, No. 9, pp (e1000191), 1553-7390

Brooks, A. N., Lamming, G. E. & Haynes, N. B. (1986). Endogenous opioid peptides and the control of gonadotrophin secretion. *Res Vet Sci* Vol. 41, No. 3, pp (285-299), 0034-5288

Bryan, M. B., Scott, A. P. & Li, W. (2007). The sea lamprey (Petromyzon marinus) has a receptor for androstenedione. *Biology of reproduction* Vol. 77, No. 4, pp (688-696), 0006-3363

Buchholz, D. R. & Hayes, T. B. (2000). Larval period comparison for the spadefoot toads Scaphiopus couchii and Spea multiplicata (Pelobatidae : Anura). *Herpetologica* Vol. 56, No. 4, pp (455-468), 0018-0831

Bull, J. J. (1980). Sex Determination in Reptiles. *Quarterly Review of Biology* Vol. 55, No. 1, pp (3-21), 0033-5770

Callard, G. V. (1983). Androgen and Estrogen Actions in the Vertebrate Brain. *American Zoologist* Vol. 23, No. 3, pp (607-620), 0003-1569

Chan, S. T. H. & Yeung, W. S. B. (1983). Sex Control and Sex Reversal in Fish Under Natural Conditions, In: *Fish Physiology*. W. S. Hoar, D. J. Randall and E. M. Donaldson, pp. (171-222), Academic Press, 1546-5098

Chang, C. Y. & Witschi, E. (1956). Genic Control and Hormonal Reversal of Sex Differentiation in Xenopus. *Proceedings of the Society for Experimental Biology and Medicine* Vol. 93, No. 1, pp (140-144), 0037-9727

Charnov, E. L., Smith, J. M. & Bull, J. J. (1976). Why Be an Hermaphrodite. *Nature* Vol. 263, No. 5573, pp (125-126), 0028-0836

Ciejek, E., Thorner, J. & Geier, M. (1977). Solid phase peptide synthesis of alpha-factor, a yeast mating pheromone. *Biochemical and biophysical research communications* Vol. 78, No. 3, pp (952-961), 0006-291X

Colborn, T. & Clement, C. (1992). Advances in Modern Environmental Toxicology, Vol. 21. Chemically-induced alterations in sexual and functional development: The wildlife-human connection; Meeting, Racine, Wisconsin, USA, July 26-28, 1991, In: *Advances in Modern Environmental Toxicology, Vol. 21. Chemically-induced alterations in sexual and functional development: The wildlife/human connection; Meeting, Racine, Wisconsin, USA, July 26-28, 1991*. T. Colborn and C. Clement, pp., Princeton Scientific Publishing Co. Inc., Princeton, New Jersey, USA

Colborn, T., Vom Saal, F. S. & Soto, A. M. (1993). Developmental effects of endocrine-disrupting chemicals in wildlife and humans. *Environmental health perspectives* Vol. 101, No. 5, pp (378-384), 0091-6765

Cole, L. A. (2009). New discoveries on the biology and detection of human chorionic gonadotropin. *Reproductive biology and endocrinology : RB&E* Vol. 7, pp (8), 1477-7827

Crain, D. A., Noriega, N., Vonier, P. M., Arnold, S. F., Mclachlan, J. A. & Guillette, L. J., Jr. (1998). Cellular bioavailability of natural hormones and environmental contaminants as a function of serum and cytosolic binding factors. *Toxicology and industrial health* Vol. 14, No. 1-2, pp (261-273), 0748-2337

Crews, D. (1982). On the origin of sexual behavior. *Psychoneuroendocrinology* Vol. 7, No. 4, pp (259-270), 0306-4530

Crews, D. (1985). Effects of Early Sex Steroid-Hormone Treatment on Courtship Behavior and Sexual Attractivity in the Red-Sided Garter Snake, Thamnophis-Sirtalis-Parietalis. *Physiology & Behavior* Vol. 35, No. 4, pp (569-575), 0031-9384

Crews, D. (1987a). Diversity and Evolution of Behavioral Controlling Mechanisms, In: *Psychobiology of reproductive behavior : an evolutionary perspective*. D. Crews, pp. (88-119), Prentice-Hall, 0137320906 (pbk.), Englewood Cliffs, N.J.

Crews, D. (1987b). *Psychobiology of reproductive behavior : an evolutionary perspective*, Prentice-Hall, 0137320906 (pbk.), Englewood Cliffs, N.J.

Crews, D. (1993). The organizational concept and vertebrates without sex chromosomes. *Brain, behavior and evolution* Vol. 42, No. 4-5, pp (202-214), 0006-8977

Crews, D., Bergeron, J. M. & Mclachlan, J. A. (1995). The role of estrogen in turtle sex determination and the effect of PCBs. *Environmental health perspectives* Vol. 103 Suppl 7, pp (73-77), 0091-6765

Crews, D., Camazine, B., Diamond, M., Mason, R., Tokarz, R. R. & Garstka, W. R. (1984). Hormonal Independence of Courtship Behavior in the Male Garter Snake. *Hormones and Behavior* Vol. 18, No. 1, pp (29-41), 0018-506X

Crews, D., Diamond, M. A., Whittier, J. & Mason, R. (1985). Small Male Body Size in Garter Snake Depends on Testes. *American Journal of Physiology* Vol. 249, No. 1, pp (R62-R66), 0002-9513

Crews, D. & Fitzgerald, K. T. (1980). Sexual-Behavior in Parthenogenetic Lizards (Cnemidophorus). *Proceedings of the National Academy of Sciences of the United States of America-Biological Sciences* Vol. 77, No. 1, pp (499-502), 0027-8424

Crews, D. & Moore, M. C. (1986). Evolution of mechanisms controlling mating behavior. *Science* Vol. 231, No. 4734, pp (121-125), 0036-8075

Cuellar, O. (1971). Reproduction and Mechanism of Meiotic Restitution in Parthenogenetic Lizard Cnemidophorus-Uniparens. *Journal of Morphology* Vol. 133, No. 2, pp (139-&), 0362-2525

Cuellar, O. (1977). Animal Parthenogenesis. *Science* Vol. 197, No. 4306, pp (837-843), 0036-8075

De Mot, R. & Parret, A. H. (2002). A novel class of self-sufficient cytochrome P450 monooxygenases in prokaryotes. *Trends in microbiology* Vol. 10, No. 11, pp (502-508), 0966-842X

De Vries, G. J., Buijs, R. M. & Van Leeuwen, F. W. (1984). Sex differences in vasopressin and other neurotransmitter systems in the brain. *Progress in brain research* Vol. 61, pp (185-203), 0079-6123

Deeming, D. C. & Ferguson, M. W. J. (1989). The Mechanism of Temperature-Dependent Sex Determination in Crocodilians - a Hypothesis. *American Zoologist* Vol. 29, No. 3, pp (973-985), 0003-1569

Demski, L., S. (1987). Diversity in Reproductive Patterns and Behavior in Teleost Fishes, In: *Psychobiology of reproductive behavior : an evolutionary perspective*. D. Crews, pp. (1-27), Prentice-Hall, 0137320906 (pbk.), Englewood Cliffs, N.J.

Di Cosmo, A., Di Cristo, C. & Paolucci, M. (2001). Sex steroid hormone fluctuations and morphological changes of the reproductive system of the female of Octopus vulgaris throughout the annual cycle. *The Journal of experimental zoology* Vol. 289, No. 1, pp (33-47), 0022-104X

Di Cosmo, A., Di Cristo, C. & Paolucci, M. (2002). A estradiol-17beta receptor in the reproductive system of the female of Octopus vulgaris: characterization and immunolocalization. *Molecular reproduction and development* Vol. 61, No. 3, pp (367-375), 1040-452X

Di Cosmo, A., Paolucci, M., Di Cristo, C., Botte, V. & Ciarcia, G. (1998). Progesterone receptor in the reproductive system of the female of Octopus vulgaris:

characterization and immunolocalization. *Molecular reproduction and development* Vol. 50, No. 4, pp (451-460), 1040-452X

Durhan, E. J., Lambright, C. S., Makynen, E. A., Lazorchak, J., Hartig, P. C., Wilson, V. S., Gray, L. E. & Ankley, G. T. (2006). Identification of metabolites of trenbolone acetate in androgenic runoff from a beef feedlot. *Environmental health perspectives* Vol. 114 Suppl 1, pp (65-68), 0091-6765

Eick, G. N. & Thornton, J. W. (2011). Evolution of steroid receptors from an estrogen-sensitive ancestral receptor. *Molecular and cellular endocrinology* Vol. 334, No. 1-2, pp (31-38), 0303-7207

Eidne, K. A., Hendricks, D. T. & Millar, R. P. (1985). Demonstration of a 60K molecular weight luteinizing hormone-releasing hormone receptor in solubilized adrenal membranes by a ligand-immunoblotting technique. *Endocrinology* Vol. 116, No. 5, pp (1792-1795), 0013-7227

Elbrecht, A. & Smith, R. G. (1992). Aromatase enzyme activity and sex determination in chickens. *Science* Vol. 255, No. 5043, pp (467-470), 0036-8075

Ernst, M., Parker, M. G. & Rodan, G. A. (1991). Functional estrogen receptors in osteoblastic cells demonstrated by transfection with a reporter gene containing an estrogen response element. *Molecular endocrinology* Vol. 5, No. 11, pp (1597-1606), 0888-8809

Fernandez-Fernandez, R., Martini, A. C., Navarro, V. M., Castellano, J. M., Dieguez, C., Aguilar, E., Pinilla, L. & Tena-Sempere, M. (2006). Novel signals for the integration of energy balance and reproduction. *Molecular and cellular endocrinology* Vol. 254-255, pp (127-132), 0303-7207

Frank, L. G., Glickman, S. E. & Powch, I. (1990). Sexual dimorphism in the spotted hyaena (Crocuta crocuta). *Journal of Zoology* Vol. 221, No. 2, pp (308-313), 1469-7998

Fukayama, S. & Takahashi, H. (1985). Changes in the serum levels of estradiol-17β and testosterone in the Japanese river lamprey, *Lampetra japonica*, in the course of sexual maturation. *Bull Fac Fish Hokkaido Univ* Vol. 36, No. 4, pp (163-169)

Gamba, M. & Pralong, F. P. (2006). Control of GnRH neuronal activity by metabolic factors: the role of leptin and insulin. *Molecular and cellular endocrinology* Vol. 254-255, pp (133-139), 0303-7207

Garstka, W. R. & Crews, D. (1981). Female Sex-Pheromone in the Skin and Circulation of a Garter Snake. *Science* Vol. 214, No. 4521, pp (681-683), 0036-8075

Gazourian, L., Deragon, K. L., Chase, C. F., Pati, D., Habibi, H. R. & Sower, S. A. (1997). Characteristics of GnRH binding in the gonads and effects of lamprey GnRH-I and -III on reproduction in the adult sea lamprey. *General and Comparative Endocrinology* Vol. 108, No. 2, pp (327-339), 0016-6480

Gibson, G. G., Plant, N. J., Swales, K. E., Ayrton, A. & El-Sankary, W. (2002). Receptor-dependent transcriptional activation of cytochrome P4503A genes: induction mechanisms, species differences and interindividual variation in man. *Xenobiotica; the fate of foreign compounds in biological systems* Vol. 32, No. 3, pp (165-206), 0049-8254

Giusti, R. M., Iwamoto, K. & Hatch, E. E. (1995). Diethylstilbestrol revisited: a review of the long-term health effects. *Annals of internal medicine* Vol. 122, No. 10, pp (778-788), 0003-4819

Glickman, S. E., Frank, L. G., Pavgi, S. & Licht, P. (1992). Hormonal correlates of 'masculinization' in female spotted hyaenas (Crocuta crocuta). 1. Infancy to sexual maturity. *Journal of reproduction and fertility* Vol. 95, No. 2, pp (451-462), 0022-4251

Goldberg, J. I., Garofalo, R., Price, C. J. & Chang, J. P. (1993). Presence and biological activity of a GnRH-like factor in the nervous system of Helisoma trivolvis. *The Journal of comparative neurology* Vol. 336, No. 4, pp (571-582), 0021-9967

Gore, A. C. (2002). *GnRH, the master molecule of reproduction / by Andrea C. Gore*, Kluwer Academic Publishers, 0792376811 (alk. paper)

Goth, A. & Booth, D. T. (2005). Temperature-dependent sex ratio in a bird. *Biology letters* Vol. 1, No. 1, pp (31-33), 1744-9561

Gray, L. E., Jr., Ostby, J., Monosson, E. & Kelce, W. R. (1999). Environmental antiandrogens: low doses of the fungicide vinclozolin alter sexual differentiation of the male rat. *Toxicol Ind Health* Vol. 15, No. 1-2, pp (48-64), 0748-2337

Gray, L. E., Jr., Ostby, J. S. & Kelce, W. R. (1994). Developmental effects of an environmental antiandrogen: the fungicide vinclozolin alters sex differentiation of the male rat. *Toxicology and applied pharmacology* Vol. 129, No. 1, pp (46-52), 0041-008X

Gray, L. E., Jr., Wilson, V., Noriega, N., Lambright, C., Furr, J., Stoker, T. E., Laws, S. C., Goldman, J., Cooper, R. L. & Foster, P. M. (2004). Use of the laboratory rat as a model in endocrine disruptor screening and testing. *ILAR journal / National Research Council, Institute of Laboratory Animal Resources* Vol. 45, No. 4, pp (425-437), 1084-2020

Guillette, L. J., Crain, D. A., Gunderson, M. P., Kools, S. a. E., Milnes, M. R., Orlando, E. F., Rooney, A. A. & Woodward, A. R. (2000). Alligators and endocrine disrupting contaminants: A current perspective. *American Zoologist* Vol. 40, No. 3, pp (438-452), 0003-1569

Guillette, L. J., Jr. (2006). Endocrine disrupting contaminants--beyond the dogma. *Environmental health perspectives* Vol. 114 Suppl 1, pp (9-12), 0091-6765

Guillette, L. J., Jr., Crain, D. A., Rooney, A. A. & Pickford, D. B. (1995). Organization versus activation: the role of endocrine-disrupting contaminants (EDCs) during embryonic development in wildlife. *Environmental health perspectives* Vol. 103 Suppl 7, pp (157-164), 0091-6765

Han, S. K., Gottsch, M. L., Lee, K. J., Popa, S. M., Smith, J. T., Jakawich, S. K., Clifton, D. K., Steiner, R. A. & Herbison, A. E. (2005). Activation of gonadotropin-releasing hormone neurons by kisspeptin as a neuroendocrine switch for the onset of puberty. *The Journal of neuroscience : the official journal of the Society for Neuroscience* Vol. 25, No. 49, pp (11349-11356), 1529-2401

Harrington, R. W., Jr. (1961). Oviparous Hermaphroditic Fish with Internal Self-Fertilization. *Science* Vol. 134, No. 3492, pp (1749-1750), 0036-8075

Harrington, R. W., Jr. & Crossman, R. A., Jr. (1976). Temperature-induced meristic variation among three homozygous genotypes (clones) of the self-fertilizing fish Rivulus marmoratus. *Canadian journal of zoology* Vol. 54, No. 7, pp (1143-1155), 0008-4301

Hayes, T., Chan, R. & Licht, P. (1993). Interactions of temperature and steroids on larval growth, development, and metamorphosis in a toad (Bufo boreas). *The Journal of experimental zoology* Vol. 266, No. 3, pp (206-215), 0022-104X

Hayes, T. B. (1997a). Hormonal mechanisms as potential constraints on evolution: Examples from the Anura. *American Zoologist* Vol. 37, No. 6, pp (482-490)

Hayes, T. B. (1997b). Steroids as potential modulators of thyroid hormone activity in anuran metamorphosis. *American Zoologist* Vol. 37, No. 2, pp (185-194), 0003-1569

Hayes, T. B. (1998). Sex determination and primary sex differentiation in amphibians: genetic and developmental mechanisms. *The Journal of experimental zoology* Vol. 281, No. 5, pp (373-399), 0022-104X

Hayes, T. B., Collins, A., Lee, M., Mendoza, M., Noriega, N., Stuart, A. A. & Vonk, A. (2002). Hermaphroditic, demasculinized frogs after exposure to the herbicide atrazine at low ecologically relevant doses. *Proc Natl Acad Sci U S A* Vol. 99, No. 8, pp (5476-5480), 0027-8424

Hayes, T. B., Khoury, V., Narayan, A., Nazir, M., Park, A., Brown, T., Adame, L., Chan, E., Buchholz, D., Stueve, T. & Gallipeau, S. (2010). Atrazine induces complete feminization and chemical castration in male African clawed frogs (Xenopus laevis). *Proc Natl Acad Sci U S A* Vol. 107, No. 10, pp (4612-4617), 0027-8424

Hayes, T. B., Stuart, A. A., Mendoza, M., Collins, A., Noriega, N., Vonk, A., Johnston, G., Liu, R. & Kpodzo, D. (2006). Characterization of atrazine-induced gonadal malformations in African clawed frogs (Xenopus laevis) and comparisons with effects of an androgen antagonist (cyproterone acetate) and exogenous estrogen (17beta-estradiol): Support for the demasculinization/feminization hypothesis. *Environmental health perspectives* Vol. 114 Suppl 1, pp (134-141), 0091-6765

Hazum, E. & Nimrod, A. (1982). Photoaffinity-labeling and fluorescence-distribution studies of gonadotropin-releasing hormone receptors in ovarian granulosa cells. *Proceedings of the National Academy of Sciences of the United States of America* Vol. 79, No. 6, pp (1747-1750), 0027-8424

Hinson, J., Raven, P. & Chew, S. L. (2010). *The endocrine system : basic science and clinical conditions* (2nd), Churchill Livingstone/Elsevier, 9780702033728 (alk. paper) 0702033723 (alk. paper), Edinburgh ; New York

Holland, C. A. & Dumont, J. N. (1975). Oogenesis in Xenopus laevis (Daudin). IV. Effects of gonadotropin, estrogen and starvation on endocytosis in developing oocytes. *Cell and tissue research* Vol. 162, No. 2, pp (177-184), 0302-766X

Howdeshell, K. L., Furr, J., Lambright, C. R., Rider, C. V., Wilson, V. S. & Gray, L. E., Jr. (2007). Cumulative effects of dibutyl phthalate and diethylhexyl phthalate on male rat reproductive tract development: altered fetal steroid hormones and genes. *Toxicological sciences : an official journal of the Society of Toxicology* Vol. 99, No. 1, pp (190-202), 1096-6080

Hughes, A. L. & Friedman, R. (2005). Loss of ancestral genes in the genomic evolution of Ciona intestinalis. *Evol Dev* Vol. 7, No. 3, pp (196-200), 1520-541X

Iwakoshi, E., Takuwa-Kuroda, K., Fujisawa, Y., Hisada, M., Ukena, K., Tsutsui, K. & Minakata, H. (2002). Isolation and characterization of a GnRH-like peptide from Octopus vulgaris. *Biochemical and biophysical research communications* Vol. 291, No. 5, pp (1187-1193), 0006-291X

Jennes, L., Eyigor, O., Janovick, J. A. & Conn, P. M. (1997). Brain gonadotropin releasing hormone receptors: localization and regulation. *Recent progress in hormone research* Vol. 52, pp (475-490; discussion 490-471), 0079-9963

Jobling, S., Reynolds, T., White, R., Parker, M. G. & Sumpter, J. P. (1995). A variety of environmentally persistent chemicals, including some phthalate plasticizers, are weakly estrogenic. *Environmental health perspectives* Vol. 103, No. 6, pp (582-587), 0091-6765

Jobling, S. & Tyler, C. R. (2003a). Endocrine disruption in wild freshwater fish. *Pure and Applied Chemistry* Vol. 75, No. 11-12, pp (2219-2234)

Jobling, S. & Tyler, C. R. (2003b). Endocrine disruption, parasites and pollutants in wild freshwater fish. *Parasitology* Vol. 126 Suppl, pp (S103-108), 0031-1820

Jobling, S., Williams, R., Johnson, A., Taylor, A., Gross-Sorokin, M., Nolan, M., Tyler, C. R., Van Aerle, R., Santos, E. & Brighty, G. (2006). Predicted exposures to steroid estrogens in U.K. rivers correlate with widespread sexual disruption in wild fish populations. *Environmental health perspectives* Vol. 114 Suppl 1, pp (32-39), 0091-6765

Kajiwara, M., Kuraku, S., Kurokawa, T., Kato, K., Toda, S., Hirose, H., Takahashi, S., Shibata, Y., Iguchi, T., Matsumoto, T., Miyata, T., Miura, T. & Takahashi, Y. (2006). Tissue preferential expression of estrogen receptor gene in the marine snail, Thais clavigera. *General and Comparative Endocrinology* Vol. 148, No. 3, pp (315-326), 0016-6480

Kanda, A., Satake, H., Kawada, T. & Minakata, H. (2005). Novel evolutionary lineages of the invertebrate oxytocin/vasopressin superfamily peptides and their receptors in the common octopus (Octopus vulgaris). *The Biochemical journal* Vol. 387, No. Pt 1, pp (85-91), 0264-6021

Kanda, A., Takahashi, T., Satake, H. & Minakata, H. (2006). Molecular and functional characterization of a novel gonadotropin-releasing-hormone receptor isolated from the common octopus (Octopus vulgaris). *The Biochemical journal* Vol. 395, No. 1, pp (125-135), 0264-6021

Kanda, A., Takuwa-Kuroda, K., Iwakoshi-Ukena, E., Furukawa, Y., Matsushima, O. & Minakata, H. (2003). Cloning of Octopus cephalotocin receptor, a member of the oxytocin/vasopressin superfamily. *The Journal of endocrinology* Vol. 179, No. 2, pp (281-291), 0022-0795

Katsu, Y., Kubokawa, K., Urushitani, H. & Iguchi, T. (2010). Estrogen-dependent transactivation of amphioxus steroid hormone receptor via both estrogen and androgen response elements. *Endocrinology* Vol. 151, No. 2, pp (639-648), 0013-7227

Kawauchi, H. & Sower, S. A. (2006). The dawn and evolution of hormones in the adenohypophysis. *General and Comparative Endocrinology* Vol. 148, No. 1, pp (3-14), 0016-6480

Kearney, M., Fujita, M. K. & Ridenour, J. (2009). Lost Sex in the Reptiles: Constraints and Correlations, In: *Lost Sex*. I. Schön, K. Martens and P. Dijk, pp. (447-474), Springer Netherlands, 978-90-481-2770-2

Keay, J., Bridgham, J. T. & Thornton, J. W. (2006). The Octopus vulgaris estrogen receptor is a constitutive transcriptional activator: evolutionary and functional implications. *Endocrinology* Vol. 147, No. 8, pp (3861-3869), 0013-7227

Kelce, W. R., Stone, C. R., Laws, S. C., Gray, L. E., Kemppainen, J. A. & Wilson, E. M. (1995). Persistent DDT metabolite p,p'-DDE is a potent androgen receptor antagonist. *Nature* Vol. 375, No. 6532, pp (581-585), 0028-0836

Kelce, W. R. & Wilson, E. M. (1997). Environmental antiandrogens: developmental effects, molecular mechanisms, and clinical implications. *J Mol Med* Vol. 75, No. 3, pp (198-207), 0946-2716

Klime, D. E. & Larsen, L. O. (1987). Effect of gonadectomy and hypophysectomy on plasma steroid levels in male and femal lampreys (*Lampetra fluviatilis*, L.). *Gen Comp Endocrinol* Vol. 68, pp (189-196)

Klotz, D. M., Beckman, B. S., Hill, S. M., Mclachlan, J. A., Walters, M. R. & Arnold, S. F. (1996). Identification of environmental chemicals with estrogenic activity using a combination of in vitro assays. *Environmental health perspectives* Vol. 104, No. 10, pp (1084-1089), 0091-6765

Kramer, C. R., Koulish, S. & Bertacchi, P. L. (1988). The effects of testosterone implants on ovarian morphology in the bluehead wrasse, Thalassoma bifasciatum (Bloch) (Teleostei: Labridae). *Journal of Fish Biology* Vol. 32, No. 3, pp (397-407), 1095-8649

Lambright, C., Ostby, J., Bobseine, K., Wilson, V., Hotchkiss, A. K., Mann, P. C. & Gray, L. E., Jr. (2000). Cellular and molecular mechanisms of action of linuron: an antiandrogenic herbicide that produces reproductive malformations in male rats. *Toxicological sciences : an official journal of the Society of Toxicology* Vol. 56, No. 2, pp (389-399), 1096-6080

Lehman, M. N., Coolen, L. M. & Goodman, R. L. (2010). Minireview: kisspeptin/neurokinin B/dynorphin (KNDy) cells of the arcuate nucleus: a central node in the control of gonadotropin-releasing hormone secretion. *Endocrinology* Vol. 151, No. 8, pp (3479-3489), 1945-7170

Levavi-Sivan, B., Bogerd, J., Mananos, E. L., Gomez, A. & Lareyre, J. J. (2010). Perspectives on fish gonadotropins and their receptors. *Gen Comp Endocrinol* Vol. 165, No. 3, pp (412-437), 0016-6480

Lewis, D. F., Watson, E. & Lake, B. G. (1998). Evolution of the cytochrome P450 superfamily: sequence alignments and pharmacogenetics. *Mutation research* Vol. 410, No. 3, pp (245-270), 0027-5107

Licht, P., Frank, L. G., Pavgi, S., Yalcinkaya, T. M., Siiteri, P. K. & Glickman, S. E. (1992). Hormonal correlates of 'masculinization' in female spotted hyaenas (Crocuta crocuta). 2. Maternal and fetal steroids. *Journal of reproduction and fertility* Vol. 95, No. 2, pp (463-474), 0022-4251

Lindeque, M., Skinner, J. D. & Millar, R. P. (1986). Adrenal and gonadal contribution to circulating androgens in spotted hyaenas (Crocuta crocuta) as revealed by LHRH, hCG and ACTH stimulation. *Journal of reproduction and fertility* Vol. 78, No. 1, pp (211-217), 0022-4251

Lombardi, J. (1998). *Comparative vertebrate reproduction*, Kluwer Academic Publishers, 0792383362 (alk. paper), Boston

Lone, K. P. (1997). Natural sex steroids and their xenobiotic analogs in animal production: growth, carcass quality, pharmacokinetics, metabolism, mode of action, residues, methods, and epidemiology. *Crit Rev Food Sci Nutr* Vol. 37, No. 2, pp (93-209), 1040-8398

Loumaye, E., Thorner, J. & Catt, K. J. (1982). Yeast mating pheromone activates mammalian gonadotrophs: evolutionary conservation of a reproductive hormone? *Science* Vol. 218, No. 4579, pp (1323-1325), 0036-8075

Maglich, J. M., Sluder, A., Guan, X., Shi, Y., Mckee, D. D., Carrick, K., Kamdar, K., Willson, T. M. & Moore, J. T. (2001). Comparison of complete nuclear receptor sets from the human, Caenorhabditis elegans and Drosophila genomes. *Genome biology* Vol. 2, No. 8, pp (RESEARCH0029), 1465-6906

Marchetti, B., Gallo, F., Farinella, Z., Tirolo, C., Testa, N., Romeo, C. & Morale, M. C. (1998). Luteinizing hormone-releasing hormone is a primary signaling molecule in the neuroimmune network. *Annals of the New York Academy of Sciences* Vol. 840, pp (205-248), 0077-8923

Marchetti, B., Guarcello, V., Morale, M. C., Bartoloni, G., Farinella, Z., Cordaro, S. & Scapagnini, U. (1989). Luteinizing hormone-releasing hormone-binding sites in the rat thymus: characteristics and biological function. *Endocrinology* Vol. 125, No. 2, pp (1025-1036), 0013-7227

Marty, M. S., Carney, E. W. & Rowlands, J. C. (2011). Endocrine disruption: historical perspectives and its impact on the future of toxicology testing. *Toxicological sciences : an official journal of the Society of Toxicology* Vol. 120 Suppl 1, pp (S93-108), 1096-0929

Mason, J. I., Carr, B. R. & Murry, B. A. (1987). Imidazole antimycotics: selective inhibitors of steroid aromatization and progesterone hydroxylation. *Steroids* Vol. 50, No. 1-3, pp (179-189), 0039-128X

Mason, R. T. & Crews, D. (1985). Female mimicry in garter snakes. *Nature* Vol. 316, No. 6023, pp (59-60), 0028-0836

Matsumoto, T., Nakamura, A. M., Mori, K., Akiyama, I., Hirose, H. & Takahashi, Y. (2007). Oyster estrogen receptor: cDNA cloning and immunolocalization. *General and Comparative Endocrinology* Vol. 151, No. 2, pp (195-201), 0016-6480

Mccarthy, M. M. & Arnold, A. P. (2007). Sex Differences in the Brain: What's Old and What's New?, In: *Sex Differences in the Brain: From genes to behavior*. J. B. Becker, K. J. Berkley, N. Gearyet al, pp. (15-33), Oxford University Press, 9780195311587, New York

Meyer, H. H. (2001). Biochemistry and physiology of anabolic hormones used for improvement of meat production. *APMIS* Vol. 109, No. 1, pp (1-8), 0903-4641

Millar, R. P., Lu, Z. L., Pawson, A. J., Flanagan, C. A., Morgan, K. & Maudsley, S. R. (2004). Gonadotropin-releasing hormone receptors. *Endocr Rev* Vol. 25, No. 2, pp (235-275)

Mittwoch, U. (1971). Sex determination in birds and mammals. *Nature* Vol. 231, No. 5303, pp (432-434)

Moore, F. L. (1978). Differential Effects of Testosterone Plus Dihydrotestosterone on Male Courtship of Castrated Newts. *American Zoologist* Vol. 18, No. 3, pp (615-615), 0003-1569

Moore, F. L. (1987). Behavioral Actions of Neurohypophysial Peptides, In: *Psychobiology of reproductive behavior : an evolutionary perspective*. D. Crews, pp. (60-87), Prentice-Hall, 0137320906 (pbk.), Englewood Cliffs, NJ

Moore, F. L. & Miller, L. J. (1983). Arginine Vasotocin Induces Sexual-Behavior of Newts by Acting on Cells in the Brain. *Peptides* Vol. 4, No. 1, pp (97-102), 0196-9781

Moore, F. L. & Miller, L. J. (1984). Stress-Induced Inhibition of Sexual-Behavior - Corticosterone Inhibits Courtship Behaviors of a Male Amphibian (Taricha-Granulosa). *Hormones and Behavior* Vol. 18, No. 4, pp (400-410), 0018-506X

Moore, F. L., Miller, L. J., Spielvogel, S. P., Kubiak, T. & Folkers, K. (1982). Luteinizing-Hormone-Releasing Hormone Involvement in the Reproductive-Behavior of a Male Amphibian. *Neuroendocrinology* Vol. 35, No. 3, pp (212-216), 0028-3835

Moore, M. C. & Kranz, R. (1983). Evidence for Androgen Independence of Male Mounting Behavior in White-Crowned Sparrows (Zonotrichia, Leucophrys, Gambelii). *Hormones and Behavior* Vol. 17, No. 4, pp (414-423), 0018-506X

Morrell, J. A. (1941). Stilbestrol - Summary of some clinical reports on stilbestrol. *Journal of Clinical Endocrinology* Vol. 1, No. 5, pp (419-423), 0368-1610

Nakabayashi, K., Matsumi, H., Bhalla, A., Bae, J., Mosselman, S., Hsu, S. Y. & Hsueh, A. J. (2002). Thyrostimulin, a heterodimer of two new human glycoprotein hormone subunits, activates the thyroid-stimulating hormone receptor. *The Journal of clinical investigation* Vol. 109, No. 11, pp (1445-1452), 0021-9738

Nakamura, M. (2009). Sex determination in amphibians. *Seminars in Cell & Developmental Biology* Vol. 20, No. 3, pp (271-282), 1084-9521

Nakamura, M. (2010). The mechanism of sex determination in vertebrates-are sex steroids the key-factor? *Journal of experimental zoology. Part A, Ecological genetics and physiology* Vol. 313, No. 7, pp (381-398), 1932-5223

Neaves, W. B. & Baumann, P. (2011). Unisexual reproduction among vertebrates. *Trends in genetics : TIG* Vol. 27, No. 3, pp (81-88), 0168-9525

Neaves, W. B., Griffin, J. E. & Wilson, J. D. (1980). Sexual dimorphism of the phallus in spotted hyaena (Crocuta crocuta). *Journal of reproduction and fertility* Vol. 59, No. 2, pp (509-513), 0022-4251

Nebert, D. W., Nelson, D. R. & Feyereisen, R. (1989). Evolution of the cytochrome P450 genes. *Xenobiotica; the fate of foreign compounds in biological systems* Vol. 19, No. 10, pp (1149-1160), 0049-8254

Nelson, D. R. (2011). Progress in tracing the evolutionary paths of cytochrome P450. *Biochimica et biophysica acta* Vol. 1814, No. 1, pp (14-18), 0006-3002

Nishimura, H. (1985). Endocrine control of renal handling of solutes and water in vertebrates. *Renal physiology* Vol. 8, No. 4-5, pp (279-300), 0378-5858

Noriega, N. C. & Hayes, T. B. (2000). DDT congener effects on secondary sex coloration in the reed frog Hyperolius argus: a partial evaluation of the Hyperolius argus endocrine screen. *Comparative biochemistry and physiology. Part B, Biochemistry & molecular biology* Vol. 126, No. 2, pp (231-237), 1096-4959

Noriega, N. C., Ostby, J., Lambright, C., Wilson, V. S. & Gray, L. E., Jr. (2005). Late gestational exposure to the fungicide prochloraz delays the onset of parturition and causes reproductive malformations in male but not female rat offspring. *Biol Reprod* Vol. 72, No. 6, pp (1324-1335), 0006-3363

Norris, D. O. & Lopez, K. H. (2011a). *Hormones and reproduction of vertebrates*, Academic Press, 9780123749321, Amsterdam

Norris, D. O. & Lopez, K. H. (2011b). *Hormones and Reproduction of Vertebrates Volume 3: Reptiles*, Academic Press, 9780123749307 Amsterdam

Norris, D. O. & Lopez, K. H. (2011c). *Hormones and Reproduction of Vertebrates Volume 4: Birds*, Academic Press, 9780123749291 Amsterdam

Nottebohm, F. & Arnold, A. P. (1976). Sexual dimorphism in vocal control areas of the songbird brain. *Science* Vol. 194, No. 4261, pp (211-213), 0036-8075

Oakley, A. E., Clifton, D. K. & Steiner, R. A. (2009). Kisspeptin signaling in the brain. *Endocrine reviews* Vol. 30, No. 6, pp (713-743), 0163-769X

Olsen, W. W. & Marsden, S. J. (1954). Natural parthenogenesis in turkey eggs. *Science* Vol. 120, No. 3118, pp (545-546), 0036-8075

Orlando, E. F. & Guillette, L. J., Jr. (2007). Sexual dimorphic responses in wildlife exposed to endocrine disrupting chemicals. *Environ Res* Vol. 104, No. 1, pp (163-173), 0013-9351

Orlando, E. F., Kolok, A. S., Binzcik, G. A., Gates, J. L., Horton, M. K., Lambright, C. S., Gray, L. E., Jr., Soto, A. M. & Guillette, L. J., Jr. (2004). Endocrine-disrupting effects of cattle feedlot effluent on an aquatic sentinel species, the fathead minnow. *Environmental health perspectives* Vol. 112, No. 3, pp (353-358), 0091-6765

Ottinger, M. A., Lavoie, E. T., Abdelnabi, M., Quinn, M. J., Jr., Marcell, A. & Dean, K. (2009). An overview of dioxin-like compounds, PCB, and pesticide exposures associated with sexual differentiation of neuroendocrine systems, fluctuating asymmetry, and behavioral effects in birds. *Journal of environmental science and health. Part C, Environmental carcinogenesis & ecotoxicology reviews* Vol. 27, No. 4, pp (286-300), 1532-4095

Owens, W., Gray, L. E., Zeiger, E., Walker, M., Yamasaki, K., Ashby, J. & Jacob, E. (2007). The OECD program to validate the rat Hershberger bioassay to screen compounds for in vivo androgen and antiandrogen responses: phase 2 dose-response studies. *Environmental health perspectives* Vol. 115, No. 5, pp (671-678), 0091-6765

Pardridge, W. M. (1987). Plasma protein-mediated transport of steroid and thyroid hormones. *The American journal of physiology* Vol. 252, No. 2 Pt 1, pp (E157-164), 0002-9513

Pardridge, W. M., Mietus, L. J., Frumar, A. M., Davidson, B. J. & Judd, H. L. (1980). Effects of human serum on transport of testosterone and estradiol into rat brain. *The American journal of physiology* Vol. 239, No. 1, pp (E103-108), 0002-9513

Paris, M., Pettersson, K., Schubert, M., Bertrand, S., Pongratz, I., Escriva, H. & Laudet, V. (2008). An amphioxus orthologue of the estrogen receptor that does not bind estradiol: insights into estrogen receptor evolution. *BMC evolutionary biology* Vol. 8, pp (219), 1471-2148

Park, J. H. & Rissman, E. F. (2011). Behavioral Neuroendocrinology of Reproduction in Mammals, In: *Hormones and Reproduction of Vertebrates Volume 5: Mammals*. D. O. Norris and K. H. Lopez, pp. (139-173), Academic Press, 9780123749284 Amsterdam

Parks, L. G., Ostby, J. S., Lambright, C. R., Abbott, B. D., Klinefelter, G. R., Barlow, N. J. & Gray, L. E., Jr. (2000). The plasticizer diethylhexyl phthalate induces malformations by decreasing fetal testosterone synthesis during sexual differentiation in the male rat. *Toxicological sciences : an official journal of the Society of Toxicology* Vol. 58, No. 2, pp (339-349), 1096-6080

Paul-Prasanth, B., Nakamura, M. & Nagahama, Y. (2011). Sex Determination in Fishes, In: *Hormones and Reproduction of Vertebrates Volume 1: Fishes*. D. O. Norris and K. H. Lopez, pp. (1-14), Academic Press, 9780123750099 Amsterdam

Pazos, A. J. & Mathieu, M. (1999). Effects of five natural gonadotropin-releasing hormones on cell suspensions of marine bivalve gonad: stimulation of gonial DNA synthesis. *General and Comparative Endocrinology* Vol. 113, No. 1, pp (112-120), 0016-6480

Phoenix, C. H., Goy, R. W., Gerall, A. A. & Young, W. C. (1959a). The Organizing Action of an Androgen Administered Prenatally on the Tissues Mediating Mating Behavior in the Guinea Pig. *Anatomical Record* Vol. 133, No. 2, pp (323-323), 0003-276X

Phoenix, C. H., Goy, R. W., Gerall, A. A. & Young, W. C. (1959b). Organizing action of prenatally administered testosterone propionate on the tissues mediating mating behavior in the female guinea pig. *Endocrinology* Vol. 65, pp (369-382), 0013-7227

Pielecka-Fortuna, J. & Moenter, S. M. (2010). Kisspeptin increases gamma-aminobutyric acidergic and glutamatergic transmission directly to gonadotropin-releasing hormone neurons in an estradiol-dependent manner. *Endocrinology* Vol. 151, No. 1, pp (291-300), 1945-7170

Pietras, R. J. & Szego, C. M. (1977). Specific binding sites for oestrogen at the outer surfaces of isolated endometrial cells. *Nature* Vol. 265, No. 5589, pp (69-72), 0028-0836

Potts, G. W., Wootton, R. J. & Fisheries Society of the British Isles. (1984). *Fish reproduction : strategies and tactics*, Academic Press, 0125636601, London ; Orlando

Powell, J. F., Reska-Skinner, S. M., Prakash, M. O., Fischer, W. H., Park, M., Rivier, J. E., Craig, A. G., Mackie, G. O. & Sherwood, N. M. (1996). Two new forms of gonadotropin-releasing hormone in a protochordate and the evolutionary implications. *Proceedings of the National Academy of Sciences of the United States of America* Vol. 93, No. 19, pp (10461-10464), 0027-8424

Raisman, G. & Field, P. M. (1973). Sexual Dimorphism in Neuropil of Preoptic Area of Rat and Its Dependence on Neonatal Androgen. *Brain Research* Vol. 54, No. May17, pp (1-29), 0006-8993

Ramenofsky, M. (2011). Hormones in Migration and Reproductive Cycles of Birds, In: *Hormones and Reproduction of Vertebrates Volume 4: Birds*. D. O. Norris and K. H. Lopez, pp. (205-237), Academic Press, 9780123749291 Amsterdam

Ravi, V. & Venkatesh, B. (2008). Rapidly evolving fish genomes and teleost diversity. *Current opinion in genetics & development* Vol. 18, No. 6, pp (544-550), 0959-437X

Riviere, J. E. & Papich, M. G. (2009). *Veterinary pharmacology and therapeutics* (9th), Wiley-Blackwell, 9780813820613, Ames, Iowa

Roa, J., Navarro, V. M. & Tena-Sempere, M. (2011). Kisspeptins in Reproductive Biology: Consensus Knowledge and Recent Developments. *Biology of reproduction*, 0006-3363

Robinson-Rechavi, M., Escriva Garcia, H. & Laudet, V. (2003). The nuclear receptor superfamily. *Journal of cell science* Vol. 116, No. Pt 4, pp (585-586), 0021-9533

Roland, A. V. & Moenter, S. M. (2011). Glucosensing by GnRH neurons: inhibition by androgens and involvement of AMP-activated protein kinase. *Molecular endocrinology* Vol. 25, No. 5, pp (847-858), 1944-9917

Roth, J., Leroith, D., Collier, E. S., Watkinson, A. & Lesniak, M. A. (1986). The evolutionary origins of intercellular communication and the Maginot Lines of the mind. *Annals of the New York Academy of Sciences* Vol. 463, pp (1-11), 0077-8923

Ruiz-Trillo, I., Riutort, M., Littlewood, D. T., Herniou, E. A. & Baguna, J. (1999). Acoel flatworms: earliest extant bilaterian Metazoans, not members of Platyhelminthes. *Science* Vol. 283, No. 5409, pp (1919-1923), 0036-8075

Sarvella, P. (1974). Environmental Effects on a Parthenogenetic Line of Chickens. *Poult Sci* Vol. 53, No. 1, pp (273-279)

Schultz, R. J. (1973). Unisexual Fish: Laboratory Synthesis of a "Species". *Science* Vol. 179, No. 4069, pp (180-181), 00368075

Schwabe, J. W. & Teichmann, S. A. (2004). Nuclear receptors: the evolution of diversity. *Science's STKE : signal transduction knowledge environment* Vol. 2004, No. 217, pp (pe4), 1525-8882

Shapiro, D. Y. (1984). Sex Reversal and Sociodemographic Processes in Coral Reef Fishes, In: *Fish reproduction : strategies and tactics*. G. W. Potts, R. J. Wootton and Fisheries Society of the British Isles., pp. (103-118), Academic Press, 0125636601, London ; Orlando

Shelton, J. N. (1990). Reproductive technology in animal production. *Rev Sci Tech* Vol. 9, No. 3, pp (825-845), 0253-1933

Simerly, R. B., Swanson, L. W. & Gorski, R. A. (1985). Reversal of the sexually dimorphic distribution of serotonin-immunoreactive fibers in the medial preoptic nucleus by treatment with perinatal androgen. *Brain Research* Vol. 340, No. 1, pp (91-98), 0006-8993

Sirinathsinghji, D. J. S. (1984). Modulation of Lordosis Behavior of Female Rats by Naloxone, Beta-Endorphin and Its Antiserum in the Mesencephalic Central Gray - Possible Mediation Via Gnrh. *Neuroendocrinology* Vol. 39, No. 3, pp (222-230), 0028-3835

Sluczewski, A. & Roth, P. (1950). [Influence of androgenic and estrogenic substances on experimental metamorphosis of hypophysectomized axalotis]. *Gynecol Obstet (Paris)* Vol. 49, No. 5, pp (504-525), 0017-601X

Smith, J. T., Coolen, L. M., Kriegsfeld, L. J., Sari, I. P., Jaafarzadehshirazi, M. R., Maltby, M., Bateman, K., Goodman, R. L., Tilbrook, A. J., Ubuka, T., Bentley, G. E., Clarke, I. J. & Lehman, M. N. (2008). Variation in kisspeptin and RFamide-related peptide (RFRP) expression and terminal connections to gonadotropin-releasing hormone neurons in the brain: a novel medium for seasonal breeding in the sheep. *Endocrinology* Vol. 149, No. 11, pp (5770-5782), 0013-7227

Smith, O. W. & Smith, G. V. (1949a). The influence of diethylstilbestrol on the progress and outcome of pregnancy as based on a comparison of treated with untreated primigravidas. *American journal of obstetrics and gynecology* Vol. 58, No. 5, pp (994-1009), 0002-9378

Smith, O. W. & Smith, G. V. (1949b). Use of diethylstilbestrol to prevent fetal loss from complications of late pregnancy. *The New England journal of medicine* Vol. 241, No. 15, pp (562-568), 0028-4793

Sodersten, P., Henning, M., Melin, P. & Ludin, S. (1983). Vasopressin Alters Female Sexual-Behavior by Acting on the Brain Independently of Alterations in Blood-Pressure. *Nature* Vol. 301, No. 5901, pp (608-610), 0028-0836

Somoza, G. M., Miranda, L. A., Strobl-Mazzulla, P. & Guilgur, L. G. (2002). Gonadotropin-releasing hormone (GnRH): from fish to mammalian brains. *Cellular and Molecular Neurobiology* Vol. 22, No. 5-6, pp (589-609), 0272-4340

Soto, A. M., Calabro, J. M., Prechtl, N. V., Yau, A. Y., Orlando, E. F., Daxenberger, A., Kolok, A. S., Guillette, L. J., Jr., Le Bizec, B., Lange, I. G. & Sonnenschein, C. (2004). Androgenic and estrogenic activity in water bodies receiving cattle feedlot effluent in Eastern Nebraska, USA. *Environmental health perspectives* Vol. 112, No. 3, pp (346-352), 0091-6765

Sower, S. A., Freamat, M. & Kavanaugh, S. I. (2009). The origins of the vertebrate hypothalamic-pituitary-gonadal (HPG) and hypothalamic-pituitary-thyroid (HPT) endocrine systems: new insights from lampreys. *General and Comparative Endocrinology* Vol. 161, No. 1, pp (20-29), 0016-6480

Stacey, N. E. (1987). Roles of Hormones and Pheromones in Fish Reproductive Behavior, In: *Psychobiology of reproductive behavior : an evolutionary perspective*. D. Crews, pp., Prentice-Hall, 0137320906 (pbk.), Englewood Cliffs, NJ

Stoker, T. E., Cooper, R. L., Lambright, C. S., Wilson, V. S., Furr, J. & Gray, L. E. (2005). In vivo and in vitro anti-androgenic effects of DE-71, a commercial polybrominated diphenyl ether (PBDE) mixture. *Toxicology and applied pharmacology* Vol. 207, No. 1, pp (78-88), 0041-008X

Stumm-Zollinger, E. & Fair, G. M. (1965). Biodegradation of steroid hormones. *Journal - Water Pollution Control Federation* Vol. 37, No. 11, pp (1506-1510), 0043-1303

Sudo, S., Kuwabara, Y., Park, J. I., Hsu, S. Y. & Hsueh, A. J. (2005). Heterodimeric fly glycoprotein hormone-alpha2 (GPA2) and glycoprotein hormone-beta5 (GPB5) activate fly leucine-rich repeat-containing G protein-coupled receptor-1 (DLGR1) and stimulation of human thyrotropin receptors by chimeric fly GPA2 and human GPB5. *Endocrinology* Vol. 146, No. 8, pp (3596-3604), 0013-7227

Sumpter, J. P. & Jobling, S. (1995). Vitellogenesis as a biomarker for estrogenic contamination of the aquatic environment. *Environmental health perspectives* Vol. 103 Suppl 7, pp (173-178), 0091-6765

Tabak, H. H., Bloomhuff, R. N. & Bunch, R. L. (1981). Steroid-Hormones as Water Pollutants .2. Studies on the Persistence and Stability of Natural Urinary and Synthetic Ovulation-Inhibiting Hormones in Untreated and Treated Wastewaters. *Developments in Industrial Microbiology* Vol. 22, pp (497-519), 0070-4563

Targonska, K. & Kucharczyk, D. (2010). The Application of hCG, CPH and Ovopel in Successful Artificial Reproduction of Goldfish (Carassius auratus auratus) Under Controlled Conditions. *Reproduction in domestic animals = Zuchthygiene*, 1439-0531

Telford, M. J. & Littlewood, D. T. J. (2009). *Animal evolution : genomes, fossils, and trees*, Oxford University Press, 9780199570300, Oxford ; New York

Tena-Sempere, M. (2008). Ghrelin as a pleotrophic modulator of gonadal function and reproduction. *Nature clinical practice. Endocrinology & metabolism* Vol. 4, No. 12, pp (666-674), 1745-8374

Thornton, J. W. (2001). Evolution of vertebrate steroid receptors from an ancestral estrogen receptor by ligand exploitation and serial genome expansions. *Proceedings of the National Academy of Sciences of the United States of America* Vol. 98, No. 10, pp (5671-5676), 0027-8424

Thornton, J. W., Need, E. & Crews, D. (2003). Resurrecting the ancestral steroid receptor: ancient origin of estrogen signaling. *Science* Vol. 301, No. 5640, pp (1714-1717), 0036-8075

Thresher, R. E. (1984). *Reproduction in reef fishes*, T.F.H. Publications ; Distributed in the U.S. by T.F.H. Publications, 0876668082, Neptune City, NJ

Tsai, P. S. & Zhang, L. (2008). The emergence and loss of gonadotropin-releasing hormone in protostomes: orthology, phylogeny, structure, and function. *Biol Reprod* Vol. 79, No. 5, pp (798-805), 0006-3363

Twan, W. H., Hwang, J. S., Lee, Y. H., Jeng, S. R., Yueh, W. S., Tung, Y. H., Wu, H. F., Dufour, S. & Chang, C. F. (2006). The presence and ancestral role of gonadotropin-releasing hormone in the reproduction of scleractinian coral, Euphyllia ancora. *Endocrinology* Vol. 147, No. 1, pp (397-406), 0013-7227

Uphouse, L. (2011). Stress and Reproduction in Mammals, In: *Hormones and Reproduction of Vertebrates Volume 5: Mammals*. D. O. Norris and K. H. Lopez, pp. (117-138), Academic Press, 9780123749284 Amsterdam

Villalpando, I. & Merchant-Larios, H. (1990). Determination of the sensitive stages for gonadal sex-reversal in Xenopus laevis tadpoles. *The International journal of developmental biology* Vol. 34, No. 2, pp (281-285), 0214-6282

Vinggaard, A. M., Nellemann, C., Dalgaard, M., Jorgensen, E. B. & Andersen, H. R. (2002). Antiandrogenic effects in vitro and in vivo of the fungicide prochloraz. *Toxicological sciences : an official journal of the Society of Toxicology* Vol. 69, No. 2, pp (344-353), 1096-6080

Walker, B. S. & Janney, J. C. (1930). Etrogenic Substnaces. II. An analysis of Plant Souces. *Endocrinology* Vol. 14, No. 6, pp (389-392)

Warner, R. R. (1982). Mating Systems, Sex Change and Sexual Demography in the Rainbow Wrasse, Thalassoma-Lucasanum. *Copeia*, No. 3, pp (653-661), 0045-8511

Warner, R. R. (1984). Mating behavior and hermaphroditism in coral reef fishes. *American Scientist* Vol. 72, No. 2, pp (128-136), 0003-0996

Whalen, R. E. & Edwards, D. A. (1967). Hormonal Determinants of Development of Masculine and Feminine Behavior in Male and Female Rats. *Anatomical Record* Vol. 157, No. 2, pp (173-&), 0003-276X

Whitfield, G. K., Jurutka, P. W., Haussler, C. A. & Haussler, M. R. (1999). Steroid hormone receptors: evolution, ligands, and molecular basis of biologic function. *Journal of cellular biochemistry* Vol. Suppl 32-33, pp (110-122), 0730-2312

Williams, R. H. & Larsen, P. R. (2003). *Williams textbook of endocrinology* (10th), Saunders, 0721691846, Philadelphia, Pa.

Wilson, V. S., Blystone, C. R., Hotchkiss, A. K., Rider, C. V. & Gray, L. E., Jr. (2008). Diverse mechanisms of anti-androgen action: impact on male rat reproductive tract development. *Int J Androl* Vol. 31, No. 2, pp (178-187), 0105-6263

Wilson, V. S., Lambright, C., Furr, J., Ostby, J., Wood, C., Held, G. & Gray, L. E., Jr. (2004). Phthalate ester-induced gubernacular lesions are associated with reduced insl3 gene expression in the fetal rat testis. *Toxicol Lett* Vol. 146, No. 3, pp (207-215), 0378-4274

Wingfield, J. C., Jacobs, J. & Hillgarth, N. (1997). Ecological constraints and the evolution of hormone-behavior interrelationships. *Annals of the New York Academy of Sciences* Vol. 807, pp (22-41), 0077-8923

Wingfield, J. C. & Moore, M. C. (1987). Hormonal, Social and Environmental Factors in the Reproductive Biology of Free-Living Male Birds, In: *Psychobiology of reproductive behavior : an evolutionary perspective*. D. Crews, pp. (148-175), Prentice-Hall, 0137320906 (pbk.), Englewood Cliffs, N.J.

Wu, J., Whittier, J. M. & Crews, D. (1985). Role of progesterone in the control of female sexual receptivity in Anolis carolinensis. *General and Comparative Endocrinology* Vol. 58, No. 3, pp (402-406), 0016-6480

Yalcinkaya, T. M., Siiteri, P. K., Vigne, J. L., Licht, P., Pavgi, S., Frank, L. G. & Glickman, S. E. (1993). A mechanism for virilization of female spotted hyenas in utero. *Science* Vol. 260, No. 5116, pp (1929-1931), 0036-8075

Young, R., Renfree, M., Mesiano, S., Shaw, G., Jenkin, G. & Smith, R. (2011). The Comparative Physiology of Parturition in Mammals: Horones and Parturition in Mammals, In: *Hormones and Reproduction of Vertebrates Volume 5: Mammals*. D. O. Norris and K. H. Lopez, pp. (95-116), Academic Press, 9780123749284 Amsterdam

Zhang, L., Wayne, N. L., Sherwood, N. M., Postigo, H. R. & Tsai, P. S. (2000). Biological and immunological characterization of multiple GnRH in an opisthobranch mollusk, Aplysia californica. *General and Comparative Endocrinology* Vol. 118, No. 1, pp (77-89), 0016-6480

2

Sex Hormone-Binding Globulin as a Modulator of the Prostate "Androgenome"

Scott M. Kahn[1,2,3,*], Nicholas A. Romas[1,2] and William Rosner[4,5]

[1]*Department of Urology St. Luke's-Roosevelt Institute for Health Sciences*

[2]*Department of Urology, Herbert Irving Comprehensive Cancer Center*

[3]*Herbert Irving Comprehensive Cancer Center*

[4]*Department of Medicine, Columbia University, New York, N.Y.*

[5]*Department of Medicine, St. Luke's-Roosevelt Institute for Health Sciences*

USA

1. Introduction

Sex hormone-binding globulin (SHBG) is a sex steroid binding protein, originally described in humans as the major binding protein for estrogens and androgens in plasma (Anderson, 1974; Avvakumov, et al, 2010). By governing equilibrium conditions in plasma between bound and free sex steroids, SHBG regulates the availability of the latter to hormonally responsive tissues. Along with regulating free steroid concentrations in plasma, it is increasingly evident that SHBG also participates in other biological processes. These include, but are not limited to- activation of a rapid, membrane based steroid signaling pathway in tissues such as the prostate and breast (Rosner et al, 2010); spermatogenesis (Selva and Hammond, 2006); and a yet to be determined consequence of co-localization with oxytosin in brain cells (Caldwell et al, 2006).

Plasma based SHBG is extensively studied, especially in the context of its regulation of free steroid concentrations and epidemiologic associations. The origin of plasma SHBG is, for all intents and purposes, the liver (Khan et al, 1981; Pugeat et al, 2010) (a differentially glycosylated isoform, androgen binding protein (ABP) is synthesized in the testis (Vigersky et al, 1976)). However, we now know that SHBG is also synthesized, albeit to a much lesser degree, in certain hormonally responsive tissues (Kahn et al, 2002). Early studies demonstrated immunoreactive SHBG in the prostate and breast (Bordin & Petra 1980; Tardivel-Lacombe et al, 1984; Sinnecker et al, 1988; 1990; Meyer et al, 1994; Germain et al, 1997), though its origin (local synthesis vs. import from plasma) was unclear. Other studies demonstrated SHBG mRNA in certain nonhepatic tissues (Larrea et al, 1993; Misao et al, 1994; 1997; Moore et al, 1996; Murayama et al, 1999), and one reported both SHBG protein and mRNA together in fallopian tube tissue (Noé, 1999). In 2002, we reported that human prostate tissue expresses both SHBG mRNA and protein, as do prostate cancer cell lines (Hryb et al, 2002), suggesting that SHBG is indeed locally

* Corresponding Author

expressed by prostate cells. We therefore set out to ascertain the biological functions associated with locally expressed SHBG in the prostate. High on our list was that locally expressed SHBG could regulate the prostate cellular response to androgen signaling by modulating the expression of androgen responsive genes, referred to herein as the "androgenome".

In this chapter, we first present an overview of human SHBG gene expression, as recent studies from our group and Pinós et al, have shown it to be far more complex than previously thought. We then review our work on the effects of SHBG on the prostate androgenome, along with our most recent findings on how SHBG modulates the expression of specific and noteworthy androgen receptor (AR) responsive genes. We conclude by addressing how SHBG, through its effects on the androgenome, might affect prostate biology, and how altered SHBG expression may influence prostate cancer progression.

2. SHBG gene structure and expression

2.1 Introduction

In plasma, SHBG exists as a homodimer, whose subunits are derived from an eight-exon long transcript as a 402 amino acid precursor protein that is glycosylated (sometimes differentially) and cleaved at its amino terminus to remove a 29 amino acid signal peptide (Hammond et al, 1987; Gershagen et al, 1989; Joseph, 1994; Avvakumov et al, 2010). The same eight-exon long transcript also encodes androgen binding protein (ABP) in the testis, an alternatively glycosylated form of SHBG (not a topic of this review). The human SHBG gene is located on chromosome 17p13.1, ~30Kb from the p53 tumor suppressor gene. As a result, in most instances where hemizygous deletions of this oft-targeted chromosomal region occur in prostate tumors, it is likely that DNA sequences involving both genes are lost.

2.2 The human SHBG gene transcription pattern.

Bolstered by recent reports (Nakhla et al, 2009; Pinós et al, 2009), we now know that transcription of the human SHBG gene is highly complex, as well as tissue dependent. The eight-exon long SHBG transcript is derived from a downstream promoter, designated here as P_L. In addition to the SHBG transcript, we found that at least five different mRNA species are generated through alternative splicing of exons 4-7 from the primary P_L derived transcript (Nakhla et al, 2009). Adding to the overall complexity of human SHBG gene transcription, we and others have detected at least five independent first exons in novel SHBG gene transcripts (Gershagen et al, 1989; Nakhla et al, 2009; Pinós et al, 2009). These additional first exon sequences are all located upstream of the P_L promoter, indicating that the SHBG gene utilizes at least six different promoters. We characterized transcripts derived from two of these upstream promoters, and found that they, too, undergo alternative splicing of exons 4-7. In total, from P_L and these two upstream promoters alone, we identified 19 different SHBG gene transcripts (Nakhla et al, 2009); Pinós et al. describe additional transcripts arising from other SHBG gene promoters (Pinós et al, 2009). However, apart from the singular transcript encoding SHBG itself, it is unclear whether any other SHBG gene transcript encodes a functional protein in humans, or whether they might act to regulate expression of the SHBG transcript.

2.3 SHBG expression in normal prostate tissue and the LNCaP prostate cancer cell line

Our analyses also included a detailed look at the SHBG expression patterns in normal human prostate tissue and the LNCaP prostate cancer cell line (Nakhla et al, 2009). Focusing on P_L, we found that only the eight exon long SHBG transcript is generated in normal prostate tissue. This suggests that alternatively spliced P_L-derived species are either not present, that they exist at levels undetectable by our RT-PCR assay, or that they are synthesized in minor cellular populations within normal prostate tissue. Compared to normal liver tissue, quantitative PCR analysis revealed that normal prostate expresses only $1/1000^{th}$ the abundance of total P_L-derived transcripts. Even taking into account the relative complexity of the P_L-transcript expression pattern in normal liver, with the SHBG transcript being most abundant, these findings are in concordance with hepatic SHBG being synthesized for global use (plasma), and prostate SHBG being synthesized for local, or intracellular use. Normal prostate revealed a low abundance of transcripts derived from the two upstream promoters we examined. In striking comparison, the LNCaP prostate cancer cell line exhibited a dramatic relative increase in both the number of alternatively spliced transcripts and transcripts from upstream promoters. The reasons behind these differences in SHBG gene transcription profiles are unclear, they could reflect the clonality of LNCaP cells vs. whole prostate tissue, dysregulation of global RNA processing in LNCaP, and/or changes in specific SHBG mRNA processing elements, among other possibilities. Taken together, the SHBG gene may be a valuable provider of diagnostic, prognostic, and predictive biomarkers for individuals with prostate cancer.

3. SHBG and its effects on the prostate "androgenome"

3.1 Introduction

Because SHBG binds androgens, we hypothesized that a major function of locally expressed SHBG in prostate cells might be to regulate the androgenome. We set out to investigate two different scenarios by which SHBG could influence androgen signaling. First was that locally synthesized SHBG could modulate the binding of androgen to the androgen receptor (AR) by acting as a steroid sequestering agent. For example, in the same way that plasma SHBG regulates the concentrations of plasma free steroids, intracellular SHBG could regulate intraprostatic free testosterone and dihydrotestosterone (DHT). Perhaps relevant to prostate cancer progression, this model predicts that diminished intracellular SHBG would allow for increased free intracellular DHT and hence increase the effect of intracellular androgens.

The second scenario envisions that locally expressed SHBG can participate, in an autocrine/paracrine manner, in a rapid, membrane based signaling pathway in prostate cells (Kahn et al, 2002; Kahn et al, 2003; Rosner et al, 2010). The initial steps of this pathway are well established biochemically, however little is understood about its biologic functions. Briefly, SHBG, in its steroid-free configuration, binds to a high affinity, but yet to be cloned membrane receptor (R_{SHBG}), forming a bipartite complex (SHBG-R_{SHBG}). Subsequently, DHT binds to and activates the SHBG-R_{SHBG} complex causing a rapid induction of cAMP and the activation of protein kinase A. This occurs independently of the AR.

3.2 Functional microarray analysis

We developed a functional microarray approach to ascertain the effects of SHBG on the androgenome of LNCaP cells (Kahn et al, 2008). Using an inducible system that enabled

SHBG overexpression in an engineered human LNCaP prostate cancer cell line, we specifically addressed the two scenarios described above. Using appropriate controls, SHBG effects on AR-mediated signaling would be evident by the altered expression of genes that are responsive to DHT treatment. And, those genes whose expression was sensitive to R_{SHBG} signaling would show changes only under conditions that activate R_{SHBG} (SHBG followed by DHT binding), but not in the presence of either SHBG or DHT alone.

3.3 Generation of the inducible L5S2 and vector control L5V4 clonal cell lines

The two clonal cell lines, L5S2 and L5V4, formed the core of our studies. The inducible L5S2 clonal cell line, which reproducibly overexpresses SHBG in response to Ponasterone A (PonA), was indirectly derived from LNCaP cells through an intermediate cell line, L5. L5 was generated by stably transfecting LNCaP cells with the plasmid, pVgRXR (Invitrogen, Carlsbad, CA). pVgRXR encodes a hybrid transactivator that is activated by PonA. This transactivator recognizes and directs transcription from a promoter within a second plasmid, pINDhygro (Invitrogen). L5S2 was generated by stably transfecting L5 cells with a pINDhygro construct that contains the full length human SHBG cDNA coding sequence cloned directly downstream of the inducible promoter. The L5V4 vector control cell line was generated by stably transfecting L5 cells with the empty vector, pINDhygro. As such, L5S2 and L5V4, both being derived directly from the L5 subclone, were considered nearly isogenic. Titration experiments revealed maximal SHBG induction was approached in L5S2 cells upon treatment with 10 μM PonA for 24 hrs, similar treatment of L5V4 cells had no effect on SHBG expression (data not shown).

Table 1 shows the effect of treatment conditions on SHBG expression in the L5S2 inducible, and L5V4 vector control cell lines. L5S2 cells treated for 24 hrs with 10 μM PonA reproducibly exhibit an 80+-fold induction over basal L5S2 levels in either the absence or presence of 10 nM DHT. The inducing agent, PonA by itself has only a very slight effect on SHBG expression.

3.4 Effects of SHBG overexpression on the LNCaP androgenome

The global effect of SHBG overexpression on gene expression in LNCaP cells following 10 nM DHT treatment is summarized in Table 2. L5S2 cells were induced with PonA for 24 hrs, then treated with 10 nM DHT for another 24 hrs (this being the same DHT treatment condition that induces R_{SHBG} signaling). Approximately 3000 genes displayed at least a 20% difference in expression when compared to similarly treated L5V4 vector control cells, with slightly over 1700 genes showing at least a 50% increase in expression, or a 33% decrease in expression. Thus, SHBG, when expressed at high levels in LNCaP cells, does affect the androgenome.

3.5 SHBG effects on c-myc, TIMP2, GPR30, and STAMP4 expression

Having demonstrated a global effect of SHBG on the androgen response of LNCaP cells, we performed a series of qPCR experiments to confirm our microarray results. We investigated a select group of four genes of potential importance in prostate cancer and hormonal signaling- c-myc, TIMP2 (tissue inhibitor of metalloproteinase 2), GPR30 (G protein-coupled receptor 30), and STEAP4 (six-transmembrane epithelial antigen of prostate 4, also known as STAMP2 (six transmembrane protein of prostate 2)), each of which displayed a sensitivity to

CELL LINE AND TREATMENT CONDITIONS	EFFECT TESTED	SHBG Fold expression change	P.Value	B value
L5S2: 10uM PonA vs. L5V4: 10uM PonA	Pon A induction	83.7	1.34E-19	38.3
L5S2: 10nM DHT, 10uM PonA vs. L5V4: 10nM DHT, 10uM PonA	Pon A induction and DHT	89.3	1.03E-19	39.8
L5V4: 10uM PonA vs. L5V4: Mock treated	Pon A effects alone	1.57	4.73E-05	7.02
L5S2: Mock treated vs. L5V4: Mock treated	Leakiness of L5S2 cells	4.82	5.53E-13	26.8
L5V4: 10nM DHT, 10uM PonA vs. L5V4: 10uM PonA	DHT on L5V4 cells	N/D	N/A	N/A
L5S2: 10nM DHT, 10uM PonA vs. L5S2: 10uM PonA	DHT on L5S2 cells	N/D	N/A	N/A

L5V4 vector control cells and inducible L5S2 cells were each seeded into two groups of multiple six well plates in RPMI-1640 medium (Mediatech, Herndon, VA) supplemented with 1mM sodium pyruvate (Mediatech), 100 units/ml of Penicillin-Streptomycin (Invitrogen), and 10% charcoal stripped fetal calf serum (Gemini Bio-Products, Woodland, CA) for 24 hours. One group was then treated with the inducing agent, PonA (10μM)(Invitrogen), and the other treated with an equal volume of carrier ethanol, for 24 hr. Triplicate wells from the PonA-treated cells were then treated for an additional 24 hr with either carrier or 10 nM DHT, giving six treatment conditions-

A. L5V4 vector control cells treated with carrier alone (mock treated)
B. L5V4 vector control cells treated with 10uM PonA 24 hrs
C. L5V4 vector control cells treated with 10uM PonA + 10nM DHT 24 hrs
D. L5S2 inducible SHBG cells treated with carrier alone (mock treated)
E. L5S2 inducible SHBG cells treated with 10uM Pon A 24 hrs
F. L5S2 inducible SHBG cells treated with 10uM PonA + 10nM DHT 24 hrs

Total RNA was isolated with Trizol (Invitrogen) followed by a Qiagen clean up procedure (Qiagen, Valencia, CA). RNA integrity was assessed using an Agilent 2100 Bioanalyzer and RNA 6000 Nano Lab Chip LabChips (Agilent, Palo Alto, CA). RNA samples showed a 260/280 ratio between 1.8 and 2.0 and 28S:18S ratio of 1.5 and higher. Each triplicate RNA preparation was used in a single microarray analysis. First-strand cDNAs were synthesized from 5 μg of each RNA sample using a T7-Oligo(dT) promoter primer and SuperScript II. After RNase H-mediated second-stranded cDNA synthesis, double-stranded cDNAs were purified using a GeneChip sample clean-up module. Biotinylated complementary RNAs (cRNAs) were generated by in vitro transcription using T7 RNA Polymerase and a biotinylated nucleotide analog/ribonucleotide mix. Biotinylated cRNAs were cleaned up, fragmented, and hybridized to Affymetrix Human Genome U133 Plus 2.0 Array chips, representing 54675 transcripts (Affymetrix, Santa Clara, CA), at 45°C for 16 h with constant rotation at 60 rpm. Chips were processed using an Affymetrix fluidics station and scanned on an Affymetrix scanner 3000 with workstation. Images were processed with GeneChip Operating Software (GCOS) and raw data were analyzed with GeneSpring 7.2 software (Silicon Genetics, Redwood City, CA) to identify differentially expressed genes between conditions. Data were normalized to the 50th percentile of measurements taken from the chip to reduce chip-wide variations in intensity. Each gene was normalized to the average measurement of the gene throughout the experiment to enable comparison of relative changes in gene expression levels between different conditions. Data filtration was performed based on flags, present or marginal. Shown are the changes in SHBG gene expression between given cell lines and treatment conditions as determined by microarray analysis. B value: Bayesian log odds score. ND= none detected; NA= not applicable

Table 1. Effect of treatment conditions on SHBG expression in L5V4 and L5S2 cells

Total Number of Induced Genes	Total Number of Repressed Genes	Genes Induced > 1.5-fold	Genes expressed <0.66-fold (repressed)
1250	1770	665	1068

L5S2 inducible and L5V4 vector control cells were treated with 10μM PonA for 24 hours, and then stimulated with 10nM DHT for an additional 24 hours. Total number of induced and repressed genes include those displaying at least a 20% difference in transcript abundance between similarly treated L5S2 and L5V4 cells, as determined by microarray analysis.

Table 2. Global effects of SHBG overexpression on DHT-treated (24 hr.) LNCaP cells

SHBG overexpression in response to DHT, as detected by microarray analysis (data not shown). The qPCR results corroborated our microarray results for these four genes. DHT treatment of induced L5S2 cells resulted in nearly a one-third decrease in c-myc gene transcript abundance compared to mock-treated L5S2 cells, whereas similar DHT treatment caused a 20% increase in L5V4 vector control cells compared to mock-treated L5V4 cells. Given that elevated c-myc gene expression is a hallmark of many prostate tumors (Gurel et al, 2008), the effect of increased SHBG serving to decrease c-myc gene expression is intriguing and warrants further investigation. We note that slightly higher levels of c-myc are seen in unstimulated L5S4 vs. L5V2 cells, this observation requires clarification. DHT treatment also caused a decrease in the abundance of TIMP2 gene transcripts in L5S2 cells, whereas there was little change in similarly treated L5V4 cells. This result is of interest, as TIMP2 expression has been correlated with advanced prostate cancer stage and recurrence (Ross et al, 2003). SHBG overexpression markedly amplified the DHT-mediated decrease in cellular levels of GPR30 gene transcripts; GPR30 is a membrane receptor for estrogen that releases epidermal growth factor-related ligands, thereby inducing signaling via the epidermal growth factor receptor (Wang et al, 2010). And, SHBG overexpression displayed a dramatic effect on STEAP4 transcript levels in LNCaP cells- DHT treatment resulted in 1000-fold higher levels in L5S2 cells than in similarly treated L5V4 cells. STEAP4 is an emerging player in metabolic syndrome and glucose transport (Wellen et al, 2007), and provocatively, SHBG has been linked to metabolic syndrome (Pugeat et al, 2007). While its expression is often elevated in prostate cancer cells (Korkmaz, et al, 2005) it is still unclear how STEAP4 expression may contribute to prostate cancer progression. This, and the exquisite responsiveness of STEAP4 expression levels to SHBG are areas that beg further investigation.

3.6 SHBG effects on the expression of AR co-regulators, including FKBP5

We next turned our attention to whether SHBG might indirectly affect AR activation by modulating the expression of AR co-regulators in response to DHT. Working with a detailed list of 186 AR co-regulators kindly provided by Dr. Donald Tindall and Dr. Hannelore Heemers (for review, see Heemers and Tindall, 2007), we examined our microarray data for those whose expression was affected by SHBG overexpression following 24 hr. DHT exposure. AR co-regulators displaying at least a 20% difference are listed in Table 3.

Of the 20 AR co-regulators whose expression was markedly changed by the presence of SHBG, eight were upregulated and 12 were downregulated. The greatest difference was in expression of the FKBP5 (FK506 binding protein 5) gene, which was elevated 3.77-fold. Because FKBP5 is a known early androgen responsive gene whose expression is rapidly induced by DHT treatment (Jääskeläinen et al, 2011), we examined its expression level in

PonA-treated L5S2 and L5V4 cells after only 4 hrs of incubation with DHT. Indeed, in L5V4 cells, FKBP5 was induced to high levels at this earlier time point, whereas its induction was dampened by the presence of SHBG in L5S2 cells (data not shown). This suggests that SHBG overexpression not only diminishes the amplitude of DHT-mediated FKBP5 induction, it also shifts the response curve to the right. This is an intriguing finding, as FKBP5 has been shown to be a limiting component of the HSP90 chaperone supercomplex that maintains the AR in its ligand binding state (Ni et al, 2010).

Gene	**Gene name**	**Fold change**
		(L5S2 vs. L5V4)
FKBP5	FK506 binding protein 5	3.77
HIPK3	homeodomain interacting protein kinase 3	1.55
APPBP2	amyloid beta precursor protein (cytoplasmic tail) binding protein 2	1.49
NCOR1	nuclear receptor co-repressor 1	1.46
RNF14	ring finger protein 14	1.45
HTATIP2	HIV-1 Tat interactive protein 2, 30kDa	1.41
NCOR1	nuclear receptor co-repressor 1	1.39
CDC37	CDC37 cell division cycle 37 homolog (S. cerevisiae)	1.36
SRA1	steroid receptor RNA activator 1	1.28
TADA3L	transcriptional adaptor 3 (NGG1 homolog, yeast)-like	0.78
CDK7	cyclin-dependent kinase 7 (MO15 homolog, Xenopus laevis, cdk-activating kinase)	0.76
BAG1	BCL2-associated athanogene	0.73
RAN	RAN, member RAS oncogene family	0.72
NONO	non-POU domain containing, octamer-binding	0.72
MMS19L	MMS19-like (MET18 homolog, S. cerevisiae)	0.69
SMARCA2	SWI/SNF related, matrix associated, actin dependent regulator of chromatin, subfamily a, member 2	0.68
UBE1C	ubiquitin-activating enzyme E1C (UBA3 homolog, yeast)	0.65
RBM9	RNA binding motif protein 9	0.63
JDP2	Jun dimerization protein 2	0.62
CRSP2	cofactor required for Sp1 transcriptional activation, subunit 2, 150kDa	0.59

Table 3. Effect of SHBG on AR Co-regulator gene expression following 24 hr. DHT treatment of LNCaP cells.

These results support the view that endogenously expressed SHBG plays a significant role in orchestrating the LNCaP androgenome. It is noted that our experimental strategy utilized unusually high SHBG concentrations, thus we need to investigate further how normal levels of SHBG expression influence the LNCaP androgenome. More detailed time course analyses are also necessary to ascertain how SHBG affects the timing of AR activation, and how perturbations in SHBG expression might affect androgen induced events. This is especially critical considering that SHBG influences the expression of specific AR co-regulators, which could impact the timing of events required for AR activation.

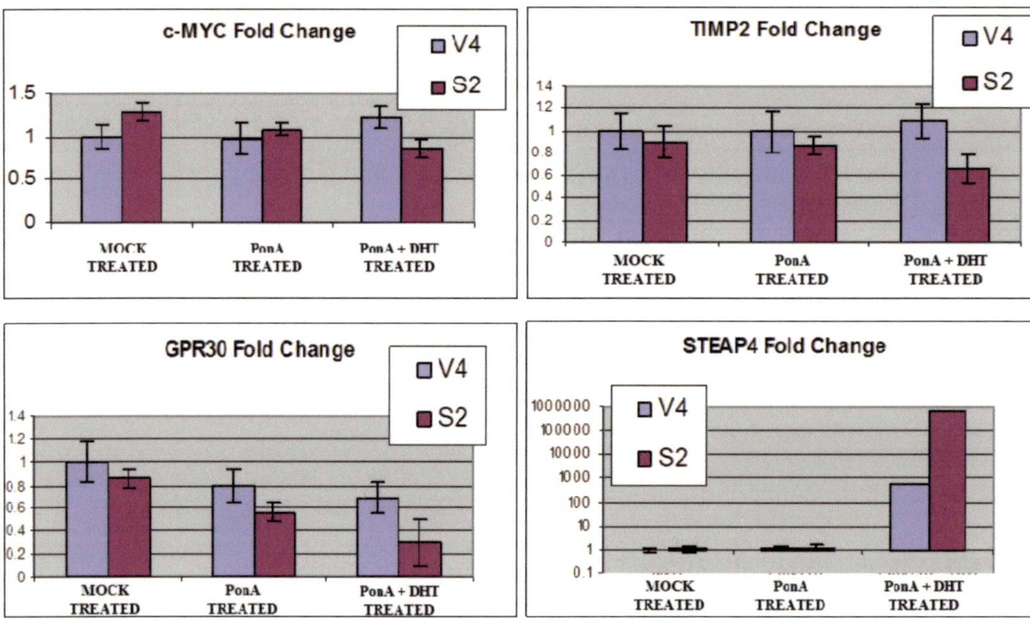

Taqman assay qPCR amplifications were performed in triplicate, using primers specific for the indicated genes. cDNA templates were generated from the same RNAs as were used for microarray analysis. Assays were run in an ABI PRISMR 7700 Sequence Detection System machine. Data were extracted and amplification plots generated with ABI SDS software. Threshold cycle (Ct) scores were averaged for subsequent calculations of relative expression values. Specific gene Ct values were normalized to GAPDH Ct values for each cell line and treatment condition, and standard deviations were calculated. Specific gene expression comparisons (fold change) are presented as the ratios of normalized Ct values for L5V4 or L5S2 cells under given treatment conditions to the normalized Ct value of the specific gene in mock-treated L5V4 vector control cells.

Fig. 1. Effect of SHBG on the expression of selected genes involved in prostate cancer progression and hormone signaling following 24 hr. DHT treatment of LNCaP cells - qPCR analysis of L5S2 and L5V4 cells.

3.7 SHBG overexpression and the R_{SHBG} pathway

Finally, our functional microarray strategy provided a means (overexpression of SHBG followed by DHT treatment) to detect genes whose altered expression is consistent with having been activated via the R_{SHBG} pathway. Just over 1000 genes displayed a pattern of not showing a significant response to either elevated SHBG expression or 24 hr. DHT treatment alone, while changing expression (a >50% induction or > 33% reduction) when SHBG was induced in L5S2 cells, followed by the addition of DHT in a manner consistent with the activation of R_{SHBG} signaling (data not shown). However, before we can assign any biologic function to R_{SHBG} signaling in prostate cells, we need to confirm these results in order to differentiate between the activation of R_{SHBG} signaling and a delay in AR mediated expression changes for specific genes in response to SHBG overexpression, as was the case for FKBP5.

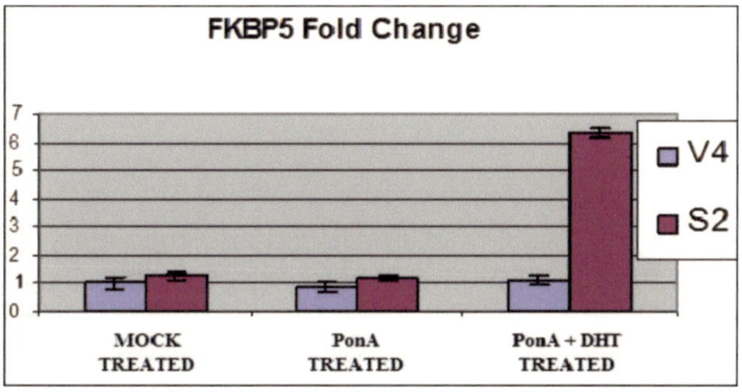

See legend to Figure 1

Fig. 2. Effect of SHBG on FKBP5 gene transcript levels following 24 hr. DHT treatment of LNCaP cells

4. Conclusions

The human SHBG gene is expressed at the mRNA and protein levels in prostate cells. Considering its sex hormone binding properties, we examined its ability to affect the androgenome of prostate cells. Using a functional microarray approach, we have obtained evidence that indeed, SHBG does affect the expression of DHT-responsive genes. In LNCaP cells, SHBG overexpression exerts global effects that include genes involved in prostate cancer (eg. c-myc and TIMP2), hormonal signaling (eg. GPR30), and the expression of AR co-regulators (eg. FKBP5), among others.

The scope of SHBG's influence on the androgenome appears to be broad and complex, involving many aspects of AR activation. Two possible mechanisms include the binding and sequestering of intracellular androgen, and the indirect modulation of AR co-regulator expression. It remains to be determined whether signaling through R_{SHBG} is also involved.

Given the ability of prostate cells to greatly ramp up their expression of endogenously synthesized SHBG (we have overexpressed SHBG in LNCaP, PC3, and DU145 cells), this raises the question of whether they regulate their androgenome by modulating intracellular SHBG levels. It is likely that a decrease in intracellular SHBG levels results in an equilibrium shift towards increased free intracellular testosterone and free intracellular DHT. We speculate that in those prostate cancer cells which undergo deletions of the SHBG/p53 locus, SHBG expression will be reduced. Deletions of the SHBG/p53 locus could thus provide a genetic means by which prostate cancer patients placed on current androgen ablation therapies can progress- enabling cells to survive under conditions of diminished androgen due to the relative increase in free intracellular androgen available to activate AR-mediated signaling. If this speculation is confirmed, it will be of interest to see how such patients respond to newer therapies that target testosterone and DHT biosynthesis, such as abiraterone.

It is intriguing to also speculate that, in addition to the prostate, locally expressed SHBG plays a functional role in the hormone response of other tissues. We have preliminary evidence that endogenously expressed SHBG can modulate the estrogen response of human breast cells (Kahn et al, 2008). And, if plasma SHBG levels provide a clue into how altered SHBG expression may contribute to the disease state at a cellular level, it will be of great interest to investigate whether there is a connection between tissue specific SHBG expression and Type 2 diabetes. This does not detract in any way from the importance of plasma SHBG levels on androgen and estrogen responsiveness in humans. Instead, it serves to broaden the scope of SHBG influence on the response to sex steroids to the individual tissue and cellular level.

5. Acknowledgements

This work is dedicated to the memory of our friend and colleague, Dr. Daniel Hryb, who devoted much of his life to understanding the biology of SHBG. The authors would like to thank Dr. Atif Nakhla and Dr. Saeed Khan for their invaluable contributions to this work. We also appreciate the terrific assistance of many collaborators, including Dr. Yu Hua Li, Dr. Richard Friedman, Dr. Zhaoying Xiang, Dr. Xinsheng Wang, Dr. Jonathan St. George, Dr. Kristina Maletz, Janice Cheong, Dr. Teri Reynolds, Dr. Amy Kappelman, Nomi Levy, Stephanie Meng, and Dr. Hisashi Koga.

6. References

Anderson DC. Sex-hormone-binding globulin. Clin Endocrinol (Oxf). 1974 Jan;3(1):69-96.

Avvakumov GV, Cherkasov A, Muller YA, Hammond GL. Structural analyses of sex hormone-binding globulin reveal novel ligands and function. Mol Cell Endocrinol. 2010 Mar 5;316(1):13-23. Epub 2009 Sep 11.

Bordin S, Petra PH. Immunocytochemical localization of the sex steroid-binding protein of plasma in tissues of the adult monkey Macaca nemestrina. Proc Natl Acad Sci U S A. 1980 Oct;77(10):5678-82.

Caldwell JD, Suleman F, Chou SH, Shapiro RA, Herbert Z, Jirikowski GF. Emerging roles of steroid-binding globulins. Horm Metab Res. 2006 Apr;38(4):206-18.

Germain P, Egloff M, Kiefer H, Metezeau P, Habrioux G. Use of confocal microscopy to localize the SHBG interaction with human breast cancer cell lines--a comparison with serum albumin interaction. Cell Mol Biol (Noisy-le-grand). 1997 Jun;43(4):501-8.

Gershagen S, Lundwall A, Fernlund P. Characterization of the human sex hormone binding globulin (SHBG) gene and demonstration of two transcripts in both liver and testis. Nucleic Acids Res. 1989;17:9245–9258

Gurel B, Iwata T, Koh CM, Yegnasubramanian S, Nelson WG, De Marzo AM. Molecular alterations in prostate cancer as diagnostic, prognostic, and therapeutic targets. Adv Anat Pathol. 2008 Nov;15(6):319-31.

Hammond GL, Underhill DA, Smith CL, Goping IS, Harley MJ, Musto NA, Cheng CY, Bardin CW. The cDNA-deduced primary structure of human sex hormone-binding globulin and location of its steroid-binding domain. FEBS Lett. 1987;215:100–104.

Heemers HV, Tindall DJ. Androgen receptor (AR) coregulators: a diversity of functions converging on and regulating the AR transcriptional complex. Endocr Rev. 2007 Dec;28(7):778-808. Epub 2007 Oct 16.

Hryb DJ, Nakhla AM, Kahn SM, St George J, Levy NC, Romas NA, Rosner W. Sex hormone-binding globulin in the human prostate is locally synthesized and may act as an autocrine/paracrine effector. J Biol Chem. 2002 Jul 19;277(29):26618-22. Epub 2002 May 15

Jääskeläinen T, Makkonen H, Palvimo JJ Steroid up-regulation of FKBP51 and its role in hormone signaling. Curr Opin Pharmacol. 2011 Aug;11(4):326-31. Epub 2011 Apr 29.

Joseph DR. Structure, function, and regulation of androgen-binding protein/sex hormone-binding globulin. Vitam Horm. 1994;49:197-280.

Kahn SM, Hryb DJ, Nakhla AM, Romas NA, Rosner W. Sex hormone-binding globulin is synthesized in target cells. J Endocrinol. 2002 Oct;175(1):113-20.

Kahn, SM, Hryb DJ, Nakhla AM, Romas NA, Rosner W. Sex Hormone Binding Globulin and steroid signaling at the cell membrane. "The Identities of Membrane Steroid Receptors- and other proteins mediating nongenomic steroid action" (2003) Cheryl S. Watson ed. Kluwer Academic Publishers pp.193-200

Kahn SM, Li YH, Hryb DJ, Nakhla AM, Romas NA, Cheong J, Rosner W. Sex hormone-binding globulin influences gene expression of LNCaP and MCF-7 cells in response to androgen and estrogen treatment. Adv Exp Med Biol. 2008;617:557-64.

Khan MS, Knowles BB, Aden DP, Rosner W. Secretion of testosterone-estradiol-binding globulin by a human hepatoma-derived cell line. J Clin Endocrinol Metab. 1981 Aug;53(2):448-9.

Korkmaz CG, Korkmaz KS, Kurys P, Elbi C, Wang L, Klokk TI, Hammarstrom C, Troen G, Svindland A, Hager GL, Saatcioglu F. Molecular cloning and characterization of STAMP2, an androgen-regulated six transmembrane protein that is overexpressed in prostate cancer. Oncogene. 2005 Jul 21;24(31):4934-45.

Larrea F, Díaz L, Cariño C, Larriva-Sahd J, Carrillo L, Orozco H, Ulloa-Aguirre A. Evidence that human placenta is a site of sex hormone-binding globulin gene expression. J Steroid Biochem Mol Biol. 1993 Oct;46(4):497-505

Meyer S, Brumm C, Stegner HE, Sinnecker GH. Intracellular sex hormone-binding globulin (SHBG) in normal and neoplastic breast tissue--an additional marker for hormone dependency? Exp Clin Endocrinol. 1994;102(4):334-40.

Misao R, Itoh N, Mori H, Fujimoto J, Tamaya T. Sex hormone-binding globulin mRNA levels in human uterine endometrium. Eur J Endocrinol. 1994 Dec;131(6):623-9

Misao R, Nakanishi Y, Fujimoto J, Tamaya T. Expression of sex hormone-binding globulin exon VII splicing variant messenger RNA in human uterine endometrial cancers. Cancer Res. 1997 Dec 15;57(24):5579-83.

Moore KH, Bertram KA, Gomez RR, Styner MJ, Matej LA. Sex hormone binding globulin mRNA in human breast cancer: detection in cell lines and tumor samples. J Steroid Biochem Mol Biol. 1996 Nov;59(3-4):297-304.

Murayama Y, Hammond GL, Sugihara K. The shbg Gene and Hormone Dependence of Breast Cancer: A Novel Mechanism of Hormone Dependence of MCF-7 Human Breast Cancer Cells Based upon SHBG. Breast Cancer. 1999 Oct 25;6(4):338-343.

Nakhla AM, Hryb DJ, Rosner W, Romas NA, Xiang Z, Kahn SM. Human sex hormone-binding globulin gene expression- multiple promoters and complex alternative splicing. BMC Mol Biol. 2009 May 5;10:37.

Ni L, Yang CS, Gioeli D, Frierson H, Toft DO, Paschal BM. FKBP51 promotes assembly of the Hsp90 chaperone complex and regulates androgen receptor signaling in prostate cancer cells. Mol Cell Biol. 2010 Mar;30(5):1243-53. Epub 2010 Jan 4

Noé G. Sex hormone binding globulin expression and colocalization with estrogen receptor in the human Fallopian tube. J Steroid Biochem Mol Biol. 1999 Feb;68(3-4):111-7

Pinós T, Barbosa-Desongles A, Hurtado A, Santamaria-Martínez A, de Torres I, Morote J, Reventós J, Munell F. Identification, characterization and expression of novel Sex Hormone Binding Globulin alternative first exons in the human prostate. BMC Mol Biol. 2009 Jun 17;10:59.

Pugeat M, Nader N, Hogeveen K, Raverot G, Déchaud H, Grenot C. Sex hormone-binding globulin gene expression in the liver: drugs and the metabolic syndrome. Mol Cell Endocrinol. 2010 Mar 5;316(1):53-9. Epub 2009 Sep 26.

Rosner W, Hryb DJ, Kahn SM, Nakhla AM, Romas NA. Interactions of sex hormone-binding globulin with target cells. Mol Cell Endocrinol. 2010 Mar 5;316(1):79-85. Epub 2009 Aug 19

Ross JS, Kaur P, Sheehan CE, Fisher HA, Kaufman RA Jr, Kallakury BV. Prognostic significance of matrix metalloproteinase 2 and tissue inhibitor of metalloproteinase 2 expression in prostate cancer. Mod Pathol. 2003 Mar;16(3):198-205.

Selva DM, Hammond GL. Human sex hormone-binding globulin is expressed in testicular germ cells and not in sertoli cells. Horm Metab Res. 2006 Apr;38(4):230-5

Sinnecker G, Hiort O, Mitze M, Donn F, Neumann S. Immunohistochemical detection of a sex hormone binding globulin like antigen in tissue sections of normal human prostate, benign prostatic hypertrophy and normal human endometrium. Steroids. 1988 Oct;52(4):335-6

Sinnecker G, Hiort O, Kwan PW, DeLellis RA. Immunohistochemical localization of sex hormone-binding globulin in normal and neoplastic breast tissue. Horm Metab Res. 1990 Jan;22(1):47-50.

Tardivel-Lacombe J, Egloff M, Mazabraud A, Degrelle H. Immunohistochemical detection of the sex steroid-binding plasma protein in human mammary carcinoma cells. Biochem Biophys Res Commun. 1984 Jan 30;118(2):488-94.

Vigersky RA, Loriaux DL, Howards SS, Hodgen GB, Lipsett MB, Chrambach A. Androgen binding proteins of testis, epididymis, and plasma in man and monkey. J Clin Invest. 1976 Nov;58(5):1061-8.

Wang D, Hu L, Zhang G, Zhang L, Chen C. G protein-coupled receptor 30 in tumor development. Endocrine. 2010 Aug;38(1):29-37. Epub 2010 Jul 8.

Wellen KE, Fucho R, Gregor MF, Furuhashi M, Morgan C, Lindstad T, Vaillancourt E, Gorgun CZ, Saatcioglu F, Hotamisligil GS. Coordinated regulation of nutrient and inflammatory responses by STAMP2 is essential for metabolic homeostasis. Cell. 2007 May 4;129(3):537-48.

3

Estrogens in the Control of Growth Hormone Actions in Liver

Leandro Fernández-Pérez[1] and Amilcar Flores-Morales[2]

[1]University of Las Palmas de Gran Canaria, Faculty of Health Sciences, Clinical Sciences Department, Pharmacology Unit, Las Palmas de G.C.,
[2]Novo Nordisk Center for Protein Research, University of Copenhagen,
[1]Spain
[2]Denmark

1. Introduction

The liver responds in a sex-specific manner to Growth Hormone (GH) and sex hormones. GH is the main regulator of body growth, somatic development, body composition, and sex-differentiated functions in liver (Butler and Le Roith, 2001; Mode and Gustafsson, 2006; LeRoith and Yakar, 2007; Lichanska and Waters, 2008; Vijayakumar et al., 2010). GH is mainly produced in the pituitary gland and acts distantly on target tissues through the activation of the transmembrane GH receptor (GHR). The liver shows the highest levels of GHR expression and, therefore, is a major target for GH, but virtually all human tissues are responsive to GH. GH regulates glucose, lipid, amino acid, and endo-xenobiotic metabolism. The sex-specific secretion release from pituitary has been shown to have a great impact on hepatic transcriptional regulation (Flores-Morales et al., 2001b; Tollet-Egnell et al., 2001; Tollet-Egnell et al., 2004; Lichanska and Waters, 2008; Waxman and Holloway, 2009). Global expression analysis of GH actions in liver using microarrays clearly indicates that most of the known physiological effects of GH can be explained through its effects on the transcription of specific genes. To this end, GH is known to activate a network of transcription factors in liver that include, among others, nuclear receptors/transcription factors such as Hepatocyte Nuclear Factors (4α, 6, 3β), Peroxisome Proliferator-Activated Receptor alpha (PPARα), Constitutive Androstane Receptor (CAR), Farnesoid X Receptor (FXR), Small Heterodimer Partner (SHP), Sterol Regulated Element-Binding Protein (SREBP), CRBP, C/EBPβ, and Signal Transducer and Activator of Transcription (STAT)-5b. The latest is of particular importance in the regulation of endocrine, metabolic, and sex-differentiated actions of GH in liver (Udy et al., 1997; Wiwi and Waxman, 2004; Waxman and O'Connor, 2006; Vidal et al., 2007).

17β-Estradiol (E2), a major natural estrogen in mammals, has physiological actions which are not limited to reproductive organs in both females and males (Simpson et al., 2005). Estrogens exert their physiological effects through two estrogen receptor (ER) subtypes, ERα and ERβ, which belong to the nuclear receptor family of ligand-activated transcription factors (Heldring et al., 2007). Moreover, together with a mechanism based in ligand-activated transcription, estrogens can modulate gene expression by a second mechanism in which ERs interact with other transcription factors through a process referred to as transcription factor cross-talk. Estrogen may also elicit effects through non-genomic mechanisms, which involve the activation of protein kinase cascades via membrane-localized ERs (Revankar et al., 2005). Recently, an orphan G protein-coupled receptor (GPR)-30 in the cell membrane was reported to mediate non-genomic and rapid estrogen signaling. Therefore, the mechanisms involved in ER signaling are influenced by cell phenotype, the target gene, and the activity or the crosstalk with other signaling networks. Biologically and clinically relevant are potential interactions of estrogens with GH-regulated endocrine, metabolic, and sex-differentiated functions in liver. Estrogens can modulate GH actions in liver by acting centrally, by regulating pituitary GH secretion, and, peripherally, modulating GH signaling. Most previous studies have focused on the influence of estrogen on pituitary GH secretion (Kerrigan and Rogol, 1992; Wehrenberg and Giustina, 1992) but there is also strong evidence that estrogen modulates GH action at the level of GHR expression and signaling. Particularly, E2 has been shown to induce Suppressor of Cytokine Signalling (SOCS)-2, a protein inhibitor for cytokine signalling, which in turn negatively regulate GHR-Janus Kinase (JAK)-2-STAT5 pathway (Leung et al., 2004). Finally, the liver is a direct target of estrogens because it expresses ERα (Heldring et al., 2007) which is connected with liver development (Fisher et al., 1984), regulation of hepatic metabolic pathways (D'Eon et al., 2005; Ribas et al., 2010; Faulds et al., 2011), growth (Vidal et al., 2000), protection from drug-induced toxicity (Yamamoto et al., 2006), hepatocarcinogenesis (Bigsby and Caperell-Grant, 2011), fertility (Della Torre et al., 2011), as well as lipid metabolism and insulin sensitivity (Simpson et al., 2005; Foryst-Ludwig and Kintscher, 2010).

Therefore, estrogen-GH interactions are relevant because physiological roles these hormones have in mammals, and the widespread use of estrogen and estrogen-related compounds in human. These have been supported from clinical observations where administration of pharmacological doses of estrogens to human impairs GH-regulated endocrine and metabolic functions in liver (Meinhardt and Ho, 2006). Thus, deficiency of GH or E2 activities as well as estrogen-GH interactions may cause a dramatic impact in liver physiology during development as well as in adulthood. In this chapter, we will address the roles of these hormones in liver physiology as well as data of how estrogens modulate GH actions in liver. A better understanding of estrogen-GH interplay will lead to improved management of children with growth and developmental disorders and of adults with GH deficiency.

2. Regulation of pituitary GH secretion

GH is a polypeptide mainly secreted from the somatotrophs within the anterior pituitary gland. In addition to the pituitary, GH is produced in extra-pituitary tissues (e.g., placenta, mammary tissue, pineal gland, brain, lymphocytes) which indicates that GH has local paracrine-autocrine effects, distinct from its classic endocrine somatotropic effects (Waters et al., 1999). The regulation of pituitary GH secretion involves a complex neuroendocrine control system that includes the participation of several neurotransmitters and the feedback of hormonal and peripheral (metabolic) factors (Le Roith et al., 2001; Kaplan and Cohen, 2007) (Figure 1).

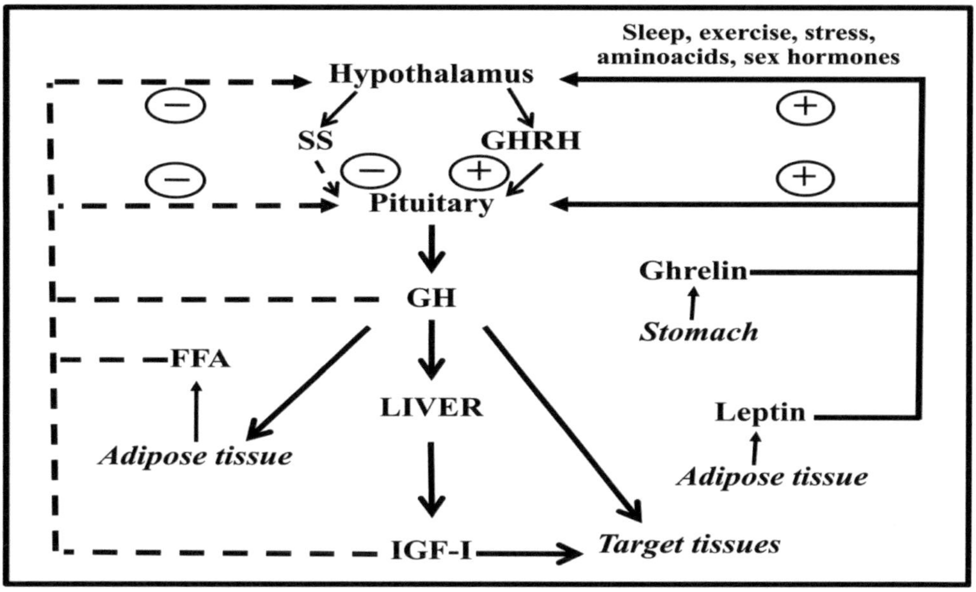

Fig. 1. **The somatotropic axis.** The synthesis and release of GH from the pituitary are controlled by two hypothalamic hormones: GHRH and SS. GHRH is negatively (dashed lines) regulated by feedback from blood GH and IGF-I concentrations. FFA also inhibits whereas leptin and ghrelin stimulate GH release. Sex hormones and other factors also act centrally to stimulate GH release. Circulating GH acts directly on many organs to stimulate IGF-I production, with IGF-I production in the liver providing the main source of blood IGF-I. As illustrated, GH also has direct effects on many target tissues (adipose, kidney, bone, pancreatic), which can be independent of IGF-I action.

GH secretion from pituitary gland is regulated by two major hypothalamic peptides: GH releasing hormone (GHRH) and the inhibitory hormone Somatostatin (SS). The balance of these stimulating and inhibiting peptides is in turn, indirectly, affected by many physiological stimulators (e.g., exercise, nutrients, sleep, thyroid hormones, and sex hormones) and inhibitors (e.g. glucocorticoids, Insulin-like Growth Factor (IGF)-I and GH). The final integration of these signals occurs in the hypothalamus. Pituitary GH secretion is mainly reduced by negative feedback of two circulating signals: pituitary GH itself and liver-derived IGF-I produced by GH. The liver-derived IGF-I is a key negative regulator of pituitary GH secretion by acting directly on the somatotroph and on hypothalamic neurones. In addition to hypothalamic (GHRS, SS) and endocrine (IGF-I, GH) factors, other peripheral (metabolic) factors influence pituitary GH release: insulin, glucose, amino acids, free fatty acids (FFA), leptin, neuropeptide Y, and ghrelin. These factors are primarily related to or derived from the metabolic status of the organism, which is consistent with the role of GH in regulating substrate metabolism, adiposity, as well as growth, and appear to coordinate the metabolic status of the organism with GH secretion. This is exemplified by adiposity which is a powerful negative regulator of GH secretion and probably contributes to the age-related decline in GH status. FFA can act directly on the pituitary to inhibit GH release, which is postulated to complete a feedback loop, since GH stimulates lipid mobilization. In addition, adipocytes produce the hormone leptin which, in contrast to FFA, stimulates GH secretion in rodents at the level of the hypothalamus (Carro et al., 1997).

Finally, ghrelin is another GH-secretory factor that is highly expressed in the endocrine cells of the stomach. Currently, synthetic analogs of ghrelin are used to induce pituitary GH secretion (Howard et al., 1996). However, endogenous ghrelin may have little effect on GH secretion in mice, given that body growth and serum IGF-I levels are largely unaffected in ghrelin and ghrelin receptor knockout (KO) mice (Zigman et al., 2005). On the other hand, selective lack of ghrelin receptor signaling in humans may lead to a syndrome characterized by short stature (Holst and Schwartz, 2006) and ghrelin analogs have been shown to be effective in enhancing serum IGF-I levels in humans (Svensson et al., 1998).

Sex steroids are also physiological regulators of pituitary GH secretion. Both neonatal and post-pubertal sex steroids control the ability of the hypothalamus to drive the sexually dimorphism of pituitary GH secretion in adulthood (Kerrigan and Rogol, 1992; Wehrenberg and Giustina, 1992). Sexually dimorphism in rodents seems to be regulated by estrogen secretion in adult females and by androgen secretion neonatally and during adulthood in males. Essentially, estrogen increases and androgen decreases basal GH levels. These effects seem to be mediated by changes in hypothalamic release of SS and GHRH. These patterns are ultimately determined by neonatal exposure to testosterone, which imprints the male program of neuroendocrine control of the pulsatile pituitary GH secretion that is first seen at puberty, when the adult pattern of GH secretion becomes evident,and continues through adulthood. If such an androgen re-programming does not occur, the secretion pattern will remain as the feminine pattern (continuous GH secretion). In post-pubertal rats, the blood male pattern consists of high amplitude pulses (near200 ng/ml) spaced near 3-4 hours apart with no measurable trough levels. In contrast, the female pattern is of lower amplitude pulses (25-50 ng/ml) and continuous; so, GH is always present. The sexually dimorphic pattern of GH secretion is also seen in humans, but not as marked as in the rat. Interestingly, depletion of liver-derived IGF-I in male mice causes a feminization of some of the GH-regulated sexually dimorphic markers of liver functions. This suggest that liver-derived IGF-I may suppress basal GH secretion in male rodents and contribute to masculinization of liver functions. Loss of the feedback effect exerted by IGF-I on the hypothalamic-pituitary system results in increased GH secretion, including elevated baseline GH levels between pulses which resemble a female pattern of pituitary GH release.

3. Positive and negative regulation of GH signaling

The GHR belongs to type I cytokine receptor, a family of receptors without intrinsic kinase activity (Lanning and Carter-Su, 2006). Figure 2 shows the traditional view of the initiation of GH signaling: one molecule of GH binds two GHR monomers and induces their dimerization. GH binding to the GHR results in activation of adjacent JAK2 molecules, cytoplasmic tyrosine kinases associated with the GHR, by trans-phosphorylation. Activated JAK2 phosphorylates the GHR on tyrosine residues, which in turn recruits members of the STAT family of transcription factors. Since the JAK family of proteins consists of only four members (JAK1, 2 and 3, and TYK2), multiple cytokines activate the same JAK. Specificity of action, accordingly, does not reside in the JAKs, but in their downstream phosphorylation targets such as the STATs. Of the various STAT proteins (STAT 1 to 4, 5a, 5b, and 6), STAT5b has been widely associated with GH biological actions; although STAT1, 3, and 5a have also been shown to be recruited by the GHR. STAT phosphorylation by JAK2 results in their dissociation from the receptor, homo- or hetero- (in the case of STAT1 and 3) dimerization, and translocation to the nucleus where they modulate the transcription of target genes such IGF-I,

ALS, or SOCS-2 (Rowland et al., 2005; Vidal et al., 2007). The STATs represent one of at least three major pathways in GH-induced signaling; others include the MAPK and PI3K pathways (Figure 3). However, to date, there is no convincing evidence linking the MAPK, ERK or PI3K pathways with GH-induced IGF-I regulation, at least in humans. Accordingly, GH-induced MAPK signaling has proven to be insufficient to compensate for the lack of STAT5b activation in patients with homozygous mutations of STAT5b or with GHR mutations, or deletions resulting in isolated failure of STAT5b activation.

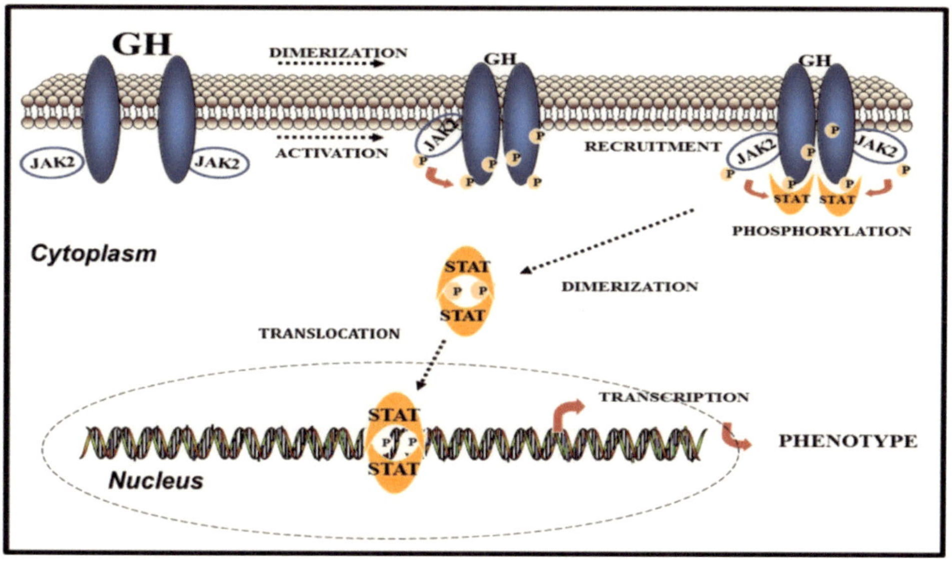

Fig. 2. Activation of GH-GHR-STAT signalling pathway.

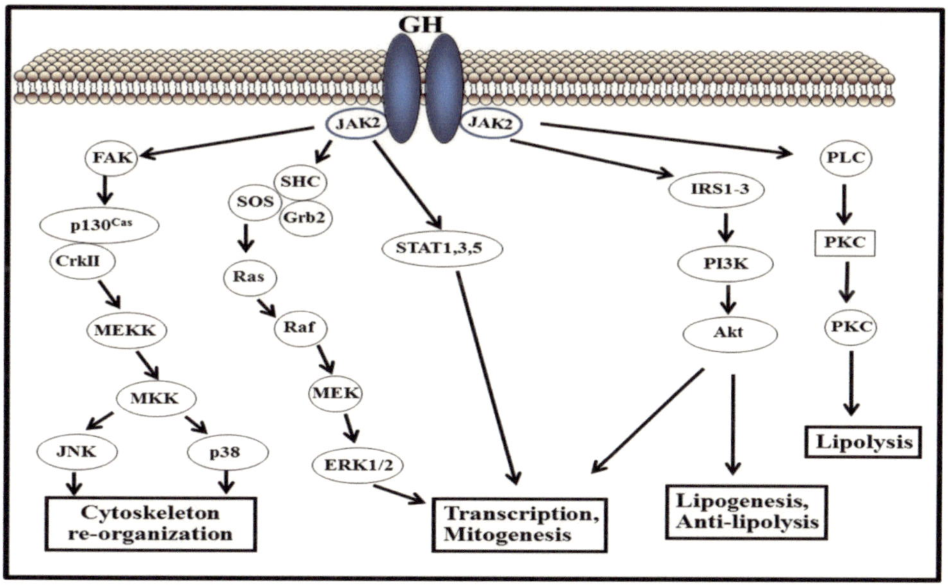

Fig. 3. Schematic representation of GH-activated signaling pathways.

The analysis of molecular mechanisms involved in inactivation of GHR signaling cascades is imperative to GH physiology. The activation of GH-signaling pathways is rapid and transient; the duration of GH-activated signals is a critical component in relation to the biological actions of this hormone. This is clearly illustrated in the case of hepatic GH actions where signal duration regulates gender differences in liver gene expression (Waxman et al., 1995). As mentioned, the male pattern of GH secretion in rats is episodic with peaks every 3-4 hours and no measurable trough levels (Jansson et al., 1985). Consequently, intracellular activation of STAT5 is also episodic and periods with low GH circulating levels are required to achieve maximal activation of STAT5. Female rats, which exhibit a more continuous GH secretion pattern with higher basal levels and smaller and irregular intermittent peaks showed reduced STAT5b activation compared with males (Waxman et al., 1995). These differences in STAT5b activation are responsible for several of the gender differences in hepatic gene expression (Waxman and O'Connor, 2006). Studies on primary hepatocytes and several cell lines have shown that GH-induced JAK2-STAT5b activation is transient, with maximal activation achieved within the first 30 min of stimulation, followed by a period of inactivation (Flores-Morales et al., 2006). This period is characterized by an inability to achieve maximal JAK2-STAT5 activation by GH in the following 3 h, unless GH is withdrawn from the media. The conserved control of GHR-JAK2 activation kinetic in multiple cell models emphasizes the importance of mechanisms of negative regulation for GH actions. Several studies already show that GH action can be modulated through interference with GHR down-regulation. Phospholipase C inhibition (Fernandez et al., 1998), induction of the unfolded protein response (Flores-Morales et al., 2001a), actin cytoskeleton depolymerization (Rico-Bautista et al., 2004), and treatment with 1α,25-dihydroxyvitamin D3 (Morales et al., 2002), prolong the duration of JAK2-STAT5 phosphorylation after GH treatment, with little or no effect on its rapid and maximal activation.

The molecular mechanisms for desensitization of GH-dependent signaling pathway play a critical role in GH physiology. Cell surface levels of GHR are the primary determinant of GH responsiveness. The coordination of extracellular and intracellular signals is achieved through inactivation of GHR signals. This mechanism is GH activated and prolonged in time (Kelly et al., 1991). The mechanisms governing GHR expression are complex (Schwartzbauer and Menon, 1998). Transcriptional, translational and posttranslational level factors can influence GHR synthesis and, thereby, regulate cell sensitivity to GH actions. These factors include nutritional status, endocrine context, developmental stage, and, relevant to this review, estrogens (Flores-Morales et al., 2006). Removal of cell surface GHRs by endocytosis is an early step in the termination of GH-dependent signaling. GHR ubiquitination is a key control mechanism in the down-regulation of GH signaling, modulating both GHR internatization and proteasomal degradation. In addition to GHR down-regulation, other mechanisms are needed to complete inactivation of GH signaling. Since activation of GH-dependent signaling pathways is critically based on protein phosphorylation on tyrosine, serine or threonine residues, the obvious mechanism for deactivation of this process is the action of protein phosphatases. Recently, several studies have resulted in the identification of three phosphatases which are involved in the specific inactivation of GHR signaling: SHP1 (SH2 domain-containing protein-tyrosine phosphatase1 or PTP-1); 2) PTP1b; and 3) PTP-H1. Second, Signal Regulatory Protein (SIRP)-α, which belongs to a family of ubiquitously expressed transmembrane glycoproteins, was identified by ability to associate with the SH2 domain of SHP-2, SHP-1, and Grb2 in response to insulin, EGF, and PDGF (Kharitonenkov et al., 1997). GH induces JAK2-

dependent phosphorylation of SIRP-α, which then enable it to bind SHP2 (Stofega et al., 1998). Overexpression of SIRP-α negatively regulates GH-activated signaling by inhibition of the phosphorylation of JAK2, STAT5b, STAT3, and ERK1-2 (Stofega et al., 1998). Finally, SOCS proteins have been shown key components of negative regulators of GHR-JAK-STAT signaling pathway. The SOCS family comprises at least eight proteins: CIS and SOCS-1 to -7 (Flores-Morales et al., 2006; Rico-Bautista et al., 2006). SOCS proteins have been shown to modify cytokine actions through a classic negative feedback loop. In general, SOCS protein levels are constitutively low, but their expression is rapidly induced by stimulation with different cytokines or growth factors including GH (Alexander, 2002). SOCS proteins bind the receptor/JAK complex and down-regulate JAK-STAT signaling pathway. Particularly, the phenotype of SOCS2 null mice (SOCS2KO) identifies SOCS2 as a key physiological player in the negative regulation of GH signaling (Rico-Bautista et al., 2006). SOCS2KO mice are 30-40% larger that their littermates, with the weight gain due to an increase in bone size and a proportionate enlargement of most organs. Similar phenotypes have been also found in animals overexpressing GH (Kopchick et al., 1999), patients with gigantism (Colao et al., 1997) and in high-growth mice, which have a spontaneous deletion within the chromosome 10 resulting in a disruption and inactivation of the socs2 locus (Horvat and Medrano, 2001). IGF-I mRNA expression in SOCS2KO mice is significantly increased in some organs, without major changes in hepatic or serum IGF-I content. Other studies have demonstrated that SOCS2 is essential for the regulation of GH actions not directly related to somatic growth. For example, SOCS2 blocks GH-dependent inhibition of neural stem cell differentiation. Consequently SOCS2KO mice have fewer neurons in the developing cortex, whereas SOCS2 overexpression results in increased neural differentiation. Recently, it has also been demonstrated that SOCS2 inhibits intestinal epithelial (Miller et al., 2004) and prostate cell proliferation (D. Iglesias et al, personal comunication), which are induced by GH in vivo. Evidence also indicates that growth factors (e.g., insulin, chemokines), xenobiotics, and steroid hormones, including estrogens, can induce SOCS expression (Rico-Bautista et al., 2006). Consequently, regulation of SOCS protein expression provides a mechanism for cross-talk where multiple factors can regulate the activity of specific cytokines (Greenhalgh and Alexander, 2004; Leung et al., 2004; Rico-Bautista et al., 2006). Particularly, SOCS2 may be a physiological mechanism by which estrogen signaling pathways influence GH activity: estrogen suppresses GH-dependent JAK2 phosphorylation by increasing the expression of SOCS2 (Leung et al., 2004).

4. Growth Hormone regulates body growth, metabolism, and sexual dimorphism

GH exerts its physiological effects through transcriptional regulation and acute changes in the catalytic activity of several enzymes (Flores-Morales et al., 2001b; Tollet-Egnell et al., 2001; Tollet-Egnell et al., 2004; Lichanska and Waters, 2008; Waxman and Holloway, 2009). Based on gene ontology analysis of liver transcript profiles from targeted disruption/mutation of signaling components of GHR-signaling pathways (Udy et al., 1997) or GHR itself (Lichanska and Waters, 2008), and GH administration to GH-deficient mice and rats (Flores-Morales et al., 2001b; Tollet-Egnell et al., 2001; Olsson et al., 2003; Tollet-Egnell et al., 2004; Rowland et al., 2005; Stahlberg et al., 2005), the main metabolic process affected by GH status is energy/fuel metabolism, particularly lipid/fat metabolism. In addition, carbohydrate, protein, steroid and drug metabolism are also strongly influenced.

These findings in animals together with clinical studies of GH-insensitive mutants have revealed the transcription factor STAT5b is a key GH signaling intermediate for the regulation of postnatal growth, lipid metabolism, and sexual dimorphism of hepatic gene expression. In addition, many transcripts are regulated independently of STAT5b, presumably as a result of GHR-dependent activation of ERK, Src, and PI3K signaling pathways.

4.1 GH and body growth

GH is predominantly linked with linear growth during childhood. The liver is a major target tissue of GH and the principal source of circulating IGF-I. GH-dependent transcription of IGF-I is regulated by STAT5 binding sites in IGF-I gene (Woelfle et al., 2003). Thus, both IGF-I and its transcriptional regulator STAT5 have key roles in mediating the actions of GH on body growth (Le Roith et al., 2001; Kaplan and Cohen, 2007). Importantly, intermittent (male pattern) GH administration to rodents is a more potent stimulus of body growth rate, IGF-I expression, and STAT5b nuclear translocation in liver than is continuous (female pattern) administration. This supports the notion that larger body growth in male compared with female rodents could be due to more effective stimulation of IGF-I and STAT5b mediated transcription. IGF-I proteins are also induced by GH in many tissues and local induction of IGF-I in chondrocytes plays an important role in longitudinal growth (Yakar et al., 1999). GH is, however, more effective that IGF-I because GH exerts additional growth-promoting actions independent of IGF-I (Lupu et al., 2001).

Global disruption of STAT5b in mice cause loss of sexually dimorphic growth characteristics, with affected males reduced to the size of females, and female mice appeared unaffected (Udy et al., 1997). Parallel observations were made with serum IGF-I concentrations, which were reduced by 30-50% in affected male mice, but not in females. However, combined disruption of STAT5a/b significantly reduced body weight gain in females and suppressed body growth more than STAT5b null mice alone in males, approaching that observed either GH or the GHR deficient mice (Rowland et al., 2005).These studies demonstrated that STAT5b is important for male-specific body growth, whereas STAT5a regulates body growth in both sexes. Experiments in mice with SOCS-2 disruption also support that STAT5b is critical for GH-regulated growth in mammals (Greenhalgh and Alexander, 2004). Importantly, SOCS2KO mice have enhanced growth whereas combined STAT5bKO and SOCS2KO mice do not, a demonstration of the necessity of STAT5b for the excess of body growth observed in SOCS2KO mice (Rico-Bautista et al., 2006). In addition to endocrine actions, paracrine involvement of STAT5a/b in the effects of GH on muscle is also evident in the loss of muscle IGF-I transcripts and mass seen with muscle-specific deletion of Stat5a/b (Klover and Hennighausen, 2007). As mentioned above, the growth of female STAT5bKO mice is normal whereas postnatal growth in female GHR-deleted mice is profoundly retarded (Zhou et al., 1997). These data suggest that in addition to STAT5b, other transcriptions factors are related with growth. This is exemplified by the glucocorticoid receptor (GR) which is a critical co-activator of STAT5b in liver: near 25% of STAT5b-regulated hepatic genes are subject to control by a GR-STAT5b transcriptional complex (Engblom et al., 2007). Importantly, these STAT5b and GR co-regulated transcripts were preferentially enriched in functional groups related to growth and maturation (i.e., IGF-1). Moreover, both direct and indirect interactions between ER and STAT5 (Bjornstrom and Sjoberg, 2005) should be added to the list of mechanisms regulated by nuclear receptors that modulate GH-dependent transcription.

4.2 GH and metabolism

Physiological effects of GH extend beyond the stimulation of linear growth. These include important metabolic actions throughout life. At all ages, GH has anabolic effects and increases muscle size in GH-deficient individuals: GH enhances amino acid uptake into skeletal muscle, increases whole body protein synthesis and enhances positive nitrogen balance, concomitant with the increase in lean body mass (LeRoith and Yakar, 2007; Lichanska and Waters, 2008; Vijayakumar et al., 2010). Thus, GH has a net metabolic effect on protein metabolism, as it stimulates protein synthesis while repressing proteolysis.

The mechanisms of GH actions on lipid metabolism are complex and involve transcriptional and acute changes in catalytic enzyme activities (Flores-Morales et al., 2001b; Tollet-Egnell et al., 2001; Tollet-Egnell et al., 2004; Lichanska and Waters, 2008; Waxman and Holloway, 2009). It is well established that human GH is a lipolytic hormone. Long-term administration of GH includes a decrease in deposition of fat and an increase in fat mobilization, increasing circulating FFA and glycerol levels. GH reduces fat mass, particularly in individuals who have accumulated excess fat during periods of GH deficiency (GHD). Obesity is clinically evident in GHD patients and a decline in GH levels correlates with age-related obesity and lack of GH or GH signaling induces obesity earlier in mice (Corpas et al., 1993; Laron et al., 2006; Cui et al., 2007). GHD in adulthood causes a syndrome characterized by increased visceral adiposity, decreased muscle mass, metabolic disturbances, and increase mortality associated with cancer or vascular complications. This syndrome closely resembles the metabolic syndrome and can be ameliorated by GH replacement (LeRoith and Yakar, 2007; Lichanska and Waters, 2008; Vijayakumar et al., 2010).

The exact mechanisms through which GH exerts lipolytic effects remain to be elicited. GH can induce hepatic LDL receptors and, therefore, increase cholesterol uptake into liver. GH deficiency associates with elevated serum cholesterol and GH replacement therapy normalizes those levels. Serum cholesterol can also be modulated by IGF-I. Specific disruption of IGF-I gene in liver (LID mice) increased circulating cholesterol levels (total and LDL cholesterol) in male and female. These findings concur with the observation that IGF-I treatment decreases serum cholesterol in humans. Interestingly, some studies have reported that LID mice show increased circulating triglycerides levels without changes in liver and muscles triglyceride content. Accumulation of FFA in the adipose tissue is dependent upon lipoprotein lipase (LPL), which hydrolyzes triglycerides into FFA. GH inhibits LPL in adipose tissue, whereas insulin increases activity of LPL. On the other hand, GH increases LPL in muscle, which leads to increased use of FFA by skeletal muscle. Additionally, GH can directly stimulate hydrolysis of triglycerides into FFA and glycerol, which stimulates FFA transport from adipose tissue into the liver and muscle. The increased release of FFA and glycerol transport from adipose tissue then affects liver insulin responsiveness, which leads to insulin resistance and induction of the gluconeogenic enzymes phosphoenol pyruvate carboxy kinase (PEPCK) and glucose-6-fosfatase (G-6-Pase). Therefore, GH increase in hepatic glucose production can be explained primarily through the effects of GH on lipolysis. Interestingly, GH treatment of both healthy and GHD individuals decreased whole-body carbohydrate oxidation and concomitantly increased whole-body lipid oxidation. This open the possibility that the GH-induced increased in FFA efflux from adipose tissue could, via the provision of substrates for gluconeogenesis, abrogate the need for amino acids and consequently proteolysis. But more direct effects of GH might also have a role in adipocytes. One of the mechanisms by which GH leads to lipolytic effects involve increased expression of β3-adrenergic receptor in adipocytes followed by activation of HSL (hormone sensitive lipase). Additional effects include uncoupling of the electron transport chain which enhances mitochondrial heat generation at the expense of energy production from ATP.

As mentioned above, GH stimulates triglyceride uptake in the skeletal muscle and induces LPL activity, thereby promoting lipid store or release energy via either lipolysis or lipid oxidation. However, several factors such as nutrition, exercise, and sex steroid hormone status could modify GH-induced triglyceride storage and lipid oxidation in skeletal muscle. GH also induces triglyceride uptake in liver by increasing LPL and/or HSL expression. GH treatment promotes a state of intrahepatic triglyceride storage. Several studies in bGH-transgenic mice, defficient GHR-JAK2-STAT-5 signaling pathway, GH-treated intact or GH-deficient rats (hypophysectomized or hypothyroid), as well as experiments in PPARα null mice, have all revealed that GH down-regulates genes involved in lipid oxidation and increases the expression of genes promoting lipogenesis in the liver (Olsson et al., 2003; Wang et al., 2007; Barclay et al., 2011; Sos et al., 2011). On the other hand, an impaired GHR-JAK2-STAT-5 signaling strongly correlates with hepatic steatosis (Fan et al., 2009; Barclay et al., 2011; Sos et al., 2011). Disruption of the hepatic GHR, JAK2 or STAT5 genes in mice resulted in hepatic steatosis due to enhanced lipogenesis and reduced triglyceride secretion. GHR-JAK2-STAT5 signaling deficiency has also been studied by mutagenesis of GHR in mice (Lichanska and Waters, 2008), a model that causes severe obesity in mature mice in proportion to loss of STAT5b activity. Collectively, these experiments have shown that STAT5 regulates several key enzymes or genes otherwise involved in lipid and energy balance. Based on altered transcript expression, several processes have been implicated. For example, up-regulation of some lipogenic genes (e.g., CD36, PPARγ, PGC*1α*/β, FAS, SCD1, LPL, VLDLR) may contribute to increased hepatic lipid storage, steatosis, and adiposity in deficient GHR-JAK2-STAT5 signaling models whereas expression of antilipogenic genes such as FGF*21* and INSIG2 are decreased. Genetically modified animals and microarray analysis have provided new insights into the long-known anti-adiposity actions of GH and highlighted a key role for STAT5 in these actions. This is supported by original findings that STAT5b-deleted male mice become obese in later life (Udy et al., 1997; Teglund et al., 1998) and that STAT5b deletion in a mature human was associated with obesity (Vidarsdottir et al., 2006). The anti-obesity actions of GH are enhanced by the pulsatility of GH secretion evident in males (Takahashi et al., 1999) because pulsatile STAT5 activation, which is, as mentioned above, so important for sexual dimorphism in hepatic gene expression (including IGF-1). Importantly, these findings suggest that despite normal plasma FFA and minimal adiposity, absent GHR activation could lead to hepatic steatosis because activated STAT5 prevents this pathology (LeRoith and Yakar, 2007).

4.3 GH and insulin sensitivity

The effects of GH on both glucose and lipid metabolism are key components in GH-dependent induction of insulin resistance (LeRoith and Yakar, 2007; Vijayakumar et al., 2010). In liver, GH has a stimulatory effect on glucose production which may be a result of its antagonism of insulin action leading to hepatic/systemic insulin resistance. GH increases glucose production by increasing glycogenolysis; however, it has either a stimulatory or no effect on gluconeogenesis. Over-expressing the human GH gene in rat increases basal hepatic glucose uptake and glycogen content (Cho et al., 2006). In contrast, GHD mice

(Ames) and the GHRKO mice have improved insulin sensitivity and an up-regulation of hepatic insulin signaling, suggesting that GH antagonizes insulin signaling in the liver (Dominici and Turyn, 2002). As mentioned above, GH-induced insulin resistance may develop by the increased FFA mobilization from adipose tissue which can then affects liver insulin sensitivity, and lead to insulin resistance and up-regulation of the PEPCK and G6Pase (Segerlantz et al., 2001; Kovacs and Stumvoll, 2005). However, LID mice showed a 75% reduction in circulating IGF-I levels, 3-4 fold increase in circulating GH levels and insulin resistance, without significant increase in circulating FFA levels. Moreover, while crossing IGF-I specific liver deficient mice with GH transgenic mice, serum FFA levels were significantly increased and there was an improvement in insulin sensitivity during a hyperinsulemic-euglycemic clamp due to higher hepatic, adipose tissue and skeletal muscle glucose uptake (Yakar et al., 2004). This suggests that, in addition to FFA, other factor(s) may also contribute to GH-induced insulin resistance. One candidate is the SOCS family of proteins whose expression is induced by GH (Rico-Bautista et al., 2006). Another mechanism by which GH may induce insulin resistance is by increasing the expression of the p85, a regulatory subunit of PI3K (Leroith and Nissley, 2005; LeRoith and Yakar, 2007). Finally, given the large homologies between the insulin and IGF-I systems, it is not surprising that IGF-I exerts profound effects on carbohydrate metabolism (e.g., insulin-like effects on glucose uptake). Alternatively, IGF-I may enhance insulin sensitivity by suppressing GH release, via negative feedback. Therefore activation of IGF-I signalling adds more complexity for understanding molecular mechanisms involved in GH-induced insulin resistance in vivo.

4.4 GH and sexual dimorphism of hepatic physiology

Five decades of research have firmly established the existence of a gonadal-hypothalamo-pituitary-liver axis determining liver sexual dimorphism and the importance of GH secretion patterns (Mode and Gustafsson, 2006). More recently, genomic and bioinformatic technologies have contributed to solve molecular mechanisms involved in hepatic gene regulation (Tollet-Egnell et al., 2000; Flores-Morales et al., 2001b; Tollet-Egnell et al., 2004; Stahlberg et al., 2005; Waxman and O'Connor, 2006; Waxman and Holloway, 2009; Wauthier et al., 2010). As mentioned above, sex hormones imprint a sex-dependent pattern of pituitary GH hormone secretion which is a major player in establishing and maintaining the sexual dimorphism of hepatic gene transcription that emerges in rodents at puberty. Sex-dependent expression and GH regulation characterizes several families of hepatic genes involved in endo- and xenobiotic metabolism as well as relevant metabolic functions (e.g., lipid metabolism); 20-30% of all hepatic genes has a sex-specific expression pattern in rodents (Tannenbaum et al., 2001; Stahlberg et al., 2004; Gustavsson et al., 2010). Most of these hepatic sex differences are explained by the female-specific secretion of GH, through the induction of female-predominant transcripts and suppression of male-predominant. A key player in this scenario is STAT5b. Results from experiments with STAT5b null mice indicated that STAT5b is responsible for the masculinization of the male liver (Udy et al., 1997; Waxman and O'Connor, 2006). STAT5b is more efficiently activated, as other transcription factors such as HNF4α, by the male GH secretion pattern. STAT5b binding sites have been found in the promoter of several sex-differentiated CYP genes in rat, including Cyp2c12, Cyp2c11, Cyp2a2 and Cyp4a2 (Waxman and Holloway, 2009). Conversely, other transcription factors (e.g., HNF6 and HNF3b) are more efficiently activated in female liver or by the continuous GH secretion pattern (Mode et al., 1998). Sex differences are not only found in hepatic genes involved in endo- and xenobiotic metabolism but they are also found in GH-regulated lipid metabolism. HNF4 and HNF3b are relevant transcription factors for regulating genes involved in glucose and lipid metabolism (Wolfrum et al., 2004; Sampath and Ntambi, 2005) and most likely they also contribute to sexual dimorphism. Continuous administration of GH has been shown to increase hepatic expression of transcription factor SREBP-1c and its downstream target genes (Tollet-Egnell et al., 2001), as well as hepatic triglyceride synthesis and VLDL secretion (Elam et al., 1988; Sjoberg et al., 1996). As mentioned above, GH actions in liver lead to increased lipogenesis (i.e., induction of SREBP1c) and decreased lipid oxidation (i.e., inhibition of PPARα), and promote anabolic growth in peripheral tissues (i.e, muscle, bone) (Flores-Morales et al., 2001b; Tollet-Egnell et al., 2004; Stahlberg et al., 2005). Relevant to this review, estrogens cause opposite effects, in comparison with GH, on hepatic lipid metabolism and insulin sensitivity which represents a relevant point of regulatory interactions between estrogens and GH (see below).

5. Estrogens and liver

Estrogens have physiological actions which are not limited to reproductive organs, in both females and males. E2 can modulate GH actions on liver by acting centrally, by regulating GH secretion, and peripherally, modulating GH responsiveness. Importantly, the liver expresses ERα which regulates development (Fisher et al., 1984), hepatic metabolic pathways (D'Eon et al., 2005; Ribas et al., 2010; Faulds et al., 2011), body growth (Vidal et al., 2000), protection from drug-induced toxicity (Yamamoto et al., 2006), hepatocarcinogenesis (Yager et al., 1994; Bigsby and Caperell-Grant, 2011), fertility (Della Torre et al., 2011), as well as lipid metabolism and insulin sensitivity (Simpson et al., 2005; Foryst-Ludwig and Kintscher, 2010).Thus, the liver is a sex steroid responsive organ and represents a site where critical interactions between estrogens and GH could be developed.

5.1 Estrogen receptor signaling

Estrogens exert their physiological effects through two ER subtypes, ERα and ERβ, which belong to the nuclear receptor family of ligand-activated transcription factors (Heldring et al., 2007). Structurally, ERs share a common framework with the other members of the nuclear receptor family. The N-terminal A/B domain is the most variable region with less that 20% amino acid identity between the two ERs, and confers subtype specific actions on target genes. This region harbors the activation function-1 (AF-1) that is ligand-independent and shows promoter- and cell-specific activity. The centrally located C-domain harbors the DNA binding domain (DBD), which is involved in DNA binding and receptor dimerization. This domain is highly conserved between ERα and ERβ with 95% amino acid identity. The D-domain is referred to as the hinge domain and shows low conservation between ERα and ERβ (30%). This domain has been shown to contain a nuclear localization signal. The C-terminal E-domain is the ligand-binding domain (LBD) and the two subtypes display 59% conservation in this region. The LBD contains a hormone-dependent activation function (AF-2) and is responsible for ligand binding and receptor dimerization. The F-domain has less that 20% amino acid identity between the two ER subtypes and the functions of this domain remain undefined. Full transcriptional activity of the ERs is mediated through a synergistic action between the two activation domains, AF-1 and AF-2. Both ERα and ERβ contain a potent AF-2 function, but unlike ERα, ERβ seems to have a weaker corresponding AF-1 function and depends more on the ligand-dependent AF-2 for its transcriptional activation function. E2 has a similar affinity for ERα and ERβ and they are activated by a wide range of ligands including selective estrogen receptor modulators (SERMS) such as raloxifen as well as many other compounds (Heldring et al., 2007). ERα is mainly expressed in reproductive tissues, kidney, bone, white adipose tissue, and liver, while ERβ is expressed in the ovary, prostate, lung, gastrointestinal tract, bladder, and hematopoietic, and the central nervous systems. Therefore, specific actions of estrogens in liver may be reached by using selective ERα agonists (e.g., propyl-pyrazole-triol, PPT) (Lundholm et al., 2008).

Classical estrogen signaling occurs through a direct binding of ER dimers to estrogen responsive elements (EREs) in the regulatory regions of estrogen target genes followed by activation of the transcriptional machinery at the transcription start site (Heldring et al., 2007) (Figure 4). Estrogen also modulates gene expression by a second mechanism in which ERs interact with other transcription factors, like STAT5, through a process referred to as transcription factor cross-talk. Estrogen may also elicit effects through non-genomic mechanisms, which involve the activation of downstream kinases pathways like PKA, PKC, and MAPK via membrane-localized ERs (Revankar et al., 2005). An orphan G protein-coupled receptor (GPR)-30 in the cell membrane has been also reported to mediate non-genomic and rapid estrogen signaling (Dahlman-Wright et al., 2006). Moreover, the mechanisms involved in ER signaling are influenced by cell phenotype, the target gene, and the activity or crosstalk with other signaling networks. Particularly relevant is E2 interaction with GH in the regulation of growth, development, body composition, hepatic metabolism, and sex-differentiated functions in liver (Stahlberg et al., 2004; Stahlberg et al., 2005; Waxman and O'Connor, 2006).

Gender-related differences in body composition are in part mediated by sex steroids modulating the GH-IGF-I axis (LeRoith, 2009; Munzer et al., 2009; Maher et al., 2010a; Maher et al., 2010b; Rogol, 2010; Barclay et al., 2011; Birzniece et al., 2011). This is supported by the observation that gender differences in body composition emerge at the time of pubertal growth. The efficiency of GH activity is also modulated by estrogens in adulthood. This is exemplified by women being less responsive than men to GH treatment (Burman et al., 1997); GH treatment induces a greater increase in lean mass and decrease in fat mass, or a greater increase in indices of bone turnover and in bone mass, in GH-deficient male compared to female patients. Furthermore, pharmacological doses of estrogens exert effects on liver that are somehow different from those caused by physiological E2. Oral administration of pharmacological doses of estrogen to hypopituitary patients inhibits GH-regulated endocrine and metabolic effects: circulating IGF-I levels, lipid oxidation, as well as protein synthesis are suppressed, with a reciprocal elevation of carbohydrate oxidation (Ho et al., 1996; Huang and O'Sullivan, 2009). These effects on metabolism and body composition are attenuated by transdermal administration, suggesting that liver is the major site of regulatory control by estrogen. Estrogens can modulate GH actions on liver by acting peripherally (Figure 4), modulating GH responsiveness, which include changes in hepatic GHR expression and crosstalk with GH-activated JAK2-STAT5 signaling pathway. In addition, direct effects through hepatic ERα play a critical role in liver physiology and pathology. However, the effect of estrogens on GHR is dependent on tissue type and species (Birzniece et al., 2009) (and references within). Estrogens reduce expression of GHR in the liver of rabbits, but exert opposite effect in rodents. In rat osteosarcoma or human osteoblast-like cells, E2 also stimulates GHR expression. Oral estrogens administration (pharmacological doses) lead to a reduction in IGF-I levels in human despite an increase in GH. This observation suggests that estrogens impair the ability of GH to stimulate hepatic IGF-I production, indicating an inhibitory effect on GHR function. As discussed above, the JAK2-STAT5 pathway is a major regulator of GH-dependent endocrine, metabolic, and sex-differentiated activities on liver. Estrogens can induce SOCS-2 expression which in turn negatively inhibits GHR-JAK2-STAT5 signalling pathway leading to reduction in transcriptional activity in liver (Leung et al., 2004; Santana-Farre, 2008).

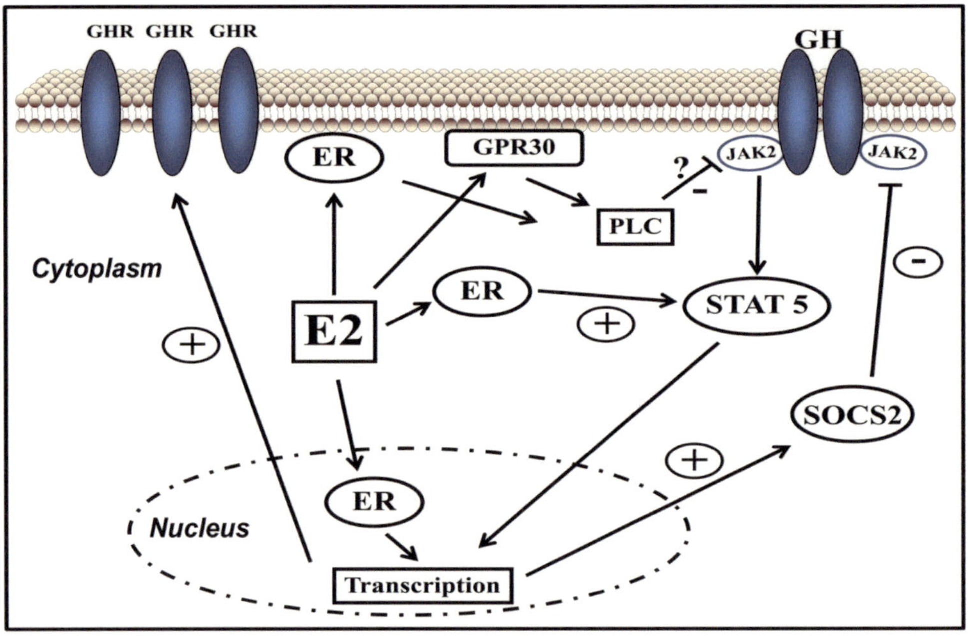

Fig. 4. Schematic representation of signalling pathways activated by E2 and its crosstalk with GH.

In summary, the effects of estrogens on GHR-JAK2-STAT5 signalling depend on tissue type, species, and route of administration. Beside E2 regulation of sex dimorphic pattern of pituitary GH secretion, induction of SOCS-2 expression and inhibition of JAK2-STAT5 signalling is a very relevant mechanism that, in part, could explain how estrogens directly inhibit the effects of GH in several STAT5-regulated actions (growth, development, body composition, metabolism, and sex-differentiated functions in liver). We have observed that long-term administration of physiological doses of E2 to GH-deficient male rats (hypothyroid) regulated several members of SOCS family by a complex interplay with GH and thyroid hormones (Santana-Farre, 2008). Our findings showed that E2 induces SOCS2 and CIS mRNA levels in liver and blocks the induction of these genes by GH, which most likely reflect an E2-dependent inhibitory effect on hepatic GHR-JAK2-STAT5 signalling. Hypothetically, other members of the negative regulators of STAT family may contribute to estrogen interaction with GH signalling in liver. In myeloma cells, IL-6-induced activation of STAT3 is blocked by pretreatment of cells with estrogen (Wang et al., 2004). This is explained by ERα stimulation of PIAS3 expression which binds to and blocks STAT3 DNA-binding activity, suggesting a possible mechanism of STAT3 inhibition requiring PIAS3 as a co-regulator modulating the crosstalk between ER and STAT3. Estrogens can also activate STAT-5 signalling not only in a pituitary but even a JAK2-independent manner. E2 activation of ER followed by direct interaction of ER with STAT5 may also inhibit STAT5-dependent transcriptional activity (Faulds et al., 2001; Wang and Cheng, 2004). Finally, via non-genomic mechanisms, E2-activation of ERα or ERβ could induce STAT5 (and STAT3)-dependent transcriptional program in endothelial cells (Bjornstrom and Sjoberg, 2005). These studies have shown a direct interaction between ER and STAT5 but also demonstrate that functional consequence of this cross-talk depends on the precise milieu of the intracellular environment.

5.2 E2 modulates GH promoting of skeletal growth

It is well known that sex steroids and GH interact closely to regulate pubertal growth (Bourguignon, 1991). Many observational studies in children have reported a correlation between IGF-I and sex steroid levels in both sexes during puberty, related closely to a concomitant increase in GH levels. Interestingly, loss of ERα (ERKO), but not ERβ, mediates important effects of estrogen in the skeleton of male mice during growth and maturation (Vidal et al., 2000). A phenotype like to ERKO mice can be found for aromatase-deficient (ArKO) male rats (Vanderschueren et al., 1997), which cannot produce estrogens. Thus, some of the effects on skeletal growth seen in ERKO mice may be caused by an inhibition of the GH-IGF-I axis. In contrast, as mentioned above, administration of pharmacological doses of estrogens results in a drastic reduction of circulating IGF-1 which most likely reflects the inhibitory effects of estrogens on hepatic GH-JAK2-STAT5 signalling pathway.

5.3 Sexually dimorphic pattern of GH secretion connects sex steroids with liver physiology

Sex steroids are physiological regulators of pituitary GH secretion and, indirectly, regulate sex-specific liver physiology. From neonatal period of life, gonadal steroids play a critical role to maintain liver response to GH in adulthood (Mode and Gustafsson, 2006) (and references herein). Neonatal exposure to androgens is crucial and the full response to androgens in adulthood is dependent on neonatal imprinting by androgens. The male characteristic metabolism in liver in adulthood is dependent on continuous androgen exposure. In female rats, gonadectomy has little impact on hepatic steroid metabolism; estrogen treatment, however, feminizes hepatic metabolism in male rats. The impact of GH secretion patterns on hepatic gene expression has become evident during last decade when DNA microarray technology has made it possible to carry out genome-wide screens of gene expression. These studies have shown that GH- and sex-dependent regulation of hepatic gene expression is not confined to steroid or drug metabolism and a number of other hepatic genes have been found to be up- and/or down-regulated by the different patterns of GH or sex-steroid exposure.GH- and sex-dependent hepatic transcripts encoding plasma proteins, enzymes, transcription factors and receptors involved in the metabolism of proteins, carbohydrates, lipids, or signalling regulation have been identified (Tollet-Egnell et al., 2000; Flores-Morales et al., 2001b; Tollet-Egnell et al., 2004; Stahlberg et al., 2005; Waxman and O'Connor, 2006; Waxman and Holloway, 2009; Wauthier et al., 2010). In addition, a proteomic approach has also been performed by Waxman's group (Wiwi and

Waxman, 2004) to identify GH and sex-dependent nuclear proteins in rat liver. Interestingly, of 165 sexually differentiated spots about 40% underwent a female-like change in male rats upon continuous treatment with GH.
The relationship among the components of GH secretion patterns (interpulse periods, GH concentration, pulse amplitude) and the characteristic sex-dependent expression of a number of genes (Mode and Gustafsson, 2006; Waxman and O'Connor, 2006) has been extensively explored during past years. In general, the GH interpulse periods constitute the major determinant of sex-specific genes; GH concentration and pulse amplitudes are also of different importance for the expression of several sex-characteristic CYP isoforms. In addition, a consensus exists that the response to sex-different GH patterns is the major cause of the "liver sexuality", it is also likely that factors other than the sexually dimorphic pattern of GH secretion are behind some sex differences in rat liver. Potential mechanisms that could contribute to "liver sexuality" are the pituitary-independent effects of estrogens through interaction with ERα or GH-JAK2-STAT5 signalling pathway in liver.

5.4 E2 is a critical regulator of lipid metabolism and insulin sensitivity: Potential crosstalk with GH

Estrogens, acting on both ERα and ERβ are recognized as important regulators of glucose homeostasis and lipid metabolism (Simpson et al., 2005; Faulds et al., 2011). Both male and female ERαKO mice develop insulin resistance and impaired glucose tolerance, similar to humans lacking ERα or aromatase. ERα mainly mediates beneficial metabolic effects of estrogens such as anti-lipogenesis, improvement of insulin sensitivity and glucose tolerance, and reduction of body weight/fat mass. In contrast, ERβ activation seems to be detrimental for the maintenance of regular glucose and lipid homeostasis. The insulin resistance in ERαKO mice is largely localized to the liver, including increased lipid content and hepatic glucose production. Interestingly, the expression of liver lipogenic genes can be decreased after E2 administration to diabetic Ob/Ob or high-fat diet fed female mice. Similarly, the aromatase knockout (ArKO) mouse, which cannot produce E2, has increased intra-abdominal adiposity and develops steatosis and an impairment of lipid oxidation in liver. Importantly, GH-GHR-JAK2-STAT5 deficiency in adults causes adiposity and hepatic steatosis suggesting that E2 and GH can regulate a common cellular network related with physiological control of lipid metabolism. In our lab, we have shown that subcutaneous administration of nearly physiological doses of E2 to male rats with GH deficiency (hypothyroid rats), dramatically influenced the hepatic transcriptional response to pulsatile GH administration (male pattern). In this model, E2 was able to increase hepatic transcriptional program in relation to lipid oxidation whereas lipid synthesis was decreased. Most relevant, expression of genes related to endocrine, metabolic, and sex-differentiated functions of GH were drastically inhibited by E2.

6. Conclusion

The liver responds in a sex-specific manner to GH and estrogens.GH is a major regulator of growth, somatic development, and body composition. Estrogens have physiological actions which are not limited to reproductive organs in both females and males, and they are recognized as key regulators of liver physiology. Physiologically and therapeutically relevant are estrogen interactions with GH-regulated endocrine (e.g., IGF-I), metabolic (e.g., lipid metabolism), and sex-differentiated (e.g., endo- and xenobiotic metabolism) functions in liver. The effects of estrogens are executed not just at the level of pituitary secretion, but also at the level of GHR signalling pathways. In addition, direct effects through hepatic ERα play a critical role in liver physiology and pathology. Thus, estrogens/GH interactions are relevant because physiological roles that these hormones have in mammals, and the widespread use of estrogen-related compounds (i.e., oral contraceptive steroids, hormone replacement therapy, SERM).This is supported from clinical observations where administration of pharmacological doses of estrogen to human impairs the GH-regulated endocrine and metabolic functions. In the general population, the endocrine and metabolic consequences of long-term treatment of women with estrogens or novel estrogen-related compounds are largely unknown. Therefore, this complex interaction deserves further research because its potential impact on GH-regulated body composition and influence on GH efficacy in GH-treated patients.

7. Acknowledgements

We thank all the authors that have made a contribution to the understanding of the crosstalk between sex hormones and GH signalling in liver. We apologize to those whose work deserves to be cited but unfortunately are not quoted because of space limitations. Research program in the author lab has been supported by grants from the Spanish Ministry of Science and Innovation with the funding of European Regional Development Fund-European Social Fund (SAF2003-02117 and SAF2006-07824).

8. References

Alexander WS (2002) Suppressors of cytokine signalling (SOCS) in the immune system. *Nat Rev Immunol*2:410-416.

Barclay JL, Nelson CN, Ishikawa M, Murray LA, Kerr LM, McPhee TR, Powell EE and Waters MJ (2011) GH-dependent STAT5 signaling plays an important role in hepatic lipid metabolism. *Endocrinology*152:181-192.

Bigsby RM and Caperell-Grant A (2011) The role for estrogen receptor-alpha and prolactin receptor in sex-dependent DEN-induced liver tumorigenesis. *Carcinogenesis*.

Birzniece V, Meinhardt UJ, Umpleby MA, Handelsman DJ and Ho KK (2011) Interaction between Testosterone and Growth Hormone on Whole-Body Protein Anabolism Occurs in the Liver. *J Clin Endocrinol Metab*96:1060-1067.

Birzniece V, Sata A and Ho KK (2009) Growth hormone receptor modulators. *Rev Endocr Metab Disord*10:145-156.

Bjornstrom L and Sjoberg M (2005) Mechanisms of estrogen receptor signaling: convergence of genomic and nongenomic actions on target genes. *Mol Endocrinol*19:833-842.

Bourguignon JP (1991) Growth and timing of puberty: reciprocal effects. *Horm Res*36:131-135.

Burman P, Johansson AG, Siegbahn A, Vessby B and Karlsson FA (1997) Growth hormone (GH)-deficient men are more responsive to GH replacement therapy than women. *J Clin Endocrinol Metab*82:550-555.

Butler AA and Le Roith D (2001) Control of growth by the somatropic axis: growth hormone and the insulin-like growth factors have related and independent roles. *Annu Rev Physiol*63:141-164.

Carro E, Senaris R, Considine RV, Casanueva FF and Dieguez C (1997) Regulation of in vivo growth hormone secretion by leptin. *Endocrinology*138:2203-2206.

Cho Y, Ariga M, Uchijima Y, Kimura K, Rho JY, Furuhata Y, Hakuno F, Yamanouchi K, Nishihara M and Takahashi S (2006) The novel roles of liver for compensation of insulin resistance in human growth hormone transgenic rats. *Endocrinology*147:5374-5384.

Colao A, Merola B, Ferone D and Lombardi G (1997) Acromegaly. *J Clin Endocrinol Metab*82:2777-2781.

Corpas E, Harman SM and Blackman MR (1993) Human growth hormone and human aging. *Endocr Rev*14:20-39.

Cui Y, Hosui A, Sun R, Shen K, Gavrilova O, Chen W, Cam MC, Gao B, Robinson GW and Hennighausen L (2007) Loss of signal transducer and activator of transcription 5 leads to hepatosteatosis and impaired liver regeneration. *Hepatology*46:504-513.

D'Eon TM, Souza SC, Aronovitz M, Obin MS, Fried SK and Greenberg AS (2005) Estrogen regulation of adiposity and fuel partitioning. Evidence of genomic and non-genomic regulation of lipogenic and oxidative pathways. *J Biol Chem*280:35983-35991.

Dahlman-Wright K, Cavailles V, Fuqua SA, Jordan VC, Katzenellenbogen JA, Korach KS, Maggi A, Muramatsu M, Parker MG and Gustafsson JA (2006) International Union of Pharmacology. LXIV. Estrogen receptors. *Pharmacol Rev*58:773-781.

Della Torre S, Rando G, Meda C, Stell A, Chambon P, Krust A, Ibarra C, Magni P, Ciana P and Maggi A (2011) Amino acid-dependent activation of liver estrogen receptor alpha integrates metabolic and reproductive functions via IGF-1. *Cell Metab*13:205-214.

Dominici FP and Turyn D (2002) Growth hormone-induced alterations in the insulin-signaling system. *Exp Biol Med (Maywood)*227:149-157.

Elam MB, Simkevich CP, Solomon SS, Wilcox HG and Heimberg M (1988) Stimulation of in vitro triglyceride synthesis in the rat hepatocyte by growth hormone treatment in vivo. *Endocrinology*122:1397-1402.

Engblom D, Kornfeld JW, Schwake L, Tronche F, Reimann A, Beug H, Hennighausen L, Moriggl R and Schutz G (2007) Direct glucocorticoid receptor-Stat5 interaction in hepatocytes controls body size and maturation-related gene expression. *Genes Dev*21:1157-1162.

Fan Y, Menon RK, Cohen P, Hwang D, Clemens T, DiGirolamo DJ, Kopchick JJ, Le Roith D, Trucco M and Sperling MA (2009) Liver-specific deletion of the growth hormone receptor reveals essential role of growth hormone signaling in hepatic lipid metabolism. *J Biol Chem*284:19937-19944.

Faulds MH, Pettersson K, Gustafsson JA and Haldosen LA (2001) Cross-talk between ERs and signal transducer and activator of transcription 5 is E2 dependent and involves two functionally separate mechanisms. *Mol Endocrinol*15:1929-1940.

Faulds MH, Zhao C, Dahlman-Wright K and Gustafsson JA (2011) Regulation of metabolism by estrogen signaling. *J Endocrinol*.

Fernandez L, Flores-Morales A, Lahuna O, Sliva D, Norstedt G, Haldosen LA, Mode A and Gustafsson JA (1998) Desensitization of the growth hormone-induced Janus kinase 2 (Jak 2)/signal transducer and activator of transcription 5 (Stat5)-signaling pathway requires protein synthesis and phospholipase C. *Endocrinology*139:1815-1824.

Fisher B, Gunduz N, Saffer EA and Zheng S (1984) Relation of estrogen and its receptor to rat liver growth and regeneration. *Cancer Res*44:2410-2415.

Flores-Morales A, Fernandez L, Rico-Bautista E, Umana A, Negrin C, Zhang JG and Norstedt G (2001a) Endoplasmic reticulum stress prolongs GH-induced Janus kinase (JAK2)/signal transducer and activator of transcription (STAT5) signaling pathway. *Mol Endocrinol*15:1471-1483.

Flores-Morales A, Greenhalgh CJ, Norstedt G and Rico-Bautista E (2006) Negative regulation of growth hormone receptor signaling. *Mol Endocrinol*20:241-253.

Flores-Morales A, Stahlberg N, Tollet-Egnell P, Lundeberg J, Malek RL, Quackenbush J, Lee NH and Norstedt G (2001b) Microarray analysis of the in vivo effects of hypophysectomy and growth hormone treatment on gene expression in the rat. *Endocrinology*142:3163-3176.

Foryst-Ludwig A and Kintscher U (2010) Metabolic impact of estrogen signalling through ERalpha and ERbeta. *J Steroid Biochem Mol Biol*122:74-81.

Greenhalgh CJ and Alexander WS (2004) Suppressors of cytokine signalling and regulation of growth hormone action. *Growth Horm IGF Res*14:200-206.

Gustavsson C, Yassin K, Wahlstrom E, Cheung L, Lindberg J, Brismar K, Ostenson CG, Norstedt G and Tollet-Egnell P (2010) Sex-different hepaticglycogen content and glucose output in rats. *BMC Biochem*11:38.

Heldring N, Pike A, Andersson S, Matthews J, Cheng G, Hartman J, Tujague M, Strom A, Treuter E, Warner M and Gustafsson JA (2007) Estrogen receptors: how do they signal and what are their targets. *Physiol Rev*87:905-931.

Ho KK, O'Sullivan AJ, Weissberger AJ and Kelly JJ (1996) Sex steroid regulation of growth hormone secretion and action. *Horm Res*45:67-73.

Holst B and Schwartz TW (2006) Ghrelin receptor mutations--too little height and too much hunger. *J Clin Invest*116:637-641.

Horvat S and Medrano JF (2001) Lack of Socs2 expression causes the high-growth phenotype in mice. *Genomics*72:209-212.

Howard AD, Feighner SD, Cully DF, Arena JP, Liberator PA, Rosenblum CI, Hamelin M, Hreniuk DL, Palyha OC, Anderson J, Paress PS, Diaz C, Chou M, Liu KK, McKee KK, Pong SS, Chaung LY, Elbrecht A, Dashkevicz M, Heavens R, Rigby M, Sirinathsinghji DJ, Dean DC, Melillo DG, Patchett AA, Nargund R, Griffin PR, DeMartino JA, Gupta SK, Schaeffer JM, Smith RG and Van der Ploeg LH (1996) A receptor in pituitary and hypothalamus that functions in growth hormone release. *Science*273:974-977.

Huang DS and O'Sullivan AJ (2009) Short-term oral oestrogen therapy dissociates the growth hormone/insulin-like growth factor-I axis without altering energy metabolism in premenopausal women. *Growth Horm IGF Res*19:162-167.

Jansson JO, Eden S and Isaksson O (1985) Sexual dimorphism in the control of growth hormone secretion. *Endocr Rev*6:128-150.

Kaplan SA and Cohen P (2007) The somatomedin hypothesis 2007: 50 years later. *J Clin Endocrinol Metab*92:4529-4535.

Kelly PA, Djiane J, Postel-Vinay MC and Edery M (1991) The prolactin/growth hormone receptor family. *Endocr Rev*12:235-251.

Kerrigan JR and Rogol AD (1992) The impact of gonadal steroid hormone action on growth hormone secretion during childhood and adolescence. *Endocr Rev*13:281-298.

Kharitonenkov A, Chen Z, Sures I, Wang H, Schilling J and Ullrich A (1997) A family of proteins that inhibit signalling through tyrosine kinase receptors. *Nature*386:181-186.

Klover P and Hennighausen L (2007) Postnatal body growth is dependent on the transcription factors signal transducers and activators of transcription 5a/b in muscle: a role for autocrine/paracrine insulin-like growth factor I. *Endocrinology*148:1489-1497.

Kopchick JJ, Bellush LL and Coschigano KT (1999) Transgenic models of growth hormone action. *Annu Rev Nutr*19:437-461.

Kovacs P and Stumvoll M (2005) Fatty acids and insulin resistance in muscle and liver. *Best Pract Res Clin Endocrinol Metab*19:625-635.

Lanning NJ and Carter-Su C (2006) Recent advances in growth hormone signaling. *Rev Endocr Metab Disord*7:225-235.

Laron Z, Ginsberg S, Lilos P, Arbiv M and Vaisman N (2006) Body composition in untreated adult patients with Laron syndrome (primary GH insensitivity). *Clin Endocrinol (Oxf)*65:114-117.

Le Roith D, Bondy C, Yakar S, Liu JL and Butler A (2001) The somatomedin hypothesis: 2001. *Endocr Rev*22:53-74.

LeRoith D (2009) Gender differences in metabolic disorders. *Gend Med*6 Suppl 1:1-3.

Leroith D and Nissley P (2005) Knock your SOCS off! *J Clin Invest*115:233-236.

LeRoith D and Yakar S (2007) Mechanisms of disease: metabolic effects of growth hormone and insulin-like growth factor 1. *Nat Clin Pract Endocrinol Metab*3:302-310.

Leung KC, Johannsson G, Leong GM and Ho KK (2004) Estrogen regulation of growth hormone action. *Endocr Rev*25:693-721.

Lichanska AM and Waters MJ (2008) How growth hormone controls growth, obesity and sexual dimorphism. *Trends Genet*24:41-47.

Lundholm L, Bryzgalova G, Gao H, Portwood N, Falt S, Berndt KD, Dicker A, Galuska D, Zierath JR, Gustafsson JA, Efendic S, Dahlman-Wright K and Khan A (2008) The estrogen receptor {alpha}-selective agonist propyl pyrazole triol improves glucose tolerance in ob/ob mice; potential molecular mechanisms. *J Endocrinol*199:275-286.

Lupu F, Terwilliger JD, Lee K, Segre GV and Efstratiadis A (2001) Roles of growth hormone and insulin-like growth factor 1 in mouse postnatal growth. *Dev Biol*229:141-162.

Maher AC, Akhtar M and Tarnopolsky MA (2010a) Men supplemented with 17beta-estradiol have increased beta-oxidation capacity in skeletal muscle. *Physiol Genomics*42:342-347.

Maher AC, Akhtar M, Vockley J and Tarnopolsky MA (2010b) Women have higher protein content of beta-oxidation enzymes in skeletal muscle than men. *PLoS One*5:e12025.

Meinhardt UJ and Ho KK (2006) Modulation of growth hormone action by sex steroids. *Clin Endocrinol (Oxf)*65:413-422.

Miller ME, Michaylira CZ, Simmons JG, Ney DM, Dahly EM, Heath JK and Lund PK (2004) Suppressor of cytokine signaling-2: a growth hormone-inducible inhibitor of intestinal epithelial cell proliferation. *Gastroenterology*127:570-581.

Mode A, Ahlgren R, Lahuna O and Gustafsson JA (1998) Gender differences in rat hepatic CYP2C gene expression--regulation by growth hormone. *Growth Horm IGF Res*8 Suppl B:61-67.

Mode A and Gustafsson JA (2006) Sex and the liver - a journey through five decades. *Drug Metab Rev*38:197-207.

Morales O, Faulds MH, Lindgren UJ and Haldosen LA (2002) 1Alpha,25-dihydroxyvitamin D3 inhibits GH-induced expression of SOCS-3 and CIS and prolongs growth hormone signaling via the Janus kinase (JAK2)/signal transducers and activators of transcription (STAT5) system in osteoblast-like cells. *J Biol Chem*277:34879-34884.

Munzer T, Harman SM, Sorkin JD and Blackman MR (2009) Growth hormone and sex steroid effects on serum glucose, insulin, and lipid concentrations in healthy older women and men. *J Clin Endocrinol Metab*94:3833-3841.

Olsson B, Bohlooly YM, Brusehed O, Isaksson OG, Ahren B, Olofsson SO, Oscarsson J and Tornell J (2003) Bovine growth hormone-transgenic mice have major alterations in hepatic expression of metabolic genes. *Am J Physiol Endocrinol Metab*285:E504-511.

Revankar CM, Cimino DF, Sklar LA, Arterburn JB and Prossnitz ER (2005) A transmembrane intracellular estrogen receptor mediates rapid cell signaling. *Science*307:1625-1630.

Ribas V, Nguyen MT, Henstridge DC, Nguyen AK, Beaven SW, Watt MJ and Hevener AL (2010) Impaired oxidative metabolism and inflammation are associated with insulin resistance in ERalpha-deficient mice. *Am J Physiol Endocrinol Metab*298:E304-319.

Rico-Bautista E, Flores-Morales A and Fernandez-Perez L (2006) Suppressor of cytokine signaling (SOCS) 2, a protein with multiple functions. *Cytokine Growth Factor Rev*17:431-439.

Rico-Bautista E, Negrin-Martinez C, Novoa-Mogollon J, Fernandez-Perez L and Flores-Morales A (2004) Downregulation of the growth hormone-induced Janus kinase 2/signal transducer and activator of transcription 5 signaling pathway requires an intact actin cytoskeleton. *Exp Cell Res*294:269-280.

Rogol AD (2010) Sex steroids, growth hormone, leptin and the pubertal growth spurt. *Endocr Dev*17:77-85.

Rowland JE, Lichanska AM, Kerr LM, White M, d'Aniello EM, Maher SL, Brown R, Teasdale RD, Noakes PG and Waters MJ (2005) In vivo analysis of growth hormone receptor signaling domains and their associated transcripts. *Mol Cell Biol*25:66-77.

Sampath H and Ntambi JM (2005) Polyunsaturated fatty acid regulation of genes of lipid metabolism. *Annu Rev Nutr*25:317-340.

Santana-Farre R, Flores-Morale A, Fernández-Pérez L (2008) Growth Hormone, Thyroid Hormones and Estradiol interplay in vivo to regulate gene expression of Suppressors of Cytokine Signalling (SOCS), in *International Proceedings 13th International Congress of Endocrinology* (A. Godoy-Matos JW ed) pp 8-12, Medimond, S.r.l., Rio de Janeiro (Brazil).

Schwartzbauer G and Menon RK (1998) Regulation of growth hormone receptor gene expression. *Mol Genet Metab*63:243-253.

Segerlantz M, Bramnert M, Manhem P, Laurila E and Groop LC (2001) Inhibition of the rise in FFA by Acipimox partially prevents GH-induced insulin resistance in GH-deficient adults. *J Clin Endocrinol Metab*86:5813-5818.

Simpson ER, Misso M, Hewitt KN, Hill RA, Boon WC, Jones ME, Kovacic A, Zhou J and Clyne CD (2005) Estrogen--the good, the bad, and the unexpected. *Endocr Rev*26:322-330.

Sjoberg A, Oscarsson J, Boren J, Eden S and Olofsson SO (1996) Mode of growth hormone administration influences triacylglycerol synthesis and assembly of apolipoprotein B-containing lipoproteins in cultured rat hepatocytes. *J Lipid Res*37:275-289.

Sos BC, Harris C, Nordstrom SM, Tran JL, Balazs M, Caplazi P, Febbraio M, Applegate MA, Wagner KU and Weiss EJ (2011) Abrogation of growth hormone secretion rescues fatty liver in mice with hepatocyte-specific deletion of JAK2. *J Clin Invest*121:1412-1423.

Stahlberg N, Merino R, Hernandez LH, Fernandez-Perez L, Sandelin A, Engstrom P, Tollet-Egnell P, Lenhard B and Flores-Morales A (2005) Exploring hepatic hormone actions using a compilation of gene expression profiles. *BMC Physiol*5:8.

Stahlberg N, Rico-Bautista E, Fisher RM, Wu X, Cheung L, Flores-Morales A, Tybring G, Norstedt G and Tollet-Egnell P (2004) Female-predominant expression of fatty acid translocase/CD36 in rat and human liver. *Endocrinology*145:1972-1979.

Stofega MR, Wang H, Ullrich A and Carter-Su C (1998) Growth hormone regulation of SIRP and SHP-2 tyrosyl phosphorylation and association. *J Biol Chem*273:7112-7117.

Svensson J, Lonn L, Jansson JO, Murphy G, Wyss D, Krupa D, Cerchio K, Polvino W, Gertz B, Boseaus I, Sjostrom L and Bengtsson BA (1998) Two-month treatment of obese subjects with the oral growth hormone (GH) secretagogue MK-677 increases GH secretion, fat-free mass, and energy expenditure. *J Clin Endocrinol Metab*83:362-369.

Takahashi J, Furuhata Y, Ikeda A, Takahashi M, Iwata H, Kazusaka A and Fujita S (1999) Characterization of hepatic cytochrome P450 isozyme composition in the transgenic rat expressing low level human growth hormone. *Xenobiotica*29:1203-1212.

Tannenbaum GS, Choi HK, Gurd W and Waxman DJ (2001) Temporal relationship between the sexually dimorphic spontaneous GH secretory profiles and hepatic STAT5 activity. *Endocrinology*142:4599-4606.

Teglund S, McKay C, Schuetz E, van Deursen JM, Stravopodis D, Wang D, Brown M, Bodner S, Grosveld G and Ihle JN (1998) Stat5a and Stat5b proteins have essential and nonessential, or redundant, roles in cytokine responses. *Cell*93:841-850.

Tollet-Egnell P, Flores-Morales A, Odeberg J, Lundeberg J and Norstedt G (2000) Differential cloning of growth hormone-regulated hepatic transcripts in the aged rat. *Endocrinology*141:910-921.

Tollet-Egnell P, Flores-Morales A, Stahlberg N, Malek RL, Lee N and Norstedt G (2001) Gene expression profile of the aging process in rat liver: normalizing effects of growth hormone replacement. *Mol Endocrinol*15:308-318.

Tollet-Egnell P, Parini P, Stahlberg N, Lonnstedt I, Lee NH, Rudling M, Flores-Morales A and Norstedt G (2004) Growth hormone-mediated alteration of fuel metabolism in the aged rat as determined from transcript profiles. *Physiol Genomics*16:261-267.

Udy GB, Towers RP, Snell RG, Wilkins RJ, Park SH, Ram PA, Waxman DJ and Davey HW (1997) Requirement of STAT5b for sexual dimorphism of body growth rates and liver gene expression. *Proc Natl Acad Sci U S A*94:7239-7244.

Vanderschueren D, van Herck E, Nijs J, Ederveen AG, De Coster R and Bouillon R (1997) Aromatase inhibition impairs skeletal modeling and decreases bone mineral density in growing male rats. *Endocrinology*138:2301-2307.

Vidal O, Lindberg MK, Hollberg K, Baylink DJ, Andersson G, Lubahn DB, Mohan S, Gustafsson JA and Ohlsson C (2000) Estrogen receptor specificity in the regulation of skeletal growth and maturation in male mice. *Proc Natl Acad Sci U S A*97:5474-5479.

Vidal OM, Merino R, Rico-Bautista E, Fernandez-Perez L, Chia DJ, Woelfle J, Ono M, Lenhard B, Norstedt G, Rotwein P and Flores-Morales A (2007) In vivo transcript profiling and phylogenetic analysis identifies suppressor of cytokine signaling 2 as a direct signal transducer and activator of transcription 5b target in liver. *Mol Endocrinol*21:293-311.

Vidarsdottir S, Walenkamp MJ, Pereira AM, Karperien M, van Doorn J, van Duyvenvoorde HA, White S, Breuning MH, Roelfsema F, Kruithof MF, van Dissel J, Janssen R, Wit JM and Romijn JA (2006) Clinical and biochemical characteristics of a male patient with a novel homozygous STAT5b mutation. *J Clin Endocrinol Metab*91:3482-3485.

Vijayakumar A, Novosyadlyy R, Wu Y, Yakar S and LeRoith D (2010) Biological effects of growth hormone on carbohydrate and lipid metabolism. *Growth Horm IGF Res*20:1-7.

Wang L, Zhang X, Farrar WL and Yang X (2004) Transcriptional crosstalk between nuclear receptors and cytokine signal transduction pathways in immunity. *Cell Mol Immunol*1:416-424.

Wang Y and Cheng CH (2004) ERalpha and STAT5a cross-talk: interaction through C-terminal portions of the proteins decreases STAT5a phosphorylation, nuclear translocation and DNA-binding. *FEBS Lett*572:238-244.

Wang Z, Masternak MM, Al-Regaiey KA and Bartke A (2007) Adipocytokines and the regulation of lipid metabolism in growth hormone transgenic and calorie-restricted mice. *Endocrinology*148:2845-2853.

Waters MJ, Shang CA, Behncken SN, Tam SP, Li H, Shen B and Lobie PE (1999) Growth hormone as a cytokine. *Clin Exp Pharmacol Physiol*26:760-764.

Wauthier V, Sugathan A, Meyer RD, Dombkowski AA and Waxman DJ (2010) Intrinsic sex differences in the early growth hormone responsiveness of sex-specific genes in mouse liver. *Mol Endocrinol*24:667-678.

Waxman DJ and Holloway MG (2009) Sex differences in the expression of hepatic drug metabolizing enzymes. *Mol Pharmacol*76:215-228.

Waxman DJ and O'Connor C (2006) Growth hormone regulation of sex-dependent liver gene expression. *Mol Endocrinol*20:2613-2629.

Waxman DJ, Ram PA, Park SH and Choi HK (1995) Intermittent plasma growth hormone triggers tyrosine phosphorylation and nuclear translocation of a liver-expressed, Stat 5-related DNA binding protein. Proposed role as an intracellular regulator of male-specific liver gene transcription. *J Biol Chem*270:13262-13270.

Wehrenberg WB and Giustina A (1992) Basic counterpoint: mechanisms and pathways of gonadal steroid modulation of growth hormone secretion. *Endocr Rev*13:299-308.

Wiwi CA and Waxman DJ (2004) Role of hepatocyte nuclear factors in growth hormone-regulated, sexually dimorphic expression of liver cytochromes P450. *Growth Factors*22:79-88.

Woelfle J, Chia DJ and Rotwein P (2003) Mechanisms of growth hormone (GH) action. Identification of conserved Stat5 binding sites that mediate GH-induced insulin-like growth factor-I gene activation. *J Biol Chem*278:51261-51266.

Wolfrum C, Asilmaz E, Luca E, Friedman JM and Stoffel M (2004) Foxa2 regulates lipid metabolism and ketogenesis in the liver during fasting and in diabetes. *Nature*432:1027-1032.

Yager JD, Zurlo J, Sewall CH, Lucier GW and He H (1994) Growth stimulation followed by growth inhibition in livers of female rats treated with ethinyl estradiol. *Carcinogenesis*15:2117-2123.

Yakar S, Liu JL, Stannard B, Butler A, Accili D, Sauer B and LeRoith D (1999) Normal growth and development in the absence of hepatic insulin-like growth factor I. *Proc Natl Acad Sci U S A*96:7324-7329.

Yakar S, Setser J, Zhao H, Stannard B, Haluzik M, Glatt V, Bouxsein ML, Kopchick JJ and LeRoith D (2004) Inhibition of growth hormone action improves insulin sensitivity in liver IGF-1-deficient mice. *J Clin Invest*113:96-105.

Yamamoto Y, Moore R, Hess HA, Guo GL, Gonzalez FJ, Korach KS, Maronpot RR and Negishi M (2006) Estrogen receptor alpha mediates 17alpha-ethynylestradiol causing hepatotoxicity. *J Biol Chem*281:16625-16631.

Zhou Y, Xu BC, Maheshwari HG, He L, Reed M, Lozykowski M, Okada S, Cataldo L, Coschigamo K, Wagner TE, Baumann G and Kopchick JJ (1997) A mammalian model for Laron syndrome produced by targeted disruption of the mouse growth hormone receptor/binding protein gene (the Laron mouse). *Proc Natl Acad Sci U S A*94:13215-13220.

Zigman JM, Nakano Y, Coppari R, Balthasar N, Marcus JN, Lee CE, Jones JE, Deysher AE, Waxman AR, White RD, Williams TD, Lachey JL, Seeley RJ, Lowell BB and Elmquist JK (2005) Mice lacking ghrelin receptors resist the development of diet-induced obesity. *J Clin Invest*115:3564-3572.

4

Somatostatin in the Periventricular Nucleus of the Female Rat: Age Specific Effects of Estrogen and Onset of Reproductive Aging

Eline M. Van der Beek, Harmke H. Van Vugt,
Annelieke N. Schepens-Franke and Bert J.M. Van de Heijning
Human and Animal Physiology Group, Dept. Animal Sciences,
Wageningen University & Research Centre
The Netherlands

1. Introduction

The functioning of the growth hormone (GH) and reproductive axis is known to be closely related: both GH overexpression and GH-deficiency are associated with dramatic decreases in fertility (Bartke, 1999; Bartke et al, 1999; 2002; Naar et al, 1991). Also, aging results in significant changes in functionality of both axes within a similar time frame.

In the rat, GH secretion patterns are clearly sexually dimorphic (Clark et al, 1987; Eden et al, 1979; Gatford et al, 1998). This has been suggested to result mainly from differences in somatostatin (SOM) release patterns from the median eminence (ME) (Gillies, 1997; Muller et al, 1999; Tannenbaum et al, 1990). SOM is synthesized in the periventricular nucleus of the hypothalamus (PeVN) and controls in concert with GH-releasing hormone (GHRH) the GH release from the pituitary (Gillies, 1987; Tannenbaum et al, 1990; Terry and Martin, 1981; Zeitler et al, 1991). An altered GH status is reflected in changes in the hypothalamic SOM system. For instance, the number of SOM cells (Sasaki et al, 1997) and pre-pro SOM mRNA levels (Hurley and Phelps, 1992) in the PeVN were elevated in animals overexpressing GH.

Several observations suggest that SOM may also affect reproductive function directly at the level of the hypothalamus. SOM synthesis in the hypothalamus and its release from the ME fluctuate over the estrous cycle. (Estupina et al, 1996, Zorrila et al, , 1991). Central injections with SOM or a SOM analog (octreotide) decreased the number of gonadotropic cells in the pituitary (Lovren et al, 1998; Nestorovic et al 2002; 2003). Also, we previously showed that a single central injection with octreotide significantly attenuated the E_2-induced Luteinizing Hormone (LH) surge and significantly decreased the activation of Gonadotropin Releasing Hormone (GnRH) cells in the hypothalamus of female rats (van Vugt et al, 2004).

Age-related changes in fertility and fecundity are associated with selective changes at the level of the ovary and uterus (Meredith and Butcher, 1985; Nass et al, 1984; te Velde et al, 1998; Wise, 1982), pituitary gland (Brito et al, 1994; DePaolo et al, 1986; Krieg et al, 1995; Nass et al, 1984; Wise, 1982), and hypothalamus (Rubin et al, 1994; Wise, 1982; Wise et al, 2002). Reproductive aging is characterized by changes in the length of the reproductive cycle. In female rats, for instance, the normal 4 or 5 day estrous cycle will lengthen with age and become irregular. This is followed by a period of repetitive pseudopregnancies and/or persistent estrus, while cyclicity ends with a state of persistent diestrus (Vom Saal, 1994). Although the general sequence of events during aging is predictable, the age at which the decline in fertility becomes evident varies considerably between individuals and rat strains (Vom Saal et al, 1994; Te Velde et al, 1998). Hence, especially during the initial stage when cyclicity is still regular, the relative contribution of the ovaries, pituitary and hypothalamus to reproductive aging is unclear.

One of the first, common changes appears to be an attenuation of the proestrous, ovulation-inducing luteinizing hormone (LH) surge (Wise et al, 2002), which can be demonstrated even before estrous cycles become irregular (DePaolo et al, 1986). The latter is strongly associated with the age at which rats become acyclic (Nass et al, 1984). Previous research suggested that changes in ovarian hormone release (DePaolo et al, 1986; Lu et al, 1985), pituitary hormone storage and/or responsiveness to ovarian or hypothalamic signaling (Brito et al, 1994; Keizer et al, 2001; Matt et al, 1998), or changes in hypothalamic signaling (Rubin et al, 2000; Downs and Wise, 2009; Wise et al, 2002) may underlie the age-related attenuation of the pituitary LH surge.

Evidence suggests that exposure to chronically elevated levels of circulating E_2 during life advances the decline in fertility with age (Lu et al, 1981; Rodrigues et al, 1993). Moreover, it is known that E_2 affects hypothalamic SOM content and release, although the literature is somewhat controversial on the precise role of E_2 on SOM cell function (Baldino et al, 1988; Estupina et al, 1996; Knuth et al, 1983; Murray et al, 1999; Werner et al, 1988; Zorilla et al, 1991). Recent studies demonstrated a clear sex difference in the number and distribution of SOM peptide containing cells in the PEVN. In the female numbers were affected by ovariectomy and gonadal steroid treatment (Van Vugt et al, 2008).

During the early phase of reproductive aging, normal (or even elevated) levels of plasma estradiol (E_2), are correlated with a decline in somatotropic axis activity (Chandrashekar and Bartke, 1993; Vom Saal et al, 1994; Wilshire et al, 1995). In 14 months old rats, hypothalamic SOM peptide content as well as basal and KCl-stimulated SOM release from the hypothalamus were increased compared to young animals (Ge et al, 1989). Compared to young female rats, SOM peptide levels in the ME are decreased at 25-29 months of age (Takahashi et al, 1987), suggesting increased SOM release from the ME with age. Altogether, these data point to the hypothalamic SOM system as a potential candidate to mediate some of the concurrent changes in the activity of the reproductive and GH axis with age.

In the light of the data described above, we set out to study the effects of E_2 exposure on hypothalamic SOM peptide levels at middle age when an attenuation of the LH surge can be found in regularly cycling females. To this end, we measured LH and P release in regularly 4-day cycling females at young (4 months) and middle-age (8.5 months) on proestrus as well as after a stimulus with a potent GnRH analog the following proestrus day. Subsequently, animals were ovariectomized to examine the effect of a physiological dose of E_2 on SOM-peptide containing cells in the PeVN at selected time points following estrogen exposure. Using this approach, we aimed to gain more insight in the mechanisms underlying the interaction between the somatotropic and gonadotropic axis, i.e. a possible role for the hypothalamic SOM system. We hypothesize that SOM plays a role in the normal, physiological regulation of LH release in the female rat and suggest that changes in the response of PeVN SOM-ir with age may contribute to the hypothalamic changes that lead to an attenuated LH surge in middle- aged rats.

2. Material & methods

2.1 Animals

Virgin female (n=60) and male (n=8) Wistar rats (HsdCpb:WU, Wistar Unilever) were obtained from Harlan (Horst, NL) at 9 to 10 weeks of age. Rats were group housed (4/cage) under regular light-dark cycles (L/D 12:12, lights on at 3:00 h defined as 'zeitgebertime' 0, ZT0) with free access to standard food pellets (Hope Farms B.V., Woerden, NL) and water. Animals were housed individually from 1 week before cannulation onwards. Young and Middle-aged females were obtained from the same batch to reduce variation between animals. All experiments were approved by the animal experimental committee (DEC) of the Wageningen University.

2.2 Experimental design

To study changes in proestrous LH and P surge characteristics with age, 4-month-old ('young') and 8.5-month-old ('middle-aged') female rats with regular 4-day cycles were used for blood sampling and hormone analyses. Hourly blood samples were taken on proestrus to measure plasma LH and P profiles. To investigate pituitary LH and FSH responsiveness, a potent GnRH analog (Ovalyse®; des-Gly^{10}-GnRH-ethylamide, Upjohn, Ede, The Netherlands) was used on the following proestrus. Ovalyse® (100 ng in 0.25 ml 0.9% NaCl (w/v) containing 1% BSA) was administered i.v. immediately after the first blood sample was drawn.

Subsequently, a group of cycling females was ovariectomized (OVX, Van der Beek et al, 1999) at 4.5 (young) or 9 mo (middle-aged) of age, and given a single s.c. injection with estrogen at ZT3 on day 13 following OVX. Animals were perfused 2, 8, 26 or 32 hrs later, i.e. at ZT5 and ZT 11. Brains sections were stained for SOM peptide as described previously (Van Vugt et al, 2008).

2.3 Estrous cycle length

Estrous cycles were monitored by daily vaginal lavage. Lavages were analyzed according to criteria described elsewhere (Freeman et al, 1994). In addition, receptive behavior (hopping and darting, ear wiggling and lordosis posture) was monitored daily. To this end, a naive male WU rat was introduced briefly in the female's home cage around ZT 11, 1 hr before dark onset to confirm a proestrous lavage typing.

Cycle length was defined by the last two monitored cycles before sampling. Most females displayed regular 4-day estrous cycles (70%). Cycle lengthening was observed in 8.5 mo old females: regular 4-day cycles decreased from 70% to 45%, while both 5-day cycles (from 10% to 24%) and acyclicity (from 0% to 10%) increased.

2.4 Cannulation and blood sampling

The right jugular vein of female rats was cannulated to obtain stress-free blood samples (Steffens, 1969, Van der Beek et al 1999, Van Vugt et al, 2004). After a recovery period of at least five days, ten hourly blood samples of 170 µl were taken on proestrus from ZT 5.5-14.5 for measurement of endogenous, preovulatory hormone profiles. To assess the amount of acutely releasable LH by the pituitary gland, ten hourly blood samples of 170 µl were drawn from ZT 5.5-14.5 on the following proestrus, following an i.v. injection of the GnRH analog Ovalyse®, just after the first sample. Blood samples were collected in heparinized, air-dried vials (25 IU heparin, Leo Pharma BV, Breda, NL) and centrifuged at 13,000 rpm for 5 minutes. Plasma was diluted 1:4 for LH and 1:20 for P analysis with PBS buffer (0.02M, pH 7.5) containing 0.1% BSA, and stored frozen at –20 °C until RIA. LH and P plasma levels were determined by validated RIAs (Van der Beek et al, 1999, Van der Meulen et al, 1988). Only samples from animals that displayed regular 4-day estrous cycles were included in the analysis. The inter- and intra-assay coefficients of variation were determined using pooled rat serum, and amounted to respectively 12.1% and 10.8 % for the LH assay and 15.8% and 6.2% for P analysis.

2.5 Tissue processing, SOM immunocytochemistry & analysis

Forty-three regularly cycling female rats aged 4.5 (n=20) or 9 (n=23) months were ovariectomized and treated with estradiol benzoate before perfusion 2, 8, 26 or 32 hours later. The brains were processed for SOM immunocytochemistry as described in detail previously (Van der Beek et al, 1991; Van Vugt et al, 2008). Staining was performed in two separate runs (4.5 and 9 mo) and intra-assay variation was controlled for by including a group of young animals at 2 and 32 h after E_2 treatment in the second run. Every third brain section containing the PeVN was stained for SOM peptide by free-floating immunocytochemistry techniques. For staining, primary polyclonal rabbit antibody raised against SOM peptide (Somaar 080289, NIN, Amsterdam, NL) (Buijs et al, 1989) was used followed by detection with biotinylated goat anti-rabbit IgG and Avidin-Biotin Complex-elite (ABC; Vector Laboratories).

SOM-immunoreactive (-ir) neurons in the PeVN of the left side of the brain were counted using computer assisted analysis as described previously (Van Vugt et al, 2008). In addition to counting SOM-ir cells, also the amount/quantity of SOM-ir fibers (expressed in μm^2) was measured in these images in the young females only. To this end, both the fibers that were located closely to the SOM cells (the "PeVN region": measured in an area that had an absolute distance from the ventricle of approximately 200 µm) and all fibers that originated from SOM cells in the PeVN, including those projecting to the ME ("total fibers": measured in an area that had an absolute distance from the ventricle of approximately 560 µm) were counted. The analysis threshold was determined in a representative selection of the images by measuring the mean gray level in an area devoid of SOM staining. Next, an upper and a lower threshold were determined (mean gray level + 3x S.D.; mean maximal gray level - 3x S.D. respectively) excluding SOM-ir cells and very light SOM-ir fibers.

2.6 Data processing

To determine the effects of age on the proestrus LH and P surge several profile characteristics were defined: i.e. basal levels, onset time, peak time, peak height and the total amount of LH and P released. Basal levels were defined as the average concentration of the first three blood samples (ZT 5.5, 6.5, and 7.5) per animal. In case of an early rise in LH levels, i.e. at ZT 7.5 (n=3), the first two blood samples were used to calculate basal levels. Onset time was defined as the sample hour (ZT; mean ± SEM expressed as h:min ± min) at which LH levels exceeded basal LH levels plus 3 x the standard deviation, while LH levels continued to rise thereafter. Peak time of the LH surge was defined as the ZT hour at which the highest LH concentration was measured. The highest amount of LH measured at that time was defined as the peak height. The total amount of LH or P was defined by the cumulative value of hormone levels during the complete sampling period. LH levels showed a clear distinction between 'early', Ovalyse® induced LH release and a second 'late' increase in LH levels resulting from endogenous proestrous GnRH release. Therefore, LH data after Ovalyse® administration were divided in ZT 5.5-8.5 ('early') and ZT 9.5-14.5 ('late'). For 'late' release, LH peak time and LH peak height were determined as described above. Finally, total LH levels during the complete sampling period were calculated. As proestrous P release continuously increased but did not peak in the time window evaluated, only basal level, preovulatory surge level, and total amount released were assessed.

2.7 Statistics

Hormone levels were expressed as mean ± SEM and analyzed using SPSS (version 12.0). Differences were considered to be significant when $P<0.05$. Basal LH levels, onset time and peak time of the LH surge, LH peak height, and basal P levels from proestrus measurements, as well as LH peak height and total LH levels following Ovalyse® were tested with the nonparametric Kruskal-Wallis test and were post-hoc tested using the Mann-Whitney test. Changes with age in the total amount of LH and P released during the proestrous surge, preovulatory P surge levels as well as LH peak height of the induced LH surge and total LH levels following Ovalyse®) were tested by one-way ANOVA. To compare the total number of SOM-ir cells between the different time points following E_2 treatment, one-way ANOVAs were used. A Bonferroni or Tukey HSD test was used as post hoc test.

3. Results

3.1 Proestrous LH profiles

The general profile of the LH surge was comparable between ages. Basal plasma LH levels averaged 0.3 to 0.4 ng/ml and onset of the surge occurred around ZT9.5, where after LH levels increased rapidly and reached peak levels around ZT12. Subsequently, LH levels gradually declined. We found a significant decrease in LH peak and total LH levels with age (P=0.041 and P = 0.035, respectively) (Table 1). Pearson correlation tests showed that the magnitude of the LH surge (i.e. total LH levels) correlated with onset and height of the LH surge (LH onset time: r=-0.527 with $P < 0.001$; LH peak levels: r=0.924 with $P < 0.001$).

age (mo)	n	LH surge					P surge		
		basal	onset time	peak time	peak height	total	basal	surge	total
4	12	0.3 ± 0.1	9:43 ± 0:30	12:06 ± 0:20	12.8 ± 1.4	40.2 ± 4.5	24.9 ± 2.6	339.4 ± 28.8	414.2 ± 35.9
8.5	9	0.4 ± 0.1	9:37 ± 0:23	11:37 ± 0:19	8.3 ± 1.4*	25.2 ± 4.6*	23.2 ± 5.0	329.0 ± 64.6	398.6 ± 78.7

Table 1. Proestrous LH and P surge characteristics of young and middle-aged 4-day cyclic WU rats. Basal levels are depicted as the average concentration ZT 5.5-7.5, onset time of the LH surge (ZT at which LH levels exceeded basal levels plus 3xSD), peak time of the LH surge (ZT at which the highest concentration was measured), peak height of the LH surge (highest concentration measured), preovulatory P surge levels (cumulative value from ZT 8.5-14.5), and the total amount of LH or P released during the surge (cumulative value during the complete sampling period). All data are expressed as group means ± SEM in ng/ml (concentrations) or h:min (time). Significant differences ($P < 0.05$) between young and middle aged with ages are indicated with an asterisk.

3.2 Proestrous P levels

Plasma P levels increased gradually during proestrus, but did not show a distinct peak during the time window evaluated. Basal P levels defined by LH release characteristics showed no significant differences between groups and age did not affect P profiles (Table 1). Total P levels correlated significantly with basal P levels (r=0.876 with $P < 0.001$) and with P surge levels (r=0.992 with $P < 0.001$), in line with the observed elevation in P levels during the entire sampling period.

3.3 Pituitary responsiveness

Administration of Ovalyse® at ZT 5.5 resulted in a rapid and consistent increase in LH plasma levels irrespective of age (Table 2). Highest plasma LH levels were measured at 1 or 2 h after Ovalyse® administration and decreased thereafter (defined as the 'early', induced LH surge). After ZT 8.5, LH levels increased again (defined as the 'late', endogenous LH surge).

LH levels were of comparable magnitude at 1 and 2 h after Ovalyse® injection between 4 and 8.5 months old females. Also, the second, endogenous LH surge was comparable in magnitude (peak height and total LH levels) between groups and accompanied by a gradual increase in P levels comparable between ages.

age (mo)	n	LH following Ovalyse®					P following Ovalyse®		
		<ZT9		>ZT9		all samples	<ZT9	>ZT9	all samples
		peak height	total	peak height	total	total	total	total	total
4	12	30.0 ± 1.6	66.9 ± 2.5	14.8 ± 1.7	48.9 ± 5.4	115.9 ± 6.0	172.9 ± 12.2	365.5 ± 30.3	538.3 ± 42.0
8.5	10	31.0 ± 3.1	63.4 ± 7.2	16.3 ± 2.2	55.0 ± 7.7	118.4 ± 12.6	157.8 ± 17.9	338.2 ± 45.6	496.0 ± 61.9

Table 2. LH and P surge characteristics following Ovalyse® administration in young and middle-aged 4-day cyclic rats on proestrus. The surge was divided into a 'early' part (ZT<9; 'induced' surge) and a 'late' surge (ZT>9; 'endogenous' surge). Measured characteristics: peak height of the 'early' and 'late' LH surge (the highest concentration measured), and the total amount of LH or P released during the 'early' and 'late' and the entire sampling period (cumulative LH or P levels during the corresponding sampling periods). All data are expressed as group means ± SEM in ng/ml (concentrations).

3.4 SOM-ir cells and fibers in the PeVN

Total numbers of SOM-ir cells were roughly comparable between age groups (Figure 1). In the young animals, SOM-ir numbers were not significantly affected by time after E_2 treatment, although they appeared to be consistently lower at ZT5 compared to ZT11 (Figure 1A). In middle-aged rats, total numbers of SOM-ir cells were significantly lower at ZT 5 on day 1 compared to day 2 (Figure 1B).

SOM-ir cells within the PeVN showed a clear rostro-caudal distribution pattern, with maximal numbers of cells appearing in the more caudal part of the PeVN. The distribution in young females varied slightly over the different time points after E_2 treatment: maximal numbers of SOM-ir cells were found consistently in PeVN section 8 at ZT5, but in PeVN section 7 at ZT11 on both days (Figure 2A and B). In middle aged female, the rostro-caudal distribution pattern in the number of SOM-ir cells at ZT 5 on day 1 (Figure 2C) was absent, e.g. the number of SOM-ir cells was comparable between PeVN sections. Distribution patterns at other time points were in general comparable with those found in the young rats, i.e. maximal numbers of SOM-ir cells in PeVN section 7 at ZT 11 and in PeVN section 8 at ZT 5 on day 2 (Figure 2D).

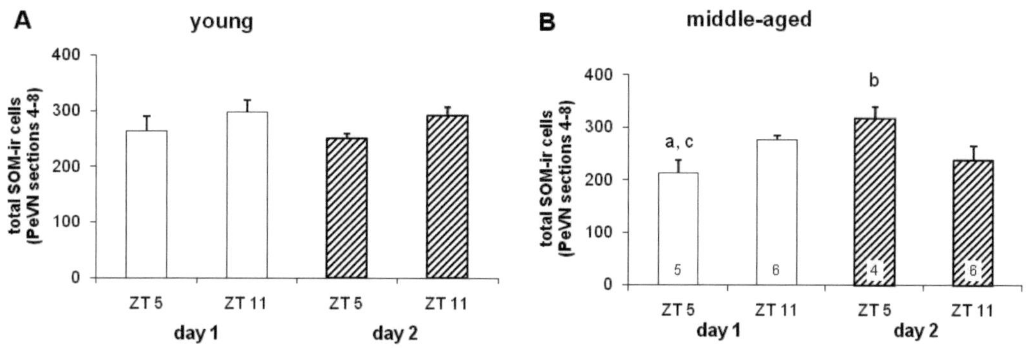

Fig. 1. Total number of SOM-ir cells (sum of PeVN sections 4-8) in young (4.5 months old) and middle aged (9 mo old) Wistar rats at different time points after E_2 treatment. ZT 5: 2 (day 1) or 26 (day 2) h after E_2 treatment, ZT 11: 8 (day 1) or 32 (day 2) h after E_2 treatment. n=5 for each young age group, numbers within base of bars indicate the number of animals.

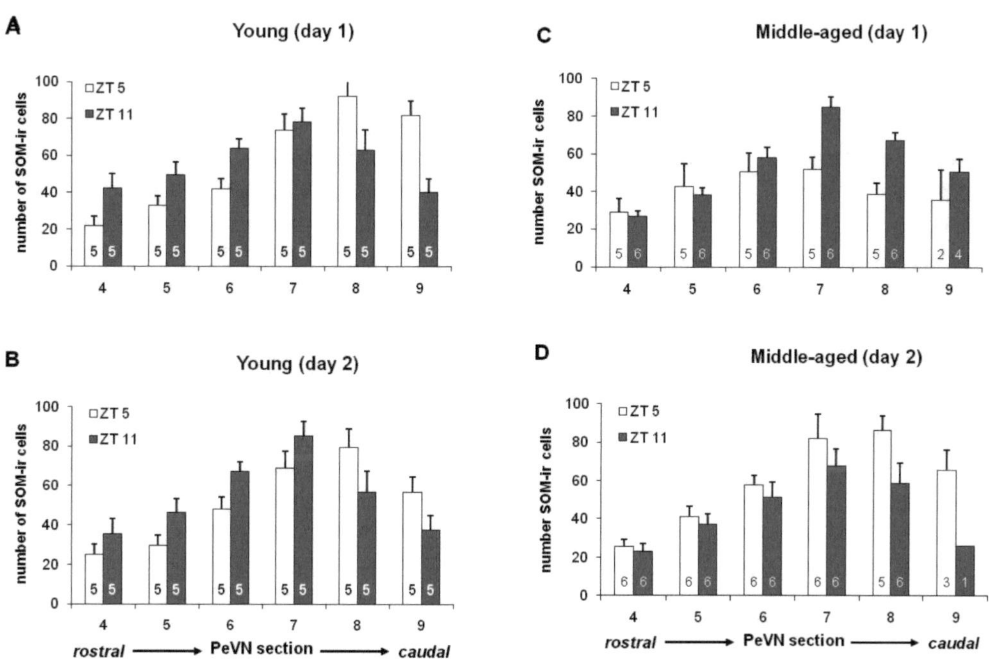

Fig. 2. Rostral to caudal distribution of SOM-ir cells in the PeVN of young (4.5 months old) (A and B) and middle aged (C and D) OVX females at different time points after E_2 treatment. Numbers within base of bars indicate the number of animals.

In young animals, the area occupied by SOM-ir fibers in the PeVN region was significantly different at ZT5 on day 1 compared to ZT11 day 2 (Figure 3A). The total area of SOM-ir fibers, i.e. including the fibers projecting to the ME, was significantly different between ZT5 and ZT11 on both days (Figure 3B).

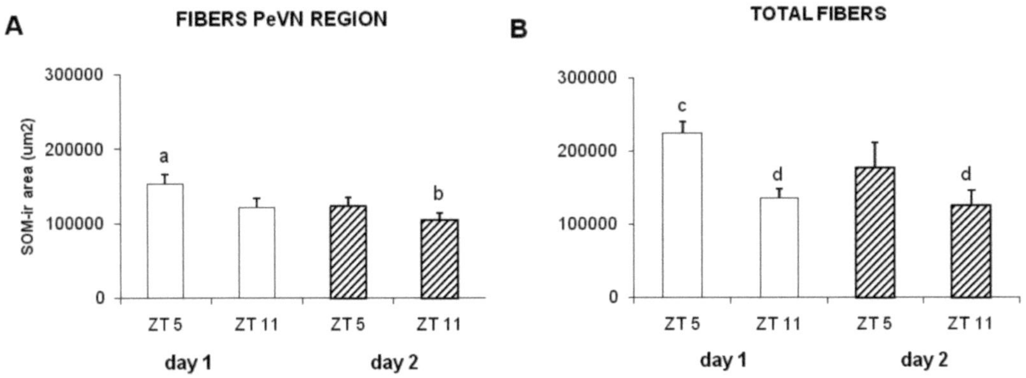

Fig. 3. Area of SOM-ir fibers in the PeVN region (A) or total SOM-ir area (B) in young (4.5 months old) OVX female Wistar rats at different time points after E_2 treatment. a significantly different from b ($p=0.047$; Bonferroni); c significantly different from d ($p \leq 0.05$; Tukey HSD). n=5 for each group.

4. Discussion

In the present study we showed that in adult female rats, the effects of E_2 on SOM-ir cell distribution and SOM-ir numbers in the PeVN were age dependent. Estrogen did not affect total numbers of SOM-ir cells in the PeVN of young female rats in line with our previous studies (Van Vugt et al, 2008) and those of others (Estupina et al, 1996). Other studies reported a decrease in SOM mRNA content in the PeVN following OVX which was reversed by E_2 treatment (Baldino et al, 1988; Zorilla et al, 1991). In these studies, however, animals were treated with E_2 for a prolonged period of time, whereas we studied the effect of a single physiological dose of E_2 on SOM peptide-containing cells on multiple time points following the estrogen exposure. Interestingly, the amount of SOM-ir fibers within the PeVN region of young females was decreased at 32 h compared to 2 h after E_2, which may suggest increased release of SOM peptide from the PeVN or decreased transport from cells to the fibers, apparently without affecting the amount of SOM peptide synthesized and/or stored in the PeVN cells. Prior to measuring SOM peptide responsiveness to an estrogen stimulus we showed that the attenuation of the LH surge at middle-age was not accompanied by a decrease in proestrus P levels or a decrease in pituitary LH responsiveness to a GnRH analog. These results clearly suggest that the attenuation of the LH surge is not initiated by alterations at the level of the ovary or pituitary gland, but rather the result of changes in response to ovarian feedback at the hypothalamic level as found for SOM peptide in this study. Subsequent experiments in the brain material obtained from these animals are now focusing on studying potential changes in hypothalamic estrogen and progesterone receptor immunoreactivity.

4.1 Reproductive aging and the pituitary gland

The attenuation of the natural LH surge at 8.5-months old is in accordance with previous reports concerning other rat strains (Brito et al, 1984; DePaolo et al, 1986; Krieg et al, 1995; Nass et al, 1984). Some studies suggested that the decrease in proestrus LH levels with age may follow changes at the level of the pituitary gland, such as changes in LH storage and/or release capacity (Matt et al, 1998; Wise et al, 1984). The results of the present study, however, suggest that this is not the case. Although the timing of GnRH analog administration was early (i.e. 3 to 4 hours before the natural LH surge occurred), no age-related differences in total and peak LH levels of the 'induced' LH surge (until ZT9) were observed. This implies that LH responsiveness to a bolus of GnRH is comparable between 4- and 8.5-month-old rats. Others did show that the acutely releasable pool of LH was reduced at the age of 9-12 months in cyclic Sprague-Dawley rats (Brann and Mahesh, 2005; Wise et al, 1984). In addition, pituitary responsiveness to GnRH in vitro is decreased in 10-12 month-old Long-Evans rats that show attenuated LH surges (Brito et al, 1994), and in pituitaries from 9- compared to 4-month-old Wistar rats that were tested in a superfusion system in our lab (Keizer et al, 2001). Since the age-related reduction in LH release after GnRH stimulation was more evident during the second and third stimulus in all studies, this suggests that the GnRH priming mechanism may be particularly affected.

Yet, we found no age-related differences in total LH levels of the 'late', 'endogenous' LH surge that results from endogenous GnRH release. Since the LH surge requires repeated pulses of GnRH to induce full pituitary priming, the absence of these age-related changes in this study suggest that GnRH priming is not significantly affected in our 8.5-month-old rats. The time between GnRH stimuli, however, differs between endogenous GnRH release (~1 hour between pulses) and our stimulus with the long-acting GnRH-analog Ovalyse® (~3 hours). Altogether, these results indicate that in our 8.5-month-old females, the attenuation of the LH surge is not caused by a diminished responsiveness of LH to initial GnRH signaling, although reproductive aging may eventually result in a decrease in the releasable pool of LH (Wise et al, 1984) and impaired GnRH priming (Brito et al,1994; Keizer et al, 2001).

4.2 Reproductive aging and the ovary

In the present study we showed that proestrous P levels were comparable between 4- and 8.5-month-old rats, and thus do not underlie the observed attenuation of the LH surge. In contrast, another study (Miller and Riegle, 1980) showed that the attenuated preovulatory LH surge was accompanied by an attenuated P surge in 12-month-old cyclic Long-Evans rats. It has been suggested that attenuated P levels result from a decrease in proestrous LH levels, although increased responsiveness of the ovary to hCG stimulation in regular cyclic middle-aged compared has been reported for Long-Evans rats (Chern et al, 2000). Consequently, the lack of concurrent changes in P and LH release in our rats could be explained by an increased responsiveness to LH stimulation.

4.3 Reproductive aging and the hypothalamus

Based on these data, we hypothesize that the initial attenuation of the LH surge is indeed initiated by alterations at the hypothalamic level (i.e. GnRH release), and not at the pituitary gland (i.e. responsiveness to GnRH, GnRH priming) or the ovary (P levels).

A previous study by Rubin (Rubin, 1992) showed that the secretory capacity of the GnRH system is still intact in middle-aged rats, but that the LH secretion per GnRH burst during the LH surge appears to decrease with age (Matt et al, 1998). This is thought to be the result of a decreased activity of the GnRH system, a reduced responsiveness to GnRH signaling, and/or a reduction in cellular LH with age (Matt et al, 1998; Rubin et al, 2000). Also, the GnRH neuroterminal-glial-capillary unit in the ME may be affected, influencing the regulation of GnRH release (Yin et al, 2009). There are no indications that the number of pituitary GnRH receptors is affected with age in female mice (Belisle et al, 1990) and our results after Ovalyse® administration suggest that the responsiveness to (robust) GnRH signaling is still intact. Indeed, several studies demonstrated that on proestrus the number of activated GnRH neurons (Wise et al, 2002; Rubin et al, 1994) and endogenous GnRH release (Rubin et al, 2000) are reduced in middle-aged female rats. The activity of GnRH neurons is regulated by many different neural signals (Smith and Jennes, 2001) and several of the systems involved in the regulation of the GnRH surge are also affected with age (Wise et al, 2002; Sahu et al, 1998; Gore et al, 2002; Mills et al, 2002). Taken together, this suggests that the input onto GnRH neurons may change with age, resulting in less activated GnRH neurons and reduced GnRH release that together with a reduction in endogenous GnRH priming could indeed lead to an attenuated LH surge. Previous studies have proposed a contribution of the suprachiasmatic nucleus (SCN) in the attenuation of the LH release surge (Wise et al, 2002; Downs and Wise 2009). Yet, we did not find any significant changes in timing of the LH surge (i.e. LH surge onset and/or peak levels) in middle-aged rats. Since a clear delay in timing of the LH surge at the age of 7-10 months has only been shown in Sprague-Dawley rats (Sahu et al, 1998; Wise, 1982), the age at which changes in SCN output influence the LH surge mechanism may be strain specific.

4.4 Effect of SOM on the reproductive axis

Previous studies provide evidence for a proposed central role of hypothalamic SOM neurons in the functional interaction between the somatotropic and gonadotropic axis. Octreotide, given during the "critical period" of the day (i.e. just prior to surge onset), completely abolished the E_2-induced LH surge and decreased GnRH cell activation (Van Vugt et al, 2004). Based on this, and the fact that SOM release may increase on proestrous afternoon (Estupina et al, 1983; Knuth et al, 1983; Zorilla et al, 1991), we hypothesize that in the cycling female rat, SOM release probably increases only after the "critical period", i.e. during the LH surge. Thus, we suggest that elevated levels of SOM on proestrous afternoon may be involved in the descending, rather than the ascending, phase of the preovulatory LH surge.

Our previous studies strongly suggest that SOM decreases LH release at least in part by decreasing hypothalamic GnRH neuron activation (Van Vugt et al 1994). However, the mechanism behind this action remains speculative. Moreover, indirect effects of SOM cannot be excluded, as SOM was demonstrated to directly affect gonadotropic cell number and morphology (Lovren et al. 1998). Here we propose three possible pathways via which SOM, originating from the PeVN, may affect GnRH neurons, resulting in a decreased LH release (see Figure 4).

The interactions between neurons in the hypothalamic areas involved in the regulation of LH (Preoptic Region, OVLT/POA) and GH (PeVN and Arcuate nucleus ARC) release are schematically depicted in Figure 4-I. GnRH neurons in the OVLT/POA are innervated by gamma-aminobutyric acid (GABA)-ergic cells, which are thought to be involved in the negative feedback of E_2 on the LH surge (Miller et al, 2003; Zhen et al, 1997). These GABA-ergic cells originating from the OVLT/POA innervate SOM neurons in the PeVN and may therefore also be involved in the regulation of GH release from the pituitary (Herbison et al, 1994; Murray et al, 1999; Rage et al, 1993; Willoughby et al, 1987). Also, within the PeVN, a small number of SOM neurons co-express GABA (Tanaka et al, 1997). GHRH neurons in the ARC are inhibited by SOM neurons originating from either the PeVN or the ARC (McCarty et al, 1992; Lanneau et al, 2000; Tannenbaum et al, 1990; Willoughby et al, 1989). Neuropeptide-Y (NPY) terminals originating from the ARC project to the preoptic region and ME, in which some of the axons make synaptic contacts with GnRH cell bodies and processes (Smith and Jennes, 2003). Also, NPY cells may project to SOM cells within the PeVN. NPY may hence be involved in the regulation of both LH and GH release from the pituitary.

4.4.1 Pathway 1: SOM projections to neurons in the OVLT/POA

We showed that a centrally injected SOM analog decreased hypothalamic GnRH cell activation (Van Vugt et al, 2004), suggesting that SOM directly affects cells in the OVLT/POA. The fact that SSTRs were demonstrated in the OVLT/POA (Helboe et al, 1998; Schindler et al, 1996), and that lesions of the anterior hypothalamic area (including the PeVN) resulted in decreased SOM peptide levels in the POA (Epelbaum et al, 1977), suggests that SOM cells originating from the PeVN project to the OVLT/POA. Possibly, GnRH neurons themselves express SSTRs, so SOM may directly inhibit GnRH cell activation, leading to the supposed decrease in GnRH release, and hence to decreased LH release from the pituitary (pathway A in Figure 4-II). Alternatively, cells, other than GnRH-producing, in the OVLT/POA may contain SSTRs. Neurons in the periventricular POA that project to GnRH neurons at the time of the preovulatory LH surge (Le et al, 1997; 1999; 2001) are a likely candidates. Although not identified yet, GABA-ergic cells may be (one of) these neurons containing SSTRs and projecting to the GnRH neurons (pathway B in Figure 4-II).

4.4.2 Pathway 2: SOM effects on LH release indirectly via NPY

NPY is very likely to influence the preovulatory LH surge: NPY synthesis and release are elevated just before the proestrous LH surge, and immunoneutralization of NPY prevents the steroid-induced LH surge. The effects of NPY on LH release may, at least in part, take place at the hypothalamic level, as NPY terminals synapse on GnRH cell bodies and processes (Smith and Jennes, 2003). As SSTRs were demonstrated on NPY cells in both the PeVN and ARC (Lanneau et al, 2000), SOM may inhibit NPY neurons activity, resulting in a decreased stimulating signal to GnRH cells, which in turn decreases GnRH cell activation and release, leading to the observed decreased LH surge (Figure 4-III).

4.4.3 Pathway 3: SOM effects pituitary LH release indirectly

Besides the decreased LH surge, we also found decreased plasma GH concentrations following the centrally injected SOM analog (Van Vugt et al, 2004). SOM was shown to directly decrease LH release (Yu et al, 1997) and affect gonadotroph cell number and morphology (Lovren et al, 1998). Moreover, both gonadotrophs and somatotrophs express SSTRs. Hence, SOM may directly decrease both LH and GH release from the pituitary. The decrease in GH release leads to decreased IGF-I release, which may subsequently result in a decreased GnRH release from the ME (Miller et al, 2003; Zhen et al, 1997) (pathway C in Figure 4-IV).

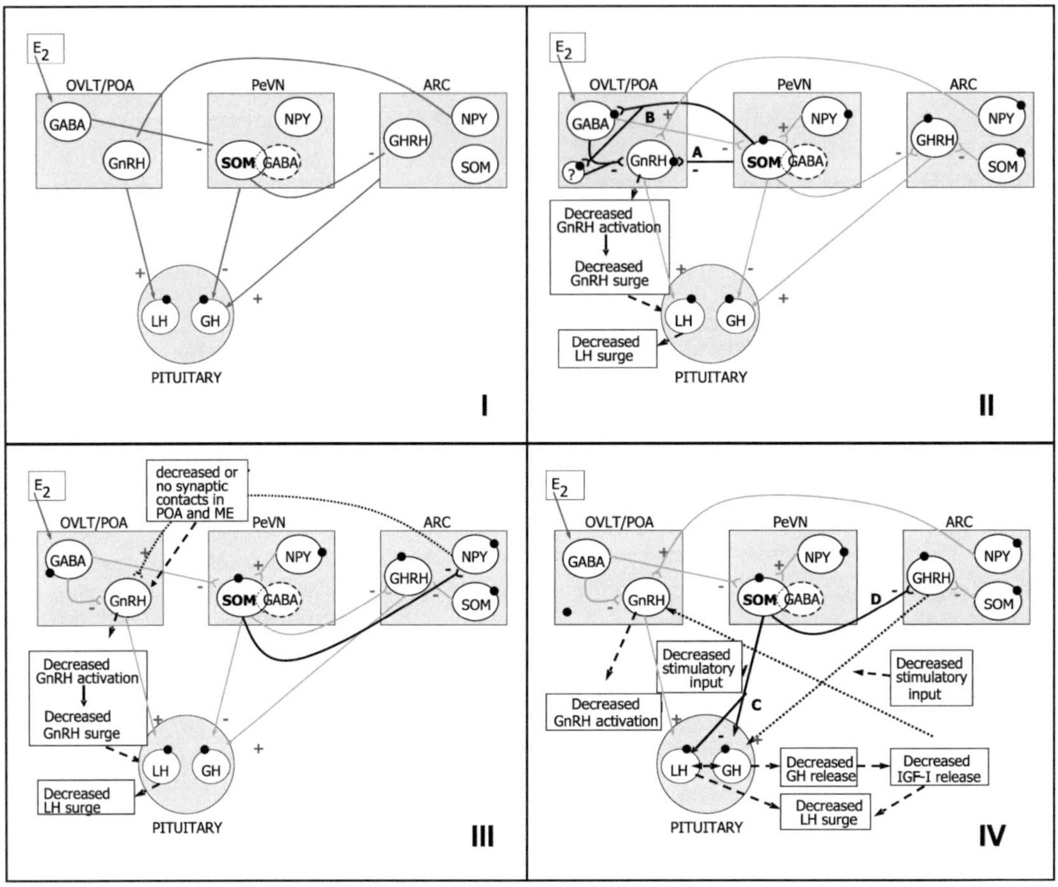

Fig. 4. Schematic drawings of the three proposed pathways via which SOM originating from the PeVN may decrease the LH surge. I: interactions between neurons in the OVLT/POA, PeVN and ARC as described in literature. II: direct effect of SOM on neurons in the OVLT/POA; A: directly on GnRH neurons; B: indirectly via cells projecting to GnRH neurons. III: indirect effect of SOM on GnRH neurons via NPY cells in the ARC. IV: indirect effect of SOM on GnRH neurons via the pituitary; C: direct effect of SOM on LH and GH cells; D: indirect effect of SOM on pituitary cells via GHRH neurons in the ARC. For more details: see text. Black circles represent SSTRs.

Alternatively, elevated SOM levels may inhibit GHRH neurons in the ARC (McCarty et al, 1992; Lanneau et al, 2000; Tannebaum et al, 1990; Willoughby et al, 1989), resulting in decreased GH release from the pituitary. As somatotroph and gonadotroph cell co-expression in the pituitary is maximal on the day of proestrus (Childs, 2000; Childs et al, 2000; 1994), a decreased activation of GH cells may lead to decreased activity of LH cells, consequently resulting in a decreased LH release. In addition, decreased IGF-I levels, due to decreased plasma GH concentrations, may lead to both decreased LH release from the pituitary (Kanematsu et al, 1991) and decreased GnRH release from the ME (Miller et al 2003; Zhen et al, 1997) (pathway D in Figure 4-IV).

Although direct effects of SOM at the pituitary level in the regulation of the LH surge (pathway 3) cannot be excluded, in the cycling female rat this pathway seems very unlikely to be the primary one with respect to hypothalamic regulation of the preovulatory LH surge. We suggest that the direct effects of SOM at the level of the pituitary may be additional to the effects at the level of the hypothalamus concerning the proposed interaction with the reproductive axis. Also, the suggested role for NPY in the hypothalamic regulation of the LH surge in the female rat (pathway 2) is probably one of the factors in a complex regulatory mechanism. In the light of our own data and data from literature, we propose that the role of SOM in the regulation of the descending phase of the LH surge, may involve, at least, a combination of pathways 1 and 2. In the cycling female rat, elevated plasma concentrations of E_2 and P on the day of proestrus may increase NPY levels in the ARC that, together with the removed inhibitory GABA-ergic tone (Smith and Jennes, 2003), stimulate GnRH cell activation, leading to the GnRH surge and, subsequently, the preovulatory LH surge. Secondly, the increased levels of gonadal steroids (Estupina et al, 1996, Van Vugt et al, 2008), and in addition, elevated levels of NPY (Rettori et al, 1990) may increase SOM release from the ME. Elevated concentrations of SOM, in turn, inhibit either neuron activity in the OVLT/POA, or NPY and its stimulating effects on GnRH neurons, or both, leading to decreased GnRH cell activation and subsequently release, finally resulting in a decrease in plasma LH levels (see figure 2).

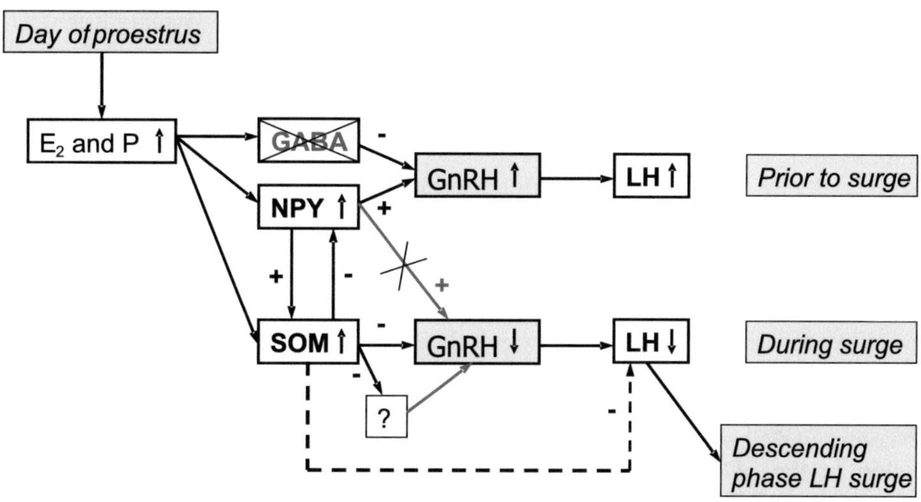

Fig. 5. Proposed mechanism via which hypothalamic SOM may be involved in the regulation of the descending phase of the preovulatory LH surge in the female rat

4.5 Age dependent effects of estrogen on PeVN SOM peptide

In young rats, the rostrocaudal distribution profiles of SOM-ir cells within the PeVN were comparable between ZT5 as well as ZT11 on the two subsequent days after E_2 treatment. In addition, the total SOM-ir fiber area, was consistently higher at ZT5 compared to ZT11 in these animals. These findings suggest that SOM peptide synthesized in the PeVN and released in the ME may be influenced by diurnal rhythms. Our data are supported by a study that reported a diurnal rhythm in SOM peptide content in the ME (Esquifino et al, 2004). Moreover, SOM peptide levels in the cortex, anterior hypothalamus and suprachiasmatic nucleus (SCN) (Fukuhara et al, 1993), and SOM release from the hypothalamus (Berelowitz et al, 1982) were demonstrated to show circadian rhythmicity and suggest that the SCN may play a role in this diurnal change in SOM peptide transport from the PeVN to the ME. Thus, our data suggest that in the young female Wistar rat SOM cells in the PeVN are influenced by at least the SCN and E_2. E_2 may affect intrahypothalamic SOM projections within the PeVN or to other hypothalamic areas that contain SOM receptors (Beaudet et al, 1995; Hervieu et al, 1999), whereas SOM release from the ME may be influenced by the SCN. SOM content and release from hypothalamic explants is influenced by sex and age (Ge et al, 1989). The rostro-caudal distribution pattern of SOM-ir cells and the total number of SOM-ir cells in the PeVN was different in the middle-aged compared to young rats, but only 2 h after E_2 treatment. These findings suggest that with age, E_2 may become more crucial for the synthesis and/or storage of SOM peptide in the PeVN and affect the diurnal change in SOM levels within the PeVN.

The function of a diurnal change in SOM levels in the PeVN remains speculative. A few studies reported more pronounced GH secretory bursts in cycling female rats after the onset of darkness (Clark et al, 1987; Pincus et al, 1996), suggesting that the shift in the rostro-caudal SOM cell distribution at ZT11, i.e. just before dark onset, may reflect this shift in GH secretion pattern. Although to our knowledge no data exist on light/dark-related GH secretory patterns during aging, mean plasma GH levels and mean peak GH levels were found to be decreased already in 11 month old compared to young females (Takahashi et al, 1987). Taking these findings into consideration, we suggest that the changes in SOM-ir levels within the PeVN may translate into changes in GH release patterns during aging in female rats.

5. Conclusion

In the present study we clearly demonstrate a significant attenuation of the LH surge at the age of 8.5 compared to 4 months old regular 4-day cycling females. This attenuation of the LH surge was not accompanied by changes in the releasable pool of LH, timing of the surge, GnRH priming or preovulatory P levels, supporting the notion that an attenuation of the LH surge may result from a change in the hypothalamic drive. Strikingly, we found clear changes in hypothalamic SOM peptide regulation following a physiological dose of estrogen in middle-aged animals. We hypothesize that the age dependent effects of an E_2 stimulus on SOM-ir cell distribution and SOM-ir numbers indicate alterations in the regulation of hypothalamic SOM peptide release in response to estrogen feedback could underlie an attenuation of the LH surge with age. These observations suggest that changes in the regulation of the GH axis with age indeed coincide with the process of reproductive aging in the female rat and suggest that the proposed interaction between these neuroendocrine axes may occur via alterations in hypothalamic somatostatin release.

6. Acknowledgements

The authors would like to thank Hans J.M. Swarts (Dept Animal Sciences, Wageningen University) for expert technical assistance and Prof Victor M. Wiegant (Dept Pharmacology, Med Fac, Utrecht University Medical Centre) for critically reviewing earlier versions of the manuscript. Current affiliations of the authors are: Danone Research, Centre for Specialised Nutrition, Singapore (EMvdB) and Wageningen, the Netherlands (BJMvdH); Notox B.V., Den Bosch, The Netherlands (HHvV) and Dept. Anatomy, Radboud University Nijmegen Medical Centre, the Netherlands (ANS-F).

7. References

Baldino F, Jr., Fitzpatrick-McElligott S, O'Kane TM, Gozes I. Hormonal regulation of somatostatin messenger RNA. Synapse 1988; 2: 317-325.

Bartke A. Role of growth hormone and prolactin in the control of reproduction: what are we learning from transgenic and knock-out animals? Steroids 1999; 64: 598-604.

Bartke A, Chandrashekar V, Bailey B, Zaczek D, Turyn D. Consequences of growth hormone (GH) overexpression and GH resistance. Neuropeptides 2002; 36: 201-208.

Bartke A, Chandrashekar V, Turyn D, Steger RW, Debeljuk L, Winters TA, Mattison JA, Danilovich NA, Croson W, Wernsing DR, Kopchick JJ. Effects of growth hormone overexpression and growth hormone resistance on neuroendocrine and reproductive functions in transgenic and knock-out mice. Proc.Soc.Exp.Biol.Med. 1999; 222: 113-123.

Beaudet A, Greenspun D, Raelson J, Tannenbaum GS. Patterns of expression of SSTR1 and SSTR2 somatostatin receptor subtypes in the hypothalamus of the adult rat: relationship to neuroendocrine function. Neuroscience 1995; 65: 551-561.

Belisle S, Bellabarba D, Lehoux JG. Hypothalamic-pituitary axis during reproductive aging in mice. Mech Ageing Dev 1990; 52:207-217.

Berelowitz M, Dudlak D, Frohman LA. Diurnal variation in release of somatostatin-like immunoreactivity from incubated, rat hypothalamus and cerebral cortex. Endocrinology 1982; 110: 2195-2197.

Brann DW, Mahesh VB. The aging reproductive neuroendocrine axis. Steroids 2005; 70:273-283

Brito AN, Sayles TE, Krieg RJ, Matt DW. Relation of attenuated proestrous luteinizing hormone surges in middle-aged female rats to in vitro pituitary gonadotropin-releasing hormone responsiveness. Eur J Endocrinol 1994; 130:540-544.

Buijs RM, Pool CW, Van Heerikhuize JJ, Sluiter AA, Van der Sluis PJ, Ramkema M, Van der Woude TP, Van der Beek E. Antibodies to small transmitter molecules and peptides: production and application of antibodies to dopamine, seretonin, GABA, vasopressin, vasoactive intestinal peptide, neuropeptide Y, somatostatin and substance P. Biomedical Research 1989; 10: 213-221.

Chandrashekar V, Bartke A. Effects of age and endogenously secreted human growth hormone on the regulation of gonadotropin secretion in female and male transgenic mice expressing the human growth hormone gene. Endocrinology 1993; 132: 1482-1488.

Chern BY, Chen YH, Hong LS, LaPolt PS. Ovarian steroidogenic responsiveness to exogenous gonadotropin stimulation in young and middle aged female rats. Proc Soc Exp Biol Med 2000; 224:285 291.

Childs GV, Unabia G, Wu P. Differential expression of growth hormone messenger ribonucleic acid by somatotropes and gonadotropes in male and cycling female rats. Endocrinology 2000; 141: 1560-1570.

Childs GV. Growth hormone cells as co-gonadotropes: partners in the regulation of the reproductive system. Trends.Endocrinol.Metab. 2000; 11: 168-175.

Childs GV, Unabia G, Rougeau D. Cells that express luteinizing hormone (LH) and follicle-stimulating hormone (FSH) beta-subunit messenger ribonucleic acids during the estrous cycle: the major contributors contain LH beta, FSH beta, and/or growth hormone. Endocrinology 1994; 134: 990-997.

Clark RG, Carlsson LM, Robinson IC. Growth hormone secretory profiles in conscious female rats. J.Endocrinol. 1987; 114: 399-407.

DePaolo LV, Chappel SC. Alterations in the secretion and production of follicle-stimulating hormone precede age-related lengthening of estrous cycles in rats. Endocrinology 1986; 118(3):1127-1133.

Downs JL, Wise PM. The role of the brain in female reproductive aging. Mol. Cell Enodcrinol. 2009; 299:32-38

Eden S. Age- and sex-related differences in episodic growth hormone secretion in the rat. Endocrinology 1979; 105: 555-560.

Epelbaum J, Willoughby JO, Brazeau P, Martin JB. Effects of brain lesions and hypothalamic deafferentation on somatostatin distribution in the rat brain. Endocrinology 1977; 101: 1495-1502.

Esquifino AI, Cano P, Jimenez V, Reyes Toso CF, Cardinali DP. Changes of prolactin regulatory mechanisms in aging: 24-h rhythms of serum prolactin and median eminence and adenohypophysial concentration of dopamine, serotonin, (gamma-aminobutyric acid, taurine and somatostatin in young and aged rats. Exp Gerontol 2004; 39: 45-52.

Estupina C, Pinter A, Belmar J, Astier H, Arancibia S. Variations in hypothalamic somatostatin release and content during the estrous cycle in the rat. Effects of ovariectomy and estrogen supplementation. Neuroendocrinology. 1996; 63: 181-187.

Freeman ME. (1994) The neuroendocrine control of the ovarian cycle of the rat. In: Knobil E, Neill JD, (eds) The physiology of reproduction. Raven Press, Ltd. New York, 2nd(46): 613-658

Fukuhara C, Shinohara K, Tominaga K, Otori Y, Inouye ST. Endogenous circadian rhythmicity of somatostatin like- immunoreactivity in the rat suprachiasmatic nucleus. Brain Res. 1993; 606: 28-35.

Gatford KL, Egan AR, Clarke IJ, Owens PC. Sexual dimorphism of the somatotrophic axis. J.Endocrinol. 1998; 157: 373-389.

Ge F, Tsagarakis S, Rees LH, Besser GM, Grossman A. Relationship between growth hormone-releasing hormone and somatostatin in the rat: effects of age and sex on content and in- vitro release from hypothalamic explants. J.Endocrinol. 1989; 123: 53-58.

Gillies G. Somatostatin: the neuroendocrine story. Trends.Pharmacol.Sci. 1997; 18: 87-95.

Gore AC, Oung T, Woller MJ. Age related changes in hypothalamic gonadotropin releasing hormone and N methyl D aspartate receptor gene expression, and their regulation by oestrogen, in the female rat. J Neuroendocrinol 2002; 14:300 309.

Helboe L, Stidsen CE, Moller M. Immunohistochemical and cytochemical localization of the somatostatin receptor subtype sst1 in the somatostatinergic parvocellular neuronal system of the rat hypothalamus. J.Neurosci. 1998; 18: 4938-4945.

Herbison AE, Augood SJ. Expression of GABAA receptor alpha 2 sub-unit mRNA by periventricular somatostatin neurones in the rat hypothalamus. Neurosci.Lett. 1994; 173: 9-13.

Hervieu G, Emson PC. Visualisation of somatostatin receptor sst(3) in the rat central nervous system. Brain Res.Mol.Brain Res. 1999; 71: 290-303.

Hurley DL, Phelps CJ. Hypothalamic preprosomatostatin messenger ribonucleic acid expression in mice transgenic for excess or deficient endogenous growth hormone. Endocrinology 1992; 130: 1809-1815.

Kanematsu T, Irahara M, Miyake T, Shitsukawa K, Aono T. Effect of insulin-like growth factor I on gonadotropin release from the hypothalamus-pituitary axis in vitro. Acta.Endocrinol. 1991; 125: 227-233.

Keizer KJ, Heijning BLM, Swarts JJM, van der Beek EM. Effect of cycle stage and age on gonadotropin releasing hormone (GnRH) induced luteinzing hormone (LH) release ex vivo. In: Program of the 31th annual meeting of the Society for Neuroscience; 2001; San Diego, LA. Abstract 731.14.

Knuth UA, Sikand GS, Casanueva FF, Friesen HG. Changes in somatostatin-like activity in discrete areas of the rat hypothalamus during different stages of proestrus and diestrus and their relation to serum gonadotropin, prolactin, and growth hormone levels. Endocrinology 1983; 112: 1506-1511.

Krieg RJ Jr, Brito AN, Sayles TE, Matt DW. Luteinizing hormone secretion by dispersed anterior pituitary gland cells from middle aged rats. Neuroendocrinology 1995; 61:318 325.

Lanneau C, Peineau S, Petit F, Epelbaum J, Gardette R. Somatostatin modulation of excitatory synaptic transmission between periventricular and arcuate hypothalamic nuclei in vitro. J.Neurophysiol. 2000; 84: 1464-1474.

Le WW, Attardi B, Berghorn KA, Blaustein J, Hoffman GE. Progesterone blockade of a luteinizing hormone surge blocks luteinizing hormone-releasing hormone Fos activation and activation of its preoptic area afferents. Brain Res 1997; 778: 272-280.

Le WW, Berghorn KA, Rassnick S, Hoffman GE. Periventricular preoptic area neurons coactivated with luteinizing hormone (LH)-releasing hormone (LHRH) neurons at the time of the LH surge are LHRH afferents. Endocrinology 1999; 140: 510-519.

Le WW, Wise PM, Murphy AZ, Coolen LM, Hoffman GE. Parallel declines in Fos activation of the medial anteroventral periventricular nucleus and LHRH neurons in middle-aged rats. Endocrinology 2001; 142: 4976-4982.

Lovren M, Sekulic M, Milosevic V, Radulovic N. Effects of somatostatins on gonadotrophic cells in female rats. Acta.Histochem. 1998; 100: 329-335.

Lu JK, Gilman DP, Meldrum DR, Judd HL, Sawyer CH. Relationship between circulating estrogens and the central mechanisms by which ovarian steroids stimulate luteinizing hormone secretion in aged and young female rats. Endocrinology 1981; 108: 836-841.

Lu JKH, LaPolt PS, Nass TE, Matt DW, Judd HL. Relation of circulating estradiol and progesterone to gonadotropin secretion and estrous cyclicity in aging female rats. Endocrinology 1985; 116(5):1953-1959.

Matt DW, Gilson MP, Sales TE, Krieg RJ, Kerbeshian MC, Veldhuis JD, Evans WS. Characterization of attenuated proestrous luteinizing hormone surges in middle-aged rats by deconvolution analysis. Biol Reprod 1998; 59:1477-1482.

McCarthy GF, Beaudet A, Tannenbaum GS. Colocalization of somatostatin receptors and growth hormone- releasing factor immunoreactivity in neurons of the rat arcuate nucleus. Neuroendocrinology. 1992; 56: 18-24.

Meredith S, Butcher RL. Role of decreased numbers of follicles on reproductive performance in young and aged rats. Biol Reprod 1985; 32: 788-94.

Miller BH, Gore AC. Alterations in hypothalamic insulin-like growth factor-I and its associations with gonadotropin releasing hormone neurones during reproductive development and ageing. J.Neuroendocrinol. 2003; 13: 728-736.

Miller AE, Riegle GD. Temporal changes in serum progesterone in aging female rats. Endocrinology 1980; 106:1579-1583.

Mills RH, Romeo HE, Lu JKH, Micevych PE. Site specific decrease of progesterone receptor mRNA expression in the hypothalamus of middle aged persistently estrus rats. Brain Res 2002; 955:200 206.

Muller EE, Locatelli V, Cocchi D. Neuroendocrine control of growth hormone secretion. Physiol.Rev. 1999; 79: 511-607.

Murray HE, Simonian SX, Herbison AE, Gillies GE. Correlation of hypothalamic somatostatin mRNA expression and peptide content with secretion: sexual dimorphism and differential regulation by gonadal factors. J.Neuroendocrinol. 1999; 11: 27-33.

Naar EM, Bartke A, Majumdar SS, Buonomo FC, Yun JS, Wagner TE. Fertility of transgenic female mice expressing bovine growth hormone or human growth hormone variant genes. Biol.Reprod. 1991; 45: 178-187.

Nass TE, LaPolt PS, Judd HL, Lu JK. Alterations in ovarian steroid and gonadotrophin secretion preceding the cessation of regular oestrous cycles in ageing female rats. J Endocrinol 1984; 100:43 50.

Nestorovic N, Lovren M, Sekulic M, Sosic-Jurjevic B, Negic N, Milosevic V. Effects of centrally applied octreotide on pituitary gonadotrophic cells in rat females. ENEA 2002 2002: PB-335.

Nestorovic N, Lovren M, Sekulic M, Filipovic B, Milosevic V. Effects of multiple somatostatin treatment on rat gonadotrophic cells and ovaries. Histochem.J. 2003; 33: 695-702.

Pincus SM, Gevers EF, Robinson IC, van den Berg G, Roelfsema F, Hartman ML, Veldhuis JD. Females secrete growth hormone with more process irregularity than males in both humans and rats. Am J Physiol 1996; 270: E107-E115.

Rage F, Jalaguier S, Rougeot C, Tapia-Arancibia L. GABA inhibition of somatostatin gene expression in cultured hypothalamic neurones. Neuroreport. 1993; 4: 320-322.

Rettori V, Milenkovic L, Aguila MC, McCann SM. Physiologically significant effect of neuropeptide Y to suppress growth hormone release by stimulating somatostatin discharge. Endocrinology 1990; 126: 2296-2301.

Rodriguez P, Fernandez-Galaz C, Tejero A. Controlled neonatal exposure to estrogens: a suitable tool for reproductive aging studies in the female rat. Biol Reprod 1993; 49: 387-392.

Rubin BS. Isolated hypothalami from aging female rats do not exhibit reduced basal or potassium stimulated secretion of luteinizing hormone releasing hormone. Biol Reprod 1992; 47:254 261.

Rubin BS. Hypothalamic alterations and reproductive aging in female rats: evidence of altered luteinizing hormone-releasing hormone neuronal function. Biol Reprod 2000; 63:968-976

Rubin BS, Lee CE, King JC. Reduced proportion of luteinizing hormone (LH) releasing hormone neurons express Fos protein during the preovulatory or steroid induced LH surge in middle aged rats. Biol Reprod 1994; 51:1264 1272.

Sahu A., Kalra SP. Absence of increased neuropeptide Y neuronal activity before and during the luteinizing hormone (LH) surge may underlie the attenuated preovulatory LH surge in middle aged rats. Endocrinology 1998; 139:696 702.

Sasaki F, Tojo H, Iwama Y, Miki N, Maeda K, Ono M, Kiso Y, Okada T, Matsumoto Y, Tachi C. Growth hormone-releasing hormone (GHRH)-GH-somatic growth and luteinizing hormone (LH)RH-LH-ovarian axes in adult female transgenic mice expressing human GH gene. J.Neuroendocrinol. 1997; 9: 615-626.

Schindler M, Humphrey PP, Emson PC. Somatostatin receptors in the central nervous system. Prog Neurobiol. 1996 Sep;50(1):9-47

Smith MJ, Jennes L. Neural signals that regulate GnRH neurones directly during the oestrous cycle. Reproduction 2003; 122:1 10.

Steffens AB. A method for frequent sampling of blood and continuous infusion of fluids in the rat without disturbing the animal. Physiol Behav 1969; 4:833 836.

Takahashi S, Gottschall PE, Quigley KL, Goya RG, Meites J. Growth hormone secretory patterns in young, middle-aged and old female rats. Neuroendocrinology. 1987; 46: 137-142.

Tanaka M, Matsuda T, Shigeyoshi Y, Ibata Y, Okamura H. Peptide expression in GABAergic neurons in rat suprachiasmatic nucleus in comparison with other forebrain structures: a double labeling in situ hybridization study. J.Histochem.Cytochem. 1997; 45: 1231-1237

Tannenbaum GS, McCarthy GF, Zeitler P, Beaudet A. Cysteamine-induced enhancement of growth hormone-releasing factor (GRF) immunoreactivity in arcuate neurons: morphological evidence for putative somatostatin/GRF interactions within hypothalamus. Endocrinology 1990; 127: 2551-2560.

Terry LC, Martin JB. The effects of lateral hypothalamic-medial forebrain stimulation and somatostatin antiserum on pulsatile growth hormone secretion in freely behaving rats: evidence for a dual regulatory mechanism. Endocrinology 1981; 109: 622-627.

Te Velde ER, Scheffer GJ, Dorland M, Broekmans FJ, Fauser BC. Developmental and endocrine aspects of normal ovarian aging. Mol Cell Endocrinol 1998; 145:67 73.

Van der Beek EM, Swarts JJM, Wiegant VM. Central administration of antiserum to vasoactive intestinal peptide delays and reduces luteinizing hormone and prolactin surges in ovariectomized, estrogen treated rats. Neuroendocrinology 1999; 69:227 237.

Van der Beek EM, van Oudheusden HJ, Buijs RM, van der Donk HA, van den Hurk R, Wiegant VM. Preferential induction of c-fos immunoreactivity in vasoactive intestinal polypeptide-innervated gonadotropin-releasing hormone neurons during a steroid-induced luteinizing hormone surge in the female rat. Endocrinology 1994; 134: 2636-2644.

Van der Meulen J, Helmond FA, Oudenaarden CPJ. Effect of flushing of blastocysts on days 10-13 on the lifespan of the corpora lutea in the pig. J Reprod Fert 1988; 84:157-162.

Van Vugt HH, Swarts HJM, Van de Heijning BJM, Van der Beek EM. Centrally applied somatostatin inhibits the estrogen-induced luteinizing hormone surge via hypothalamic gonadotropin-releasing hormone cell activation in female rats. Biol. Reprod. 2004; 71: 813-819.

Van Vugt HH, Van de Heijning BJM, Van der Beek EM. Somatostatin in the rat periventicular nucleau: sex differences and effects of gonadal steroids. Exp. Brain Res. 2008; 188: 483-491

Vom Saal FS, Finch CE, Nelson JF. Natural history and mechanisms of reproductive aging in humans, laboratory rodents, and other selected vertebrates. In: Knobil E, Neill JD (eds.), The Physiology of Reproduction, vol. 2, 2nd ed. New York: Raven Press; 1994: 1213-1314.

Werner H, Koch Y, Baldino F, Jr., Gozes I. Steroid regulation of somatostatin mRNA in the rat hypothalamus. J.Biol.Chem. 1988; 263: 7666-7671.

Willoughby JO, Beroukas D, Blessing WW. Ultrastructural evidence for gamma aminobutyric acid- immunoreactive synapses on somatostatin-immunoreactive perikarya in the periventricular anterior hypothalamus. Neuroendocrinology. 1987; 46: 268-272.

Willoughby JO, Brogan M, Kapoor R. Intrahypothalamic actions of somatostatin and growth hormone releasing factor on growth hormone secretion. Neuroendocrinology. 1989; 50: 592-596.

Wilshire GB, Loughlin JS, Brown JR, Adel TE, Santoro N. Diminished function of the somatotropic axis in older reproductive-aged women. J.Clin.Endocrinol.Metab. 1995; 80: 608-613.

Wise PM. Alterations in the proestrous pattern of median eminence LHRH, serum LH, FSH, estradiol and progesterone concentrations in middle-aged rats. Life Sciences 1982; 31:165-173.

Wise PM. Estradiol induced daily luteinizing hormone and prolactin surges in young and middle aged rats: correlations with age related changes in pituitary responsiveness and catecholamine turnover rates in microdissected brain areas. Endocrinology 1984; 115:801 809.

Wise PM, Smith MJ, Dubal DB, Wilson ME, Rau SW, Cashion AB, Böttner M, Rosewell KL. Neuroendocrine modulation and repercussions of female reproductive aging. Rec Prog Horm Res 2002; 235-256.

Yin W, Wu D, Noel ML, Gore AC. Gonadotropin-Releasing Hormone neuroterminals and their microenvironment in the median eminence: effects of aging and estradiol treatment. Endocrinology, 2009; 150: 5498-5508

Yu WH, Kimura M, McCann SM. Effect of somatostatin on the release of gonadotropins in male rats. Proc.Soc.Exp.Biol.Med. 1997; 214: 83-86.

Zeitler P, Tannenbaum GS, Clifton DK, Steiner RA. Ultradian oscillations in somatostatin and growth hormone- releasing hormone mRNAs in the brains of adult male rats. Proc.Natl.Acad.Sci.U.S.A. 1991; 88: 8920-8924.

Zhen S, Zakaria M, Wolfe A, Radovick S. Regulation of gonadotropin-releasing hormone (GnRH) gene expression by insulin-like growth factor I in a cultured GnRH-expressing neuronal cell line. Mol.Endocrinol. 1997; 11: 1145-1155.

Zorilla R, Simard J, Labrie F, Pelletier G. Variations of Pre-prosomatostatin mRNA Levels in the Hypothalamic periventricular Nucleus during the Rat Estrous Cycle. Mol.and Cel.Neurosciences 1991; 2: 294-298.

Zorrilla R, Simard J, Rheaume E, Labrie F, Pelletier G. Multihormonal control of pre-pro-somatostatin mRNA levels in the periventricular nucleus of the male and female rat hypothalamus. Neuroendocrinology. 1990; 52: 527-536.

5

Telocytes in Human Fallopian Tube and Uterus Express Estrogen and Progesterone Receptors

Sanda M. Cretoiu[1,2], Dragos Cretoiu[1,2],
Anca Simionescu[3] and Laurentiu M. Popescu[1,2]
[1]*Carol Davila University of Medicine and Pharmacy*
[2]*Victor Babes National Institute of Pathology*
[3]*Filantropia Hospital*
Romania

1. Introduction

Evidence has accumulated over a number of years for the existence of a new cell type found in cavitary and parenchimatous organs - called telocytes (TCs). The cell biology of TCs, and especially their function is a rapidly growing area of biomedical research (Figure 1) (free-access data is available at www.telocytes.com). TCs are also present in fallopian tube (Popescu et al., 2005a) and uterine walls (Ciontea et al., 2005).
Progress in cellular and molecular techniques led to the identification of subtypes and isoforms of estrogen receptors (ER) (Green et al., 1986; Kuiper et al., 1996; Tremblay et al., 1997) and progesterone receptors (PR) (Kastner et al., 1990; Giangrande & McDonnell, 1999) in the female reproductive tract, two for each receptor (ERα and β, and PR A and B). Cells of the female reproductive tract are subject to hormonal control via sex steroids receptors. Subsequently, we investigated the expression of estrogen receptor (ER) and progesterone receptor (PR) in cell cultures enriched in TCs, obtained from the muscle coat of both the fallopian tube and uterus.

2. The concept of telocytes

In 2005, we described a new cell type which we called interstitial Cajal-like cells (ICLC) due to their similarity with canonical gastrointestinal interstitial cells of Cajal (ICC). By using electron microscopy, immunohistochemstry and cell cultures, we revealed that ICLC have particular features that distinguish and separate them from the ICC and/or other interstitial cells. Given these new findings, Popescu renamed ICLC to TELOCYTES (TCs) (Popescu & Faussone-Pellegrini, 2010) by using the Greek affix 'telos', meaning "goal", "end", and "fulfilment", suggesting cells with a particular goal, accomplished through their extremely long prolongations. The new term aims to avoid any confusion between these cells and other interstititial cells such as fibroblasts, mesenchymal cells, and myofibroblasts. The very long and thin prolongations emitted by TCs were re-defined as telopodes (TPs). TPs are built of alternating thin segments known as podomers (≤ 200 nm, below the resolving power of light microscope) and dilated segments called podoms (with a mean width of 462.31 nm), which accommodate mitochondria, rough endoplasmic reticulum and caveolae.

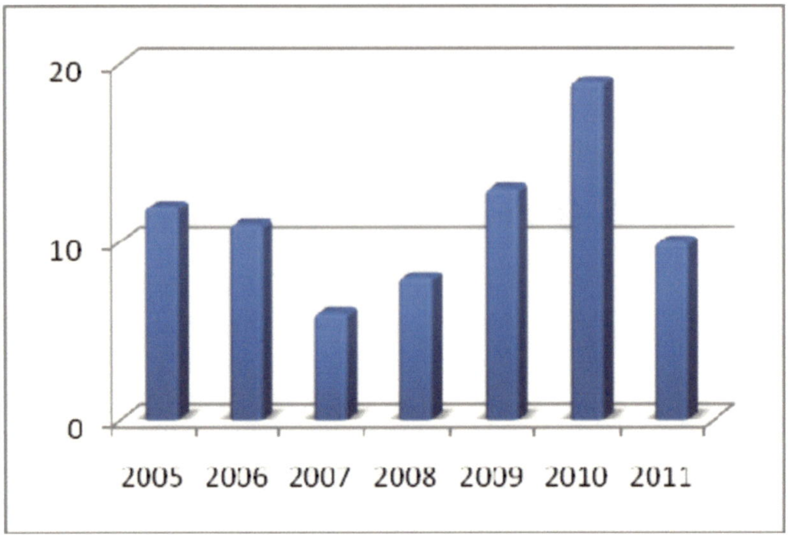

Fig. 1. Graph showing the ascending trend of the number of articles retrieved from www.pubmed.gov using key words "telocytes", "interstitial Cajal-like cell", or "ICC-like". The number of published papers is increasing exponentially.

TPs are a distinctive feature of TCs and are characterized by the following main features:

- **Number**: can vary between 1 and 5. Frequently, only 2–3 telopodes are observed on a single section, depending on site and angle of section (Figure 2, 3), since their 3D convolutions prevent them from being observed at their full length in a very thin 2D section (Figure 4);

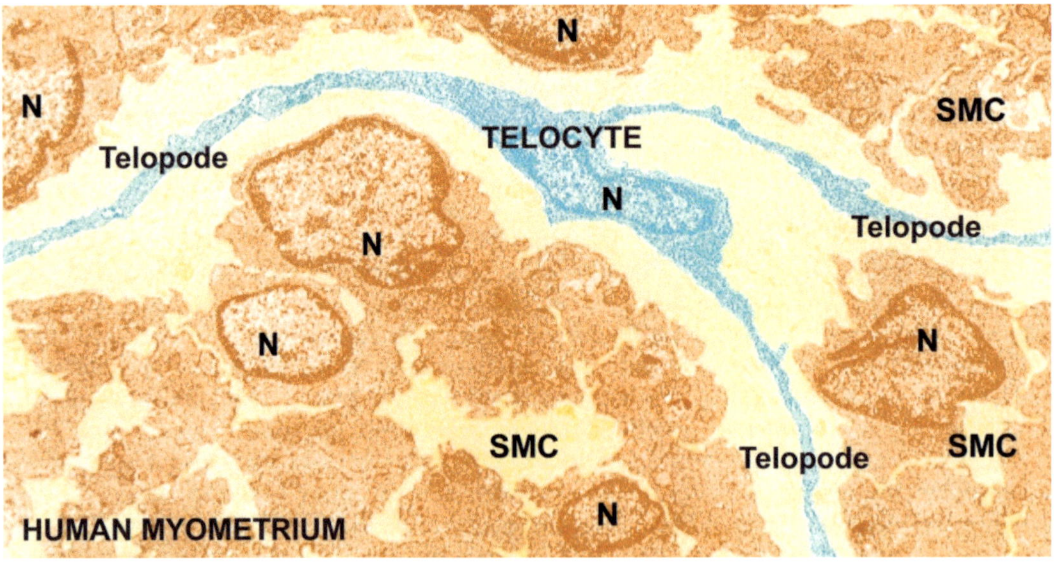

Fig. 2. Non-pregnant myometrium. Digitally coloured TC (blue) with 3 TPs that encircle bundles of cross-cut smooth muscle cells (SMC, Sienna brown); N - nuclei. Reproduced, with permission, from Ciontea et al., 2005.

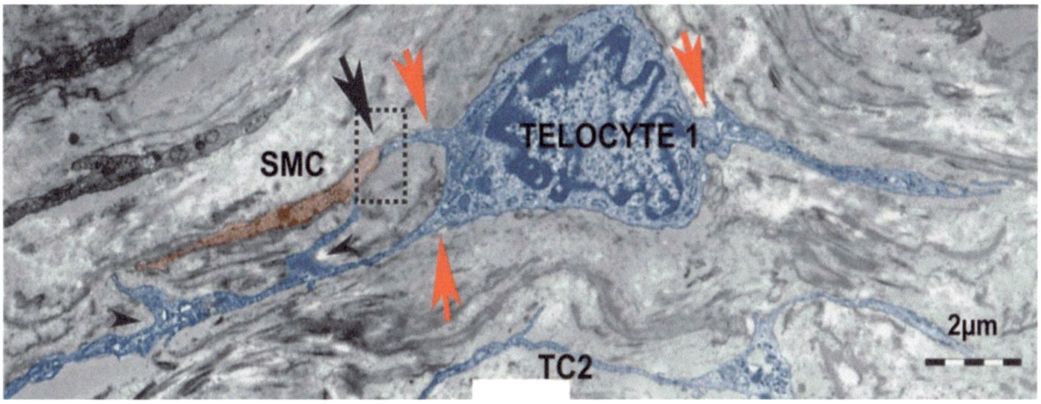

Fig. 3. Human term placenta. Telocyte 1 (blue) has few organelles in the perinuclear area and three emerging TPs (red arrows); black arrowheads mark the dichotomic branching points. Note the podoms and podomeres. The black arrow indicates the junction between TPs and a smooth muscle cell (SMC, coloured in brown). Reproduced, with permission, from Suciu et al., 2010.

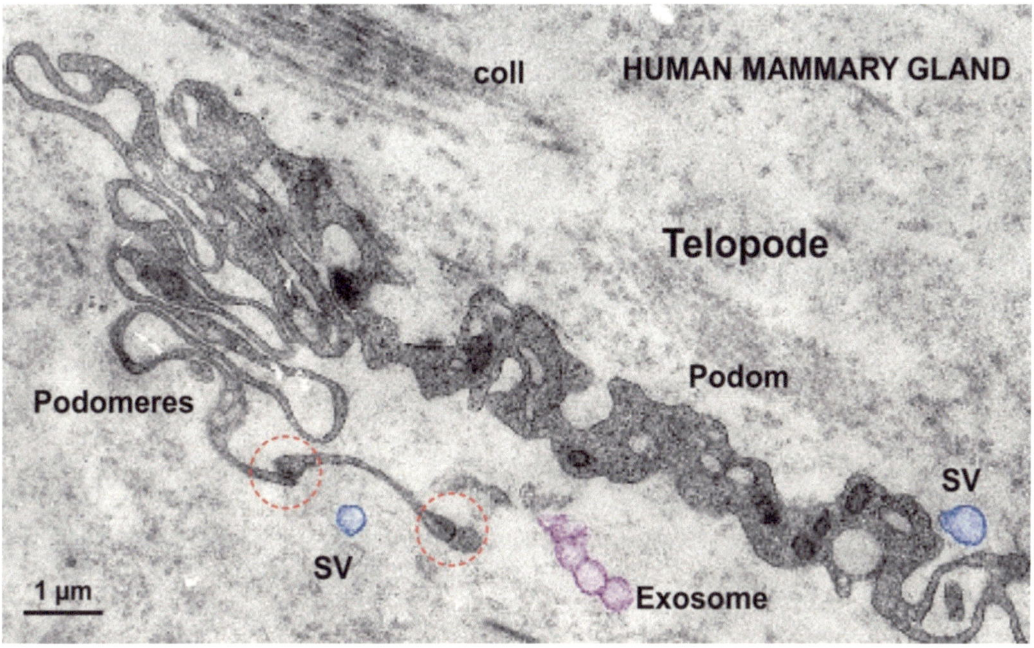

Fig. 4. Human resting mammary gland stroma. One TC hallmark, namely TPs, appears quite long and convoluted. Note homocellular junctions marked by red circles, as well as shed vesicles (blue) and an exosome (violet). Reproduced, with permission, from Gherghiceanu & Popescu, 2005.

- **Length**: tens to hundreds of µm, as measured on EM images (Figure 5). However, under favorable cell culture conditions, their entire length can be captured in several successive images (Figure 6);

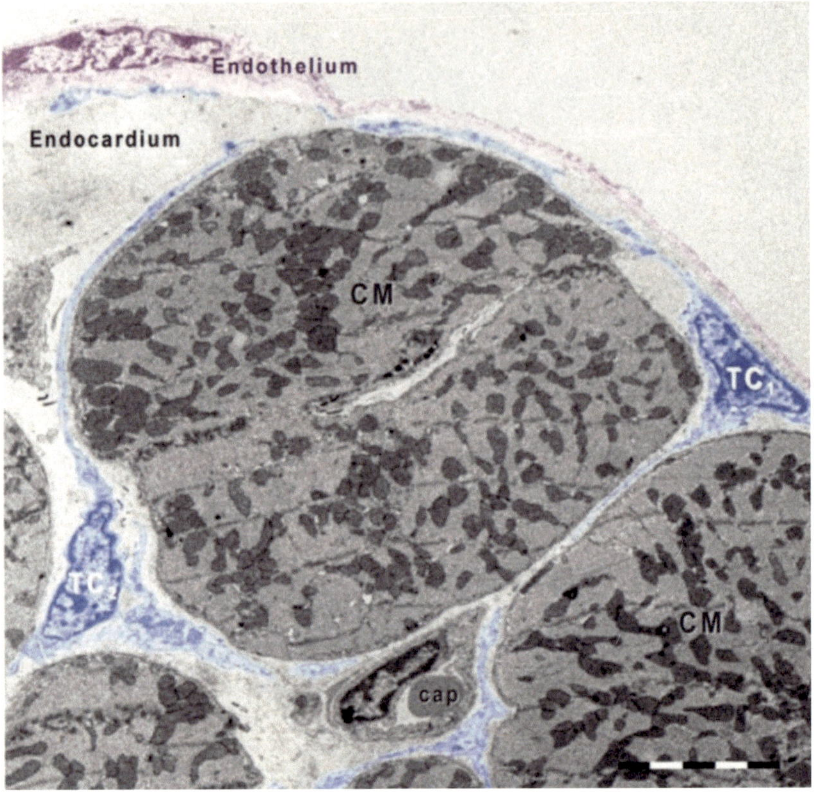

Fig. 5. Digitally coloured electron micrograph of mouse ventricular endocardium (burgundy). TCs (blue) form an interstitial network in the heart. A subendocardial telocyte (TC_1) sends TPs between cardiomyocytes (CM) and communicates with TC_2. Cap, blood capillary. Scale bar 5 μm. Reproduced, with permission, from Gherghiceanu et al., 2010.

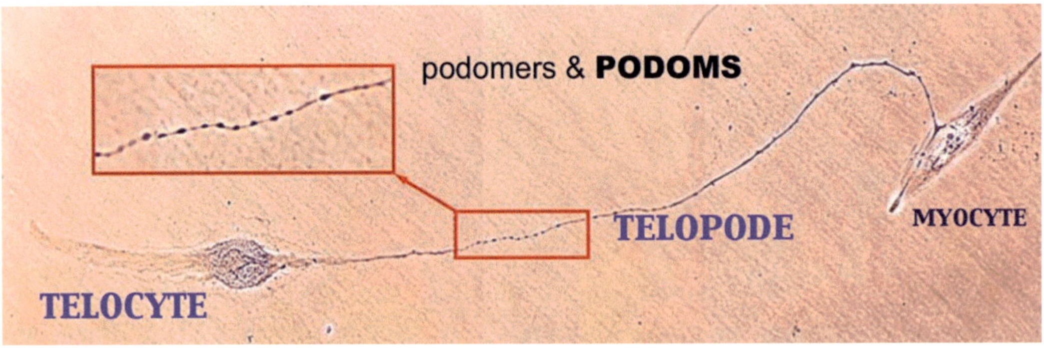

Fig. 6. Non-pregnant human myometrium in cell culture, day 3, the first passage. Giemsa staining. TC establishing contacts with a myocyte by a TP of about 65 μm long. Photographic composition of 4 serial phase contrast images; original magnification 40x. A higher magnification of TP (rectangles) clearly shows a moniliform aspect: at least 40 specific dilations (podoms) connected by thin segments (podomers) are visible in a 'beadlike' fashion. Reproduced, with permission, from Ciontea et al., 2005.

- **Thickness**: uneven caliber, mostly below 0.2 μm (below the resolving power of light microscopy), visible under electron microscopy;
- **Moniliform aspect**: podoms and podomeres (Figures 7, 8); average caliber of podomeres: 0.1 μm ± 0.05 μm, min. = 0.003 μm; max. = 0.24 μm; Podoms accommodate: mitochondria, (rough) endoplasmic reticulum, caveolae, a trio called 'Ca^{2+}-uptake/release units' (Figure 9);

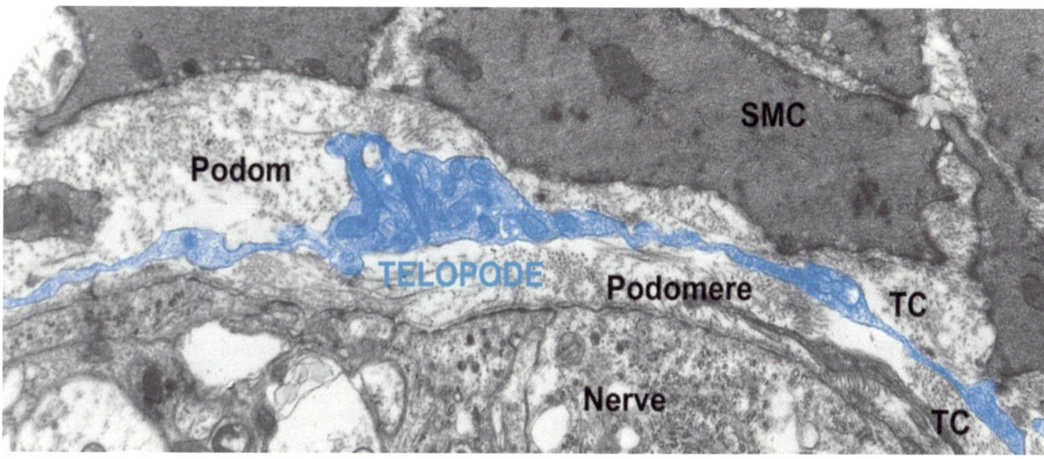

Fig. 7. Rat jejunum. A typical TP (blue) located between smooth muscle cells (SMC) and nerve endings. Note a large podom and the corresponding podomeres. TC body is not captured in the image.

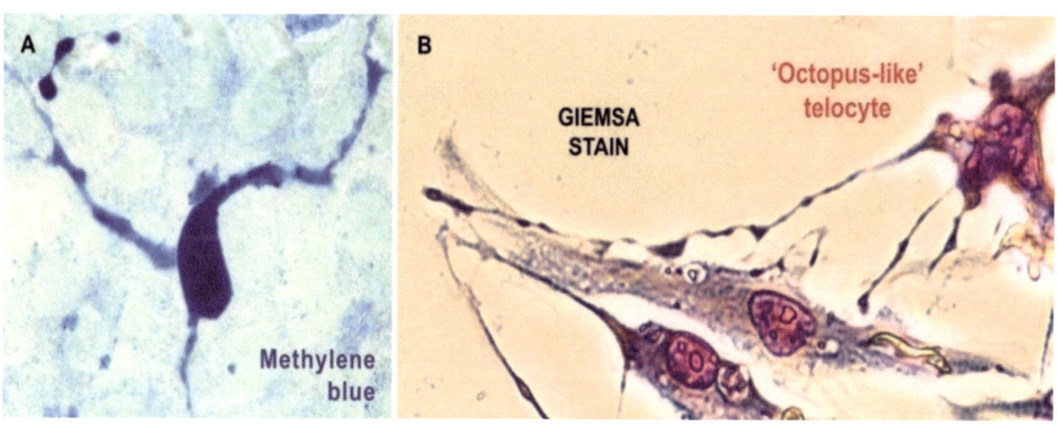

Fig. 8. A. Human pregnant myometrium. Primary confluent cultures (day 8) showing a telocyte with at least seven 'beads' per process. B. Human fallopian tube, preconfluent primary cell cultures. Conventional light microscopy, Giemsa staining. Original magnification 40x (A), 100x, oil immersion (B). Reproduced, with permission, from Ciontea et al., 2005 and Popescu et al., 2005a.

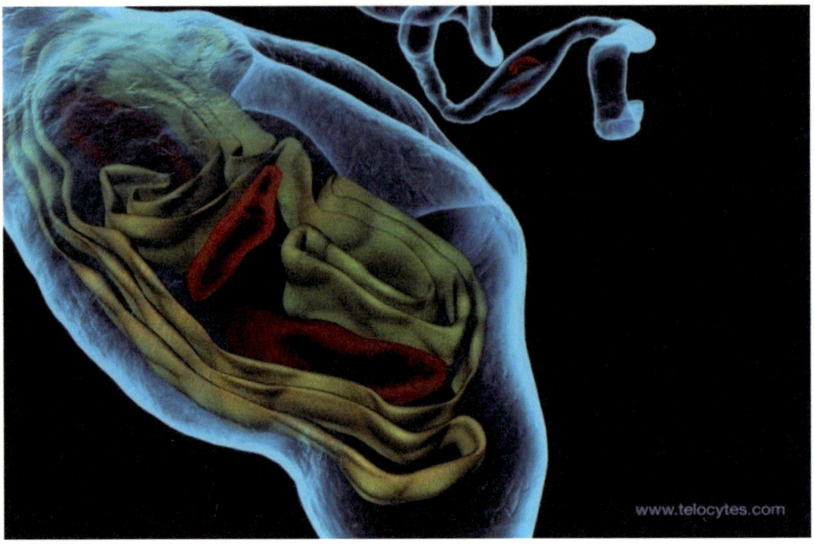

Fig. 9. The schematic drawing of a podom (blue), the dilated portion of a telopode. Note the podomic endoplasmic reticulum in yellow and the mitochondria in red.

- **Branching**, with a dichotomous pattern (Figure 10);

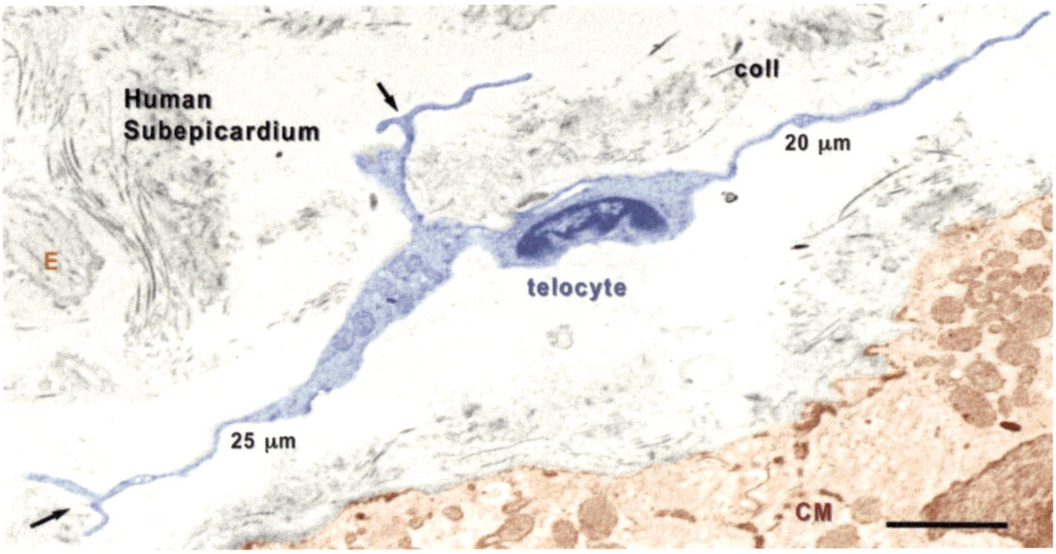

Fig. 10. Digitally coloured TEM image shows TC (blue) in human subepicardium, bordering the peripheral cardiomyocytes (CM, highlighted in brown). The TC has three telopodes, illustrating: a) the distinctive dichotomous pattern of branching (arrows); b) Tp are very thin at the emergence from the cell body; c) alternating podoms and podomeres. Note that some portions of podomeres have the same thickness as collagen fibrils, which makes observation under light microscopy impossible. E – elastin. Scale bar - 2 μm. Reproduced, with permission, from Popescu et al., 2010b.

- Organization in a labyrinthine system, forming a 3D network anchored by hetero- and homocellular junctions.

The concept of TC was soon embraced by other laboratories as well (Bani et al., 2010; Cantarero et al., 2011; Carmona et al., 2011; Eyden et al., 2010; Kostin, 2010; Zhou et al., 2010).

3. Sex steroids and TCs

The "sex hormones"— estrogens, progesterone, and androgens—are a special category of steroids. Their actions are mediated by intracellular receptors, generally known as nuclear receptors, acting as ligand regulating transcription factors (slow genomic mechanisms) as well as by membrane-associated receptors and signaling cascades (fast nongenomic mechanism) (Giretti & Simoncini, 2008; Tetel et al., 2009). Sex steroids are involved in the regulation of many functions in human organism, including reproduction and behaviour.
Female genital organs, especially those directly involved in ovum fertilization and embryo implantation - fallopian tubes and uterus - are highly influenced by sex steroids.

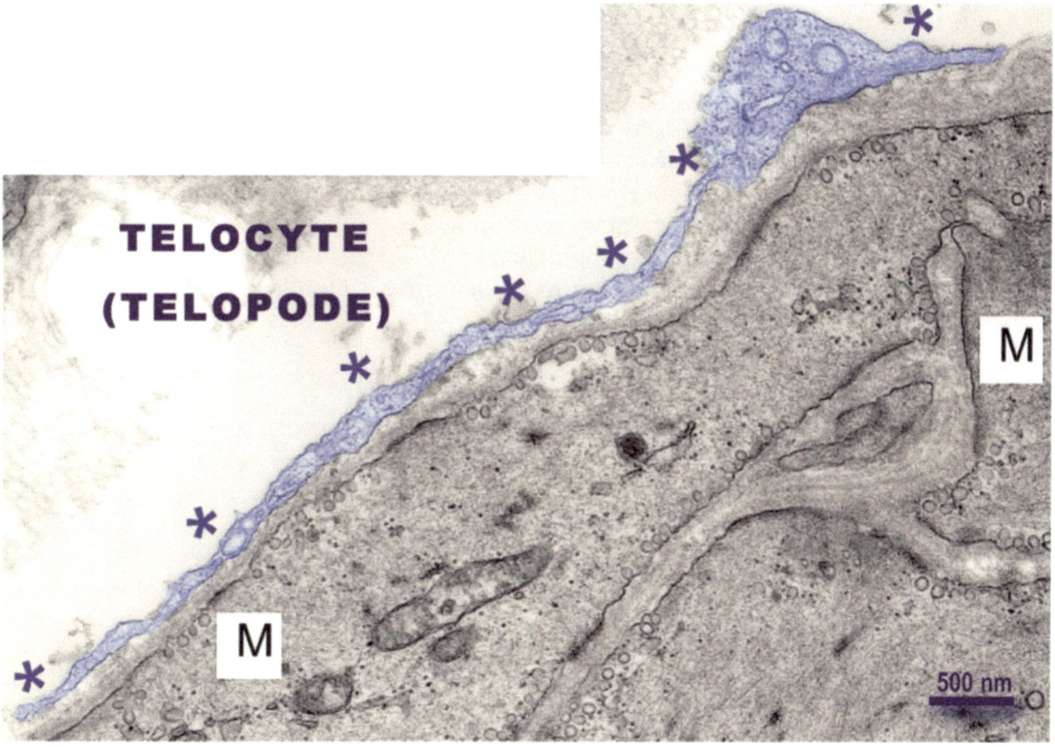

Fig. 11. Electron microscopy of non-pregnant human uterus. Note the telocyte covering smooth muscle cells (M). The telopode is digitally coloured in blue, marked with asterisks. Image obtained in 2006. Courtesy of Prof. M. Taggart (Newcastle University, UK) and Dr. Carolyn J.P. Jones (Manchester University, UK).

Connective tissue filling the space between epithelial, muscular and nerve tissue, found in the walls of these organs, abound in different cells. They are generally referred to as stromal cells and are subclassified into fibroblasts, fibrocytes, myofibroblasts, interstitial cells, and mesenchymal cells. In recent years we describe a novel cell type - TCs - with a completely different silhouette. TCs are unequivocally recognized under transmission electron microscope on the basis of their most peculiar feature: TCs have extremely long prolongations, with a very thin and moniliform aspect (Figure 11).

Our laboratory was the first to describe the presence of sex steroid hormone receptors in TCs (D. Cretoiu et al., 2006, S.M. Cretoiu et al., 2009). TCs for cell cultures were obtained from the muscle coat of the fallopian tube and uterus, and analyzed by immunohistochemistry using monoclonal antibodies to determine the presence of estrogen receptor alpha (ERα) and progesterone receptor (PR). TCs were enriched in primary culture by magnetically-activated cell sorting. The magnetic beads conjugated with goat anti-mouse IgG were incubated with monoclonal anti human CD117, considered to be specific for TCs. The cell suspension was then incubated with the magnetic beads and the supernatant was collected as the negative fraction. Culture medium was added to collect the remaining cells and the tube was removed from the magnet. This was considered as the positive fraction. We obtained 1.8×10^5 cells in the positive fraction and 4.8×10^6 cells in the negative fraction. After 9 days, cells grown on coverslips, in primary culture underwent subsequent examination.

3.1 TCs as steroid hormone sensors in human myometrium

TCs have been described in human uterine tissue under different names since 2004 : c-kit-positive cells (Shafik et al., 2004), m-CLIC (Ciontea et al., 2005), Vimentin-positive, c-kit-negative interstitial cells (Duquette et al., 2005), ICLC (Popescu et al., 2007; Hutchings et al., 2009). Our group found that myometrial TCs possessed very long cytoplasmic processes which, by *in vitro* Janus green B staining, were shown to contain numerous mitochondria. (Ciontea et al., 2005). TCs represented approximately 7% of the total cell number on random semi-thin myometrial tissue sections (Figure 12) stained with toluidin blue (Popescu et al., 2006).

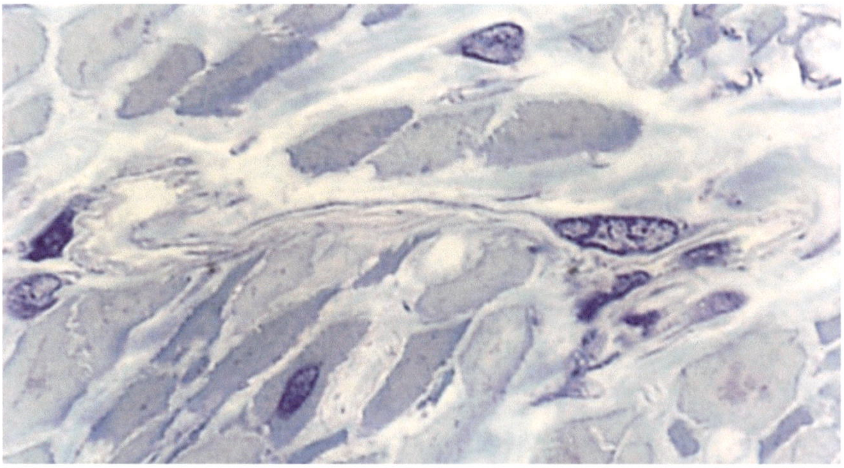

Fig. 12. Pregnant human myometrium (39 weeks of gestation). Semi-thin sections (0.5 - 1 μm thick) of uterine muscular layer embedded in Epon resin and stained with toluidine blue. Note the very long process of the TC squeezing between obliquely cut smooth muscle cells. Original magnification 100x. Reproduced, with permission, from Hutchings *et al.*, 2009.

Uterine TCs display distinct features which avoid possible confusion with other types of interstitial cells. Methylene blue staining and Golgi impregnation, which was used for the first time by Cajal in 1892 (for ICC identification) are also necessary for identification of TC presence at tissue level or in cell culture (Figures 13, 14).

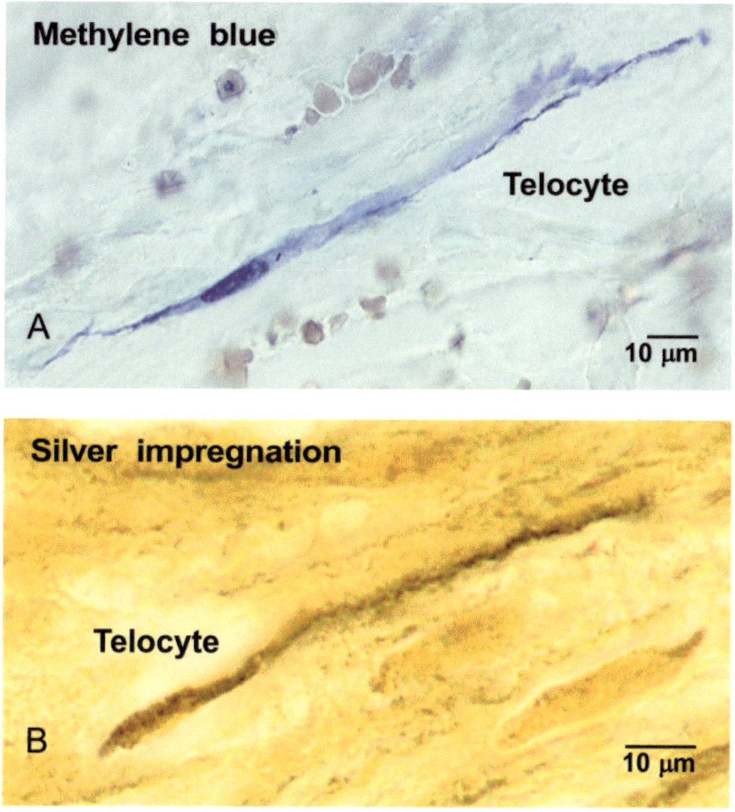

Fig. 13. Human myometrium. A. Methylene blue vital staining, before cryofixation (cryosectioning). Note the selective affinity of a telocyte for the blue dye. B. Silver impregnation after fixation and paraffin embedding. A pyriform telocyte with a very long, moniliform process. Original magnification: 1000x. Reprinted from European Journal of Pharmacology, 546, L. M. Popescu, C. Vidulescu, A. Curici,L. Caravia, A. A. Simionescu, S. M. Ciontea, S. Simion, Imatinib inhibits spontaneous rhythmic contractions of human uterus and intestine, 177-181, Copyright (2006), with permission from Elsevier..

At the myometrial level, TCs establish, through their TPs, vicinity relationships with capillaries and nerve fibers, as well as specialized contacts with other interstitial cells (e.g. macrophages, mast cells, lymphocytes, eosinophils) (Popescu et al., 2005b) (Figure 15). TCs interconnect with each other and with smooth muscle cells (SMC) through cell-to-cell point contacts or gap junctions. Interestingly, we found in uterine myocytes typical 'Ca^{2+} release units (caveolae, sarcoplasmic reticulum and mitochondria) in the vicinity of gap junctions (Figure 16).

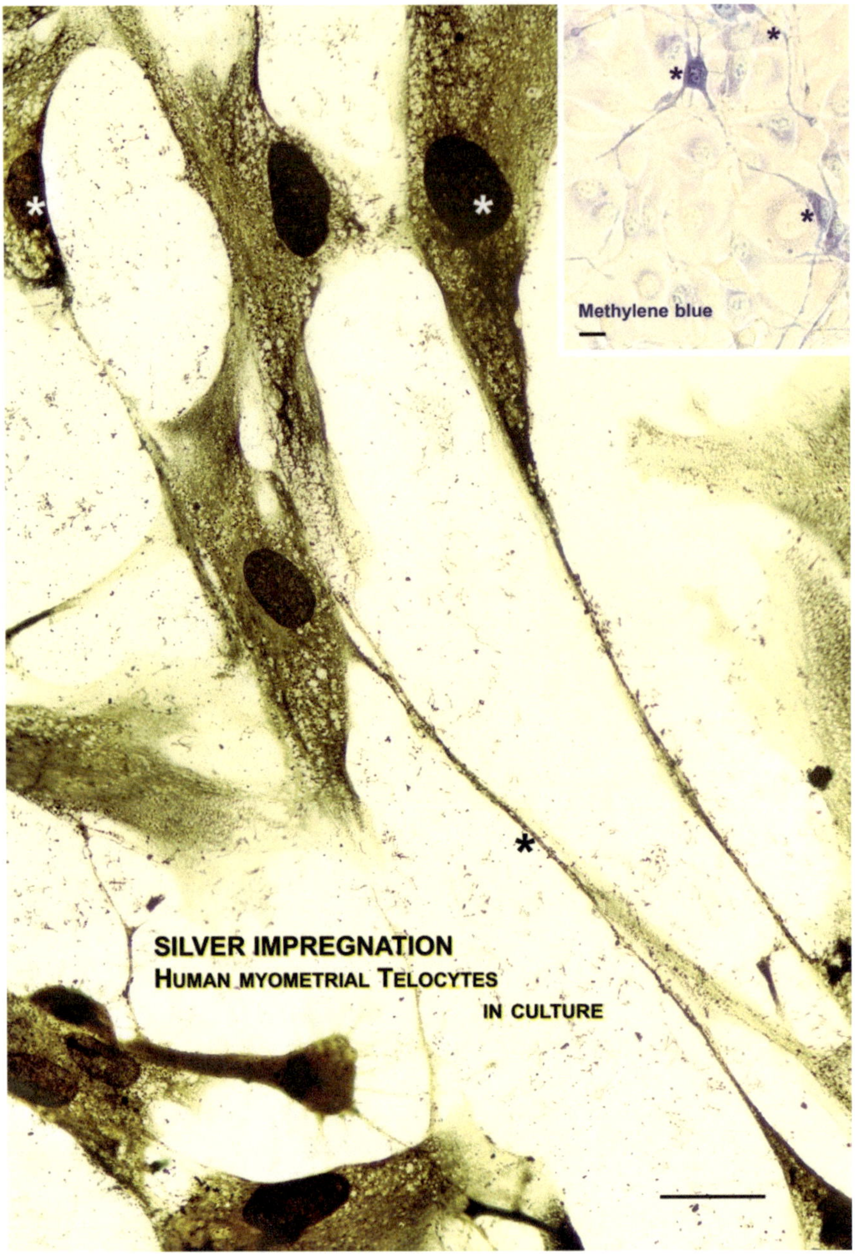

Fig. 14. Photographic reconstruction of human TCs in culture establishing contact with smooth muscle cells. From our experience, silver impregnation is one of the choice methods for revealing the typical moniliform aspect of TCs in culture. Inset- the same interlaced distribution of TCs (*) using methylene blue vital staining. Both methods reveal weaker myocyte staining. Scale bar 10 μm. Reproduced, with permission, from Cretoiu et al., 2006.

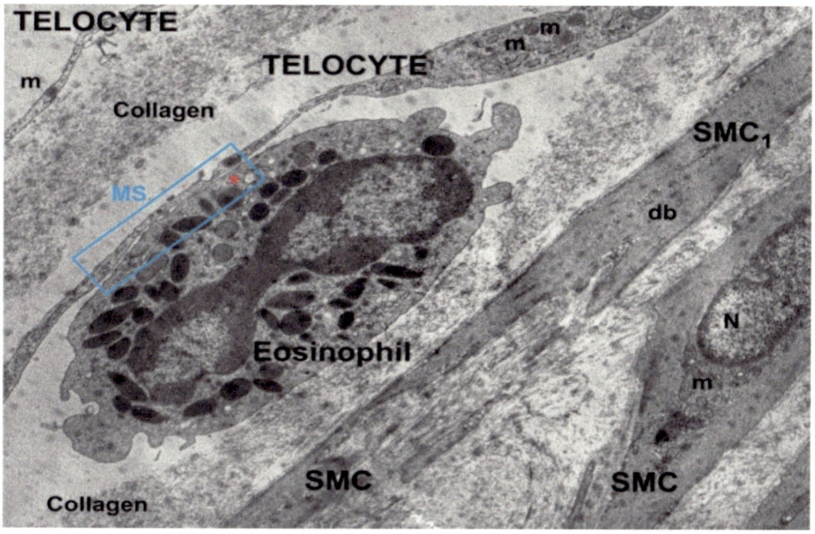

Fig. 15. Rat myometrium: TEM; original magnification 7100x. A multi-contact synapse (MS) between a telocyte and an eosinophil, in the neighbourhood of smooth muscle cells (SMC); m, mitochondria; N, nucleus; db, dense bodies; Note presence of mitochondria (*) in the synaptic vicinity, typical of chemical synapses. Reproduced, with permission, from Popescu et al., 2005b.

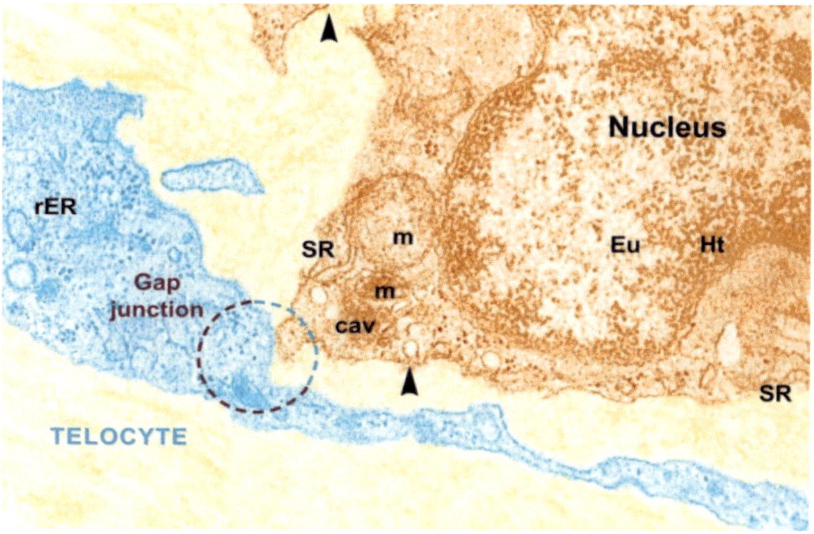

Fig. 16. Digitally-coloured TEM image of a TC in rat myometrium: TC (blue), smooth muscle cells (Sienna brown). Note the 'Ca^{2+}-release units' (caveolae, sarcoplasmic reticulum and mitochondria) in the cytoplasmic region where smooth muscle sarcolemma comes into close contact with TC plasmalemma. Original magnification: x15000. SMC = smooth muscle cells; Ht = heterochromatin; Eu = euchromatin; rER = rough endoplasmic reticulum; SR = sarcoplasmic reticulum; m = mitochondria; cav = caveolae (arrowheads). Reproduced from Ciontea et al., 2005.

Currently, there is no established panel of antibodies for TC immunophenotyping. We previously reported that antibodies against CD117/c-kit result in weak and sometimes inconsistent TC immunostaining. Most of CD117 positive cells co-express CD34 and vimentin (Ciontea et al., 2005, Popescu et al., 2006) (Figure 17).

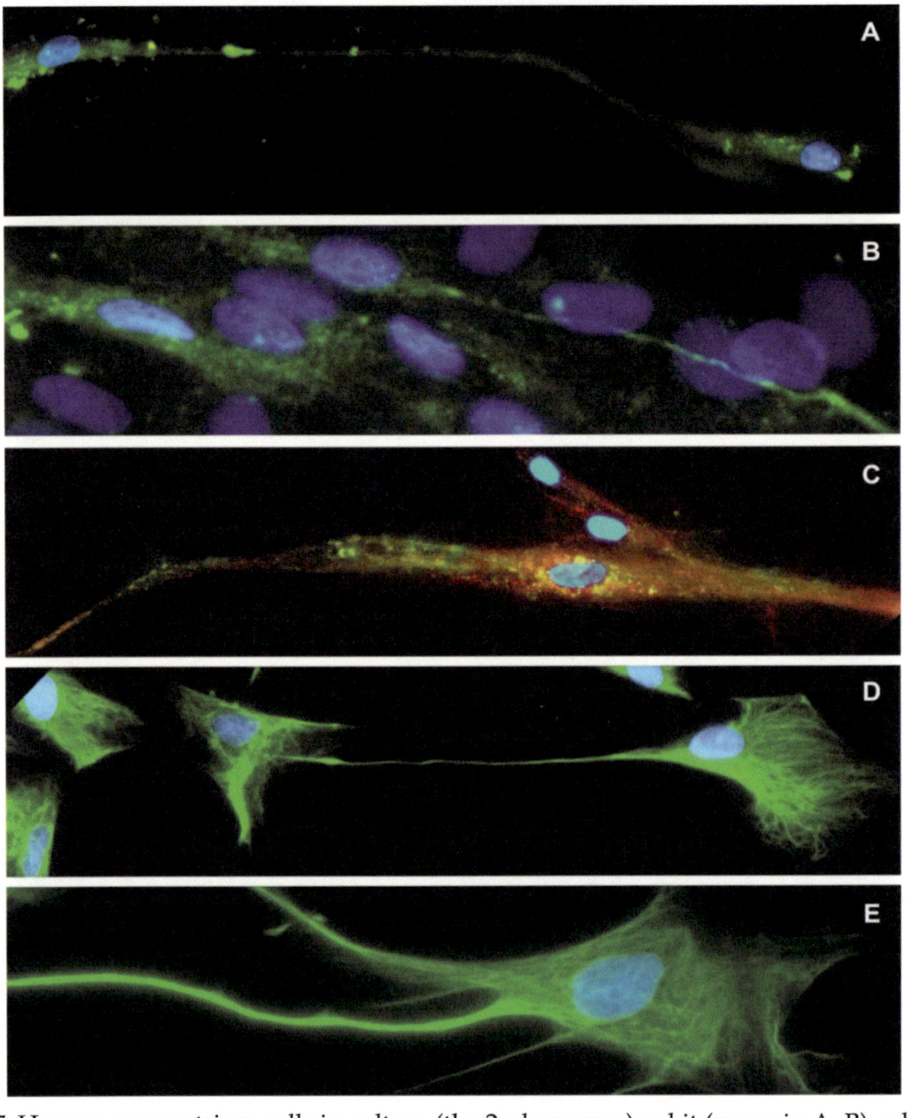

Fig. 17. Human myometrium cells in culture (the 2nd passage): c-kit (green in A, B), c-kit and CD34 (red and green, respectively, in C) and vimentin (green in D, E). Cells which display the morphologic TC feature (long, moniliform processes) express c-kit and contact adjacent cells (A–C). Some cells suggestive of TCs co-express c-kit and CD34 (C). The characteristic cell processes are immunoreactive for vimentin and establish connections with nearby cells (D and E). Original magnification 60x, nuclear counterstaining with Hoechst 33342 (blue). Reproduced, with permission, from Ciontea et al., 2005.

However, using immunohistochemistry alone, we cannot differentiate between interstitial cells since. For instance, c-kit positive cells could be stem cells, mast cells (Terada, 2009; Cinel et al., 2009), or TCs. TCs have a thin rim of cytoplasm. Their TPs (often up to 100 nm thick) can be undetectable under an immunofluorescence microscope, falling below light microscopy resolution. Electron microscopy is fundamental in identifying TCs with their peculiar appearance, having extremely long and moniliform processes with a dichotomous branching pattern which sometimes gave them a dendritic aspect. Table 1 distinctively draws a demarcation line between TCs, canonical ICC and fibroblasts.

Once TCs were established as cellular components of the hormonally responsive uterine tissue, we addressed whether they might express steroid receptors. Because, *in situ,* it may be difficult to observe morphological differences between the tightly packed myometrial cells and TCs, we chose to dissociate myometrial tissue to determine which cell type(s) expresses ER-α or PR-A. By Immunocytochemistry, we identified two cell types on the basis of their ER and PR immunoreactivity: a. TCs, which showed intense nuclear and weak cytoplasmic immunostaining for both ER and PR, (Figure 18 A, B); b. myocytes and/or fibroblasts which remained relatively unstained (Figure 18 A). Using double immunostaining for CD117/c-kit, we confirmed that cells which stained positive for ER and PR were TCs, (Figure 18 C, D). Double immunofluorescence confirmed the same distribution of PR and ER in c-kit positive cells, intense at nuclear level and weak in the cytoplasm (Figure 19 A-H).

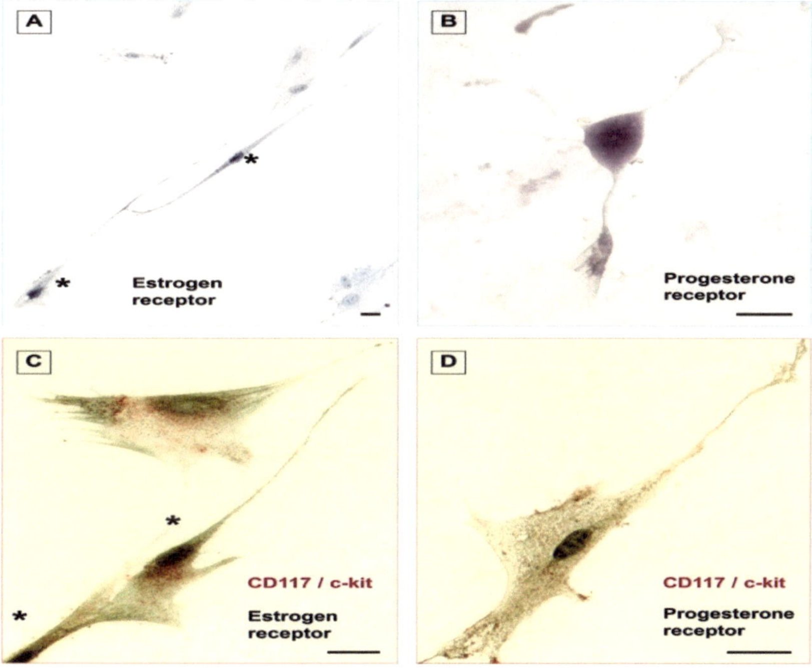

Fig. 18. A-D. Human myometrial cell culture, fourth passage. Immunocytochemical staining for estrogen and progesterone receptors. A. Immunocytochemical detection of estrogen receptor - dark stained nuclei (*), counterstaining with methyl green for negative nuclei. B. TCs stained positive for progesterone receptor. C. Doublestaining (*) for CD117/c-kit (red) and estrogen receptor (black). D. Double staining for CD117/c-kit (red) and progesterone receptor (black). Scale bar = 10 µm. Reproduced, with permission, from Cretoiu et al., 2006.

		Interstitial cells of Cajal (ICC)	**Myometrial telocytes**	**Fallopian tube telocytes**	**Fibroblasts**
Cell shape		Oval or spindle-shaped body	Spindle or stellate body		Polymorphic body
Nucleus		Oval, mostly euchromatic	Oval, heterochromatic under nuclear membrane		Oval, euchromatic with 1-2 visible nucleoli
Cytoplasm	Smooth ER	++	+	+	+-
	Rough ER	+	+	+	+++
	Golgi apparatus	+	+		+++
	Mitochondria	+++	++	+	+
	Intermediate filaments	++	+	+	+
	Microtubules	+	+	+	+
	Thin filaments	+	+	+	+
	Calcium releasing units	n.a.	present	n.a.	n.a.
Other structures	Caveolae	+	+	++	-
	Basal lamina	0	+-	+-	-
Immunohisto-chemical markers		c-kit	Co-localiza-tion of c-kit, CD34 and connexin 43, lack of prolyl 4-hydroxlase		Prolyl 4-hydroxylase
Intercellular contacts	Nerve endings	++	+	+	-
	Blood vessels	n.a.	+		-
	Immune cells	n.a.	+++		-
	Smooth muscle cells	+	+	+	-
	Other interstitial cells	+	+	+	-
	Gap junctions	+	+		-

Table 1. Morphological aspects, semi-quantitative data concerning the ultrastructural elements (transmission electron microscopy) and specific markers of telocytes compared to archetypal enteric interstitial cells of Cajal (ICC) and fibroblasts. Adapted from Hutchings et al., 2009.

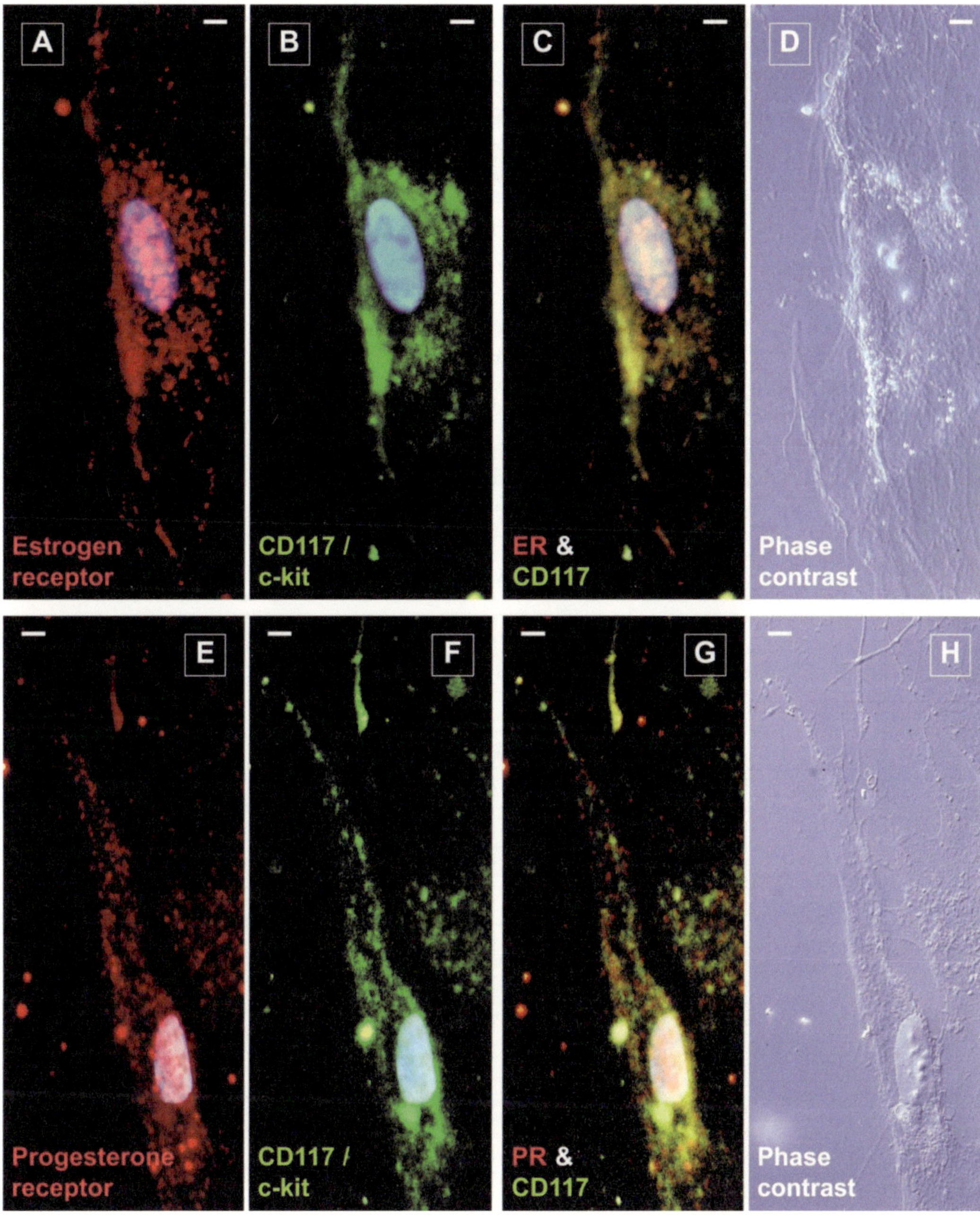

Fig. 19. A-H.Human myometrial cell culture, fourth passage. Immunofluorescent labeling for estrogen (A) and progesterone (E) receptor (red) which appear both inside the nucleus and in cytoplasm. c-kit/CD117 only (green) found in the cytoplasm (B, F) and double labeling for both markers (C, G), where co-expression appears as yellow areas. Hoechst 33342 (blue) for nuclear counterstaining. Phase contrast microscopy focused on the same cells, typical TCs with long, moniliform prolongations (D, H). Scale bar = 2 µm. Reproduced, with permission, from Cretoiu et al., 2006

3.2 TCs of human fallopian tube express ER and PR

Fallopian tubes are very important in human reproductive medicine playing active roles in such as gamete transport and final maturation, capacitation of sperm, ovum fertilization, early embryo development and delivery of embryo to the uterus. Each anatomic region (infundibulum with fimbria, ampulla, isthmus and intramural segment) seem to perform specific functions. Our discovery of novel interstitial cells in Fallopian tube tissue in 2005 (Popescu, 2005), which we now know to be TCs, has brought more attention to studies of this tissue. TCs are resident (dominantly) in fallopian tube lamina propria and in between smooth muscular fibres. The TCs percentage in the fallopian tube wall discloses the following areas of interest, starting from the basement membrane toward the serosa: area in the lamina propria found in close vicinity of the basement membrane (18±2%); area containing the entire lamina propria thickness (~8%); muscularis per se (7.8±1.2%) and the remaining zone beneath serosa (was not assessed). We concluded that the TC spatial distribution gradient decreases from the sub-epithelial area to the serosa. In lamina propria the percentage of TCs represent on average 11.0±0.6% of all cells. TC cellular bodies can take on various shapes: pyriform (having only one prolongation), (50%); spindle (with two opposite prolongations), (30%), triangular (15%) and other shapes with more than three prolongations (5%).

Tubal TC immunophenotyping was performed by correlating morphology with immunohistochemistry using a panel of 15 antibodies (Table 2).

Antibody	Clone	Dilution	Source	IHC positivity
CD117/c-kit	polyclonal	1:100	DAKO	+ + + +
CD34	QBEnd10	1:100	Biogenex	+ + +
S-100	polyclonal	1:500	DAKO	+ +
α-SMA	1A4	1:1500	Sigma	+
CD57	NK1	1:50	DAKO	+
nestin	5326	1:100	Santa Cruz	+
desmin	D33	1:50	DAKO	–
vimentin	V9	1:50	DAKO	+
NSE	BBS/NC/VI-H14	1:50	DAKO	+
GFAP	6F2	1:50	DAKO–	
CD68	PG-M1	1:50	DAKO	+
CD62P	1E3	1:25	DAKO	–
CD1a	CD1a-235	1:30	Novocastra	–
Chromo A	LK2H10	1:50	Novocastra	–
PGP9.5	10A1	1:40	Novocastra	–

Table 2. Summary of immunohistochemical results for telocytes from human fallopian tube. The intensity of telocyte reactivity was assessed semi-quantitatively using an adaptation of the Quick score method. Intensity: Negative (no staining of any cellular part at high magnification):–; Occasionally weak positive: +; Low (only visible at high magnification):+; Medium (readily visible at low magnification):+ +; High (strikingly positive at high magnification):+ + +; Strong (strikingly positive even at low magnification):+ + + +.

TCs with characteristic morphology (one or more very long, thin processes, sometimes with 'beads-on-a-string' appearance, that arise from pyriform, stellate or spindle shaped cell bodies) were found to express c-kit. Some of the TCs co-express CD34, desmin, vimentin and even α-SMA. TCs in the fallopian tube fulfill the ultrastructural identification criteria and are definitely distinct from fibroblasts (Figure 20).

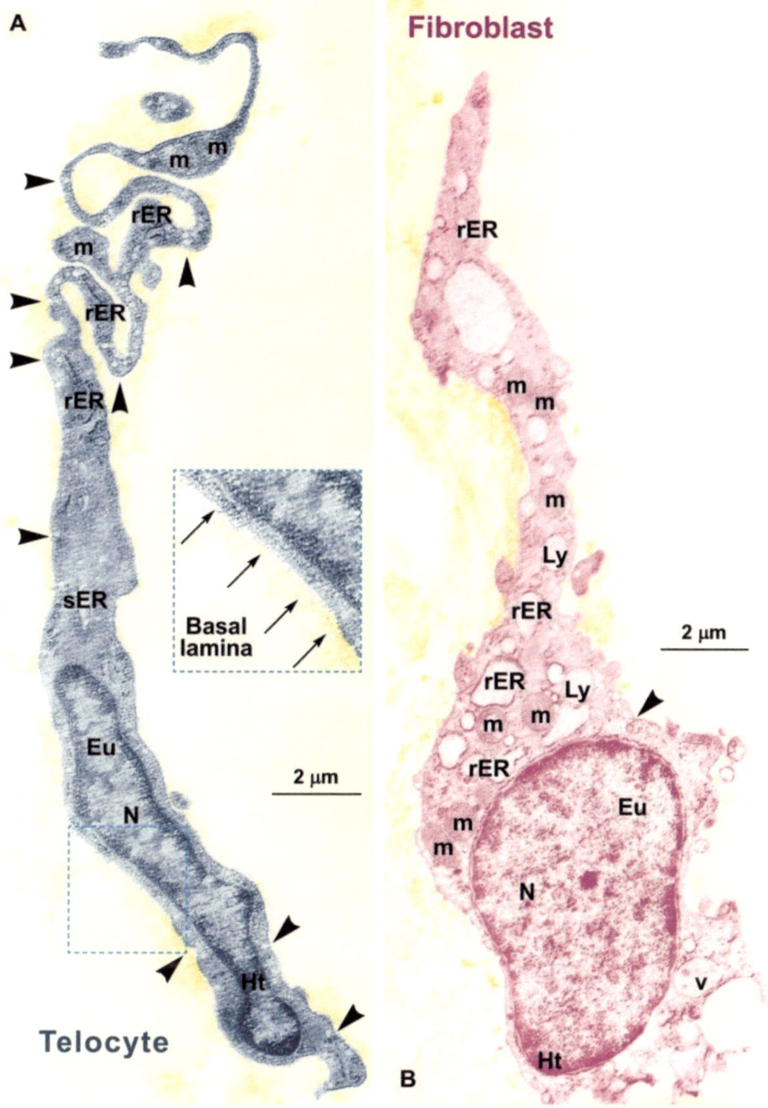

Fig. 20. (A) A telocyte compared to (B) a fibroblast from the same TEM ultrathin section of human fallopian tube (digitally coloured images). N = nucleus; Eu = euchromatin; Ht = heterochromatin; rER = rough endoplasmic reticulum; sER = smooth endoplasmic reticulum; m = mitochondria; v = vacuolae; Ly = lysosomes; arrowheads indicate caveolae. At least 29 caveolae can be counted in the TC's convoluted process (A, upper part). Reproduced, with permission, from Popescu et al., 2005a.

TCs were enriched in primary culture by magnetically-activated cell sorting, after being identified as c-kit positive cells with characteristic morphology. Indeed TCs were found in a higher percentage after magnetic cell sorting: approximately 30 ± 0.8% (n = 516) compared to 9.9 ± 0.9% (n = 324) (Popescu, 2005). The sorted populations underwent subsequent passages, because according to our previous experience, the number of TCs increases with each passage.

In vitro double staining on Fallopian tube samples showed that desmin-positive cells (SMC) tested negative for ER-α or PR-A and c-kit-positive cells (telocytes) tested positive for ER-α or PR-A (Fig. 21 A,B). Moreover, double staining for c-kit (green fluorescence) and PR-A or ER-α (red fluorescence) revealed that only cells positive for c-kit were also positive for ER-α and PR-A at nuclear level (Fig. 22 A-F). PR-A expression at nuclear level was more intense than for ER-α. SMC were weakly positive or completely negative.

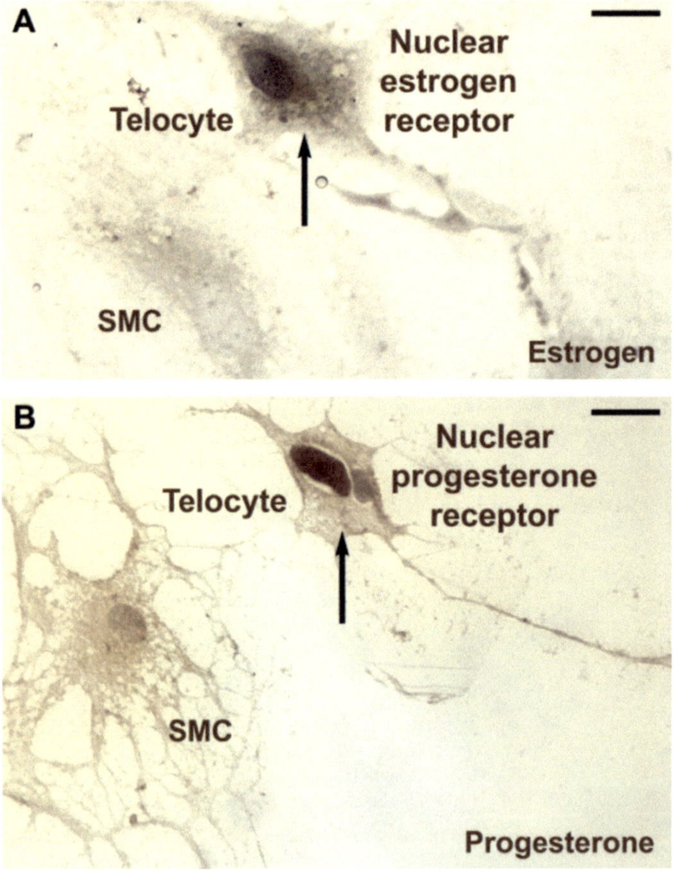

Fig. 21. A,B. Human Fallopian tube cell culture, fourth passage. The expression of ER-α (A) and PR-A (B) demonstrated by immunocytochemical staining. TCs (arrows) stained positive for ER and PR (brown nuclei). Scale bar = 5 μm. With kind permission from Springer Science+Business Media: Journal of Molecular Histology, Interstitial Cajal-like cells of human Fallopian tube express estrogen and progesterone receptors, 40, 2009, 387-394, Cretoiu, S.M.;Cretoiu, D.;Suciu, L.&Popescu, L.M., figure 4.

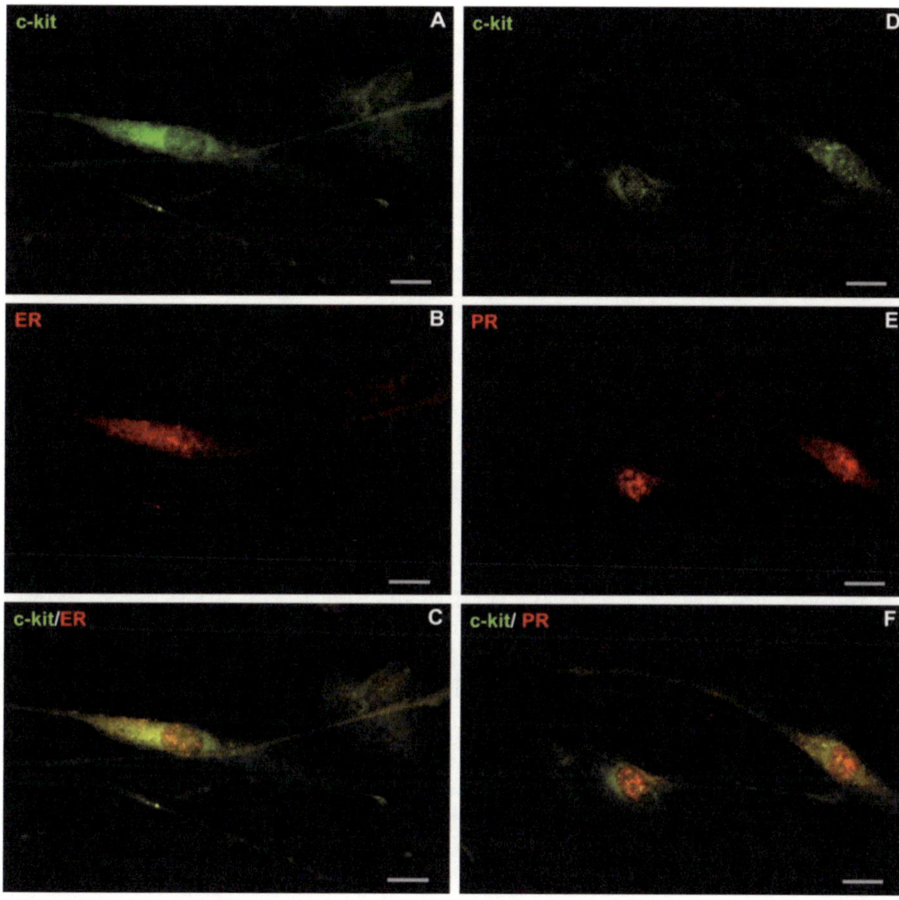

Fig. 22. A-F. Human Fallopian tube cell culture, sixth passage. Immunofluorescent labeling for c-kit/FITC (A) and ER-α/Alexa Fluor 546 (B), and superimposed images to show colocalization (C). c-kit fluorescence of TC (D) and PR-A fluorescence (E). Superimposed labeling for both markers (F), where c-kit (green) is localized only in the cytoplasm and PR-A is expressed in the TC nuclei (red). Scale bar = 5 µm. With kind permission from Springer Science+Business Media: Journal of Molecular Histology, Interstitial Cajal-like cells of human Fallopian tube express estrogen and progesterone receptors, 40, 2009, 387-394, Cretoiu, S.M.;Cretoiu, D.;Suciu, L.&Popescu, L.M., figure 5.

4. Possible TC roles

4.1 TCs and signaling processes

Recently, some of the TCs located on the extracellular matrix of blood vessels were described as having a primary cilium (Cantarero et al., 2011). The presumed functions of such a non-motile cilium could be:- organizer of the mitotic spindle (Alieva et al., 2004), sensory organelle involved in signal transduction - hedgehog pathway (Singla et al., 2006), mechanical sensing and mechano-chemical conversion in endothelial cells (Egorova et al., 2011; Nauli et al., 2008). By analogy, we can presume that TCs could be involved in the signaling process if located near the stromal colony-forming cells/units in human endometrium or might act as stretch sensors if located near smooth muscle structures in both Fallopian tubes and uterus.

TPs usually form and release vesicles (or exosomes) which might indicate the possible involvement of TCs in intercellular communication. For example, in the heart, heterocellular communication between TCs and cardiomyocytes seems to occur by shed vesicles and close apposition (Gherghiceanu et al., 2011). Intercellular signaling can occur by two mechanisms: a paracrine and/or juxtacrine secretion of small signaling molecules and shedding microvesicles which transport 'horizontal' "packets" of macromolecules to the target cells, modifying their physiology. These vesicles can even transport DNA or RNA among neighbouring cells, inducing epigenetic changes (Akao et al., 2010; Zomer et al., 2010). We suspect a complex interplay between TCs, immune cells, cells involved in epithelial or even myometrial regeneration and cancer spreading (Pap et al., 2011).

4.2 TCs and stem cells

It is known that the remodeling events which take place in the uterus (endo- and myometrium) during implantation and pregnancy are coordinated by sequential actions of estrogen and progesterone (Szotek et al., 2007). TCs, as a special type of stromal cells, could be involved in uterine remodeling since they express ER and PR, and are also located in the lamina propria, beneath the epithelium and in between myocytes. There are fundamental studies that provide evidence that both epithelial and stromal stem/progenitor cells are found in human and mouse uterus (Gargett et al., 2008). The discovery of relationships between TCs and these uterine stem cells could provide new insights into the pathophysiology of various gynecological and obstetrical disorders. In 2009, Shynlova et al. proposed a new model of phenotypic modulation of uterine myocytes during pregnancy. These changes evolve in an early proliferative phase, an intermediate phase of cellular hypertrophy and matrix elaboration, a third phase in which the cells assume a contractile phenotype and the final phase in which cells become highly active and committed to labour. The final phase of myometrial differentiation is postpartum uterine involution. These stages are in fact the result of integration of endocrine signals and mechanical stimulation of the uterus by the growing fetus (Shynlova et al., 2009). In our opinion, TCs could be themselves stem cells (Popescu et al., 2011b), playing a part in muscle regeneration (Popescu et al., 2011a), these processes possibly depending on steroid hormones receptors.

4.3 TCs and immune cells

TCs often establish contacts with targets, such as smooth muscle cells, nerve fibres, and capillaries (Popescu et al., 2011). Over time, we also described close contact between TCs and cells of the immune system, found in the interstitial space (e.g. eosinophils, plasma cell, etc.). We considered that this is a new type of synapse - the stromal synapse - in addition to the existing neuronal and immunological synapse (Popescu et al., 2005b). The intercellular contact can either be "plain" uniform or "kiss-and-run" multicontact, based on synaptic cleft tracing.

5. Perspectives

TCs can be putative cellular mechanotransducers in smooth muscle tissue. They may sense and translate stretch information for the nucleus, and activate genes responsible for protein synthesis which can influence the surrounding cells by juxta- or paracrine mechanisms.
TCs could also be 'hormonal sensors' in human myometrium and the Fallopian tube since they express estrogen and progesterone receptors *in vitro*. The presence of steroid hormone receptors suggests that TCs could also be responsible for myogenic contractility modulation under hormonal control, either by transferring bioactive molecules (towards cells from an

endometrial stem cell colony), either by direct stimulation of target cells (immunoreactive cells). Recent evidence suggests that TCs may play a role as putative actors in neo-angiogenesis (Manole et al., 2011).

6. Conclusions

In conclusion, the presence of steroid hormone receptors suggests that TCs could behave as sensors controlling the Fallopian tube peristalsis by signaling mechanisms (para- or juxtacrine), depending on ovarian hormone levels, by opposite effects (accelerated by estrogens and delayed by progesterone). Our findings might even explain infertility in patients without any proven Fallopian tube abnormalities. At uterine level, the discovery of TCs is fundamental for a totally new approach regarding the mechanisms controlling myometrial contractility during and outside pregnancy. The evidence for steroid hormone receptors at the level of myometrial TCs might open a path towards the understanding of contractility modulation using steroid hormones. This effect could be the result of intercellular connections between TCs and myocytes. The particular structure of the podoms with energetic (mitochondria) and functional (proteins from ER) resources favours the extension of Tp in the extracellular environment for signalling purposes of for intercellular communication. The steroid receptors occurrence in TCs could also suggest that these cells participate in the exchange of genetic information with other cells (myocytes, immune cells, nerve fibres) or for sensing changes in stromal microenvironment. If some of the supposed functions will be proven, TCs could be used in the future as molecular tools for delivering biological drugs at genital organs level.

7. Acknowledgment

This work was partially supported by the "Sectorial Operational Programme" Human Resources Development, financed from the European Social Fund and by the Romanian Government under the contract number POSDRU/89/1.5/S/64109.

8. References

Akao, Y.; Iio, A.; Itoh, T.; Noguchi, S.; Itoh, Y.; Ohtsuki, Y. & Naoe, T. (2011).Microvesicle-mediated RNA molecule delivery system using monocytes/macrophages.*Molecular therapy*, Vol.19, No.2, (February 2011), pp. 395-399, ISSN 1525-0024

Alieva, I.B. & Vorobjev, I.A. (2004).Vertebrate primary cilia: a sensory part of centrosomal complex in tissue cells, but a "sleeping beauty" in cultured cells? *Cell biology international*, Vol.28, No.2, (April 2004), pp. 139-150, ISSN 1095-8355

Bani, D.; Formigli, L.; Gherghiceanu, M. & Faussone-Pellegrini, M.S. (2010).Telocytes as supporting cells for myocardial tissue organization in developing and adult heart.*Journal of cellular and molecular medicine*,Vol.14, No.10, (October 2010) pp. 2531-2538, ISSN 1582-4934

Cantarero, C.I.; Luesma, B.M.J. & Junquera, E.C. (2011).The primary cilium of telocytes in the vasculature: electron microscope imaging. *Journal of cellular and molecular medicine*, doi: 10.1111/j.1582-4934.2011.01312.x, ISSN 1582-4934

Carmona, I.C.; Bartolomé, M.J. & Escribano, C.J. (2011).Identification of telocytes in the lamina propria of rat duodenum: transmission electron microscopy. *Journal of cellular and molecular medicine*, Vol.15, No.1, (January 2011), pp. 26-30, ISSN 1582-4934

Cinel, L.; Aban, M.; Basturk, M.; Ertunc, D.; Arpaci, R.; Dilek, S. & Camdeviren, H. (2009).The association of mast cell density with myometrial invasion in endometrial carcinoma: a preliminary report. *Pathology, research and practice,* Vol.205, No.4, (April 2009), pp. 255-258, ISSN 1618-0631

Ciontea, S.M.; Radu, E.; Regalia, T.; Ceafalan, L.; Cretoiu, D.; Gherghiceanu, M.; Braga, R.I.; Malincenco, M.; Zagrean, L.; Hinescu, M.E. & Popescu, L.M. (2005). C-kit immunopositive interstitial cells (Cajal-type) in human myometrium.*Journal of cellular and molecular medicine*, Vol.9, No.2, (June 2005), pp. 407-420, ISSN 1582-4934

Cretoiu, D.; Ciontea, S.M.; Popescu, L.M.; Ceafalan, L. & Ardeleanu, C.(2006).Interstitial Cajal-like cells (ICLC) as steroid hormone sensors in human myometrium: immunocytochemical approach. *Journal of cellular and molecular medicine*, Vol.10, No.3, (September 2006), pp. 789-795, ISSN 1582-4934

Cretoiu, S.M.; Cretoiu, D.; Suciu, L. & Popescu, L.M. (2009).Interstitial Cajal-like cells of human Fallopian tube express estrogen and progesterone receptors. *Journal of molecular histology*,Vol.40, No.5-6, (October 2009), pp. 387-394, ISSN 1567-2387

Duquette, R.A.; Shmygol, A.; Vaillant, C.; Mobasheri, A.; Pope, M.; Burdyga, T. & Wray, S. (2005). Vimentin-positive, c-kit-negative interstitial cells in human and rat uterus: a role in pacemaking?*Reproductive biology*,Vol.72, No.2, (February 2005), pp. 276-283, ISSN 1642-431X

Egorova, A.D.; Khedoe, P.P.; Goumans, M.J.; Yoder, B.K.; Nauli, S.M.; Ten Dijke, P.; Poelmann, R.E. & Hierck, B.P. (2011). Lack of Primary Cilia Primes Shear-Induced Endothelial-to-Mesenchymal Transition.*Circulation research*, Vol.108, No.9, (April 2011), ISSN 1524-4571

Eyden, B.; Curry, A. & Wang, G. (2011).Stromal cells in the human gut show ultrastructural features of fibroblasts and smooth muscle cells but not myofibroblasts. *Journal of cellular and molecular medicine*, Vol.15, No.7,(July 2011), ISSN 1582-4934

Gargett, C.E.; Chan, R.W. & Schwab, K.E. (2008). Hormone and growth factor signaling in endometrial renewal: role of stem/progenitor cells.*Molecular and cellular endocrinology*, Vol.288, No.1-2, (June 2008), pp. 22-29, ISSN 1872-8057

Gherghiceanu, M. & Popescu, L.M. (2011).Heterocellular communication in the heart: electron tomography of telocyte-myocyte junctions. *Journal of cellular and molecular medicine*, Vol.15, No.4, (April 2011), pp. 1005-1011,ISSN 1582-4934

Gherghiceanu, M. & Popescu, L.M. (2005).Interstitial Cajal-like cells (ICLC) in human resting mammary gland stroma.Transmission electron microscope (TEM) identification.*Journal of cellular and molecular medicine*, Vol. 9, No. 4, (December 2005), pp. 893-910, ISSN 1582-4934

Gherghiceanu, M.; Manole, C.G. & Popescu, L.M. (2010).Telocytes in endocardium: electron microscope evidence. *Journal of cellular and molecular medicine*, Vol.14, No.9, (September 2010), pp. 2330-2334, ISSN 1582-4934

Giangrande, P.H. & McDonnell, D.P. (1999).The A and B isoforms of the human progesterone receptor: two functionally different transcription factors encoded by a single gene.*Recent progress in hormone research*, Vol.54, pp. 291-313; ISSN 0079-9963

Giretti, M.S. & Simoncini, T. (2008).Rapid regulatory actions of sex steroids on cell movement through the actin cytoskeleton.*Steroids*.Vol.73, No.9-10, (October 2008), pp. 895-900, ISSN 1878-5867

Green, S.; Walter, P.; Greene, G.; Krust, A.; Goffin, C.; Jensen, E.; Scrace, G.; Waterfield, M. & Chambon, P.(1986). Cloning of the human oestrogen receptor cDNA.*Journal of steroid biochemistry*,Vol.24, No.1, (January 1986), pp. 77-83, ISSN 0022-4731

Hinescu, M.E.; Gherghiceanu, M.; Mandache, E.; Ciontea, S.M. & Popescu, L.M.(2006). Interstitial Cajal-like cells (ICLC) in atrial myocardium: ultrastructural and immunohistochemical characterization. *Journal of cellular and molecular medicine*, Vol.10, No.1, (March 2006), pp. 243-257, ISSN 1582-4934

Hutchings, G.; Williams, O.; Cretoiu, D. & Ciontea, S.M. (2009).Myometrial interstitial cells and the coordination of myometrial contractility.*Journal of cellular and molecular medicine*, Vol.13, No.10, (October 2009), pp. 4268-4282, ISSN 1582-4934

Kastner, P.; Bocquel, M.T.; Turcotte, B.; Garnier, J.M.; Horwitz, K.B.; Chambon., P. & Gronemeyer, H.(1990). Transient expression of human and chicken progesterone receptors does not support alternative translational initiation from a single mRNA as the mechanism generating two receptor isoforms.*Journal of chemical biology*, Vol.265, No.21, (July 1990), pp. 12163-12167, ISSN 1864-6166

Kostin S.(2010). Myocardial telocytes: a specific new cellular entity. *Journal of cellular and molecular medicine*,Vol.14, No.7, (July 2010), pp. 1917-1921, ISSN 1582-4934

Kuiper, G.G.; Enmark, E.; Pelto-Huikko, M.; Nilsson, S. & Gustafsson, J.A.(1996).Cloning of a novel receptor expressed in rat prostate and ovary.*Proceedings of the National Academy of Sciences of the United States of America*, Vol.93, No.12, (June 1996), pp. 5925-5930, ISSN 1091-6490

Manole C.G.; Cismasiu V.; Gherghiceanu M.; Popescu L.M. (2011). Experimental acute myocardial infarction: telocytes involvement in neo-angiogenesis. Journal of cellular and molecular medicine, (September 2011) doi: 10.1111/j.1582-4934.2011.01449.x, ISSN 1582-4934

Nauli, S.M.; Kawanabe, Y.; Kaminski, J.J.; Pearce, W.J.; Ingber, D.E. & Zhou, J. (2008).Endothelial cilia are fluid shear sensors that regulate calcium signaling and nitric oxide production through polycystin-1. *Circulation*,Vol.117, No.9, (March 2008), pp. 1161-1171, ISSN 1524-4539

Pap E.(2011).The role of microvesicles in malignancies.*Advances in experimental medicine and biology*, Vol.714, pp. 183-199, ISSN 0065-2598

Popescu, L.M.; Gherghiceanu, M.; Kostin, S. & Faussone-Pellegrini, M.S. (2011).Telocytes and Heart Renewing. In:*Adaptation Biology and Medicine(Volume 6: Cell Adaptations and Challenges)*. P. Wang, C.-H. Kuo, N. Takeda and P.K. Singal, pp.17-39, Narosa Publishing House Pvt. Ltd., ISBN 978-81-7319-935-6, New Delhi, India

Popescu, L.M.; Ciontea, S.M.; Cretoiu, D.; Hinescu, M.E.; Radu, E.; Ionescu, N.; Ceausu, M.; Gherghiceanu, M.; Braga, R.I.; Vasilescu, F.; Zagrean, L. & Ardeleanu, C. (2005a). Novel type of interstitial cell (Cajal-like) in human fallopian tube. *Journal of cellular and molecular medicine*, Vol.9, No.2, (June 2005), pp. 479-523, ISSN 1582-4934

Popescu, L.M.; Gherghiceanu, M.; Cretoiu, D. & Radu, E. (2005b).The connective connection: interstitial cells of Cajal (ICC) and ICC-like cells establish synapses with immunoreactive cells. Electron microscope study in situ. *Journal of cellular and molecular medicine*, Vol.9, No.3, (September 2005), pp. 714-730, ISSN 1582-4934

Popescu, L.M.; Vidulescu, C.; Curici, A.; Caravia, L.; Simionescu, A.A.; Ciontea, S.M. & Simion, S. (2006). Imatinib inhibits spontaneous rhythmic contractions of human uterus and intestine.*European journal of pharmacology*, Vol.546, No.1-3, (September 2006), pp. 177–181, ISSN 1879-0712

Popescu, L.M.; Ciontea, S.M. & Cretoiu, D. (2007). Interstitial Cajal-like cells in human uterus and fallopian tube.*Annals of the New York Academy of Sciences*,(April 2007), Vol.1101, pp. 139-165, ISSN 1749-6632

Popescu, L.M. & Faussone-Pellegrini, M.S. (2010a).TELOCYTES - a case of serendipity: the winding way from Interstitial Cells of Cajal (ICC), via Interstitial Cajal-Like Cells

(ICLC) to TELOCYTES. *Journal of cellular and molecular medicine*, (April 2010), Vol.14, No.4, pp. 729-740, ISSN 1582-4934

Popescu, L.M.; Manole, C.G.; Gherghiceanu, M.; Ardelean, A..; Nicolescu, M.I.; Hinescu, M.E. & Kostin, S. (2010b). Telocytes in human epicardium.*Journal of cellular and molecular medicine*,Vol.14, No.8, (August 2010), pp. 2085-2093, ISSN 1582-4934

Popescu, L.M.; Manole E.; Serboiu C.S.; Manole C.G.; Suciu L.C.; Gherghiceanu M. & Popescu B.O. (2011a). Identification of telocytes in skeletal muscle interstitium: implication for muscle regeneration. Journal of cellular and molecular medicine, Vol.15, No.6, (June 2011) pp. 1379-1392, ISSN 1582-4934

Popescu, L.M.; Gherghiceanu M.; Suciu L.C.; Manole C.G. & Hinescu M.E. (2011b). Telocytes and putative stem cells in the lungs: electron microscopy, electron tomography and laser scanning microscopy. Cell And Tissue Research, (August 2011), doi: 10.1007/s00441-011-1229-z, ISSN 1432-0878

Shafik, A.; El-Sibai, O. & Shafik, I. (2004).Identification of c-kit-positive cells in the uterus.*International journal of gynaecology and obstetrics: the official organ of the International Federation of Gynaecology and Obstetrics*,Vol.87, No.3, (December 2004), pp. 254-255, ISSN 1879-3479

Shynlova, O.; Tsui, P.; Jaffer, S. & Lye, S.J. (2009).Integration of endocrine and mechanical signals in the regulation of myometrial functions during pregnancy and labour.*European journal of obstetrics, gynecology, and reproductive biology*,Vol.144, Suppl.1, (May 2009), pp. S2-10, ISSN 1872-7654

Singla, V. & Reiter, J.F. (2006).The primary cilium as the cell's antenna: signaling at a sensory organelle. *Science*, Vol.313, No.5787, (August 2006), pp. 629-633, ISSN 1095-9203

Suciu L., Popescu L.M., Gherghiceanu M., Regalia T., Nicolescu M.I., Hinescu M.E. & Faussone-Pellegrini M.S. (2010). Telocytes in human term placenta: morphology and phenotype. *Cells Tissues Organs*, Vol.192, No.5, pp. 325-339, ISSN 1422-6421

Szotek, P.P.; Chang, H.L.; Zhang, L.; Preffer, F.; Dombkowski, D.; Donahoe, P.K. & Teixeira, J.(2007).Adult mouse myometrial label-retaining cells divide in response to gonadotropin stimulation. *Stem Cells*,Vol.25, No.5, (May 2007), pp. 1317-1325, ISSN 0250-6793

Terada, T. (2009).Gastrointestinal stromal tumor of the uterus: a case report with genetic analyses of c-kit and PDGFRA genes.*International journal of gynecological pathology*, Vol.28, No.1, (January 2009), pp. 29-34, ISSN 1538-7151

Tetel, M.J.; Auger, A.P. & Charlier, T.D. (2009).Who's in charge? Nuclear receptor coactivator and corepressor function in brain and behavior. *Frontiers in neuroendocrinology*,Vol.30, No.3, (August 2009), pp. 328-342, ISSN 1095-6808

Tremblay, G.B.; Tremblay, A.; Copeland, N.G.; Gilbert, D.J.; Jenkins, N.A.; Labrie, F. & Giguère, V. (1997). Cloning, chromosomal localization, and functional analysis of the murine estrogen receptor beta.*Molecular endocrinology*,Vol.11, No.3, (March 1997), pp. 353-365, ISSN 1944-9917

Zhou, J.; Zhang, Y.; Wen, X.; Cao, J.; Li, D.; Lin, Q.; Wang, H.; Liu, Z.; Duan, C.; Wu, K. & Wang, C. (2010). Telocytes accompanying cardiomyocyte in primary culture: two- and three-dimensional culture environment. *Journal of cellular and molecular medicine*, Vol.14, No.11, (November 2010), pp. 2641-2645, ISSN 1582-4934

Zomer, A.; Vendrig, T.; Hopmans, E.S.; van Eijndhoven, M.; Middeldorp, J.M. & Pegtel, D.M. (2010).Exosomes: Fit to deliver small RNA. *Communicative & integrative biology*,Vol.3, No.5, (September 2010), pp. 447-50, ISSN 1942-0889

6

Sex Differences and the Role of Sex Steroids in Sympatho-Adrenal Medullary System and Hypothalamo-Pituitary Adrenal Axis Responses to Stress

Anne I. Turner[1], Charlotte L. Keating[2] and Alan J. Tilbrook[3]
[1]*Centre for Physical Activity and Nutrition Research, School of Exercise and Nutrition Sciences, Deakin University, Burwood, Victoria,*
[2]*Monash Alfred Psychiatry Research Centre, Monash University, The Alfred Hospital, Prahran, Victoria,*
[3]*Department of Physiology, Monash University, Victoria, Australia*

1. Introduction

We have undertaken a critical analysis of the role of sex and sex steroids in influencing stress responsiveness. We have reviewed the current literature regarding the manner in which the stress-induced activation of the sympatho-adrenal medullary system and the hypothalamo-pituitary adrenal axis are influenced by the sex of individuals and the sex steroids that are present and how these vary with different types of stress and in different physiological conditions. The chapter focuses predominantly on sheep and human research, although research in rodents is introduced where pertinent. Where appropriate, we draw on our extensive research published over the last two decades using sheep as an experimental model and consider how these data inform and compliment the current findings in human studies. It is clear from the literature reviewed here that there is a major need for research to understand stress responsiveness. The gaps in knowledge requiring this research are highlighted.

2. What is stress and what are the physiological responses to stress?

For a term used frequently in everyday language, stress has proven surprisingly difficult to define. Stress is a term that can appear diffuse, lacking in rigor and certainty of meaning. Nevertheless, most published definitions of stress are concerned with challenges to, or disruptions of, homeostasis. Indeed, our own working definition of stress is "a complex physiological state that embodies a range of integrative physiological and behavioral processes that occur when there is a real or perceived threat to homeostasis" [1, 2]. Certainly, the importance of the maintenance of homeostasis has long been recognized. For example, the ancient Greek philosopher Empedocles (500-430 BC) acknowledged the concept of a steady or harmonious state [3] and, in the 19th century, the work of French physiologist Claude Bernard (1813-1878) laid the groundwork for appreciating the importance of adaptive internal mechanisms to challenges [3]. Bernard developed the concept that organisms maintain a stable internal environment (*milieu intérieur*). This concept and understanding was substantially extended by the groundbreaking research of American physiologist Walter Cannon (1871-1945) [3]. It was Cannon who devised the term "homeostasis" and who noted that animals and humans in dangerous situations showed adaptive responses in which they may choose to fight or to escape, termed the "fight or flight" syndrome [4]. Clearly, this requires rapid responses of the body and the physiological system primarily responsible for these adaptive responses is the sympatho-adrenal medullary system. The work of Cannon inspired another researcher, Hans Selye (1907 Vienna-1982, Montreal), whose seminal work during the 1930's at McGill University in Montreal, Canada, led to the development of a theory to describe the concept of stress. He developed the "General Adaptation Syndrome", defined as "the sum of all non-specific, systemic reactions of the body which ensue upon long continued exposure to stress" [5]. He depicted three stages in this response: 1) the alarm reaction, which involved activation of the hypothalamo-pituitary adrenal axis, 2) the period of resistance, where the organism "coped" with the challenge and 3) the stage of exhaustion, where the organism's ability to resist or adapt to the challenge declined [5]. A premise of this theory is that organisms have a generalized and non-specific response to all noxious stimuli [5]. While it is now recognized that there may be different types of physiological responses to different stressful environments [1], Selye unquestionably founded the field of stress physiology and provided the framework to define and understand stress. His work continues to stimulate debate and research. Importantly, his work demonstrated the paramount role of the hypothalamo-pituitary adrenal axis in adaption to stressful situations [5].

It follows from the work of Cannon and Selye that the two most common physiological responses to stress are activation of the sympatho-adrenal medullary system and the hypothalamo-pituitary adrenal axis (Figure 1). The former is activated immediately upon threat or detection of a noxious stimulus and the response is transient, whereas the latter is activated less rapidly and the response is more prolonged. It is common practice to define threats and noxious stimuli that cause stress responses as stressors [1, 2]. While the sympatho-adrenal medullary system and hypothalamo-pituitary adrenal axis are considered the primary means of dealing with stressors, there are other responses, mostly of a neural and neuroendocrine nature, such as the opioidergic system [2], which contribute to an integrated stress response.

The sympatho-adrenal medullary system consists of the sympathetic nervous system and the adrenal medulla (Figure 1). The catecholamines epinephrine and norepinephrine induce the actions of the sympatho-adrenal medullary system which are primarily to stimulate rapid and vigorous neural, behavioral and muscular activity, to stimulate the cardiovascular system to increase cardiac output and redistribute blood flow to the pulmonary blood system and appropriate organs to deal with the stressor [6]. The catecholamines bind to adrenergic receptors, of which there are different subtypes, termed α and β, and this allows for divergent effects in target tissues [6]. The sympathetic component, or "arm", of the sympatho-adrenal medullary system, comprises pre-ganglionic neurons that project from the spinal cord to the various ganglia in the body where they synapse with post-ganglionic neurons that project to, and innervate, target tissues. Acetylcholine from the pre-ganglionic neurons stimulates the post-ganglionic neurons which release norepinephrine into the target tissue. In the adrenal arm of the sympatho-adrenal medullary system, pre-ganglionic

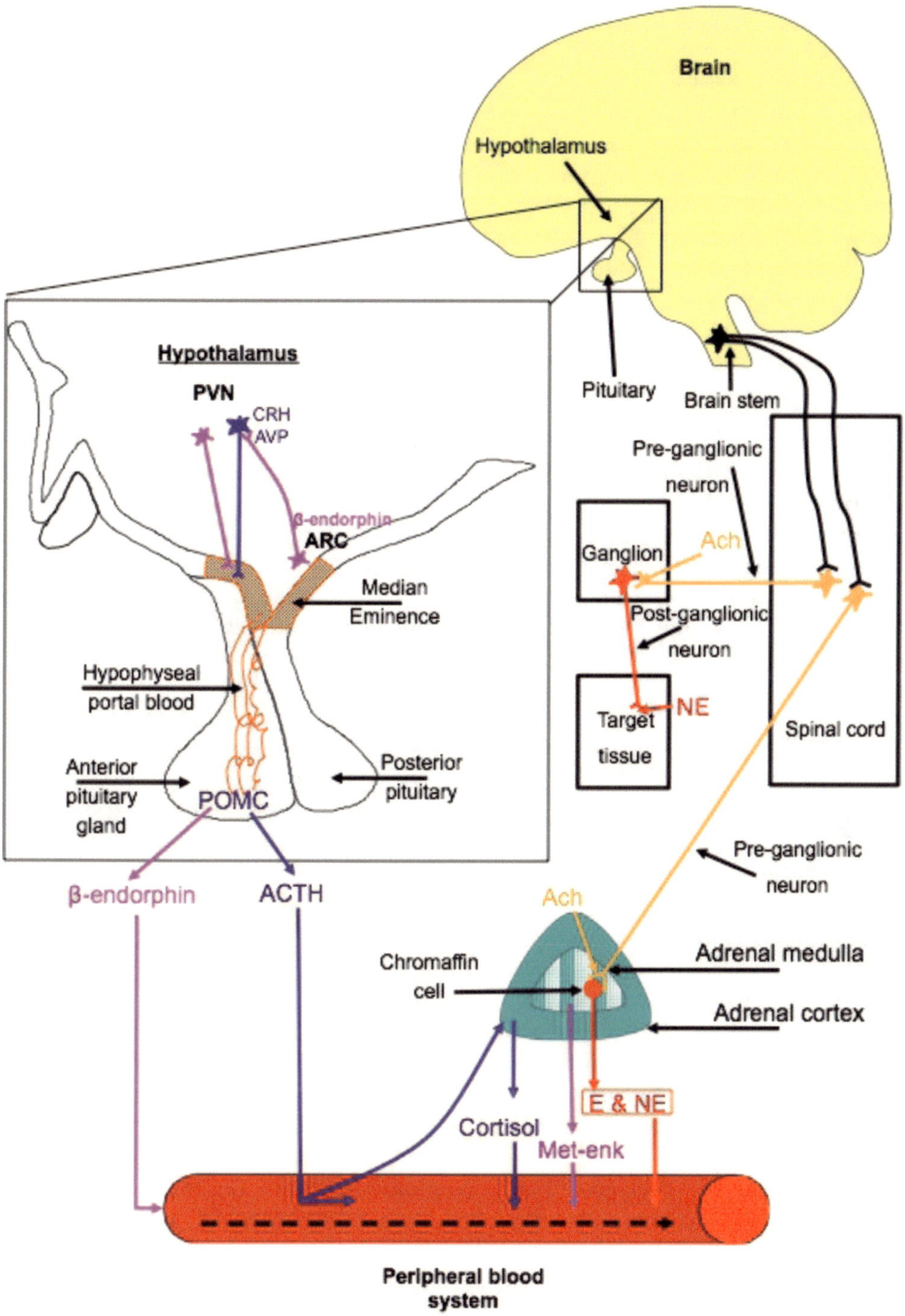

Fig. 1. Schematic diagram of the sympatho-adrenal medullary system, hypothalamo-pituitary adrenal axis and some opioidergic pathways. The sympatho-adrenal medullary system consists of the sympathetic nervous system and adrenal medulla. Pre-ganglionic neurons

extend from the spinal cord to ganglia and to the adrenal medulla. When activated the preganglionic neurons release the neurotransmitter acetylcholine (Ach) that stimulates postganglionic neurons to release norepinephrine (NE) directly into target tissue and endocrine cells called chromaffin cells in the adrenal medulla to release epinephrine (E) and NE into the peripheral blood system. The hypothalamo-pituitary adrenal axis is regulated by corticotropin releasing hormone (CRH) and arginine vasopressin (AVP) in the paraventricular nucleus (PVN) of the hypothalamus which are released into the hypophyseal portal blood system and transported to the anterior pituitary. They stimulate the synthesis of pro-opiomelanocortin (POMC) resulting in various products including adrenocorticotropic hormone (ACTH) and the opioid β-endorphin, which are secreted into the peripheral blood system. ACTH acts at the adrenal cortex to stimulate synthesis of the glucocorticoids which are cortisol in humans and non-rodent species (shown here) and corticosterone in rodents and avian species. β-endorphin is also synthesized in the arcuate nucleus (ARC) and the opioid met-enkephalin (Met-enk) in the adrenal medulla in response to stress.

neurons innervate endocrine cells, called chromaffin cells, in the adrenal medulla, stimulating them to synthesize epinephrine and norepinephrine, and to secrete both catecholamines into the systemic circulation. These catecholamines then act as classic hormones, affecting target tissues throughout the body. It is generally considered that more epinephrine than norepinephrine is released from the adrenal medulla into the systemic circulation [7] because norepinephrine is converted to epinephrine [6]. While this may be the case in various species, possibly including humans, in sheep the adrenal medulla secretes substantially more norepinephrine than epinephrine [8].

The hypothalamo-pituitary adrenal axis is often referred to as the "Stress System" and one might imagine that this is a result of the work of Selye that effectively identified the importance of the adrenal glands in coping with stress. This is a classic neuroendocrine axis where the hypothalamus of the brain controls the activity of the adrenal glands via the anterior pituitary gland (Figure 1). The adrenals are located in the visceral cavity superior to the kidneys. Neurons in each paraventricular nucleus of the hypothalamus synthesize the neuropeptides that are released when stressors activate the hypothalamo-pituitary adrenal axis. These are referred to as hypophysiotropic hormones [9] and in the case of the hypothalamo-pituitary adrenal axis are corticotropic releasing hormone (CRH) [10] and, in all species studied except the pig, arginine vasopressin (AVP) [11]. In the pig, lysine substitutes for arginine to form lysine vasopressin [2]. CRH and AVP are secreted from the terminals of neurons directly into the primary capillary bed of a specialized portal blood system that communicates between the hypothalamus and anterior pituitary gland. This is the hypophyseal portal blood system [9]. CRH and AVP are transported by portal vessels to the secondary capillary bed where they exit and act upon corticotropes, the endocrine cells that produce peptides derived from pro-opiomelanocortin (POMC). These include adrenocorticotropic hormone (ACTH), the opioid β-endorphin and α-melanocyte stimulating hormone [12-16]. Of these, ACTH is of major importance when it comes to regulation of the hypothalamo-pituitary adrenal axis. ACTH acts on the cortex of the adrenal glands to stimulate the synthesis of steroids, including the glucocorticoids, which are essential in responding to stress. In many species, including humans, the predominant glucocorticoid released from the adrenal glands is cortisol. In rodents and avian species it is corticosterone [1]. As the name suggests, glucocorticoids have glucoregulatory actions, evident as widespread effects to mobilize energy stores throughout the body [17-24]. Furthermore, these hormones have far reaching effects on most tissues, organs and systems with the objective of re-establishing homeostasis [17-24].

The hypothalamo-pituitary adrenal axis is regulated by various neural inputs and negative feedback by the glucocorticoids. There are extensive neuronal pathways within the central nervous system that are activated during stress and there are multiple interactions between these systems (for review see [1]). For example, there are reciprocal connections between noradrenergic neurons located in the brain stem (A_1, A_2 and A_6 noradrenergic cell groups) and CRH and AVP neurons in the paraventricular nuclei of the hypothalamus that are important in mounting a stress response [1]. There are also reciprocal interactions between CRH and AVP neurons and cells in the arcuate nucleus, particularly those expressing peptides derived from POMC, including β-endorphin [1]. It has been shown in rats that serotonergic neurons project from the raphe nucleus of the midbrain to the hypothalamus, and there are interactions between serotoninergic cells, the hypothalamo-pituitary adrenal axis and the sympathetic nervous system [1]. There are also neurons that produce the opioid peptide enkephalin in the paraventricular nucleus but the significance of these with respect to stress responses are unknown [1].

The negative feedback effects of glucocorticoids on the brain are mediated via high affinity mineralocorticoid receptors (MR) and low affinity glucocorticoid receptors (GR). MR are present in the hippocampus and other regions of the limbic system, including the amygdala and lateral septum, and in the hypothalamus [1, 2]. Glucocorticoids act via MR to maintain the basal activity of the hypothalamo-pituitary adrenal axis [25, 26]. The distribution of GR within the brain is much more widespread than for MR and they are found extensively within the hypothalamus and also the anterior pituitary gland [27]. GR are involved in the negative feedback actions of both basal and stress-induced levels of glucocorticoids, particularly the latter and facilitate homeostasis when stress levels of glucocorticoids prevail [25, 26, 28]. The hypothalamo-pituitary adrenal undergoes a circadian rhythm of regulation and this is evident in the negative feedback actions of the glucocorticoids [17-24].

While the sympatho-adrenal medullary system and the hypothalamo-pituitary adrenal axis are acknowledged as the front-line physiological systems to deal with stress, the opioids (Figure 1) also have a diverse range of stress-related actions [2]. There are three classes of opioids: β-endorphin, the enkephalins (met-enkephalin and leu-enkephalin) and dynorphin. The opioids act via different receptor subtypes (termed μ, δ and κ) and β-endorphin is the opioid most studied in terms of responses to stress (for review see [2]). As indicated above, β-endorphin is involved in the regulation of the hypothalamo-pituitary adrenal axis and the opioids are generally considered to attenuate and terminate stress responses [2]. Furthermore, these neuropeptides regulate sympathetic, cardiovascular and neural control systems and are involved in the regulation of pain, reinforcement and reward, the release of neurotransmitters and other autonomic and neuroendocrine functions [2].

Although the opioids clearly play various roles in responses to stress, and in regulating hypothalamo-pituitary adrenal axis responses to stress, it remains the case that most research on stress, particularly with respect to responses to, and impact of, different stressors has been on the sympatho-adrenal medullary system and the hypothalamo-pituitary adrenal axis. Consequently, we focus on these systems here, while acknowledging the need for a greater understanding of the roles of the opioidergic and other central systems in stress responses, and in the impact of stress on physiology and behaviour.

3. Stress and health

Irrespective of the precise definition of stress that one chooses, it is clear that stress embodies a range of physiological and behavioral processes that occur when there is a real or perceived threat to homeostasis. These adaptive responses are designed to re-establish homeostasis and allow coping. For the most part, this is what they do but if the various stress systems are repeatedly or continuously activated over long periods the effects can be deleterious for health [18, 20-24, 29-33]. This is not surprising when one considers the actions of catecholamines and glucocorticoids, as well as other stress hormones and neuropeptides like the opioids. For example, stimulation of the cardiovascular system and mobilization of energy have clear benefits in the short term in dealing with stress but the longer term effects will likely have harmful outcomes, increasing the chance of cardiovascular disease and energy deficits. This premise holds for most body systems as all tissues are affected by stress hormones. Initial benefits can become serious drawbacks, with the stress response becoming pathological.

Severe stress is associated with the increased prevalence of devastating conditions such as major depression, dementia and impaired cognition; cardiovascular disease; impaired immune function with increased vulnerability to disease; impaired growth and reproductive function; osteoporosis; diabetes, the metabolic syndrome and reduced life expectancy [18, 20-24, 29-47]. Some of the conditions associated with severe stress, such as major depression and cardiovascular disease, are amongst the most serious and costly to treat [17][48]. As with most areas of stress research, it is the hypothalamo-pituitary adrenal axis that has received most attention in terms of the impact on health. Nevertheless, as indicated, repeated and chronic activation of the sympatho-adrenal medullary system can lead to disorders and the increased prevalence of ill-health. In addition to stress, there are clinical conditions where the concentrations of glucocorticoids are pathologically high, and this is associated with physiological and behavioral dysfunction similar to that seen during chronic stress. These conditions include Cushing's Syndrome [35, 36], Cushing's Disease [35, 36] obesity [37], metabolic syndrome [37], functional hypothalamic amenorrhea [38, 39], hyperthyroidism [24], Diabetes Mellitus type II [37], hypertension [37] and major depression [37].

It follows that understanding stress responses is important if preventions and treatments of the deleterious effects of stress are to be established. This understanding will need to encompass the mechanisms of responses under a range of conditions, and in response to various stressors, as well as the effects of these responses on the body. The latter is not the focus of the current discussion but the former is. Individuals react to stressors in different ways and various physiological conditions including the sex of an individual will influence stress responses [1, 49]. Given that physiological responses to stress are important determinants for health, we will consider different types of stressors, sex differences in response to stress and the importance of physiological state, particularly reproductive state, in influencing responses to stress.

4. Different types of stressors

There are many different stressors that we encounter in our daily lives. It is commonly considered that stressors can be categorized as physical stressors or psychological stressors [1]. Physical stressors are those that pose a real threat to homeostasis and which result in "reactive" glucocorticoid responses to stress, whereas psychological stressors are those that are perceived to pose a threat to homeostasis and which result in "anticipatory" glucocorticoid responses to stress. Herman and colleagues [50] asserted that "reactive" glucocorticoid responses to stress are those induced by a genuine challenge to physiological homeostasis that is recognized by sensory pathways. Such challenges may include a change in cardiovascular tone, respiratory distress, pain or circulating cytokines. In such cases, there is a direct neuronal pathway to CRH neurons in the paraventricular nucleus via the brain stem to activate the hypothalamo-pituitary adrenal axis. In contrast, "anticipatory" glucocorticoid responses to stress are not mounted in response to an actual disruption to physiological homeostasis but to the anticipation of such a disruption. These responses require some higher cortical processing involving limbic pathways [50].

Physiological responses to physical stressors may be considered appropriate since the body is being prepared for a real threat and the elevated heart rate and blood pressure and energy stores mobilised by catecholamines and glucocorticoids (see Section 2) are required to deal with the stressor. For example, a direct physical threat may require vigorous skeletal muscle activity in order to avert detrimental consequences imposed by the stressor. Conversely, physiological responses to psychological stressors are potentially more harmful since the body does not usually need to respond with a physical use of energy, certainly not for a prolonged period. This would be evident where there may be a stressful environment induced without the need for physical exercise, such as being caught in traffic on the way to an important appointment. Heart rate and blood pressure may be elevated, and energy stores mobilized, but with no obvious benefit to dealing with the stressor. An exception would be the possible beneficial effects of increased mental acuity. Nevertheless, it follows that psychological stress may be detrimental to health, particularly if it is prolonged or repeated frequently, because it unnecessarily elevates heart rate and blood pressure and mobilizes energy stores placing unnecessary strain on essential physiological systems. It is important to appreciate that excessive activation of the stress systems can have a negative impact on normal physiological functioning [19, 20, 32].

Since different types of stressors activate the physiological stress systems via different mechanisms, it is important to consider different types of stressors when considering the roles of sex and the sex steroids in influencing the responsiveness of the sympatho-adrenal medullary system and the hypothalamo-pituitary adrenal axis.

5. Sex differences in responses to stress

Men and women differ in the prevalence of chronic diseases. For example, men have a higher risk of infectious disease [51] and incidence of cardiovascular disease than women [52, 53] whereas women have a higher incidence of major depression and anxiety [54-56] and autoimmune disorders, including rheumatoid arthritis, systemic lupus erythematosus and multiple sclerosis [57] than men. Since there are also sex differences in the response to stress, the response to stress poses a potential candidate in the etiology of the chronic disease progression. As indicated above, we will focus on the sympatho-adrenal medullary system and hypothalamo-pituitary adrenal axis when considering sex differences in response to stress.

There has been relatively little research on sex differences in the response of the sympatho-adrenal medullary system to stress compared to the hypothalamo-pituitary adrenal axis, where most of the effort has been concentrated. We conducted one study comparing plasma catecholamine concentrations in gonadectomized sheep subjected to isolation and restraint stress [58]. Plasma concentrations of epinephrine were significantly elevated above pretreatment concentrations for longer in rams (2-180 minutes after the commencement of stress) than in ewes (2-25 minutes after the commencement of stress). Nevertheless, there were no consistent significant differences between rams and ewes in plasma concentrations of epinephrine [58]. Interestingly, plasma concentrations of norepinephrine were not influenced by the isolation/restraint stress in either sex [58]. The reasons for this are not apparent given that the source of both catecholamines in plasma would have been the adrenal medulla.

In humans, the issue of sex differences in responses of the sympatho-adrenal medullary system to stress has been extensively reviewed [49] and sex differences are evident, although they do not always appear consistent. One reason for this is that physiological state influence these responses [49] and only a small number of studies have standardized the stage of the menstrual cycle thereby standardizing the sex steroid milieu of females. For example, one study reported that women in both the luteal and follicular phases of the menstrual cycle had a higher increase in heart rate in response to a psychological stress (mental arithmetic) compared to men but this sex difference was not present for a physical stress (cold pressor test) [59]. Women also tended to have a higher increase in diastolic blood pressure following the mental arithmetic stress compared to men ($p<0.07$) but, again, this was not the case for the physical stress and there were no differences between the sexes for systolic blood pressure [59]. In a different study, it was found that heart rate response to a psychosocial stress (Trier Social Stress Test) was significantly higher in luteal phase women compared to men [60]. Collectively, these findings indicate that sex differences in response of the sympatho-adrenal medullary system to stress will vary with different stressors, and this has also been apparent in various other studies [49]. This is not surprising and is also the case with respect to the hypothalamo-pituitary adrenal axis (see below). Furthermore, sex differences in the response of the sympatho-adrenal medullary system to stress in humans are influenced by age and reproductive hormonal status of the women [49].

We have demonstrated sex differences in the responsiveness of the hypothalamo-pituitary adrenal axis to stress in sheep. This was quantified on the basis of plasma concentrations of cortisol and it is evident that sex differences in responses to stress vary with the stressor. For instance, female sheep had a greater cortisol response to isolation/restraint stress (Figure 2)[61], an audiovisual stress (Figure 3)[62] and a wetting stress (Figure 4)[63] compared with male sheep, whereas male sheep had a greater cortisol response to insulin induced hypoglycaemia compared with female sheep (Figure 5) [61]. It is tempting to speculate that the direction of differences between females and males in cortisol responses to stress may be explained on the basis of psychosocial compared to metabolic stressors but further research is required to ascertain this. Besides, not all stressors elicit sex differences in cortisol responses, there being no differences between the sexes in the cortisol response to exercise stress (Figure 6) [63] or to endotoxin (Figure 7) [63]. Nevertheless, when sex differences do occur in sheep, it appears that the mechanisms for this are in place early in life, at least for some stressors. In lambs, we found that females had a significantly higher cortisol response to tail docking compared to males and that this sex difference developed between one and eight weeks of age [64]. We have also investigated the mechanisms for sex differences in hypothalamo-pituitary adrenal axis responses to stress and have found various differences between males and females at each level of the axis, some of which depend on gonadal factors [65, 66], which are discussed in the next section. These include differences in neuropeptide distribution in the paraventricular nucleus of the hypothalamus [66] as well as adrenal size and adrenal responsiveness to ACTH [65].

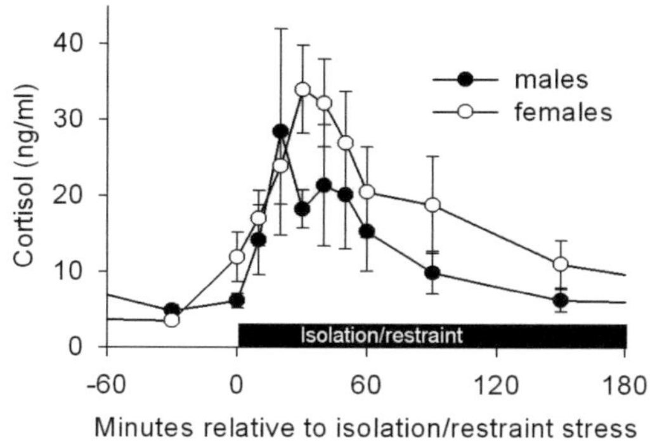

Fig. 2. Mean (±SEM) plasma concentrations of cortisol in gonadectomized male and female sheep before and during exposure to 180 min of isolation/restraint stress (indicated by the black bar). From [61].

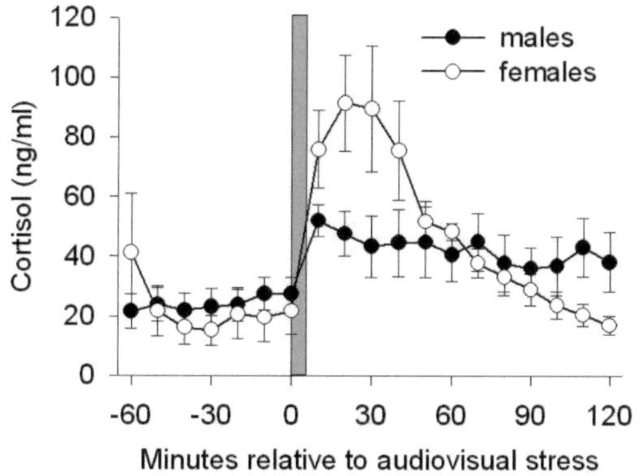

Fig. 3. Mean (±SEM) plasma concentrations of cortisol in gonadectomized male and female sheep before, during and after exposure to 5 min of audiovisual stress (barking dog; indicated by the grey bar). From [62]. *Copyright S. Karger AG, Basel*

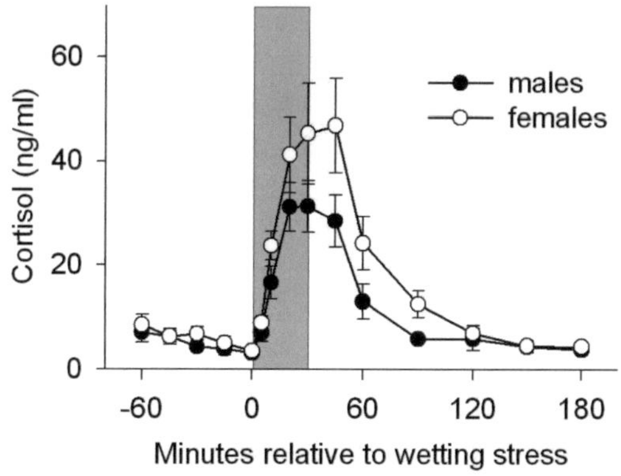

Fig. 4. Mean (±SEM) plasma concentrations of cortisol in gonadectomized male and female sheep before, during and after exposure to 30 min of wetting stress (indicated by the grey bar). From [63]. *Copyright 2010, The Endocrine Society.*

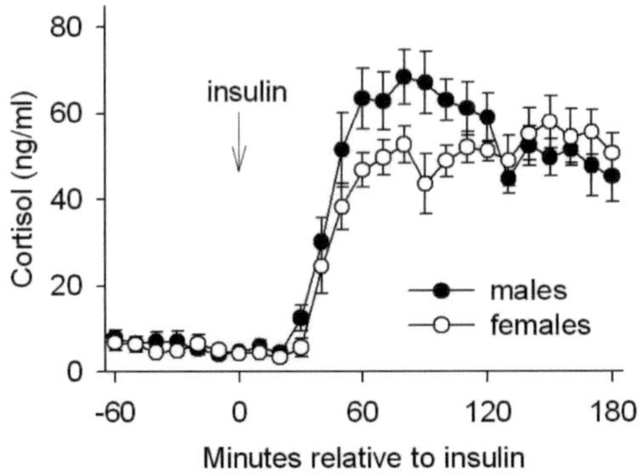

Fig. 5. Mean (±SEM) plasma concentrations of cortisol in gonadectomized male and female sheep before and after injection of insulin (indicated by the arrow). From [61].

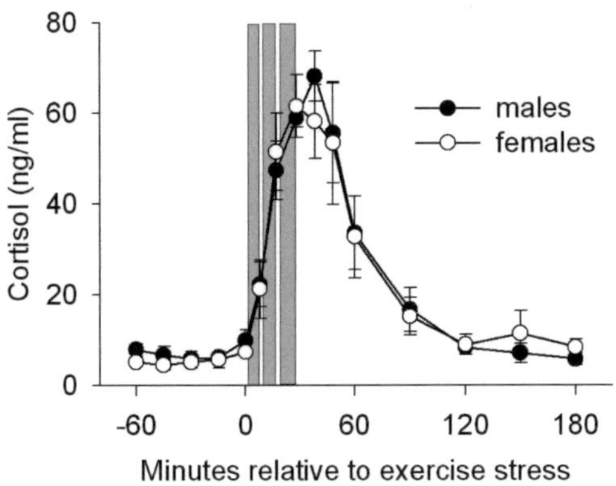

Fig. 6. Mean (±SEM) plasma concentrations of cortisol in gonadectomized male and female sheep before, during and after exercise stress, which consisted of running 3 x 0.6 km (indicated by the grey bars). From [63]. *Copyright 2010, The Endocrine Society.*

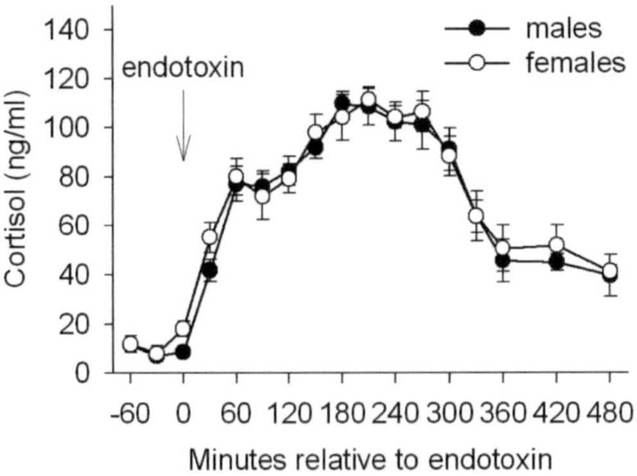

Fig. 7. Mean (±SEM) plasma concentrations of cortisol in gonadectomized male and female sheep before, during and after injection of endotoxin (indicated by the arrow). From [63]. *Copyright 2010, The Endocrine Society.*

In humans, there is also evidence that hypothalamo-pituitary adrenal axis responses to stress differ between adult men and women (see [49] for an extensive review of the literature). The initial research effort in humans was hampered by a lack of treatments that adequately activated the hypothalamo-pituitary adrenal axis [49]. More recent research has shown that there are only subtle sex differences in the basal activity of the hypothalamo-pituitary adrenal axis but these become more pronounced with the imposition of a psychological stressor. In general, it seems that between puberty and menopause, cortisol responses to psychosocial stress are lower in women compared with aged matched men [49, 67]. Nevertheless, as in our sheep studies, there is also some evidence from human studies that sex differences in cortisol responses to stress may depend on the stressor encountered since men had significantly greater cortisol responses to achievement challenges than women and women had significantly greater cortisol responses to social rejection challenges than men [49]. In contrast to studies in post-pubertal humans, few studies have found sex differences in stress responsiveness during infancy and childhood [49]. Unlike sheep where a window of development of sex differences has been identified [64], the precise stage of development of sex differences is unknown in humans. Nonetheless, there is a prolonged activation of the hypothalamo-pituitary adrenal axis to stress during adolescence (for review see [68, 69]).

While there has been various research across a range of species to try and understand the mechanisms for sex differences in responses to stress, with a large emphasis on the role of gonadal factors such as the sex steroids (see Section 6), there has been little attention paid to understanding the physiological importance of these sex differences. This needs to be considered from both an adaptive perspective, and from consideration of the impact of stress on health. With regard to the former, if one considers that stress responses are designed to re-establish homeostasis, to ward off the detrimental effects of noxious stimuli (Section 2), then one could argue that the sex with the greater catecholamine and cortisol responses to a particular stressor is the better equipped to deal with the stress. On the other hand, if one considers that prolonged or repeated activation of stress systems can be damaging to health (Section 3), then the sex with the greater response may be in the greater danger of the deleterious effects of the response. Unfortunately, these hypotheses have hitherto not been tested and this highlights an important issue requiring research. There is a need to determine the salience of stressors when undertaking sex comparisons, and there is a need to undertake sex comparisons over extended periods, and under conditions of repeated stress, to ascertain the relative impact of stress on each sex.

6. The role of sex steroids and reproductive state on stress responsiveness

It is apparent that there are interactions between the stress systems and sex steroid producing systems. This is most marked with the interactions between the hypothalamo-pituitary adrenal axis and reproductive axis, which are bidirectional. Activation of the stress systems can impact the reproductive axis [16, 70-75] and sex steroids can affect activation of the stress systems. When it comes to trying to appreciate the role of sex steroids in influencing the stress systems one is compelled to consider research in rodents because this is where the majority of investigation has been. Furthermore, most research concerning the effects of steroids on stress systems has concentrated on the hypothalamo-pituitary adrenal axis, with relatively little attention paid to the sympatho-adrenal medullary system. Nevertheless, there are actions of sex steroids on catecholaminergic neurons in various brain regions [76-80]. For example, it has been demonstrated that estradiol benzoate treatment of ovariectomized rats increased extracellular levels of norepinephrine and dopamine in the pre-optic area of the hypothalamus during the dark phase [81], although this is not considered the predominant locus in regulating the sympatho-adrenal medullary system. Furthermore, sexually dimorphic responses in activation of the locus coeruleus-norepinephrine system have been shown in rats [82] although it is possible that this is more important to regulation of the hypothalamo-pituitary adrenal axis than the sympatho-adrenal medullary system. An *in vitro* study showed that estradiol-17β stimulated catecholamine synthesis from adrenal medullary cells, which is direct evidence that this steroid is capable of influencing the sympatho-adrenal medullary system [83]. In human females, one study found that sympathetic nervous activity in response to mental stress was similar between the early follicular phase and mid-luteal phase but the recovery was prolonged during the mid-luteal phase [84]. A number of other investigations in women have reported that estrogen attenuates sympathetic activity in response to stress although this has not been found in all studies (for review see [49]). An attenuating effect on sympathetic activity in response to mental arithmetic was also demonstrated in young men treated with estradiol [85]. Nonetheless, these were not extended to the complete sympatho-adrenal medullary system and little is known about the effects of progesterone and testosterone on this stress system.

The body of work in rodents and humans has generally suggested that females have higher basal glucocorticoid levels than males [86, 87]. In rodents, females also have higher stress-induced ACTH and glucocorticoid responses [88-90] than males and this is due, at least in part, to a stimulatory effect of estradiol on the hypothalamo-pituitary adrenal axis [91-93]. One possible mechanism for this may involve enhanced CRH expression because there are estrogen-responsive elements on the 5′ regulatory region of the CRH gene [93]. Estradiol has also been shown to act directly on neurons within the paraventricular nucleus via estrogen receptor α [94]. Given this effect of estradiol it follows that reproductive state will affect the hypothalamo-pituitary adrenal axis and variations in activity occur across the estrous cycle of the rat [95, 96] and menstrual cycle of the monkey [97]. In contrast to estrogens, in rodents androgens are considered to inhibit the activity of the hypothalamo-pituitary adrenal axis [88, 92, 94, 98], possibly via a mechanism that involves direct actions of testosterone on neurons within the paraventricular nucleus via estrogen receptor β (for extensive review see [94]). It has been proposed that testosterone is converted to an androgenic metabolite, 5α-androstane-3β,17β-diol, that binds estrogen receptor β to regulate oxytocinergic neurons in the paraventricular nucleus [94]. Despite these opposing actions of estrogens and androgens on the activity of the hypothalamo-pituitary adrenal axis in rodents, the roles of sex steroids in influencing stress responses are less clear-cut in other species, and it is unknown if similar mechanism of action exist in non-rodent species.

We have not directly addressed the effects of steroids on the sympatho-adrenal medullary system in sheep but have considered sex differences and the importance of the gonads when it comes to the hypothalamo-pituitary adrenal axis. In adult sheep we identified a range of differences between males and females in the hypothalamo-pituitary adrenal axis and some, but not all, of these differences depended on gonadal factors [99]. Of significance in this study was an enhanced adrenocortical response to ACTH in females compared to males, and this occurred irrespective of the presence or absence of gonads. Males had higher AVP in the median eminence than females and gonadectomy increased this in both sexes [99].

Gonadectomy also elevated median eminence content of CRH but there was no difference between sexes. There was no effect of *in vitro* ACTH secretion in response to treatment with AVP, CRH and the two in combination [99]. Our research in prepubertal sheep has also shown that some sex differences in the activity of the hypothalamo-pituitary adrenal axis endure in the absence of the sex steroids [64]. Consistent with these findings, we also showed that sex and gonadal status affect the distribution of CRH, AVP and enkephalin in the paraventricular nucleus of sheep, providing a neuroanatomical basis for sex differences in the central regulation of the hypothalamo-pituitary adrenal axis [66]. Others have shown that steroids and reproductive state can affect the activity of the hypothalamo-pituitary adrenal axis in female sheep [100], but there were no comparisons with males. In a series of studies in ewes it was shown that progesterone inhibits ACTH stimulation of cortisol [101, 102, 103] and stress, induced secretion of cortisol estrogens and androgens influence hypothalamic concentrations of CRH and AVP [104], and that ovariectomy affects hypothalamo-pituitary adrenal axis responses to stress [105, 106]. While it is clear that gonadal factors, such as the sex steroids, and reproductive state, influence the activity of the hypothalamo-pituitary adrenal axis in sheep, there is a need for more extensive research to establish the precise roles of steroids and reproductive state, including with regard to different stressors.

In women the stage of the reproductive cycle has been shown to affect the hypothalamo-pituitary adrenal axis responses to stress (for an extensive review see [49]). It has been consistently reported that cortisol responses to psychosocial stress were lower in women in the follicular phase of the menstrual cycle compared with women in the luteal phase of the menstrual cycle [49]. This suggests that there is attenuation of the hypothalamo-pituitary adrenal axis in response to psychosocial stress in an estrogenic environment (i.e. the follicular phase), and this is supported by studies showing that women taking a synthetic estrogen as an oral contraceptive had similar cortisol responses to psychosocial stress compared to women in the follicular phase of the menstrual cycle and lower than those in the luteal phase [49]. An attenuating action of estradiol on stress-induced hypothalamo-pituitary adrenal axis activity in women is similar to the effects of estrogen on the autonomic nervous system but contrasts with the situation in rodents, where estradiol generally has facilitatory actions (see above). There has been considerably less research on the role of the other principal ovarian steroid, progesterone, in influencing the hypothalamo-pituitary adrenal axis. In rodents, progesterone has been reported to suppress the hypothalamo-pituitary adrenal axis response to stress [107-109] and there is now direct evidence to suggest that this is also the case in men, although there may be divergent effects on the sympatho-adrenal medullary system [110]. Administration of progesterone to men attenuated cortisol responses to the Trier Social Stress Test and reduced negative mood and alertness after stress but increased plasma norepinephrine and systolic blood pressure [110]. A similar approach has not been undertaken in women although in a study that utilised positive emotion-arousing there was a positive correlation between salivary progesterone and cortisol in men and in women taking hormonal contraceptives but not in women undergoing natural menstrual cycles, prompting the authors to suggest that progesterone may play a role in down-regulating the stress response [111]. Testosterone may also have a down regulating effect on the stress systems in humans because administration of testosterone to women resulted in decreased stress responsiveness [112-114], which is similar to the case in rodents (see above). While a role for testosterone in regulating the activity of the hypothalamo-pituitary adrenal axis was suggested [112], the collective work of these authors (e.g. [112-114]) also implicates a regulatory role for testosterone on the autonomic nervous system and, possibly, the sympatho-adrenal medullary system. Further research is necessary to confirm this and the research needs to be extended to males.

Lactation is a physiological state that can have profound effects on both the basal and stress-induced activity of the hypothalamo-pituitary adrenal axis. In many species, including humans, ungulates and rodents, it has been consistently found that lactating females show attenuated neuroendocrine responses to stress (for reviews see [115-117]) and anxiety-related behaviours (for reviews see [116, 118, 119]). The alterations in the hypothalamo-pituitary adrenal axis that result in reduced responses to stress begin to emerge in late pregnancy and occur in a continuum throughout lactation (for reviews see [116, 118, 120, 121]). Although the mechanisms for attenuated hypothalamo-pituitary adrenal axis responses to stress during lactation are not fully known, it appears that they include reduced synthesis and secretion of CRH and AVP due to enhanced negative feedback by glucocorticoids and/or reduced noradrenergic stimulatory input from the brain stem, reduced pituitary responsiveness to CRH and AVP and, possibly, inhibition by oxytocin and prolactin [1]. We have shown in sheep that the greatest attenuation of the hypothalamo-pituitary adrenal axis is achieved when the lactating mother is suckled [122] and this is likely to also be the case for humans when breastfeeding [1]. Despite the many published reports of attenuated stress responses in lactating females this has not always been the case and the nature of the stressor seems to be important. It has been shown in both sheep [123] and humans [87] that the there is activation of the hypothalamo-pituitary adrenal axis in response to a stressor that may threaten the welfare of the infant by virtue of harming the mother. This makes perfect sense given that the mother would require a stress response in order to dispose of the threat posed to herself and her offspring. This underscores the importance of being able to mount stress responses so that homeostasis can be restored (Section 1).

7. Conclusions

Although there are various ways to define stress there is generally acceptance that stress responses occur in response to noxious stimuli, whether perceived or real, commonly called stressors. A range of physiological systems are activated with the two of the most prominent being the sympatho-adrenal medullary system and the hypothalamo-pituitary adrenal axis. The catecholamines and glucocorticoids, released by each system respectively, have far-reaching effects within the body to re-establish the homeostasis that was disrupted by stressors. Such stress responses are vital for a healthy life. Nevertheless, when the stress systems are frequently or continually activated, the on-going action of the catecholamines and glucocorticoids can be destructive and lead to pathological conditions. An inability to mount an appropriate stress response may also result in illness. Therefore, it follows that understanding stress responses, and the factors that affect stress responses, is paramount to develop strategies and treatments to avoid or cure stress-induced disorders and pathologies. These factors include sex, sex steroids and physiological state, particularly reproductive state. There are differences between males and females in various illnesses and pathological states and many of these are those induced or exacerbated by frequent or chronic stress. Males and females respond differently to some stressors and not others. The implications for health and survival of these different stress responses are unknown and research is required to determine this. At least some of the mechanisms for sex differences in stress responses are due to gonadal factors, such as the sex steroids, but others are not. There also appear to be differences between species in the impact of sex steroids on the stress systems. For example, whereas estrogens appear to facilitate and androgens abrogate stress responses in rodents, the actions of estrogens on stress responses in humans may be the opposite, at least in some cases, and the effects of androgens have received insufficient research in non-rodent species to draw definitive conclusions. Nevertheless, since there are effects of sex steroids on stress responsiveness, there are differences in stress responsiveness at different stages of the female reproductive cycle. Furthermore, during lactation, stress responses are generally attenuated, unless the stressor threatens the well-being of the mother and, in turn, the offspring.

This review has highlighted substantial gaps in knowledge that are required to fully appreciate the field of stress physiology. These include understanding mechanisms of stress responses to different types of stressors, between sexes and in different physiological states. They also include the mechanisms by which different stressors impact the body of males and females in different physiological states.

8. Acknowledgements

We acknowledge Deakin University and Monash University for their support. We are grateful to the Australian Research Council and National Health and Medical Research Council of Australia for funding the research that generated the data presented in this chapter. We also thank Sara Drew for proof reading this manuscript.

9. References

[1] Tilbrook, A.J. and I.J. Clarke, *Neuroendocrine mechanisms of innate states of attenuated responsiveness of the hypothalamo-pituitary adrenal axis to stress.* Frontiers in Neuroendocrinology, 2006. 27(3): p. 285-307.

[2] Tilbrook, A.J., *Neuropeptides, Stress-Related,* in *Encyclopedia of stress*, G. Fink, Editor. 2007, Academic Press: Oxford. p. 903-908.

[3] Johnson, E.O., et al., *Mechanisms of stress: a dynamic overview of hormonal and behavioral homeostasis. [Review] [218 refs].* Neuroscience & Biobehavioral. Reviews., 1992. 16(2): p. 115-130.

[4] Cannon, W., *The Wisdom of the Body*. 1932, New York: Norton.

[5] Selye, H., *The general adaptation syndrome and the diseases of adaption.* Journal of Clinical Endocrinology and Metabolism, 1946. 6: p. 117-230.

[6] Goldstein, D.S. and A. Grossman, *Stress-induced activation of the sympathetic nervous system,* in *Neuroendocrinology of Stress*. 1987, Bailliere Tindall: London. p. 253-278.

[7] Axelrod, J. and T.D. Reisine, *Stress hormones: their interaction and regulation.* Science, 1984. 224: p. 452-459.

[8] Stackpole, C.A., et al., Seasonal differences in the effect of isolation and restraint stress on the luteinizing hormone response to gonadotropin-releasing hormone in hypothalamopituitary disconnected, gonadectomized rams and ewes. Biology of Reproduction, 2003. 69(4): p. 1158-1164.

[9] Harris, G.W., Neural control of the pituitary gland. 1955, London: Arnold.

[10] Vale, W., et al., *Characterization of a 41-residue ovine hypothalamic peptide that stimulates secretion of corticotropin and β-endorphin.* Science, 1981. 213: p. 1394-1397.

[11] Antoni, F.A., *Vasopressinergic control of pituitary adrenocorticotropin secretion comes of age.* Frontiers in Neuroendocrinology, 1993. 14: p. 76-122.
[12] Delitala, G. and M. Motta, *Opioid peptides and pituitary function Basic and clinical aspects, in Brain Endocrinology.* 1991, Ravenh Press: New York. p. 217-244.
[13] Duclos, M., et al., *Corticosterone-dependent metabolic and neuroendocrine abnormalities in obese Zucker rats in relation to feeding.* Am.J.Physiol Endocrinol.Metab, 2005. 288(1): p. E254-E266.
[14] Engler, D., et al., *Corticotropin-release inhibitory factor Evidence for dual stimulatory and inhibitory hypothalamic regulation over adrenocorticotropin secretion and biosynthesis.* Trends in Endocrinology and Metabolism, 1994. 5: p. 2-13.
[15] Bohus, B., et al., *Neuroendocrine states and behavioral and physiological stress responses.* Prog.Brain Res., 1987. 72: p. 57-70.
[16] Rivier, C. and S. Rivest, *Effect of stress on the activity of the hypothalamic-pituitary- gonadal axis: peripheral and central mechanisms.* Biology of Reproduction, 1991. 45: p. 523-532.
[17] Chrousos, G.P., *The HPA axis and the stress response.* Endocrine Research, 2000. 26(4): p. 513-514.
[18] Chrousos, G.P., *Stress, chronic inflammation, and emotional and physical well-being: concurrent effects and chronic sequelae.* J.Allergy Clin.Immunol., 2000. 106(5 Suppl): p. S275-S291.
[19] Chrousos, G.P., *The role of stress and the hypothalamic-pituitary-adrenal axis in the pathogenesis of the metabolic syndrome: neuro-endocrine and target tissue-related causes.* International Journal of Obesity, 2000. 24: p. S50-S55.
[20] Chrousos, G.P., *Stress and disorders of the stress system.* Nature Reviews Endocrinology, 2009. 5(7): p. 374-381.
[21] Chrousos, G.P., *Regulation and dysregulation of the hypothalamic-pituitary-adrenal axis. The corticotropin-releasing hormone perspective.* Endocrinol.Metab Clin.North Am., 1992. 21(4): p. 833-858.
[22] Chrousos, G.P., *Stressors, stress, and neuroendocrine integration of the adaptive response. The 1997 Hans Selye Memorial Lecture.* Annals.of the.New York.Academy.of Sciences., 1998. 851: p. 311-335.
[23] Chrousos, G.P., *The role of stress and the hypothalamic-pituitary-adrenal axis in the pathogenesis of the metabolic syndrome: neuro-endocrine and target tissue-related causes.* Int.J.Obes.Relat Metab Disord., 2000. 24 Suppl 2: p. S50-S55.
[24] Sapolsky, R.M., L.M. Romero, and A.U. Munck, *How do glucocorticoids influence stress responses? Integrating permissive, suppressive, stimulatory, and preparative actions [Review].* Endocrine Reviews, 2000. 21(1): p. 55-89.
[25] Miller, A.H., et al., *Adrenal steroid receptor activation in rat brain and pituitary following dexamethasone: implications for the dexamethasone suppression test.* Biol.Psychiatry, 1992. 32(10): p. 850-869.
[26] Reul, J.M. and E.R. de Kloet, *Two receptor systems for corticosterone in rat brain: microdistribution and differential occupation.* Endocrinology, 1985. 117(6): p. 2505-2511.
[27] de Kloet, E.R., N.Y. Rots, and A.R. Cools, *Brain-corticosteroid hormone dialogue: slow and persistent.* Cell Mol.Neurobiol., 1996. 16(3): p. 345-356.
[28] Kim, P.J., et al., *Evaluation of RU28318 and RU40555 as selective mineralocorticoid receptor and glucocorticoid receptor antagonists, respectively: receptor measures and functional studies.* J.Steroid Biochem.Mol.Biol., 1998. 67(3): p. 213-222.

[29] Sapolsky, R.M., *Stress-induced suppression of testicular function in the wild baboon: Role of glucocorticoids.* Endocrinology, 1985. 116: p. 2273-2278.

[30] Sapolsky, R.M. and L.C. Krey, *Stress-induced suppression of luteinizing hormone concentrations in wild baboons: role of opiates.* Journal of Clinical Endocrinology & Metabolism, 1988. 66(4): p. 722-726.

[31] Sapolsky, R.M. and G.E. Mott, *Social subordinance in wild baboons is associated with suppressed high density lipoprotein-cholesterol concentrations: the possible role of chronic social stress.* Endocrinology, 1987. 121(5): p. 1605-1610.

[32] Sapolsky, R.M., *Glands, Gooseflesh and Hormones*, in *Why zebra's don't get ulcers: a guide to stress, stress-related diseases and coping*. 1994, W.H. Freeman and Company: New York. p. 20-36.

[33] Tombaugh, G.C. and R.M. Sapolsky, *Endocrine features of glucocorticoid endangerment in hippocampal astrocytes.* Neuroendocrinology., 1993. 57: p. 7-13.

[34] Stoney, C.M., et al., *Influences of the normal menstrual cycle on physiologic functioning during behavioral stress.* Psychophysiology, 1990. 27(2): p. 125-135.

[35] Schobel, H.P., et al., *Preeclampsia -- a state of sympathetic overactivity.* N Engl J Med, 1996. 335(20): p. 1480-5.

[36] Phillips, D.I., et al., *Elevated plasma cortisol concentrations: a link between low birth weight and the insulin resistance syndrome?* J Clin Endocrinol Metab, 1998. 83(3): p. 757-60.

[37] Phillips, D.I., et al., *Low birth weight predicts elevated plasma cortisol concentrations in adults from 3 populations.* Hypertension, 2000. 35(6): p. 1301-6.

[38] Heim, C., U. Ehlert, and D.H. Hellhammer, *The potential role of hypocortisolism in the pathophysiology of stress-related bodily disorders.* Psychoneuroendocrinology, 2000. 25(1): p. 1-35.

[39] Yang, C.C., et al., *Preeclamptic pregnancy is associated with increased sympathetic and decreased parasympathetic control of HR.* Am J Physiol Heart Circ Physiol, 2000. 278(4): p. H1269-73.

[40] Kajantie, E., et al., *Placental 11 beta-hydroxysteroid dehydrogenase-2 and fetal cortisol/cortisone shuttle in small preterm infants.* J Clin Endocrinol Metab, 2003. 88(1): p. 493-500.

[41] Kajantie, E., et al., *Pre-eclampsia is associated with increased risk of stroke in the adult offspring: the Helsinki birth cohort study.* Stroke, 2009. 40(4): p. 1176-80.

[42] Kajantie, E., et al., *Size at birth as a predictor of mortality in adulthood: a follow-up of 350 000 person-years.* Int J Epidemiol, 2005. 34(3): p. 655-63.

[43] Tsigos, C. and G.P. Chrousos, *Hypothalamic-pituitary-adrenal axis, neuroendocrine factors and stress.* J.Psychosom.Res., 2002. 53(4): p. 865-871.

[44] Treiber, F.A., et al., *Cardiovascular reactivity and development of preclinical and clinical disease states.* Psychosom Med, 2003. 65(1): p. 46-62.

[45] Kreier, F., et al., *Hypothesis: shifting the equilibrium from activity to food leads to autonomic unbalance and the metabolic syndrome.* Diabetes, 2003. 52(11): p. 2652-6.

[46] Schwartz, A.R., et al., *Toward a causal model of cardiovascular responses to stress and the development of cardiovascular disease.* Psychosom Med, 2003. 65(1): p. 22-35.

[47] Brown, E.S., F.P. Varghese, and B.S. McEwen, *Association of depression with medical illness: does cortisol play a role?* Biol Psychiatry, 2004. 55(1): p. 1-9.

[48] Licinio, J. and M.L. Wong, *Depression, antidepressants and suicidality: a critical appraisal.* Nat Rev Drug Discov, 2005. 4(2): p. 165-71.

[49] Kajantie, E. and D.I. Phillips, *The effects of sex and hormonal status on the physiological response to acute psychosocial stress.* Psychoneuroendocrinology, 2006. 31(2): p. 151-78.

[50] Herman, J.P., et al., *Central mechanisms of stress integration: hierarchical circuitry controlling hypothalamo-pituitary-adrenocortical responsiveness.* Front Neuroendocrinol., 2003. 24(3): p. 151-180.

[51] Klein, S.L., *The effects of hormones on sex differences in infection: from genes to behavior.* Neurosci Biobehav Rev, 2000. 24(6): p. 627-38.

[52] Pilote, L., et al., *A comprehensive view of sex-specific issues related to cardiovascular disease.* Canadian Medical Association Journal, 2007. 176(6): p. S1-S44.

[53] Tunstall-Pedoe, H., et al., *Contribution of trends in survival and coronary-event rates to changes in coronary heart disease mortality: 10-year results from 37 WHO MONICA Project populations.* Lancet, 1999. 353(9164): p. 1547-1557.

[54] Bekker, M.H.J. and J. van Mens-Verhulst, *Anxiety disorders: Sex differences in prevalence, degree, and background, but gender-neutral treatment.* Gender Medicine, 2007. 4: p. S178-S193.

[55] Breslau, N., H. Chilcoat, and L.R. Schultz, *Anxiety disorders and the emergence of sex differences in major depression.* J Gend Specif Med, 1998. 1(3): p. 33-9.

[56] Earls, F., *SEX-DIFFERENCES IN PSYCHIATRIC-DISORDERS - ORIGINS AND DEVELOPMENTAL INFLUENCES.* Psychiatric Developments, 1987. 5(1): p. 1-23.

[57] Beeson, P.B., *Age and sex associations of 40 autoimmune diseases.* Am J Med, 1994. 96(5): p. 457-62.

[58] Stackpole, C.A., et al., *Seasonal differences in the effect of isolation and restraint stress on the luteinizing hormone response to gonadotropin-releasing hormone in hypothalamopituitary disconnected, gonadectomized rams and ewes.* Biology of Reproduction, 2003. 69: p. 1158-1164.

[59] Tersman, Z., A. Collins, and P. Eneroth, *Cardiovascular responses to psychological and physiological stressors during the menstrual cycle.* Psychosom.Med., 1991. 53(2): p. 185-197.

[60] Kudielka, B.M., et al., *Differential heart rate reactivity and recovery after psychosocial stress (TSST) in healthy children, younger adults, and elderly adults: The impact of age and gender.* International Journal of Behavioral Medicine, 2004. 11(2): p. 116-121.

[61] Turner, A.I., et al., *Influence of sex and gonadal status of sheep on cortisol secretion in response to ACTH and on cortisol and LH secretion in response to stress: importance of different stressors.* Journal of Endocrinology, 2002. 173: p. 113-121.

[62] Turner, A.I., et al., *Noradrenaline, but not neuropeptide Y, is elevated in cerebrospinal fluid from the third cerebral ventricle following audiovisual stress in gonadectomised rams and ewes.* Neuroendocrinology, 2002. 76: p. 373-380.

[63] Turner, A.I., et al., *Stressor specificity of sex differences in hypothalamo-pituitary-adrenal axis activity: cortisol responses to exercise, endotoxin, wetting, and isolation/restraint stress in gonadectomized male and female sheep.* Endocrinology, 2010. 151(9): p. 4324-31.

[64] Turner, A.I., et al., *A sex difference in the cortisol response to tail docking and ACTH develops between 1 and 8 weeks of age in lambs.* Journal of Endocrinology, 2006. 188(3): p. 443-449.

[65] Canny, B.J., et al., *Influence of sex and gonadal status on the hypothalamo-pituitary-adrenal (HPA) axis of the sheep.* Proceedings of the International Congress on Endocrinology, 1996. 10: p. P3-3.

[66] Rivalland, E.T.A., et al., *Co-localization and distribution of corticotrophin-releasing hormone, arginine vasopressin and enkephalin in the paraventricular nucleus of sheep: A sex comparison.* Neuroscience, 2005. 132(3): p. 755-766.
[67] Maestripieri, D., et al., *Between- and within-sex variation in hormonal responses to psychological stress in a large sample of college students.* Stress, 2010. 13(5): p. 413-24.
[68] McCormick, C.M. and I.Z. Mathews, *HPA function in adolescence: role of sex hormones in its regulation and the enduring consequences of exposure to stressors.* Pharmacol Biochem Behav, 2007. 86(2): p. 220-33.
[69] McCormick, C.M., C. Smith, and I.Z. Mathews, *Effects of chronic social stress in adolescence on anxiety and neuroendocrine response to mild stress in male and female rats.* Behav Brain Res, 2008. 187(2): p. 228-38.
[70] Tilbrook, A.J., A.I. Turner, and I.J. Clarke, *Effects of stress on reproduction in non-rodent mammals: the role of glucocorticoids and sex differences.* Reviews of Reproduction, 2000. 5(2): p. 105-113.
[71] Tilbrook, A.J., A.I. Turner, and I.J. Clarke, *Stress and reproduction: central mechanisms and sex differences in non-rodent species.* Stress, 2002. 5: p. 83-100.
[72] Turner, A.I., P.H. Hemsworth, and A.J. Tilbrook, *Susceptibility of reproduction in female pigs to impairment by stress and the role of the hypothalamo-pituitary-adrenal axis.* Reproduction Fertility and Development, 2002. 14(6): p. 377-391.
[73] Turner, A.I. and A.J. Tilbrook, *Stress, cortisol and reproduction in female pigs.* Society Of Reproduction And Fertility Supplement, 2006. 62: p. 191-203.
[74] Breen, K.M. and F.J. Karsch, *New insights regarding glucocorticoids, stress and gonadotropin suppression.* Front Neuroendocrinol, 2006. 27(2): p. 233-45.
[75] Moberg, G.P., *Influence of the adrenal axis upon the gonads.* Oxford Reviews of Reproductive Biology, 1987. 9: p. 456-496.
[76] Crowley, W.R., *Effects of ovarian hormones on norepinephrine and dopamine turnover in individual hypothalamic and extrahypothalamic nuclei.* Neuroendocrinology, 1982. 34(6): p. 381-6.
[77] Deecher, D.C., et al., *Alleviation of thermoregulatory dysfunction with the new serotonin and norepinephrine reuptake inhibitor desvenlafaxine succinate in ovariectomized rodent models.* Endocrinology, 2007. 148(3): p. 1376-83.
[78] Etgen, A.M., M.A. Ansonoff, and A. Quesada, *Mechanisms of ovarian steroid regulation of norepinephrine receptor-mediated signal transduction in the hypothalamus: implications for female reproductive physiology.* Horm Behav, 2001. 40(2): p. 169-77.
[79] Renner, K.J., D.L. Allen, and V.N. Luine, *Monoamine levels and turnover in brain: relationship to priming actions of estrogen.* Brain Res Bull, 1986. 16(4): p. 469-75.
[80] Weiland, N.G. and P.M. Wise, *Estrogen alters the diurnal rhythm of alpha 1-adrenergic receptor densities in selected brain regions.* Endocrinology, 1987. 121(5): p. 1751-8.
[81] Alfinito, P.D., et al., *Estradiol increases catecholamine levels in the hypothalamus of ovariectomized rats during the dark-phase.* Eur J Pharmacol, 2009. 616(1-3): p. 334-9.
[82] Curtis, A.L., T. Bethea, and R.J. Valentino, *Sexually dimorphic responses of the brain norepinephrine system to stress and corticotropin-releasing factor.* Neuropsychopharmacology, 2006. 31(3): p. 544-54.
[83] Yanagihara, N., et al., *Stimulation of catecholamine synthesis through unique estrogen receptors in the bovine adrenomedullary plasma membrane by 17beta-estradiol.* Biochem Biophys Res Commun, 2006. 339(2): p. 548-53.

[84] Carter, J.R. and J.E. Lawrence, *Effects of the menstrual cycle on sympathetic neural responses to mental stress in humans.* J Physiol, 2007. 585(Pt 2): p. 635-41.

[85] Del Rio, G., et al., *Effect of estradiol on the sympathoadrenal response to mental stress in normal men.* J Clin Endocrinol Metab, 1994. 79(3): p. 836-40.

[86] Critchlow, V., et al., *Sex difference in resting pituitary-adrenal function in the rat.* American Journal of Physiology, 1963. 205: p. 807-815.

[87] Kaye, J., et al., *Responses to the 35% CO challenge in postpartum women.* Clin.Endocrinol.(Oxf), 2004. 61(5): p. 582-588.

[88] Handa, R.J., et al., *Gonadal steroid hormone receptors and sex differences in the hypothalamo-pituitary-adrenal axis.* Hormones and Behavior, 1994. 28: p. 464-476.

[89] Kant, G.J., et al., *Comparison of stress response in male and female rats: pituitary cyclic AMP and plasma prolactin, growth hormone and corticosterone.* Psychoneuroendocrinology, 1983. 8(4): p. 421-428.

[90] Mitsushima, D., J. Masuda, and F. Kimura, *Sex differences in the stress-induced release of acetylcholine in the hippocampus and corticosterone from the adrenal cortex in rats.* Neuroendocrinology, 2003. 78(4): p. 234-240.

[91] Bohler, H.C., Jr., et al., *Corticotropin releasing hormone mRNA is elevated on the afternoon of proestrus in the parvocellular paraventricular nuclei of the female rat.* Brain Res.Mol.Brain Res., 1990. 8(3): p. 259-262.

[92] Patchev, V.K. and O.F. Almeida, *Gender specificity in the neural regulation of the response to stress: new leads from classical paradigms.* Molecular Neurobiology, 1998. 16(1): p. 63-77.

[93] Vamvakopoulos, N.C. and G.P. Chrousos, *Evidence of direct estrogenic regulation of human corticotropin-releasing hormone gene expression. Potential implications for the sexual dimophism of the stress response and immune/inflammatory reaction.* J.Clin.Invest, 1993. 92(4): p. 1896-1902.

[94] Handa, R.J., M.J. Weiser, and D.G. Zuloaga, *A role for the androgen metabolite, 5alpha-androstane-3beta,17beta-diol, in modulating oestrogen receptor beta-mediated regulation of hormonal stress reactivity.* J Neuroendocrinol, 2009. 21(4): p. 351-8.

[95] Buckingham, J.C., K.D. Dohler, and C.A. Wilson, *Activity of the pituitary-adrenocortical system and thyroid gland during the oestrous cycle of the rat.* Journal of Endocrinology, 1978. 78: p. 359-366.

[96] Viau, V. and M.J. Meaney, *Variations in the hypothalamic-pituitary-adrenal response to stress during the estrous cycle in the rat.* Endocrinology, 1991. 129(5): p. 2503-2511.

[97] Smith, C.J. and R.L. Norman, *Influence of the gonads on cortisol secretion in female rhesus macaques.* Endocrinology, 1987. 121: p. 2192-2198.

[98] Bingaman, E.W., et al., *Androgen inhibits the increase in hypothalamic corticotropin-releasing hormone (CRH) and CRH-immunoreactivity following gonadectomy.* Neuroendocrinology, 1994. 59: p. 228-234.

[99] Canny, B.J., et al., *Inlfuence of sex and gonadal status on the hypothalamo-pituitary- adrenal (HPA) axis of the sheep.* Proceedings of the 10th International Congress of Endocrinology, 1996. 1: p. P1-368.

[100] Bell, M.E., C.E. Wood, and M. Keller-Wood, *Influence of reproductive state on pituitary-adrenal activity in the ewe.* Domestic Animal Endocrinology, 1991. 8: p. 245-254.

[101] Keller-Wood, M., J. Silbiger, and C.E. Wood, *Progesterone attenuates the inhibition of adrenocorticotropin responses by cortisol in nonpregnant ewes.* Endocrinology, 1988. 123: p. 647-651.

[102] Keller-Wood, M. and C.E. Wood, *Pregnancy alters cortisol feedback inhibition of stimulated ACTH: studies in adrenalectomized ewes.* Am.J.Physiol Regul.Integr.Comp Physiol, 2001. 280(6): p. R1790-R1798.

[103] Pecins-Thompson, M. and M. Keller-Wood, *Effects of progesterone on blood pressure, plasma volume, and responses to hypotension.* Am.J.Physiol, 1997. 272(1 Pt 2): p. R377-R385.

[104] Wood, C.E., et al., *Estrogen and androgen influence hypothalamic AVP and CRF concentrations in fetal and adult sheep.* Regul.Pept., 2001. 98(1-2): p. 63-68.

[105] Keller-Wood, M. and C.E. Wood, *Effect of ovariectomy on vasopressin, ACTH, and renin activity responses to hypotension.* American Journal of Physiology, 1991. 261: p. R223-R230.

[106] Pecins-Thompson, M. and M. Keller-Wood, *Prolonged absence of ovarian hormones in the ewe reduces the adrenocorticotropin response to hypotension, but not to hypoglycemia or corticotropin-releasing factors.* Endocrinology, 1994. 134: p. 678-684.

[107] Genazzani, A.R., et al., *Evidence for a role for the neurosteroid allopregnanolone in the modulation of reproductive function in female rats.* Eur.J.Endocrinol., 1995. 133(3): p. 375-380.

[108] Patchev, V.K., et al., *The neurosteroid tetrahydroprogesterone counteracts corticotropin-releasing hormone-induced anxiety and alters the release and gene expression of corticotropin-releasing hormone in the rat hypothalamus.* Neuroscience, 1994. 62(1): p. 265-71.

[109] Patchev, V.K., et al., *The neurosteroid tetrahydroprogesterone attenuates the endocrine response to stress and exerts glucocorticoid-like effects on vasopressin gene transcription in the rat hypothalamus.* Neuropsychopharmacology, 1996. 15(6): p. 533-40.

[110] Childs, E., N.T. Van Dam, and H. de Wit, *Effects of acute progesterone administration upon responses to acute psychosocial stress in men.* Exp Clin Psychopharmacol. 18(1): p. 78-86.

[111] Wirth, M.M., et al., *Relationship between salivary cortisol and progesterone levels in humans.* Biological Psychology, 2007. 74(1): p. 104-107.

[112] Hermans, E.J., et al., *Exogenous testosterone attenuates the integrated central stress response in healthy young women.* Psychoneuroendocrinology, 2007. 32(8-10): p. 1052-61.

[113] Hermans, E.J., N.F. Ramsey, and J. van Honk, *Exogenous testosterone enhances responsiveness to social threat in the neural circuitry of social aggression in humans.* Biol Psychiatry, 2008. 63(3): p. 263-70.

[114] Wirth, M.M. and O.C. Schultheiss, *Basal testosterone moderates responses to anger faces in humans.* Physiol Behav, 2007. 90(2-3): p. 496-505.

[115] Lightman, S.L., et al., *Peripartum plasticity within the hypothalamo-pituitary-adrenal axis.* Prog.Brain Res., 2001. 133: p. 111-129.

[116] Tu, M.T., S.J. Lupien, and C.D. Walker, *Measuring stress responses in postpartum mothers: perspectives from studies in human and animal populations.* Stress., 2005. 8(1): p. 19-34.

[117] Walker, C.D., D.J. Toufexis, and A. Burlet, *Hypothalamic and limbic expression of CRF and vasopressin during lactation: implications for the control of ACTH secretion and stress hyporesponsiveness.* Prog.Brain Res., 2001. 133: p. 99-110.

[118] Neumann, I.D., *Alterations in behavioral and neuroendocrine stress coping strategies in pregnant, parturient and lactating rats.* Prog.Brain Res., 2001. 133: p. 143-152.

[119] Uvnas-Moberg, K., *Oxytocin linked antistress effects--the relaxation and growth response.* Acta Physiol Scand.Suppl, 1997. 640: p. 38-42.

[120] Douglas, A.J. and J.A. Russell, *Endogenous opioid regulation of oxytocin and ACTH secretion during pregnancy and parturition.* Prog.Brain Res., 2001. 133: p. 67-82.

[121] Russell, J.A., A.J. Douglas, and C.D. Ingram, *Brain preparations for maternity--adaptive changes in behavioral and neuroendocrine systems during pregnancy and lactation. An overview.* Prog.Brain Res., 2001. 133: p. 1-38.

[122] Tilbrook, A.J., et al., *Activation of the hypothalamo-pituitary-adrenal axis by isolation and restraint stress during lactation in ewes: Effect of the presence of the lamb and suckling.* Endocrinology, 2006. 147(7): p. 3501-3509.

[123] Cook, C.J., *Oxytocin and prolactin suppress cortisol responses to acute stress in both lactating and non-lactating sheep.* J.Dairy Res., 1997. 64(3): p. 327-339.

Part 2

Sex Steroids, Memory and the Brain

7

Estrogen and Brain Protection

Xiaohua Ju, Daniel Metzger and Marianna Jung
University of North Texas Health Science Center
USA

1. Introduction

In 1931, estrogen was originally discovered as a female sex hormone by Marrian and Butenandt (1931). Estrogen is responsible for maintaining female reproductive organs and functions. Beyond the effects on reproductive organs, the neuroprotective activities of estrogen have been identified by Simpkins et al. (1994) and thereafter by numerous other researchers (Viscoli et al., 2001). The simple classification of the mechanisms of estrogen is genomic and non-genomic processes. The genomic mechanisms of estrogen involve estrogen receptors located in DNA. Upon binding its receptors, estrogen stimulates the synthesis of a variety of neuro-modulatory proteins. A body of evidence indicates that estrogen receptors are not necessary for certain neuroprotective effects of estrogen. For example, estrogen scavenges harmful reactive free radical species (Dhandapani & Brann, 2002), inhibits apoptotic process (a certain type of cell death), and modulates signal transduction, all of which do not require nucleic estrogen receptors. Estrogen's neuroprotective properties may be the end result of well-orchestrated genomic and non-genomic processes.

There are three major forms of endogenous estrogens; 17β-estradiol, estrone, and estriol based on the hydroxyl or ketone ligand attached to the C17 position of the rightmost ring (D ring). Among these estrogens, 17β-estradiol (Figure 1) is the most potent, naturally occurring estrogen. Accordingly, 17β-estradiol has been the subject for neuroprotective properties in major neurodegenerative disorders such as stroke, Alzheimer's disease, Parkinson's disease, and ethanol withdrawal, and thus a topic of this book chapter.

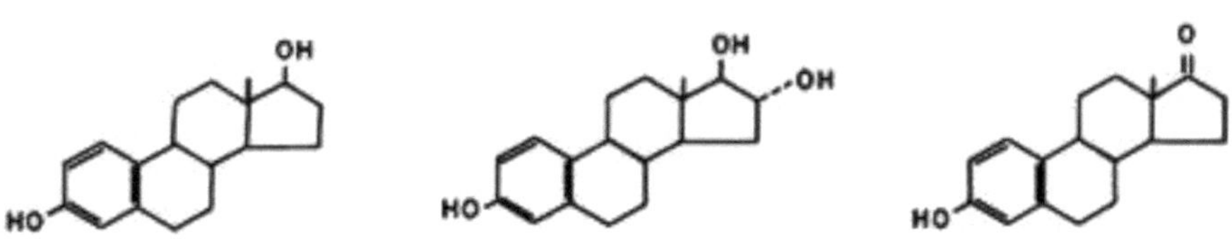

17β-Estradiol Estriol Estrone

Fig. 1. Chemical structures of 17β-estradiol, estriol, and estrone. Notice that 17β-estradiol has two hydroxyl (OH) groups, estriol has three hydroxyl groups, and estrone has one hydroxyl and one ketone group.

2. Estrogen and ischemia

2.1 Introduction

Stroke is the sudden loss of brain function that is attributed to ischemia which indicates a disturbance in the blood supply to the brain. The affected brain area is unable to function, resulting in an inability to move limbs, understand or formulate speech, or an inability to see the visual field. It is the leading cause of adult disability in the United States and Europe and the second leading cause of death worldwide (Feigin, 2005). Women have a higher risk, due to their longer lifespan and are also more likely to have fatal strokes than men (Bushnell, 2008). Especially women in the 45−54 age range (perimenopause) are reportedly at a higher risk for stroke (Towfighi et al., 2007). This study suggests that declining levels of ovarian hormones perpetuate the risk for this neurovascular disease. The depletion of ovarian hormones also alters stroke outcomes. In postmenopausal women, stroke-associated disability and fatality are worse compared to men (Niewada et al., 2005). If ovarian hormones influence stroke, it is not surprising to see sex differences in the severity of stroke. For instance, a smaller area of tissue death was found in young adult female mice (Park et al., 2006) compared to their age-matched males. Furthermore, the sex difference in stroke infarct (area of tissue death) was abolished when the female mice were ovariectomized, suggesting that ovarian steroids mediate the neuroprotection seen in younger females (Selvamani et al., 2010).

Among ovarian hormones, 17β-estradiol seems to possess greater protective properties than other ovarian hormones. 17β-estradiol mitigated brain inflammation (Suzuki et al., 2009) and blood-brain barrier dysfunction (R. Liu et al., 2005). 17β-estradiol increased the blood flow of the cerebrum (Pelligrino et al., 1998), the ability of neurons to transmit signals (synaptic plasticity), and cognitive function (Sherwin, 2007). By comparison to these protections in animal studies, human studies showed somewhat inconsistent results. In large clinical trials, such as the Women Estrogen Stroke Trial and the Women's Health Initiative, estrogen treatment failed to exert the beneficial effects on stroke incidence (Viscoli et al., 2001). Rather, the clinical study showed that estrogen treatment increased the stroke risk and worsened neurological outcomes in postmenopausal women (Viscoli et al., 2001). Similarly, the Women's Health Initiative study reported an increased risk for stroke following the treatment with estrogen or another female hormone progestin (synthetic progesterone) (Wassertheil-Smoller et al., 2003). Notably, many women in these clinical trials were postmenopausal for several years prior to the hormone treatment. The unexpected negative results might have been due to prolonged estrogen-withdrawal before estrogen was reintroduced (De et al., 2009). Other researchers suggested that differences in the duration of treatment, timing of administration, sex, age, and an ischemia model contributed to the inconsistent outcome of estrogen therapy (J. Li, 2011; Sherwin, 2009).

2.2 Apoptosis

Apoptosis is a type of cell death that normally occurs to replace aged or injured cells with newer cells. However, excessive or defective apoptosis is often present at regions affected by stroke (Dirnagl et al., 1999). Fas is a receptor protein that triggers apoptotic cell death upon the binding of its ligand (Fas ligand). The structure of Fas contains a particular region, called 'death domain'. There is a cytoplasmic protein that favors to associate with the death domain of Fas. Therefore, it is called Fas-associated death domain adaptor protein. When this adaptor protein binds to the death domain of Fas, it subsequently activates another apoptotic protein, caspase-8. An increasing body of work has shown that Fas and Fas Ligand play an important role in the pathology of ischemic stroke (L. Liu et al., 2008; Rosenbaum et al., 2000). Both Fas and Fas ligand were upregulated by cerebral ischemia in brains of developing, as well as adult mice (Felderhoff-Mueser et al., 2000, 2003). Intriguingly, estrogen significantly reduced the level of Fas and the adaptor protein in mice undergoing post-ischemic stress (Jia et al., 2009). Furthermore, estrogen reduced the downstream apoptotic effectors such as caspase-8 and caspase-3. These findings suggest that estrogen protects against ischemia, in part, through its inhibitory effects on apoptosis associated with Fas (Jia et al., 2009).

Estrogen also protects neurons from ischemia (Petito et al., 1987). Estrogen administered at physiological levels for two weeks before ischemia rescued the hippocampal neurons and ameliorated ischemia-induced cognitive deficits in female rats (Lebesgue, 2009). This study provides direct evidence that estrogen is neuroprotective against ischemia. There are at least two estrogen receptors in the brain, estrogen receptor-α and -β (Shughrue, 2004). Estrogen receptors are intracellular proteins which activate genomic as well as nongenomic effectors in neural cells (Maggi et al., 2004). Selective agonists for estrogen receptor-α or estrogen receptor-β was to were able to spare hippocampal neurons following ischemia. In addition, ICI 182780, a competitive antagonist for both estrogen receptors-α and -β, completely blocked estrogen's protection against post-ischemic stress (Miller et al., 2005). On the other hand, Lebesgue et al. (2009) found that a single injection of estrogen into the brain ventricle immediately after an ischemic event reduced both neuronal death and cognitive deficits. The genomic mechanism of estrogen is typically a slow process because it involves estrogen's receptors in the nuclei, affecting protein synthesis. Therefore, the rapid protection achieved by acute estrogen in Lebesgue's study may indicate the non-genomic effects of estrogen.

Above studies suggest that estrogen exerts neuroprotection against ischemia through its anti-apoptotic property and the mechanisms associated with estrogen receptors.

2.3 Oxidative stress

When ischemic patients receive blood supply (reperfusion), the introducing blood itself can induce significant damage to the brain. The damage is largely attributable to very active harmful oxygen species such as the reactive superoxide anion (Peters et al., 1998; Sugawara et al., 2005). These oxygen species give rise to other damaging oxygen species, for example, hydroxyl ion and peroxynitrite (Mattson et al., 2000). Estrogen contains profound antioxidant properties that mediate its protective effects on neurons. Estrogen directly scavenges free radicals by oxidizing its hydroxyl group attached to the C3 position of A ring (left most ring) through an enzyme, NADPH. The A ring then becomes the phenoxyl radical ring, a certain type of a ring structure containing free radicals. The phenoxyl radical ring is converted to para-quinol ring by scavenging further free radicals like -OH. This para-quinol ring structure finally becomes the original A ring of 17β-estradiol through NADPH (Prokai et al., 2003; Prokai-Tatrai et al., 2008). The important point of this cyclic reaction is that 17β-estradiol is rejuvenated after it absorbs harmful free radicals (Figure 2). Indeed, estrogen attenuated superoxide production in hippocampal neurons after stroke (Q.G. Zhang et al., 2009). In addition to this directly scavenging of free radicals, estrogen upregulates antioxidant enzymes and chelates redox-active metal ions. In terms of estrogen receptor, Zhang et al. (2009) suggested that the antioxidant effect of estrogen is independent of estrogen receptor-α. They found that estrogen deprivation abolished the antioxidant and neuroprotective effects on the hippocampus without affecting estrogen receptor-α mediated effect on the uterus. At the very least, these findings indicate that estrogen protects against ischemia through antioxidant properties.

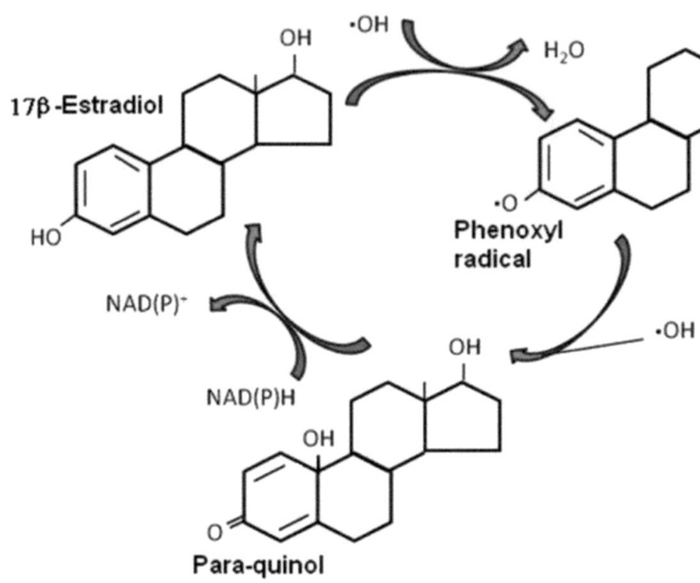

Fig. 2. Schematic illustration of the free radical scavenging antioxidant activity of 17β-estradiol. 17β-estradiol captures •OH, producing the phenoxyl radical and then bioreversible quinol. The quinol is rapidly converted to the parent estrogen via a NAD(P)H-dependent reductive aromatization to perpetuate the antioxidant action. During this process, •OH is detoxified to H_2O (Prokai et al., 2003; Prokai-Tatrai et al., 2008).

2.4 Inflammation\Immune response

Inflammation is a critical event that occurs upon ischemic insults. Post-stroke events include the stimulation and subsequent degeneration of lymphoid organs such as the spleen and thymus (Offner et al., 2009). The activation of these lymphoid organs likely leads to immunocyte translocation into brain, exacerbating the evolving brain ischemia (Ajmo et al., 2008). Proinflammatory genes are rapidly induced in brain after ischemic injury, including genes synthesizing TNF-α (X. Wang et al., 1994), IL-6 (X. Wang et al., 1995), IL-1β (X. Wang et al., 1994), and interferon inducible protein-10 (IP-10) (X. Wang et al., 1998). The subsequent degeneration of lymphoid organs leads to immunodepression. Humans who survive the initial brain insult, may succumb to fatal infection due to the immunodepression (Dirnagl et al., 2007; Meisel et al., 2005).

Estrogen deficiency during menopause is associated with a proinflammatory phenotype, namely 'T cell expansion' in bone marrow that secretes inflammatory proteins such as IL-1, TNF-α, and IL-6 (Pfeilschifter et al., 2002). In a study done by Zhang et al. (2010), estrogen partially restored immune reactivity in ovariectomized females by increasing spleen cell population and cytokine responses (B. Zhang et al., 2010). In agreement, estrogen induced anti-inflammatory cytokines in the spleen after traumatic brain injury (Bruce-Keller et al.,

2007). In lipopolysaccharide-induced brain inflammation, estrogen suppressed both resident microglial activation and the recruitment of peripheral T and B cells (Vegeto et al., 2001). These studies provide empirical evidence that the anti-inflammatory effect of estrogen plays a protective role in immune responses to stroke.

Collectively, cumulative evidence indicates that the convergence of endocrine changes, especially estrogen, impacts the pathophysiology of stroke and ischemic injury. It appears that estrogen protects against ischemia through multiple factors associated with apoptosis, inflammation, redox, and estrogen receptors. Understanding these mechanisms may ultimately contribute to better research and therapeutic strategies for stroke therapy.

3. Estrogen and Alzheimer's disease

3.1 Introduction

Alzheimer's disease is characterized as a gradual failure of memory, cognition, and bodily functions, ultimately leading to death. Although the exact etiology and mechanisms are unknown, the abnormal accumulation of a particular protein, called Amyloid β, has long been proposed as the most likely culprit in the pathogenesis of this disease (Hardy & Selkoe, 2002; Tanzi & Bertram, 2005). In a healthy brain, Amyloid β remains at a steady-state level as a result of the metabolic balance between production of Amyloid β from amyloid precursor protein and removal by cellular uptake and proteolytic degradation (Saido, 1998; Selkoe, 2000). Such a dynamic equilibrium, however, could be altered by genetic or environmental factors that may lead to Alzheimer's disease. It has been hypothesized that Amyloid β is folded into a oligomeric form or a fibrillar (cable-like strings) form (Yamin et al., 2008), both of which are more neurotoxic than Amyloid β itself. Of several different Amyloid β peptides produced, products of Amyloid β-40 and Amyloid β-42 residues are the most common constituents of amyloid plaques, and are widely accepted as the primary trigger for Alzheimer's disease (St George-Hyslop, 2000). In brains with early onset Alzheimer's disease, Amyloid β excessively accumulates. This may be due to the mutations of presenelin genes, which provoke the overproduction of Amyloid β from amyloid precursor protein (Hardy, 2004). In late-onset Alzheimer's disease, which constitutes more than 90% of the disease, the excess accumulation of Amyloid β has been associated with abnormal Amyloid β degrading proteases (Nalivaeva et al., 2008).

Women are more likely to develop Alzheimer's disease after adjusting for age (Andersen et al., 1999). After menopause, the decline of estrogen levels in the brain may render neurons more susceptible to age-related neurodegenerative processes (Coffey et al., 1998). Estrogen therapy, when initiated at the onset of menopause, has reduced the risk or delayed the onset of Alzheimer's disease in women (LeBlanc et al., 2001; Zandi et al., 2002). A recent randomized control trial indicated that estrogen treatment had a beneficial effect on verbal memory in men with mild cognitive impairment (Sherwin et al., 2011 in press). However, clinical studies of estrogen therapy in non-demented and menopausal women have yielded inconclusive results (Craig & Murphy, 2010; Sano et al., 2008). In addition, estrogen administration induced beneficial effects on neuronal function and survival through improving mitochondrial function in healthy neurons (Brinton, 2008). When neurons became unhealthy, estrogen exposure had a detrimental effect (Brinton, 2008). This discrepancy may be due to differences in neurological health, age, hormonal status, the severity of symptoms, the type of menopause (surgical vs. natural), and the type of estrogen compound used (Brinton, 2009). Also, the age when estrogen therapy is initiated, may in part determine the outcome of estrogen therapy and probably estrogen treatment during the peri-menopause has the highest efficacy (Craig & Murphy, 2010; Genazzani et al., 2007).

In diverse animal models of Alzheimer's disease, estrogen has prevented or delayed the development of Alzheimer's disease pathology in particular Amyloid β accumulation and plaque formation (Carroll et al., 2007; Zheng et al., 2002). Mechanistically, estrogen may regulate the production of Amyloid β and in turn, sustain an improved Amyloid β homeostasis by increasing the metabolism of amyloid precursor protein and destabilization of Amyloid β fibrils (Greenfield et al., 2002; Morinaga et al., 2007). Estrogen's bioenergetic protection may also influence Alzheimer's disease. For instance, estrogen prevented the brain from using alternative fuel sources, such as the ketones (Brinton, 2008, 2009). Aromatase catalyzes the conversion of testosterone to estrogen. Not surprisingly, mice lacking aromatase genes (low estrogen production) showed the loss of hippocampal neurons in response to neurotoxins more severely than wild type mice (Azcoitia et al., 2001), suggesting that estrogen spared those neurons. Indeed, the levels of estrogen and aromatase were significantly reduced in the brains of Alzheimer's disease women (Yue et al., 2005). The view of brain estrogen deficiency as a risk factor for developing Alzheimer's disease pathology is consistent with genetic studies showing an association between the aberration of aromatase gene and the risk for Alzheimer's disease (Iivonen et al., 2004). All these studies suggest that estrogen may have the capacity to interfere with the pathways mediating Alzheimer's disease.

3.2 Estrogen synthesis in Alzheimer's disease

Since estrogen has a potential capacity to control Alzheimer's disease, one therapeutic strategy might be to target the biosynthesis of estrogen. Indeed, numerous studies have tested whether Alzheimer's disease alters the endogenous synthesis of estrogen. While the levels of estrogens were unchanged in the prefrontal cortex of Alzheimer's disease patients (Rosario et al., 2011), the estrogen biosynthetic enzymes such as aromatase and 17β-hydroxysteroid dehydrogenase type 1 were upregulated in the late stages of Alzheimer's disease (Luchetti et al., 2011). Studies using immunohistochemistry showed that aromatase expression was upregulated in astrocytes in later stages of Alzheimer's disease (Azcoitia et al., 2003). Another immunochemistry study also detected an increase in the level of aromatase in the hypothalamic neurons of Alzheimer's patients (Ishunina et al., 2005). The increase was especially profound in the Nucleus basalis of Meynert, a nucleus that is strongly affected in Alzheimer's disease (Ishunina et al., 2005). These findings suggest that during Alzheimer's disease, there is an attempt to increase the biosynthesis of estrogen. The aromatase upregulation may be a defense mechanism of brain areas that undergo neurodegeneration. In support of this notion, the reduced levels of testosterone were found in the aging brain of male and female Alzheimer's patients (Rosario et al., 2011; Weill-Engerer et al., 2002). This seems in line with the idea of a compensatory mechanism, since testosterone is used up after it is locally metabolized into neuroprotective estrogen.

3.3 Amyloid β

Cumulative evidence indicates that estrogen protects against Amyloid β and its toxicity through mechanisms involving Amyloid β degradation and signaling changes. Estrogen deficiency accelerated the formation of Amyloid β plaque in mice (Yue et al., 2005). Estrogen treatment reduced the level of Amyloid β (Jaffe et al., 1994; Xu et al., 1998) and its availability through enhancing the uptake of Amyloid β by microglia (R. Li et al., 2000). In vitro estrogen treatment inhibited the formation of toxic Amyloid β oligomers (Morinaga et al., 2007). Finally, estrogen activated Neprilysin, the primary enzyme that degrades Amyloid β, thereby facilitating Amyloid β degradation in human neuroblastoma cells (Liang et al., 2010). It is possible that this effect of estrogen is preceded by estrogen's action on amyloid precursor protein. Several studies support this notion that estrogen treatment profoundly decreased the levels of amyloid precursor protein by enhancing the degradation of this precursor through the α- and β-secretase pathways (Amtul et al., 2010). Alternatively, estrogen may reduce available amyloid precursor protein by stimulating the formation of vesicles that uptake this precursor-protein, thereby precluding maximal generation of Amyloid β (Greenfield et al., 2002). These findings suggest another mechanism underlying estrogen's protection against Alzheimer's disease involving Amyloid β degredation (Liang et al., 2010). Estrogen may also protect the signaling function of protein kinases from Amyloid β. For example, Amyloid β oligomer inhibited the activity of calcium/calmodulin-dependent protein kinase II and extracellular signal-regulated kinase in a manner ameliorated by estrogen treatment (Logan et al., 2011). In agreement with the protective effect of estrogen on protein kinase, Szego et al. (2011) reported that the function of protein kinases correlated with avoidance learning behavior. In that study, the treatment with Amyloid β oligomers impeded the learning in a manner that was protected by estrogen. These studies suggest a diverse mechanism by which estrogen protects against Amyloid β as an attempt to cope with Alzheimer's disease.

3.4 Neuroinflammation

The neurotoxicity of Alzheimer's disease is in part mediated by inflammatory processes (McGeer et al., 2006). Glial cells (non neuronal cells) are involved in this process such that Amyloid β activates glial cells to produce pro-inflammatory cytokines like IL-1β, IL-6, and TNF-α. Activated glial cells have the potential to produce large amounts of reactive oxygen species/nitrogen species by various mechanisms (Zhu et al., 2007). Activated astrocytes produced excessive nitric oxide, which reacted with superoxide to form harmful peroxynitrite (Smith et al., 1997). Excess nitric oxide synthetase was also detected in astrocytes surrounding plaques in Alzheimer's disease (Luth et al., 2001). Estrogen interfered with this process by limiting astroglial cells and inhibiting chronic inflammation associated with Alzheimer's disease (Vegeto et al., 2003). The anti-inflammatory effects of estrogen were shown in a primary culture study; estrogen treatment decreased the expression of pro-inflammatory molecules, such as TNF-α and IL-1β, as well as nitric oxide synthase and cyclooxygenase-2 in astrocytes (Valles et al., 2010).

Vegeto et al. (2006) conducted a study further supporting the protective effects of estrogen on inflammation associated with Alzheimer's disease. They used the APP23 mouse model, a model of Alzheimer's disease that creates chronic neuroinflammation resembling that in Alzheimer's disease. They found that the number of plaques associated with reactive microglia was increased with age (Vegeto et al., 2006). Interestingly, ovariectomy accelerated microglial activation surrounding Amyloid β plaques, whereas estrogen replacement delayed this process. In parallel, they showed that estrogen reduced the expression of inflammatory mediators, such as monocyte chemoattractant protein-1, macrophage inflammatory protein-2, and TNF-α. That study indicates that microglia is a direct target of estrogen action in the brain. All of these findings reinforce the hypothesis that inflammatory mechanisms significantly contribute to the pathogenesis of Alzheimer's disease and support the use of estrogen in the fight against Alzheimer's disease.

Collectively, animal studies on Alzheimer's disease have shown beneficial effects of estrogen through inhibiting the synthesis of amyloid β, facilitating its metabolisms, modulating protein kinases, and inhibiting inflammatory pathways. Human studies on the effects of estrogen on Alzheimer's disease have resulted in both positive and negative effects. It is unclear what causes the inconsistent results. Nevertheless, it seems clear that estrogen influences Alzheimer's disease pathology, if not etiology. How to identify and adjust factors underlying the discrepancies seems to be an essential task.

4. Estrogen and Parkinson's disease

4.1 Introduction

Parkinson's disease is the second most common neurodegenerative movement disorder. It is mainly characterized by the slow and gradual emergence of motor disorders such as tremor, rigidity, bradykinesia, and postural instability (Lang, 2007). Parkinson's disease is less prevalent in women than in men by an approximate 2:3 ratio and evidence suggests that estrogen influences the onset and severity of disease-associated symptoms (Currie, 2004; Shulman, 2006). Women with Parkinson's disease tend to have an earlier menopause, are more likely to have undergone hysterectomy, and used estrogen therapy less frequently than control subjects (Benedetti et al., 2001). Ragonese et al. (2004) suggested that factors reducing estrogen contribute to the development of Parkinson's disease (Ragonese et al., 2004). This was recently supported by the Observational Study of the Women's Health Initiative (WHI-OS) that employed 83,482 women. The study showed association between the number of women with longer fertile lifespan and a reduced risk of Parkinson's disease (Saunders-Pullman et al., 2009). In another human study, women with Parkinson's disease were less likely to have used postmenopausal estrogen therapy (Currie et al., 2004), suggesting that estrogen produces a beneficial effect on Parkinson's disease.

4.2 Dopamine neurotransmission

Dopamine is a neurotransmitter that has multiple functions in the brain such as cognition, reward, mood, and voluntary movement. The substantia nigra is a brain area that governs these functions. So far, this neurotransmitter has been the major player in Parkinson's disease such that dopamine synthesizing neurons are progressively depleted in the substantia nigra of Parkinson's patients (Emborg, 2004). Aberrant dopamine transmission is implicated in Parkinson's disease, particularly because the symptoms are ameliorated by a drug which increases dopamine signaling. Dopamine is actively eliminated from the extracellular space by astrocytes and neurons through dopamine transporters. Afterwards, dopamine is either recycled into vesicles or metabolized. In previous studies, estrogen increased the availability of dopamine by inhibiting uptake and by decreasing the affinity of the transporter for dopamine (Disshon et al., 1998). Estrogen also increases the synthesis of dopamine in the substantia nigra and the release of dopamine from axon terminals. In rodents and in neuronal cell culture studies, estrogen protected dopaminergic neurons from injury (B. Liu & Dluzen, 2006; Arvin et al., 2000). Given this, the beneficial effect of estrogen on Parkinson's disease may be mediated through estrogen's action on dopamine.

Studies have further identified how estrogen acts on the dopamine system. Estrogen modulates the development of dopaminergic neurons and neurotransmission (Bourque,

2009) by promoting neurite plasticity (Beyer et al., 2000). These effects are either mediated through a direct action on dopaminergic neurons or interactions with local astroglia (Ivanova et al., 2001, 2002). Alternatively, estrogen may act on genetic levels to modulate dopamine. For instance, estrogen regulates dopamine gene expression by activating transcriptional factors (DonCarlos et al., 2009). Estrogen also exerts non-genomic membrane effects, interaction with neurotransmitter receptors, and ionic channel regulation (Garcia-Segura et al., 2009). These studies suggest that estrogen protects against Parkinson's disease through genomic and non-genomic effects on the dopamine system.

Dopamine transporters mediate the uptake of dopamine from synapses to presynaptic vesicles, thereby restoring depleted vesicular dopamine levels (Jourdain et al., 2005). Estrogen stimulated dopamine uptake by nerve cells through neuronal dopamine transporter (D'Astous et al., 2004). On the other hand, estrogen decreased astroglial dopamine uptake, increasing the available levels of synaptic dopamine. This allowed more synaptic dopamine to be taken up by neurons. These studies suggest a few important points: first, not only dopamine neurons but also nigrostriatal astroglia contribute to the metabolic processes of dopamine (Karakaya et al., 2007); second, astroglia are implicated in estrogen-transmitted neuroprotection during dopamine neuro-degeneration (Morale et al, 2006), and finally, as the complementary action of estrogen on neurons, astrocyte and microglia may represent a potential pharmacological target for Parkinson's disease management (Vegeto et al., 2008).

4.3 Oxidative stress

In the process of dopamine being catalyzed by monoamine oxidase, a large amount of reactive oxygen species is produced, resulting in cell death (Hastings et al., 1996; Luo et al., 1998). In addition, dopamine aldehyde generated in the oxidative deamination reaction is 1000-fold more toxic than dopamine (Burke, 2003). Dopamine neurons in Parkinson's disease become vulnerable to oxidative stress (Dexter et al., 1989; Sian et al., 1994) perhaps due to lower levels of glutathione (endogenous antioxidant) than other cell types.

The brain has a predominant defense mechanism against superoxide radicals through antioxidant enzymes such as superoxide dismutase. Studies have demonstrated that superoxide dismutase is implicated in dopamine and Parkinson's disease. Mutant mice that over-expressed or lacked superoxide dismutase were more resistant to (Przedborski et al., 1992) or vulnerable to (Andreassen et al., 2001; J. Zhang et al., 2000) dopamine neurotoxin than wild type mice, respectively. The expression of superoxide dismutase was upregulated in the substantia nigra following the dopamine neurotoxin insult, yet the loss of dopaminergic neurons still occurred (Tripanichkul et al., 2007). These results suggest that there is an attempt to combat the oxidative stress in nigral neurons but not sufficient to spare neurons. The implication of superoxide dismutase in the antioxidant effect of estrogen has been shown in a study done by Tripanichkul et al. (2007). In that study, estrogen treatment increased the expression of superoxide dismutase in the substantia nigra of animals that were treated with the dopamine neurotoxin. This study suggests that estrogen up-regulates superoxide dismutase in critical brain areas, thereby exerting protection against dopamine neurotoxin or Parkinson's disease.

4.4 Neuroinflammation

Neuroinflammation and microglial activation are often seen in Parkinson's disease (McGeer et al., 1988; Hunot et al., 2003) and anti-inflammatory drugs reduce the risk of this disease

(H. Chen et al., 2003; Wahner et al., 2007). A positive correlation was found between antecedent brain injuries, such as trauma or exposure to infectious agents and the development of Parkinson's disease (B. Liu et al., 2003). This correlation implies that the brain inflammatory response to these noxious events, and specifically microglial activation, plays a critical role in Parkinson's disease. In support of this view, researchers have detected pro-inflammatory molecules (e.g. TNF-α) and excessive reactive oxygen species in the nervous system of Parkinson's disease patients (Hunot et al., 1996; Knott et al., 2000). The inflammatory molecules seem to amplify neuroinflammation as well as neuro-toxicity, ultimately leading to a slow and irreversible destruction of dopaminergic neurons. Using estrogen receptor-null mice, several studies have demonstrated that estrogen receptor-α is involved in the anti-inflammatory activity of estrogen (Dubal et al., 2001; Vegeto et al., 2003). Although estrogen receptor-β is expressed widely in brain, it does not seem to mediate the protective effect of estrogen. Or the effects of estrogen receptors on inflammation depend on the brain area (Harris et al., 2003). Whether or which receptor mediates estrogen's protection against inflammatory response still remains unclear.

Collectively, the protective effects of estrogen on Parkinson's disease appear to involve dopaminergic neuroprotection, anti-oxidant activities, anti-inflammatory activities, and estrogen receptors. Considering that Parkinson's disease is more prevalent in male than female patients, how these effects of estrogen can be implemented to clinical usages is an open question. At the very least, estrogen can be used as an interventional tool for a new mechanistic insight into this neurodegenerative disease.

5. Estrogen and ethanol withdrawal

5.1 Introduction

The distress of alcohol (ethanol) withdrawal is initiated by abruptly removing the inhibitory stimulus of ethanol and thus, is associated with rebound hyper-excitatory stimuli. In general, the overt initial signs of ethanol withdrawal include anxiety, ataxia, muscle incoordination, seizures, coma, and even death (American Psychiatric Association, 2000). While repeating unsuccessful attempts to quit heavy drinking, the brain undergoes random exposure to ethanol and withdrawal, damaging cellular and neuronal integrity (Wober et al., 1998).

The neuronal activity of the brain tends to be hyper-excitable during ethanol withdrawal due to an increase in the level of glutamate, a major excitatory neurotransmitter (Rossetti & Carboni, 1995). This can result in neuronal damage to vulnerable brain areas such as the cortex, hippocampus, and cerebellum. In addition to this well known glutamate neurotransmission, ethanol withdrawal perturbs the homeostasis of redox balance and signaling mechanisms. For instance, ethanol withdrawal provokes the intense generation of reactive oxygen species and activates stress-responding protein kinases (Jung et al., 2009). In addition, ethanol withdrawal inflicts mitochondrial membranes/membrane potential and suppresses mitochondrial enzymes such as cytochrome c oxidase, all of which impair fundamental functions of mitochondria (Jung et al., 2007, 2009). In our recent study, brain aging occurred earlier in ethanol withdrawn animals than in control-diet animals (Jung et al., 2010). These studies indicate that mal-managed ethanol withdrawal can clearly provoke neurodegenerative disorders.

5.2 Oxidative stress

Chronic ethanol consumption and ethanol withdrawal both generate oxidative free radicals and subsequent lipid peroxidation (Nordmann et al., 1990; Montoliu et al., 1994). Lipid peroxidation reflects the interaction between oxygen and the polyunsaturated fatty acids of membrane lipids, generating deteriorating breakdown products. Since the brain consists of a high content of unsaturated membrane lipids, it is a preferred target of both reactive oxygen species and ethanol (Hernandez-Munoz et al., 2000). Ethanol withdrawal-induced oxidative stress was associated with an increase in glutamatergic neurotransmission (Rossetti & Carboni, 1995), the upregulation of calcium channels, and the accumulation of intracellular calcium (Rewal et al., 2005). The functional consequence of prooxidant ethanol withdrawal is shown in several animal and human studies. For instance, enhanced reactive oxygen species concurred with ethanol withdrawal-induced seizure activity in rats (Vallett et al., 1997). The cerebrospinal fluid of patients who underwent ethanol withdrawal showed higher concentrations of excitatory neurotransmitters and oxidative markers (Marotta et al., 1997; Tsai et al., 1998) than control subjects. Higher levels of lipid peroxide and lower levels of superoxide dismutase (antioxidant enzyme) activity were also seen in those patients (Tsai et al., 1998). These studies indicate that the redox imbalance has a causative relationship with ethanol withdrawal insults.

If ethanol withdrawal is a prooxidant stimulus, estrogen treatment should be able to mitigate the stress through its antioxidant property. Our recent findings essentially confirmed the hypothesis using the in vivo and in vitro model of ethanol withdrawal. Estrogen treatment mitigated reactive oxygen species generation, lipid peroxidation, and protein oxidation (Jung et al. 2004, 2006). Estrogen protection against the prooxidant effect of ethanol withdrawal may involve glutamate transmission because glutamate-induced oxidative stress is attenuated by estrogen (Behl & Manthey, 2000) and the quinol derived from estrogen (Prokai et al., 2003). It is also possible that estrogen elevates the levels of endogenous antioxidants, such as glutathione, so that a favorable redox potential for an antioxidant environment is created (Prokai et al., 2003). Since oxidative molecules are generated mainly from mitochondria, these studies suggest that the antioxidant protection of estrogen against ethanol withdrawal is linked to the mitoprotective activity of estrogen.

5.3 Mitochondria

Indeed, the mitoprotective effects of estrogen are interactive with the antioxidant effect by virtue of the fact that mitochondria are the major source and target of oxidative free radicals. The mitoprotective effect of estrogen has been extended to the ethanol withdrawal model in our recent study in which ethanol withdrawal provokes the oxidation of mitochondrial proteins in rats, in a manner mitigated by estrogen. Since cellular energy ATP is mainly generated in mitochondria, it is not surprising that estrogen protects against mitochondrial respiratory deficit during ethanol withdrawal (Jung et al., 2011). Presumably, estrogen plays a role in alleviating the oxidative burden in mitochondria, thus increasing mitochondrial respiration efficiency (J.Q. Chen & Yager 2004; Jung et al., 2011).

5.4 Signaling pathways

P38 is referred to as a stress-activated protein kinase because it is often activated in response to a variety of stress. A transient, moderate activation of P38 normally occurs in association with cell survival or differentiation. However, excess activation generally correlates with pathological conditions (Barca et al., 2008). P38 is activated upon phosphorylation (Moriguchi et al., 1996) and thus, pP38 is often measured as an indicator of P38 activation. A previous study reported that the P38 inhibitor SB203580 attenuated ethanol-induced cell death (Ku et al., 2007), suggesting that P38 activation mediates cytotoxic ethanol. Acute ethanol treatment led to P38 activation (Norkina et al., 2007) and augmented endotoxin-induced pP38 levels in a manner attenuated by P38 inhibitor in human monocytes (Drechsler et al., 2006). Recently, we have demonstrated that estrogen protected against ethanol withdrawal-induced hyperactivation of P38, suggesting that there is a crucial link between estrogen, P38, and ethanol withdrawal (Jung et al., 2010). In that study, middle-age female rats (12-15 month old) were more vulnerable to the ethanol withdrawal-induced P38 activation than young or older rats (Jung et al., 2010). Importantly, chronic estrogen treatment abolished the age difference in P38 activation. These studies indicate that ethanol withdrawal interferes with signaling pathways, including P38, in a manner that depends on age and that is protected by estrogen.

In conclusion, findings from our and others' laboratories suggest that ethanol withdrawal distress is more than a neurotransmitter disorder. It is attributed to the perturbation of redox balance, protein kinase signaling, and mitochondria, all of which can be mitigated by estrogen treatment. Understanding the interaction between ethanol withdrawal and estrogen may contribute to the improvement of the pharmacological treatment of ethanol withdrawal.

6. Conclusion

There are some lingering controversies in the neuroprotective effects and underlying mechanisms of estrogen. Nevertheless, numerous studies indicate the profound neuroprotective effects of 17β-estradiol on neurodegenerative diseases including ischemia, Alzheimer's disease, Parkinson's disease, and ethanol withdrawal syndromes. Diverse mechanisms mediate estrogen's protection through neurotrophic, neuroprotective, antiapoptotic, and antioxidant activities. Furthermore, estrogen exerts its neuroprotection through inhibiting inflammation and preserving the homeostasis of neurotransmitters. Estrogen receptors appear to mediate some of estrogen's protection, although it is not yet entirely clear whether it is estrogen receptor-α, estrogen receptor-β, or membrane estrogen receptors. At the mitochondrial level, estrogen inhibits peroxidation, eliminates reactive oxygen species, and maintains the homeostasis of mitochondrial membranes/respiration.

The extent to which estrogen can actually ameliorate neurodegenerative diseases in clinical settings may depend on well controlled systematic clinical studies that are largely absent in current situations. Nevertheless, it may be a matter of time that this amazing molecule alleviates the human burden of devastating brain diseases.

7. Acknowledgment

This work was supported by National Institute on Alcohol Abuse and Alcoholism (AA015982 and AA018747). We wish to thank Claudia Martinez and David Julovich for their editorial assistance.

8. References

Ajmo, C. T., Jr.; Vernon, D. O.; Collier, L.; Hall, A. A.; Garbuzova-Davis, S.; Willing, A. & Pennypacker, K. R. (2008). The Spleen Contributes to Stroke-Induced Neurodegeneration. *J Neurosci Res*, Vol. 86, No. 10, pp. 2227-34, ISSN 1097-4547

Amtul, Z.; Wang, L.; Westaway, D. & Rozmahel, R. F. (2010). Neuroprotective Mechanism Conferred by 17beta-Estradiol on the Biochemical Basis of Alzheimer's Disease. *Neuroscience*, Vol. 169, No. 2, pp. 781-6, ISSN 1873-7544

Andersen, K.; Launer, L. J.; Dewey, M. E.; Letenneur, L.; Ott, A.; Copeland, J. R.; Dartigues, J. F.; Kragh-Sorensen, P.; Baldereschi, M.; Brayne, C.; Lobo, A.; Martinez-Lage, J. M.; Stijnen, T. & Hofman, A. (1999). Gender Differences in the Incidence of Alzheimer's Disease and Vascular Dementia: The Eurodem Studies. Eurodem Incidence Research Group. *Neurology*, Vol. 53, No. 9, pp. 1992-7, ISSN 0028-3878

Andreassen, O. A.; Ferrante, R. J.; Dedeoglu, A.; Albers, D. W.; Klivenyi, P.; Carlson, E. J.; Epstein, C. J. & Beal, M. F. (2001). Mice with a Partial Deficiency of Manganese Superoxide Dismutase Show Increased Vulnerability to the Mitochondrial Toxins Malonate, 3-Nitropropionic Acid, and MPTP. *Exp Neurol*, Vol. 167, No. 1, pp. 189-95, ISSN 0014-4886

Arvin, M.; Fedorkova, L.; Disshon, K. A.; Dluzen, D. E. & Leipheimer, R. E. (2000). Estrogen Modulates Responses of Striatal Dopamine Neurons to Mpp(+): Evaluations Using in Vitro and in Vivo Techniques. *Brain Res*, Vol. 872, No. 1-2, pp. 160-71, ISSN 0006-8993

Association, American Psychiatric. (2000). *Diagnostic and Statistical Manual of Mental Disorders Dsm-Iv-Tr*. 4th ed. (Washington, DC: Amer Psychiatric Pub).

Azcoitia, I.; Sierra, A.; Veiga, S. & Garcia-Segura, L. M. (2003). Aromatase Expression by Reactive Astroglia Is Neuroprotective. *Ann N Y Acad Sci*, Vol. 1007 pp. 298-305, ISSN 0077-8923

Azcoitia, I.; Sierra, A.; Veiga, S.; Honda, S.; Harada, N. & Garcia-Segura, L. M. (2001). Brain Aromatase Is Neuroprotective. *J Neurobiol*, Vol. 47, No. 4, pp. 318-29, ISSN 0022-3034

Barca, O.; Costoya, J. A.; Senaris, R. M. & Arce, V. M. (2008). Interferon-Beta Protects Astrocytes against Tumour Necrosis Factor-Induced Apoptosis Via Activation of P38 Mitogen-Activated Protein Kinase. *Exp Cell Res*, Vol. 314, No. 11-12, pp. 2231-7, ISSN 1090-2422

Bastide, M.; Ouk, T.; Plaisier, F.; Petrault, O.; Stolc, S. & Bordet, R. (2007). Neurogliovascular Unit after Cerebral Ischemia: Is the Vascular Wall a Pharmacological Target. *Psychoneuroendocrinology*, Vol. 32 Suppl 1 pp. S36-9, ISSN 0306-4530

Behl, C. & Manthey, D. (2000). Neuroprotective Activities of Estrogen: An Update. *J Neurocytol*, Vol. 29, No. 5-6, pp. 351-8, ISSN 0300-4864

Benedetti, M. D.; Maraganore, D. M.; Bower, J. H.; McDonnell, S. K.; Peterson, B. J.; Ahlskog, J. E.; Schaid, D. J. & Rocca, W. A. (2001). Hysterectomy, Menopause, and Estrogen Use Preceding Parkinson's Disease: An Exploratory Case-Control Study. *Mov Disord*, Vol. 16, No. 5, pp. 830-7, ISSN 0885-3185

Beyer, C. & Karolczak, M. (2000). Estrogenic Stimulation of Neurite Growth in Midbrain Dopaminergic Neurons Depends on cAMP/Protein Kinase a Signaling. *J Neurosci Res*, Vol. 59, No. 1, pp. 107-16, ISSN 0360-4012

Bourque, M.; Dluzen, D. E. & Di Paolo, T. (2009). Neuroprotective Actions of Sex Steroids in Parkinson's Disease. *Front Neuroendocrinol*, Vol. 30, No. 2, pp. 142-57, ISSN 1095-6808

Brinton, R. D. (2009). Estrogen-Induced Plasticity from Cells to Circuits: Predictions for Cognitive Function. *Trends Pharmacol Sci*, Vol. 30, No. 4, pp. 212-22, ISSN 0165-6147

Brinton, R. D. (2008). The Healthy Cell Bias of Estrogen Action: Mitochondrial Bioenergetics and Neurological Implications. *Trends Neurosci*, Vol. 31, No. 10, pp. 529-37, ISSN 0166-2236

Bruce-Keller, A. J.; Dimayuga, F. O.; Reed, J. L.; Wang, C.; Angers, R.; Wilson, M. E.; Dimayuga, V. M. & Scheff, S. W. (2007). Gender and Estrogen Manipulation Do Not Affect Traumatic Brain Injury in Mice. *J Neurotrauma*, Vol. 24, No. 1, pp. 203-15, ISSN 0897-7151

Burke, W. J. (2003). 3,4-Dihydroxyphenylacetaldehyde: A Potential Target for Neuroprotective Therapy in Parkinson's Disease. *Curr Drug Targets CNS Neurol Disord*, Vol. 2, No. 2, pp. 143-8, ISSN 1568-007X

Bushnell, C. D. (2008). Stroke and the Female Brain. *Nat Clin Pract Neurol*, Vol. 4, No. 1, pp. 22-33, ISSN 1745-8358

Carroll, J. C.; Rosario, E. R.; Chang, L.; Stanczyk, F. Z.; Oddo, S.; LaFerla, F. M. & Pike, C. J. (2007). Progesterone and Estrogen Regulate Alzheimer-Like Neuropathology in Female 3xtg-Ad Mice. *J Neurosci*, Vol. 27, No. 48, pp. 13357-65, ISSN 1529-2401

Chen, H.; Zhang, S. M.; Hernan, M. A.; Schwarzschild, M. A.; Willett, W. C.; Colditz, G. A.; Speizer, F. E. & Ascherio, A. (2003). Nonsteroidal Anti-Inflammatory Drugs and the Risk of Parkinson Disease. *Arch Neurol*, Vol. 60, No. 8, pp. 1059-64, ISSN 0003-9942

Chen, J. Q. & Yager, J. D. (2004). Estrogen's Effects on Mitochondrial Gene Expression: Mechanisms and Potential Contributions to Estrogen Carcinogenesis. *Ann N Y Acad Sci*, Vol. 1028 pp. 258-72, ISSN 0077-8923

Coffey, C. E.; Lucke, J. F.; Saxton, J. A.; Ratcliff, G.; Unitas, L. J.; Billig, B. & Bryan, R. N. (1998). Sex Differences in Brain Aging: A Quantitative Magnetic Resonance Imaging Study. *Arch Neurol*, Vol. 55, No. 2, pp. 169-79, ISSN 0003-9942

Craig, M. C. & Murphy, D. G. (2010). Estrogen Therapy and Alzheimer's Dementia. *Ann N Y Acad Sci*, Vol. 1205 pp. 245-53, ISSN 1749-6632

Currie, L. J.; Harrison, M. B.; Trugman, J. M.; Bennett, J. P. & Wooten, G. F. (2004). Postmenopausal Estrogen Use Affects Risk for Parkinson Disease. *Arch Neurol*, Vol. 61, No. 6, pp. 886-8, ISSN 0003-9942

D'Astous, M.; Morissette, M. & Di Paolo, T. (2004). Effect of Estrogen Receptor Agonists Treatment in MPTP Mice: Evidence of Neuroprotection by an ER Alpha Agonist. *Neuropharmacology*, Vol. 47, No. 8, pp. 1180-8, ISSN 0028-3908

De Butte-Smith, M.; Gulinello, M.; Zukin, R. S. & Etgen, A. M. (2009). Chronic Estradiol Treatment Increases CA1 Cell Survival but Does Not Improve Visual or Spatial Recognition Memory after Global Ischemia in Middle-Aged Female Rats. *Horm Behav*, Vol. 55, No. 3, pp. 442-53, ISSN 1095-6867

del Zoppo, G. J. & Mabuchi, T. (2003). Cerebral Microvessel Responses to Focal Ischemia. *J Cereb Blood Flow Metab*, Vol. 23, No. 8, pp. 879-94, ISSN 0271-678X

Dexter, D. T.; Carter, C. J.; Wells, F. R.; Javoy-Agid, F.; Agid, Y.; Lees, A.; Jenner, P. & Marsden, C. D. (1989). Basal Lipid Peroxidation in Substantia Nigra Is Increased in Parkinson's Disease. *J Neurochem*, Vol. 52, No. 2, pp. 381-9, ISSN 0022-3042

Dhandapani, K. M. & Brann, D. W. (2002). Estrogen-Astrocyte Interactions: Implications for Neuroprotection. *BMC Neurosci*, Vol. 3 pp. 6, ISSN 1471-2202

Dirnagl, U.; Iadecola, C. & Moskowitz, M. A. (1999). Pathobiology of Ischaemic Stroke: An Integrated View. *Trends Neurosci*, Vol. 22, No. 9, pp. 391-7, ISSN 0166-2236

Dirnagl, U.; Klehmet, J.; Braun, J. S.; Harms, H.; Meisel, C.; Ziemssen, T.; Prass, K. & Meisel, A. (2007). Stroke-Induced Immunodepression: Experimental Evidence and Clinical Relevance. *Stroke*, Vol. 38, No. 2 Suppl, pp. 770-3, ISSN 1524-4628

Disshon, K. A.; Boja, J. W. & Dluzen, D. E. (1998). Inhibition of Striatal Dopamine Transporter Activity by 17beta-Estradiol. *Eur J Pharmacol*, Vol. 345, No. 2, pp. 207-11, ISSN 0014-2999

DonCarlos, L. L.; Azcoitia, I. & Garcia-Segura, L. M. (2009). Neuroprotective Actions of Selective Estrogen Receptor Modulators. *Psychoneuroendocrinology*, Vol. 34 Suppl 1 pp. S113-22, ISSN 1873-3360

Drechsler, Y.; Dolganiuc, A.; Norkina, O.; Romics, L.; Li, W.; Kodys, K.; Bach, F. H.; Mandrekar, P. & Szabo, G. (2006). Heme Oxygenase-1 Mediates the Anti-Inflammatory Effects of Acute Alcohol on IL-10 Induction Involving P38 MAPK Activation in Monocytes. *J Immunol*, Vol. 177, No. 4, pp. 2592-600, ISSN 0022-1767

Dubal, D. B.; Zhu, H.; Yu, J.; Rau, S. W.; Shughrue, P. J.; Merchenthaler, I.; Kindy, M. S. & Wise, P. M. (2001). Estrogen Receptor Alpha, Not Beta, Is a Critical Link in Estradiol-Mediated Protection against Brain Injury. *Proc Natl Acad Sci U S A*, Vol. 98, No. 4, pp. 1952-7, ISSN 0027-8424

Emborg, M. E. (2004). Evaluation of Animal Models of Parkinson's Disease for Neuroprotective Strategies. *J Neurosci Methods*, Vol. 139, No. 2, pp. 121-43, ISSN 0165-0270

Feigin, V. L. (2005). Stroke Epidemiology in the Developing World. *Lancet*, Vol. 365, No. 9478, pp. 2160-1, ISSN 1474-547X

Felderhoff-Mueser, U.; Buhrer, C.; Groneck, P.; Obladen, M.; Bartmann, P. & Heep, A. (2003). Soluble Fas (Cd95/Apo-1), Soluble Fas Ligand, and Activated Caspase 3 in the Cerebrospinal Fluid of Infants with Posthemorrhagic and Nonhemorrhagic Hydrocephalus. *Pediatr Res*, Vol. 54, No. 5, pp. 659-64, ISSN 0031-3998

Felderhoff-Mueser, U.; Taylor, D. L.; Greenwood, K.; Kozma, M.; Stibenz, D.; Joashi, U. C.; Edwards, A. D. & Mehmet, H. (2000). Fas/Cd95/Apo-1 Can Function as a Death Receptor for Neuronal Cells in Vitro and in Vivo and Is Upregulated Following Cerebral Hypoxic-Ischemic Injury to the Developing Rat Brain. *Brain Pathol*, Vol. 10, No. 1, pp. 17-29, ISSN 1015-6305

Garcia-Segura, L. M. & Balthazart, J. (2009). Steroids and Neuroprotection: New Advances. *Front Neuroendocrinol*, Vol. 30, No. 2, pp. v-ix, ISSN 1095-6808

Genazzani, A. R.; Pluchino, N.; Luisi, S. & Luisi, M. (2007). Estrogen, Cognition and Female Aging. *Hum Reprod Update*, Vol. 13, No. 2, pp. 175-87, ISSN 1355-4786

Greenfield, J. P.; Leung, L. W.; Cai, D.; Kaasik, K.; Gross, R. S.; Rodriguez-Boulan, E.; Greengard, P. & Xu, H. (2002). Estrogen Lowers Alzheimer Beta-Amyloid Generation by Stimulating Trans-Golgi Network Vesicle Biogenesis. *J Biol Chem*, Vol. 277, No. 14, pp. 12128-36, ISSN 0021-9258

Hardy, J. (2004). Toward Alzheimer Therapies Based on Genetic Knowledge. *Annu Rev Med*, Vol. 55 pp. 15-25, ISSN 0066-4219

Hardy, J. & Selkoe, D. J. (2002). The Amyloid Hypothesis of Alzheimer's Disease: Progress and Problems on the Road to Therapeutics. *Science*, Vol. 297, No. 5580, pp. 353-6, ISSN 1095-9203

Harris, H. A.; Albert, L. M.; Leathurby, Y.; Malamas, M. S.; Mewshaw, R. E.; Miller, C. P.; Kharode, Y. P.; Marzolf, J.; Komm, B. S.; Winneker, R. C.; Frail, D. E.; Henderson, R. A.; Zhu, Y. & Keith, J. C., Jr. (2003). Evaluation of an Estrogen Receptor-Beta Agonist in Animal Models of Human Disease. *Endocrinology*, Vol. 144, No. 10, pp. 4241-9, ISSN 0013-7227

Hastings, T. G.; Lewis, D. A. & Zigmond, M. J. (1996). Role of Oxidation in the Neurotoxic Effects of Intrastriatal Dopamine Injections. *Proc Natl Acad Sci U S A*, Vol. 93, No. 5, pp. 1956-61, ISSN 0027-8424

Hawkins, B. T. & Davis, T. P. (2005). The Blood-Brain Barrier/Neurovascular Unit in Health and Disease. *Pharmacol Rev*, Vol. 57, No. 2, pp. 173-85, ISSN 0031-6997

Hernandez-Munoz, R.; Montiel-Ruiz, C. & Vazquez-Martinez, O. (2000). Gastric Mucosal Cell Proliferation in Ethanol-Induced Chronic Mucosal Injury Is Related to Oxidative Stress and Lipid Peroxidation in Rats. *Lab Invest*, Vol. 80, No. 8, pp. 1161-9, ISSN 0023-6837

Hunot, S.; Boissiere, F.; Faucheux, B.; Brugg, B.; Mouatt-Prigent, A.; Agid, Y. & Hirsch, E. C. (1996). Nitric Oxide Synthase and Neuronal Vulnerability in Parkinson's Disease. *Neuroscience*, Vol. 72, No. 2, pp. 355-63, ISSN 0306-4522

Hunot, S. & Hirsch, E. C. (2003). Neuroinflammatory Processes in Parkinson's Disease. *Ann Neurol*, Vol. 53 Suppl 3 pp. S49-58; discussion S58-60, ISSN 0364-5134

Iivonen, S.; Corder, E.; Lehtovirta, M.; Helisalmi, S.; Mannermaa, A.; Vepsalainen, S.; Hanninen, T.; Soininen, H. & Hiltunen, M. (2004). Polymorphisms in the CYP19 Gene Confer Increased Risk for Alzheimer Disease. *Neurology*, Vol. 62, No. 7, pp. 1170-6, ISSN 1526-632X

Ishunina, T. A.; van Beurden, D.; van der Meulen, G.; Unmehopa, U. A.; Hol, E. M.; Huitinga, I. & Swaab, D. F. (2005). Diminished Aromatase Immunoreactivity in the Hypothalamus, but Not in the Basal Forebrain Nuclei in Alzheimer's Disease. *Neurobiol Aging*, Vol. 26, No. 2, pp. 173-94, ISSN 0197-4580

Ivanova, T.; Kuppers, E.; Engele, J. & Beyer, C. (2001). Estrogen Stimulates Brain-Derived Neurotrophic Factor Expression in Embryonic Mouse Midbrain Neurons through a Membrane-Mediated and Calcium-Dependent Mechanism. *J Neurosci Res*, Vol. 66, No. 2, pp. 221-30, ISSN 0360-4012

Ivanova, T.; Mendez, P.; Garcia-Segura, L. M. & Beyer, C. (2002). Rapid Stimulation of the PI3K/Akt Signalling Pathway in Developing Midbrain Neurones by Oestrogen. *J Neuroendocrinol*, Vol. 14, No. 1, pp. 73-9, ISSN 0953-8194

Jaffe, A. B.; Toran-Allerand, C. D.; Greengard, P. & Gandy, S. E. (1994). Estrogen Regulates Metabolism of Alzheimer Amyloid Beta Precursor Protein. *J Biol Chem*, Vol. 269, No. 18, pp. 13065-8, ISSN 0021-9258

Jia, J.; Guan, D.; Zhu, W.; Alkayed, N. J.; Wang, M. M.; Hua, Z. & Xu, Y. (2009). Estrogen Inhibits Fas-Mediated Apoptosis in Experimental Stroke. *Exp Neurol*, Vol. 215, No. 1, pp. 48-52, ISSN 1090-2430

Jourdain, S.; Morissette, M.; Morin, N. & Di Paolo, T. (2005). Oestrogens Prevent Loss of Dopamine Transporter (DAT) and Vesicular Monoamine Transporter (VMAT2) in

Substantia Nigra of 1-Methyl-4-Phenyl-1,2,3,6-Tetrahydropyridine Mice. *J Neuroendocrinol*, Vol. 17, No. 8, pp. 509-17, ISSN 0953-8194

Jung, M. E.; Agarwal, R. & Simpkins, J. W. (2007). Ethanol Withdrawal Posttranslationally Decreases the Activity of Cytochrome C Oxidase in an Estrogen Reversible Manner. *Neurosci Lett*, Vol. 416, No. 2, pp. 160-4, ISSN 0304-3940

Jung, M. E.; Ju, X.; Metzger, D. B. & Simpkins, J. W. (2011). Ethanol Withdrawal Hastens the Aging of Cytochrome C Oxidase. *Neurobiol Aging*, pp. 1558-1497, ISSN 1558-1497

Jung, M. E.; Ju, X.; Simpkins, J. W.; Metzger, D. B.; Yan, L. J. & Wen, Y. (2010). Ethanol Withdrawal Acts as an Age-Specific Stressor to Activate Cerebellar P38 Kinase. *Neurobiol Aging* pp. 1558-1497, ISSN 1558-1497

Jung, M. E. & Metzger, D. B. (2010). Alcohol Withdrawal and Brain Injuries: Beyond Classical Mechanisms. *Molecules*, Vol. 15, No. 7, pp. 4984-5011, ISSN 1420-3049

Jung, M. E.; Rewal, M.; Perez, E.; Wen, Y. & Simpkins, J. W. (2004). Estrogen Protects against Brain Lipid Peroxidation in Ethanol-Withdrawn Rats. *Pharmacol Biochem Behav*, Vol. 79, No. 3, pp. 573-86, ISSN 0091-3057

Jung, M. E.; Wilson, A. M.; Ju, X.; Wen, Y.; Metzger, D. B. & Simpkins, J. W. (2009). Ethanol Withdrawal Provokes Opening of the Mitochondrial Membrane Permeability Transition Pore in an Estrogen-Preventable Manner. *J Pharmacol Exp Ther*, Vol. 328, No. 3, pp. 692-8, ISSN 1521-0103

Jung, M. E.; Wilson, A. M. & Simpkins, J. W. (2006). A Nonfeminizing Estrogen Analog Protects against Ethanol Withdrawal Toxicity in Immortalized Hippocampal Cells. *J Pharmacol Exp Ther*, Vol. 319, No. 2, pp. 543-50, ISSN 0022-3565

Karakaya, S.; Kipp, M. & Beyer, C. (2007). Oestrogen Regulates the Expression and Function of Dopamine Transporters in Astrocytes of the Nigrostriatal System. *J Neuroendocrinol*, Vol. 19, No. 9, pp. 682-90, ISSN 0953-8194

Knott, C.; Stern, G. & Wilkin, G. P. (2000). Inflammatory Regulators in Parkinson's Disease: iNOS, Lipocortin-1, and Cyclooxygenases-1 and -2. *Mol Cell Neurosci*, Vol. 16, No. 6, pp. 724-39, ISSN 1044-7431

Ku, B. M.; Lee, Y. K.; Jeong, J. Y.; Mun, J.; Han, J. Y.; Roh, G. S.; Kim, H. J.; Cho, G. J.; Choi, W. S.; Yi, G. S. & Kang, S. S. (2007). Ethanol-Induced Oxidative Stress Is Mediated by P38 MAPK Pathway in Mouse Hippocampal Cells. *Neurosci Lett*, Vol. 419, No. 1, pp. 64-7, ISSN 0304-3940

Lang, A. E. (2007). The Progression of Parkinson Disease: A Hypothesis. *Neurology*, Vol. 68, No. 12, pp. 948-52, ISSN 1526-632X

Lebesgue, D.; Chevaleyre, V.; Zukin, R. S. & Etgen, A. M. (2009). Estradiol Rescues Neurons from Global Ischemia-Induced Cell Death: Multiple Cellular Pathways of Neuroprotection. *Steroids*, Vol. 74, No. 7, pp. 555-61, ISSN 0039-128X

LeBlanc, E. S.; Janowsky, J.; Chan, B. K. & Nelson, H. D. (2001). Hormone Replacement Therapy and Cognition: Systematic Review and Meta-Analysis. *JAMA*, Vol. 285, No. 11, pp. 1489-99, ISSN 0098-7484

Li, J.; Siegel, M.; Yuan, M.; Zeng, Z.; Finnucan, L.; Persky, R.; Hurn, P. D. & McCullough, L. D. (2011). Estrogen Enhances Neurogenesis and Behavioral Recovery after Stroke. *J Cereb Blood Flow Metab*, Vol. 31, No. 2, pp. 413-25, ISSN 1559-7016

Li, R.; Shen, Y.; Yang, L. B.; Lue, L. F.; Finch, C. & Rogers, J. (2000). Estrogen Enhances Uptake of Amyloid Beta-Protein by Microglia Derived from the Human Cortex. *J Neurochem*, Vol. 75, No. 4, pp. 1447-54, ISSN 0022-3042

Liang, K.; Yang, L.; Yin, C.; Xiao, Z.; Zhang, J.; Liu, Y. & Huang, J. (2010). Estrogen Stimulates Degradation of Beta-Amyloid Peptide by up-Regulating Neprilysin. *J Biol Chem*, Vol. 285, No. 2, pp. 935-42, ISSN 1083-351X

Liu, B. & Dluzen, D. E. (2006). Effect of Estrogen Upon Methamphetamine-Induced Neurotoxicity within the Impaired Nigrostriatal Dopaminergic System. *Synapse*, Vol. 60, No. 5, pp. 354-61, ISSN 0887-4476

Liu, B. & Hong, J. S. (2003). Role of Microglia in Inflammation-Mediated Neurodegenerative Diseases: Mechanisms and Strategies for Therapeutic Intervention. *J Pharmacol Exp Ther*, Vol. 304, No. 1, pp. 1-7, ISSN 0022-3565

Liu, F.; Day, M.; Muniz, L. C.; Bitran, D.; Arias, R.; Revilla-Sanchez, R.; Grauer, S.; Zhang, G.; Kelley, C.; Pulito, V.; Sung, A.; Mervis, R. F.; Navarra, R.; Hirst, W. D.; Reinhart, P. H.; Marquis, K. L.; Moss, S. J.; Pangalos, M. N. & Brandon, N. J. (2008). Activation of Estrogen Receptor-Beta Regulates Hippocampal Synaptic Plasticity and Improves Memory. *Nat Neurosci*, Vol. 11, No. 3, pp. 334-43, ISSN 1097-6256

Liu, L.; Kim, J. Y.; Koike, M. A.; Yoon, Y. J.; Tang, X. N.; Ma, H.; Lee, H.; Steinberg, G. K.; Lee, J. E. & Yenari, M. A. (2008). FasL Shedding Is Reduced by Hypothermia in Experimental Stroke. *J Neurochem*, Vol. 106, No. 2, pp. 541-50, ISSN 1471-4159

Liu, R.; Wen, Y.; Perez, E.; Wang, X.; Day, A. L.; Simpkins, J. W. & Yang, S. H. (2005). 17beta-Estradiol Attenuates Blood-Brain Barrier Disruption Induced by Cerebral Ischemia-Reperfusion Injury in Female Rats. *Brain Res*, Vol. 1060, No. 1-2, pp. 55-61, ISSN 0006-8993

Logan, S. M.; Sarkar, S. N.; Zhang, Z. & Simpkins, J. W. (2011). Estrogen-Induced Signaling Attenuates Soluble Aβ Peptide-Mediated Dysfunction of Pathways in Synaptic Plasticity. *Brain Res*, Vol. 1383 pp. 1-12, ISSN 1872-6240

Luchetti, S.; Huitinga, I. & Swaab, D. F. (2011). Neurosteroid and GABA-a Receptor Alterations in Alzheimer's Disease, Parkinson's Disease and Multiple Sclerosis. *Neuroscience* pp. 1873-7544, ISSN 1873-7544

Luo, Y.; Umegaki, H.; Wang, X.; Abe, R. & Roth, G. S. (1998). Dopamine Induces Apoptosis through an Oxidation-Involved SAPK/JNK Activation Pathway. *J Biol Chem*, Vol. 273, No. 6, pp. 3756-64, ISSN 0021-9258

Luth, H. J.; Holzer, M.; Gartner, U.; Staufenbiel, M. & Arendt, T. (2001). Expression of Endothelial and Inducible NOS-isoforms Is Increased in Alzheimer's Disease, in APP23 Transgenic Mice and after Experimental Brain Lesion in Rat: Evidence for an Induction by Amyloid Pathology. *Brain Res*, Vol. 913, No. 1, pp. 57-67, ISSN 0006-8993

Maggi, A.; Ciana, P.; Belcredito, S. & Vegeto, E. (2004). Estrogens in the Nervous System: Mechanisms and Nonreproductive Functions. *Annu Rev Physiol*, Vol. 66 pp. 291-313, ISSN 0066-4278

Marotta, F.; Reizakovic, I.; Tajiri, H.; Safran, P. & Ideo, G. (1997). Abstinence-Induced Oxidative Stress in Moderate Drinkers Is Improved by Bionormalizer. *Hepatogastroenterology*, Vol. 44, No. 17, pp. 1360-6, ISSN 0172-6390

Marrian, G. F. & Butenandt, A. (1931). Oestrus-Producing Hormones. *Science*, Vol. 74, No. 1926, pp. 547, ISSN 0036-8075

Mattson, M. P.; Culmsee, C. & Yu, Z. F. (2000). Apoptotic and Antiapoptotic Mechanisms in Stroke. *Cell Tissue Res*, Vol. 301, No. 1, pp. 173-87, ISSN 0302-766X

McGeer, P. L.; Itagaki, S.; Boyes, B. E. & McGeer, E. G. (1988). Reactive Microglia Are Positive for HLA-DR in the Substantia Nigra of Parkinson's and Alzheimer's Disease Brains. *Neurology*, Vol. 38, No. 8, pp. 1285-91, ISSN 0028-3878

McGeer, P. L.; Rogers, J. & McGeer, E. G. (2006). Inflammation, Anti-Inflammatory Agents and Alzheimer Disease: The Last 12 Years. *J Alzheimers Dis*, Vol. 9, No. 3 Suppl, pp. 271-6, ISSN 1387-2877

Meisel, C.; Schwab, J. M.; Prass, K.; Meisel, A. & Dirnagl, U. (2005). Central Nervous System Injury-Induced Immune Deficiency Syndrome. *Nat Rev Neurosci*, Vol. 6, No. 10, pp. 775-86, ISSN 1471-003X

Miller, N. R.; Jover, T.; Cohen, H. W.; Zukin, R. S. & Etgen, A. M. (2005). Estrogen Can Act Via Estrogen Receptor Alpha and Beta to Protect Hippocampal Neurons against Global Ischemia-Induced Cell Death. *Endocrinology*, Vol. 146, No. 7, pp. 3070-9, ISSN 0013-7227

Montoliu, C.; Valles, S.; Renau-Piqueras, J. & Guerri, C. (1994). Ethanol-Induced Oxygen Radical Formation and Lipid Peroxidation in Rat Brain: Effect of Chronic Alcohol Consumption. *J Neurochem*, Vol. 63, No. 5, pp. 1855-62, ISSN 0022-3042

Morale, M. C.; Serra, P. A.; L'Episcopo, F.; Tirolo, C.; Caniglia, S.; Testa, N.; Gennuso, F.; Giaquinta, G.; Rocchitta, G.; Desole, M. S.; Miele, E. & Marchetti, B. (2006). Estrogen, Neuroinflammation and Neuroprotection in Parkinson's Disease: Glia Dictates Resistance Versus Vulnerability to Neurodegeneration. *Neuroscience*, Vol. 138, No. 3, pp. 869-78, ISSN 0306-4522

Moriguchi, T.; Toyoshima, F.; Gotoh, Y.; Iwamatsu, A.; Irie, K.; Mori, E.; Kuroyanagi, N.; Hagiwara, M.; Matsumoto, K. & Nishida, E. (1996). Purification and Identification of a Major Activator for P38 from Osmotically Shocked Cells. Activation of Mitogen-Activated Protein Kinase Kinase 6 by Osmotic Shock, Tumor Necrosis Factor-Alpha, and H_2O_2. *J Biol Chem*, Vol. 271, No. 43, pp. 26981-8, ISSN 0021-9258

Morinaga, A.; Hirohata, M.; Ono, K. & Yamada, M. (2007). Estrogen Has Anti-Amyloidogenic Effects on Alzheimer's Beta-Amyloid Fibrils *in vitro*. *Biochem Biophys Res Commun*, Vol. 359, No. 3, pp. 697-702, ISSN 0006-291X

Nalivaeva, N. N.; Fisk, L. R.; Belyaev, N. D. & Turner, A. J. (2008). Amyloid-Degrading Enzymes as Therapeutic Targets in Alzheimer's Disease. *Curr Alzheimer Res*, Vol. 5, No. 2, pp. 212-24, ISSN 1567-2050

Niewada, M.; Kobayashi, A.; Sandercock, P. A.; Kaminski, B. & Czlonkowska, A. (2005). Influence of Gender on Baseline Features and Clinical Outcomes among 17,370 Patients with Confirmed Ischemic Stroke in the International Stroke Trial. *Neuroepidemiology*, Vol. 24, No. 3, pp. 123-8, ISSN 0251-5350

Nordmann, R.; Ribiere, C. & Rouach, H. (1990). Ethanol-Induced Lipid Peroxidation and Oxidative Stress in Extrahepatic Tissues. *Alcohol Alcohol*, Vol. 25, No. 2-3, pp. 231-7, ISSN 0735-0414

Norkina, O.; Dolganiuc, A.; Shapiro, T.; Kodys, K.; Mandrekar, P. & Szabo, G. (2007). Acute Alcohol Activates STAT3, AP-1, and SP-1 Transcription Factors Via the Family of Src Kinases to Promote IL-10 Production in Human Monocytes. *J Leukoc Biol*, Vol. 82, No. 3, pp. 752-62, ISSN 0741-5400

Offner, H.; Vandenbark, A. A. & Hurn, P. D. (2009). Effect of Experimental Stroke on Peripheral Immunity: CNS Ischemia Induces Profound Immunosuppression. *Neuroscience*, Vol. 158, No. 3, pp. 1098-111, ISSN 0306-4522

Oldendorf, W. H.; Cornford, M. E. & Brown, W. J. (1977). The Large Apparent Work Capability of the Blood-Brain Barrier: A Study of the Mitochondrial Content of Capillary Endothelial Cells in Brain and Other Tissues of the Rat. *Ann Neurol*, Vol. 1, No. 5, pp. 409-17, ISSN 0364-5134

Park, E. M.; Cho, S.; Frys, K. A.; Glickstein, S. B.; Zhou, P.; Anrather, J.; Ross, M. E. & Iadecola, C. (2006). Inducible Nitric Oxide Synthase Contributes to Gender Differences in Ischemic Brain Injury. *J Cereb Blood Flow Metab*, Vol. 26, No. 3, pp. 392-401, ISSN 0271-678X

Pelligrino, D. A.; Santizo, R.; Baughman, V. L. & Wang, Q. (1998). Cerebral Vasodilating Capacity During Forebrain Ischemia: Effects of Chronic Estrogen Depletion and Repletion and the Role of Neuronal Nitric Oxide Synthase. *Neuroreport*, Vol. 9, No. 14, pp. 3285-91, ISSN 0959-4965

Peters, O.; Back, T.; Lindauer, U.; Busch, C.; Megow, D.; Dreier, J. & Dirnagl, U. (1998). Increased Formation of Reactive Oxygen Species after Permanent and Reversible Middle Cerebral Artery Occlusion in the Rat. *J Cereb Blood Flow Metab*, Vol. 18, No. 2, pp. 196-205, ISSN 0271-678X

Petito, C. K.; Kraig, R. P. & Pulsinelli, W. A. (1987). Light and Electron Microscopic Evaluation of Hydrogen Ion-Induced Brain Necrosis. *J Cereb Blood Flow Metab*, Vol. 7, No. 5, pp. 625-32, ISSN 0271-678X

Pfeilschifter, J.; Koditz, R.; Pfohl, M. & Schatz, H. (2002). Changes in Proinflammatory Cytokine Activity after Menopause. *Endocr Rev*, Vol. 23, No. 1, pp. 90-119, ISSN 0163-769X

Polanczyk, M.; Zamora, A.; Subramanian, S.; Matejuk, A.; Hess, D. L.; Blankenhorn, E. P.; Teuscher, C.; Vandenbark, A. A. & Offner, H. (2003). The Protective Effect of 17beta-Estradiol on Experimental Autoimmune Encephalomyelitis Is Mediated through Estrogen Receptor-Alpha. *Am J Pathol*, Vol. 163, No. 4, pp. 1599-605, ISSN 0002-9440

Pozzilli, C.; Falaschi, P.; Mainero, C.; Martocchia, A.; D'Urso, R.; Proietti, A.; Frontoni, M.; Bastianello, S. & Filippi, M. (1999). MRI in Multiple Sclerosis During the Menstrual Cycle: Relationship with Sex Hormone Patterns. *Neurology*, Vol. 53, No. 3, pp. 622-4, ISSN 0028-3878

Prokai-Tatrai, K.; Perjesi, P.; Rivera-Portalatin, N. M.; Simpkins, J. W. & Prokai, L. (2008). Mechanistic Investigations on the Antioxidant Action of a Neuroprotective Estrogen Derivative. *Steroids*, Vol. 73, No. 3, pp. 280-8, ISSN 0039-128X

Prokai, L.; Prokai-Tatrai, K.; Perjesi, P.; Zharikova, A. D.; Perez, E. J.; Liu, R. & Simpkins, J. W. (2003). Quinol-Based Cyclic Antioxidant Mechanism in Estrogen Neuroprotection. *Proc Natl Acad Sci U S A*, Vol. 100, No. 20, pp. 11741-6, ISSN 0027-8424

Przedborski, S.; Kostic, V.; Jackson-Lewis, V.; Naini, A. B.; Simonetti, S.; Fahn, S.; Carlson, E.; Epstein, C. J. & Cadet, J. L. (1992). Transgenic Mice with Increased Cu/Zn-Superoxide Dismutase Activity Are Resistant to N-Methyl-4-Phenyl-1,2,3,6-Tetrahydropyridine-Induced Neurotoxicity. *J Neurosci*, Vol. 12, No. 5, pp. 1658-67, ISSN 0270-6474

Ragonese, P.; D'Amelio, M.; Salemi, G.; Aridon, P.; Gammino, M.; Epifanio, A.; Morgante, L. & Savettieri, G. (2004). Risk of Parkinson Disease in Women: Effect of Reproductive Characteristics. *Neurology*, Vol. 62, No. 11, pp. 2010-4, ISSN 1526-632X

Rewal, M.; Wen, Y.; Wilson, A.; Simpkins, J. W. & Jung, M. E. (2005). Role of Parvalbumin in Estrogen Protection from Ethanol Withdrawal Syndrome. *Alcohol Clin Exp Res*, Vol. 29, No. 10, pp. 1837-44, ISSN 0145-6008

Rosario, E. R.; Chang, L.; Head, E. H.; Stanczyk, F. Z. & Pike, C. J. (2011). Brain Levels of Sex Steroid Hormones in Men and Women During Normal Aging and in Alzheimer's Disease. *Neurobiol Aging*, Vol. 32, No. 4, pp. 604-13, ISSN 1558-1497

Rosenbaum, D. M.; Gupta, G.; D'Amore, J.; Singh, M.; Weidenheim, K.; Zhang, H. & Kessler, J. A. (2000). Fas (CD95/APO-1) Plays a Role in the Pathophysiology of Focal Cerebral Ischemia. *J Neurosci Res*, Vol. 61, No. 6, pp. 686-92, ISSN 0360-4012

Rossetti, Z. L. & Carboni, S. (1995). Ethanol Withdrawal Is Associated with Increased Extracellular Glutamate in the Rat Striatum. *Eur J Pharmacol*, Vol. 283, No. 1-3, pp. 177-83, ISSN 0014-2999

Saido, T. C. (1998). Alzheimer's Disease as Proteolytic Disorders: Anabolism and Catabolism of Beta-Amyloid. *Neurobiol Aging*, Vol. 19, No. 1 Suppl, pp. S69-75, ISSN 0197-4580

Sano, M.; Jacobs, D.; Andrews, H.; Bell, K.; Graff-Radford, N.; Lucas, J.; Rabins, P.; Bolla, K.; Tsai, W. Y.; Cross, P.; Andrews, K.; Costa, R. & Xiaodong, Luo. (2008). A Multi-Center, Randomized, Double Blind Placebo-Controlled Trial of Estrogens to Prevent Alzheimer's Disease and Loss of Memory in Women: Design and Baseline Characteristics. *Clin Trials*, Vol. 5, No. 5, pp. 523-33, ISSN 1740-7745

Saunders-Pullman, R.; Derby, C.; Santoro, N.; Bressman, S.; Chiu, R.B.; Lipton, R.B.; Wassertheil-Smoller, S. (2009). Role of Endogenous and Exogenous Hormone Exposure on the Risk of Parkinson Disease: Results from the Women's Health Initiative Observational Study. *American Academy of Neurology*

Selkoe, D. J. (2000). The Genetics and Molecular Pathology of Alzheimer's Disease: Roles of Amyloid and the Presenilins. *Neurol Clin*, Vol. 18, No. 4, pp. 903-22, ISSN 0733-8619

Selvamani, A. & Sohrabji, F. (2010). Reproductive Age Modulates the Impact of Focal Ischemia on the Forebrain as Well as the Effects of Estrogen Treatment in Female Rats. *Neurobiol Aging*, Vol. 31, No. 9, pp. 1618-28, ISSN 1558-1497

Sherwin, B. B. (2007). The Clinical Relevance of the Relationship between Estrogen and Cognition in Women. *J Steroid Biochem Mol Biol*, Vol. 106, No. 1-5, pp. 151-6, ISSN 0960-0760

Sherwin, B. B. (2009). Estrogen Therapy: Is Time of Initiation Critical for Neuroprotection? *Nat Rev Endocrinol*, Vol. 5, No. 11, pp. 620-7, ISSN 1759-5037

Sherwin, B.B.; Chertkow, H.; Schipper, H.; Nasreddine, Z. (2011). A Randomized Controlled Trial of Estrogen Treatment in Men with Mild Cognitive Impairment. . *Neurobiol Aging*

Shughrue, P. J. (2004). Estrogen Attenuates the MPTP-Induced Loss of Dopamine Neurons from the Mouse SNC Despite a Lack of Estrogen Receptors (Eralpha and Erbeta). *Exp Neurol*, Vol. 190, No. 2, pp. 468-77, ISSN 0014-4886

Shulman, L. M. & Bhat, V. (2006). Gender Disparities in Parkinson's Disease. *Expert Rev Neurother*, Vol. 6, No. 3, pp. 407-16, ISSN 1744-8360

Sian, J.; Dexter, D. T.; Lees, A. J.; Daniel, S.; Agid, Y.; Javoy-Agid, F.; Jenner, P. & Marsden, C. D. (1994). Alterations in Glutathione Levels in Parkinson's Disease and Other Neurodegenerative Disorders Affecting Basal Ganglia. *Ann Neurol*, Vol. 36, No. 3, pp. 348-55, ISSN 0364-5134

Simpkins, J. W.; Singh, M. & Bishop, J. (1994). The Potential Role for Estrogen Replacement Therapy in the Treatment of the Cognitive Decline and Neurodegeneration Associated with Alzheimer's Disease. *Neurobiol Aging*, Vol. 15 Suppl 2 pp. S195-7, ISSN 0197-4580

Smith, M. A.; Richey Harris, P. L.; Sayre, L. M.; Beckman, J. S. & Perry, G. (1997). Widespread Peroxynitrite-Mediated Damage in Alzheimer's Disease. *J Neurosci*, Vol. 17, No. 8, pp. 2653-7, ISSN 0270-6474

St George-Hyslop, P. H. (2000). Genetic Factors in the Genesis of Alzheimer's Disease. *Ann N Y Acad Sci*, Vol. 924 pp. 1-7, ISSN 0077-8923

Sugawara, T.; Kinouchi, H.; Oda, M.; Shoji, H.; Omae, T. & Mizoi, K. (2005). Candesartan Reduces Superoxide Production after Global Cerebral Ischemia. *Neuroreport*, Vol. 16, No. 4, pp. 325-8, ISSN 0959-4965

Suzuki, S.; Brown, C. M. & Wise, P. M. (2009). Neuroprotective Effects of Estrogens Following Ischemic Stroke. *Front Neuroendocrinol*, Vol. 30, No. 2, pp. 201-11, ISSN 1095-6808

Szego, E. M.; Csorba, A.; Janaky, T.; Kekesi, K. A.; Abraham, I. M.; Morotz, G. M.; Penke, B.; Palkovits, M.; Murvai, U.; Kellermayer, M. S.; Kardos, J. & Juhasz, G. D. (2011). Effects of Estrogen on Beta-Amyloid-Induced Cholinergic Cell Death in the Nucleus Basalis Magnocellularis. *Neuroendocrinology*, Vol. 93, No. 2, pp. 90-105, ISSN 1423-0194

Tanzi, R. E. & Bertram, L. (2005). Twenty Years of the Alzheimer's Disease Amyloid Hypothesis: A Genetic Perspective. *Cell*, Vol. 120, No. 4, pp. 545-55, ISSN 0092-8674

Towfighi, A.; Saver, J. L.; Engelhardt, R. & Ovbiagele, B. (2007). A Midlife Stroke Surge among Women in the United States. *Neurology*, Vol. 69, No. 20, pp. 1898-904, ISSN 1526-632X

Tripanichkul, W.; Sripanichkulchai, K.; Duce, J. A. & Finkelstein, D. I. (2007). 17beta-Estradiol Reduces Nitrotyrosine Immunoreactivity and Increases SOD1 and SOD2 Immunoreactivity in Nigral Neurons in Male Mice Following MPTP Insult. *Brain Res*, Vol. 1164 pp. 24-31, ISSN 0006-8993

Tsai, G. E.; Ragan, P.; Chang, R.; Chen, S.; Linnoila, V. M. & Coyle, J. T. (1998). Increased Glutamatergic Neurotransmission and Oxidative Stress after Alcohol Withdrawal. *Am J Psychiatry*, Vol. 155, No. 6, pp. 726-32, ISSN 0002-953X

Valles, S. L.; Dolz-Gaiton, P.; Gambini, J.; Borras, C.; Lloret, A.; Pallardo, F. V. & Vina, J. (2010). Estradiol or Genistein Prevent Alzheimer's Disease-Associated Inflammation Correlating with an Increase PPAR Gamma Expression in Cultured Astrocytes. *Brain Res*, Vol. 1312 pp. 138-44, ISSN 1872-6240

Vallett, M.; Tabatabaie, T.; Briscoe, R. J.; Baird, T. J.; Beatty, W. W.; Floyd, R. A. & Gauvin, D. V. (1997). Free Radical Production During Ethanol Intoxication, Dependence, and Withdrawal. *Alcohol Clin Exp Res*, Vol. 21, No. 2, pp. 275-85, ISSN 0145-6008

Vegeto, E.; Belcredito, S.; Etteri, S.; Ghisletti, S.; Brusadelli, A.; Meda, C.; Krust, A.; Dupont, S.; Ciana, P.; Chambon, P. & Maggi, A. (2003). Estrogen Receptor-Alpha Mediates the Brain Antiinflammatory Activity of Estradiol. *Proc Natl Acad Sci U S A*, Vol. 100, No. 16, pp. 9614-9, ISSN 0027-8424

Vegeto, E.; Belcredito, S.; Ghisletti, S.; Meda, C.; Etteri, S. & Maggi, A. (2006). The Endogenous Estrogen Status Regulates Microglia Reactivity in Animal Models of Neuroinflammation. *Endocrinology*, Vol. 147, No. 5, pp. 2263-72, ISSN 0013-7227

Vegeto, E.; Benedusi, V. & Maggi, A. (2008). Estrogen Anti-Inflammatory Activity in Brain: A Therapeutic Opportunity for Menopause and Neurodegenerative Diseases. *Front Neuroendocrinol*, Vol. 29, No. 4, pp. 507-19, ISSN 1095-6808

Vegeto, E.; Bonincontro, C.; Pollio, G.; Sala, A.; Viappiani, S.; Nardi, F.; Brusadelli, A.; Viviani, B.; Ciana, P. & Maggi, A. (2001). Estrogen Prevents the Lipopolysaccharide-Induced Inflammatory Response in Microglia. *J Neurosci*, Vol. 21, No. 6, pp. 1809-18, ISSN 1529-2401

Viscoli, C. M.; Brass, L. M.; Kernan, W. N.; Sarrel, P. M.; Suissa, S. & Horwitz, R. I. (2001). A Clinical Trial of Estrogen-Replacement Therapy after Ischemic Stroke. *N Engl J Med*, Vol. 345, No. 17, pp. 1243-9, ISSN 0028-4793

Wahner, A. D.; Bronstein, J. M.; Bordelon, Y. M. & Ritz, B. (2007). Nonsteroidal Anti-Inflammatory Drugs May Protect against Parkinson's Disease. *Neurology*, Vol. 69, No. 19, pp. 1836-42, ISSN 1526-632X

Wang, X.; Ellison, J. A.; Siren, A. L.; Lysko, P. G.; Yue, T. L.; Barone, F. C.; Shatzman, A. & Feuerstein, G. Z. (1998). Prolonged Expression of Interferon-Inducible Protein-10 in Ischemic Cortex after Permanent Occlusion of the Middle Cerebral Artery in Rat. *J Neurochem*, Vol. 71, No. 3, pp. 1194-204, ISSN 0022-3042

Wang, X.; Yue, T. L.; Barone, F. C.; White, R. F.; Gagnon, R. C. & Feuerstein, G. Z. (1994). Concomitant Cortical Expression of TNF-alpha and IL-1 beta mRNAs Follows Early Response Gene Expression in Transient Focal Ischemia. *Mol Chem Neuropathol*, Vol. 23, No. 2-3, pp. 103-14, ISSN 1044-7393

Wang, X.; Yue, T. L.; Young, P. R.; Barone, F. C. & Feuerstein, G. Z. (1995). Expression of Interleukin-6, C-Fos, and Zif268 mRNAs in Rat Ischemic Cortex. *J Cereb Blood Flow Metab*, Vol. 15, No. 1, pp. 166-71, ISSN 0271-678X

Wassertheil-Smoller, S.; Hendrix, S. L.; Limacher, M.; Heiss, G.; Kooperberg, C.; Baird, A.; Kotchen, T.; Curb, J. D.; Black, H.; Rossouw, J. E.; Aragaki, A.; Safford, M.; Stein, E.; Laowattana, S. & Mysiw, W. J. (2003). Effect of Estrogen Plus Progestin on Stroke in Postmenopausal Women: The Women's Health Initiative: A Randomized Trial. *JAMA*, Vol. 289, No. 20, pp. 2673-84, ISSN 0098-7484

Weill-Engerer, S.; David, J. P.; Sazdovitch, V.; Liere, P.; Eychenne, B.; Pianos, A.; Schumacher, M.; Delacourte, A.; Baulieu, E. E. & Akwa, Y. (2002). Neurosteroid Quantification in Human Brain Regions: Comparison between Alzheimer's and Nondemented Patients. *J Clin Endocrinol Metab*, Vol. 87, No. 11, pp. 5138-43, ISSN 0021-972X

Wober, C.; Wober-Bingol, C.; Karwautz, A.; Nimmerrichter, A.; Walter, H. & Deecke, L. (1998). Ataxia of Stance in Different Types of Alcohol Dependence--a Posturographic Study. *Alcohol Alcohol*, Vol. 33, No. 4, pp. 393-402, ISSN 0735-0414

Xu, H.; Gouras, G. K.; Greenfield, J. P.; Vincent, B.; Naslund, J.; Mazzarelli, L.; Fried, G.; Jovanovic, J. N.; Seeger, M.; Relkin, N. R.; Liao, F.; Checler, F.; Buxbaum, J. D.; Chait, B. T.; Thinakaran, G.; Sisodia, S. S.; Wang, R.; Greengard, P. & Gandy, S. (1998). Estrogen Reduces Neuronal Generation of Alzheimer Beta-Amyloid Peptides. *Nat Med*, Vol. 4, No. 4, pp. 447-51, ISSN 1078-8956

Yamin, G.; Ono, K.; Inayathullah, M. & Teplow, D. B. (2008). Amyloid Beta-Protein Assembly as a Therapeutic Target of Alzheimer's Disease. *Curr Pharm Des*, Vol. 14, No. 30, pp. 3231-46, ISSN 1873-4286

Yue, X.; Lu, M.; Lancaster, T.; Cao, P.; Honda, S.; Staufenbiel, M.; Harada, N.; Zhong, Z.; Shen, Y. & Li, R. (2005). Brain Estrogen Deficiency Accelerates Aβ Plaque Formation in an Alzheimer's Disease Animal Model. *Proc Natl Acad Sci U S A*, Vol. 102, No. 52, pp. 19198-203, ISSN 0027-8424

Zandi, P. P.; Carlson, M. C.; Plassman, B. L.; Welsh-Bohmer, K. A.; Mayer, L. S.; Steffens, D. C. & Breitner, J. C. (2002). Hormone Replacement Therapy and Incidence of Alzheimer Disease in Older Women: The Cache County Study. *JAMA*, Vol. 288, No. 17, pp. 2123-9, ISSN 0098-7484

Zhang, B.; Subramanian, S.; Dziennis, S.; Jia, J.; Uchida, M.; Akiyoshi, K.; Migliati, E.; Lewis, A. D.; Vandenbark, A. A.; Offner, H. & Hurn, P. D. (2010). Estradiol and G1 Reduce Infarct Size and Improve Immunosuppression after Experimental Stroke. *J Immunol*, Vol. 184, No. 8, pp. 4087-94, ISSN 1550-6606

Zhang, J.; Graham, D. G.; Montine, T. J. & Ho, Y. S. (2000). Enhanced N-Methyl-4-Phenyl-1,2,3,6-Tetrahydropyridine Toxicity in Mice Deficient in Cu Zn-Superoxide Dismutase or Glutathione Peroxidase. *J Neuropathol Exp Neurol*, Vol. 59, No. 1, pp. 53-61, ISSN 0022-3069

Zhang, Q. G.; Raz, L.; Wang, R.; Han, D.; De Sevilla, L.; Yang, F.; Vadlamudi, R. K. & Brann, D. W. (2009). Estrogen Attenuates Ischemic Oxidative Damage Via an Estrogen Receptor Alpha-Mediated Inhibition of NADPH Oxidase Activation. *J Neurosci*, Vol. 29, No. 44, pp. 13823-36, ISSN 1529-2401

Zheng, H.; Xu, H.; Uljon,S.N.; Gross, R.; Hardy,K.;Gaynor, J.; Lafrancois, J.; Simpkins, J.; Refolo,L.M.; Petanceska,S.; Wang, R.; Duff, K. (2002). Modulation of Aβ Peptides by Estrogen in Mouse Models. *J Neurochem*, Vol. 80, No. 1, pp. 191-6, ISSN

Zhu, X.; Su, B.; Wang, X.; Smith, M. A. & Perry, G. (2007). Causes of Oxidative Stress in Alzheimer Disease. *Cell Mol Life Sci*, Vol. 64, No. 17, pp. 2202-10, ISSN 1420-682X

8

Estrogen Influences on Cognition

Antonella Gasbarri[1] and Carlos Tomaz[2]

[1]*Department of Biomedical Sciences and Technologies, University of L'Aquila, L'Aquila,*

[2]*Department of Physiological Sciences, Laboratory of Neurosciences and Behavior,Institute of Biology, University of Brasília, Brasília, DF,*

[1]*Italy*

[2]*Brazil*

1. Introduction

Sex steroids are hormones produced mainly by the reproductive glands, either the ovaries or testes, which share a similar basic structure of three hexane rings and a pentane ring. They include estrogens, androgens, and progestogens, and each has major effects on reproductive physiology (Henderson, 2009; Osterlund & Hurd, 2001). Estrogens are required for normal female sexual maturation; they promote growth and differentiation of the breast, uterus, fallopian tubes, vagina, and ovaries (Carr, 1998). Male reproductive tissues, such as testis and prostate, are also estrogen target tissues (Clark et al., 1992). In addition, estrogens have an important role in bone maintenance (Turner et al., 1994), and protection of the cardiovascular system (Farhat et al., 1996) .

Even though estrogens (e.g., 17β-estradiol) and progestogens (e.g., progesterone) are classified as female sex hormones and androgens (e.g., testosterone) as male sex hormones, this categorization is misleading. In fact, for example, estrogens are found both in men and women, and they have effects in both sexes; besides, they arise in tissues other than the ovaries (Osterlund & Hurd, 2001).

Among the sex steroids, estrogens are the best studied with respect to human non-reproductive behaviors. They exert a broad range of effects throughout the body, including the central nervous system (CNS), where their actions are not limited to the regulation of reproductive neuroendocrinology and sexual behavior (Henderson 2009, 2010, 2011; Ziegler & Gallagher, 2005). In fact, accumulating evidence points to their involvement in influencing the function of numerous neural systems and, presumably, different behavioral domains (McEwen & Alves, 1999; McEwen et al, 2001; McEwen, 2010; Ziegler & Gallagher, 2005). Recent studies have highlighted a number of important, global issues regarding the influence of estrogen on cognitive functions (Lacreuse, 2006; Luine, 2007, 2008; Markou et al., 2007).

A possible explanation for this effect can be represented by the modulator role exerted by estrogens on several neurotransmitter systems (such as acetylcholine, catecholamines, serotonin, and GABA), both in animals and humans (Amin et al, 2006; Dumas et al 2006). Another reason may lie in the widespread presence of estrogen receptors (ERs) in many regions involved in cognitive processes, such as learning and memory, including the

hippocampal formation (HF), amygdala, and cerebral cortex (Genazzani et al 2007; Sherwin, 2003; Shughrue & Merchenthaler, 2000) .
Sex-related differences in cognitive abilities, such as verbal, memory and spatial tasks, have been reported; in addition, several estrogen effects differ qualitatively or quantitatively between the sexes, suggesting that they could be subject to sexual differentiation during pre- or early postnatal development (Gasbarri et al, 2009). Ovarian hormones affect cognition and neural substrates subserving learning and memory functions, in both rodents (Daniel, 2006; Warren & Juraska, 1997) and humans (Janowski et al, 2000), as it was evidenced by studies assessing performances across the estrous and menstrual cycles. Sex-related differences in brain function are also observed in the incidence of some psychopathology, such as depressive illness, which is more frequent in women, antisocial behavior and substance abuse, which are more common in men (McEwen, 2002). The variety of these effects confirms that other brain structures are implicated, besides the hypothalamus, which has been the traditional site for the study of ovarian steroid receptors and their role in the control of reproductive function. For example, the hormonal influences on motor activity involve brain areas such as the nucleus accumbens, striatum, substantia nigra and ventral tegmental area, while the effects on memory processes imply actions on brain structures such as basal forebrain and HF, and those on mood involve, at least in part, the serotonergic system of the midbrain raphe nuclei.
Postmenopausal alterations of the limbic system are related to mood changes, anxiety, depression, insomnia, headaches/migraine, alterations of cognitive functions (Genazzani et al 2002).
Even though there is currently a substantial literature on the putative neuroprotective effects of estrogen on cognitive functions in postmenopausal women, some discrepancy still exists. The critical period hypothesis, validated several years ago, attempts to account for the literature inconsistencies by positing that estrogen treatment can protect aspects of cognition in older women only if treatment starts soon after the menopause. Although it is not totally clear why estrogen administered to women over 65 does not provide any neuroprotection and may even impair cognition, it could be possible that the events characterizing brain aging (such as alterations in neurotransmitter systems and decrease of brain volume, neuronal size, dendritic spine number) represent an adverse background preventing the neuroprotective effect of exogenous estrogen on the brain. Other factors that could have contributed to the discrepancies in the literature include differences in the type of estrogen compounds used, their route of administration, cyclic versus continuous regimens, and the concomitant administration of progestins (Sherwin & Henry, 2008).

2. Neurobiology of estrogen

The identification and mapping of ERs in the brain led to the discovery that they are concentrated in the hypothalamus, hypophysis, HF, cerebral cortex, midbrain, and brainstem (Micevych & Mermelstein, 2008).
Even though a complete description is beyond the scope of the present paper, the mechanisms that are likely the most relevant to explain the cognitive function of estrogen are briefly described here (see McEwen, 2002, for a review).
The nuclear ERs are ligands activated transcription factors belonging to the steroid hormone receptors, included in the nuclear receptor superfamily (Osterlund & Hurd, 2001). Two types of ERs are known: ERα and ERβ, which are similar in their structural organization into

domains, but differ in their binding affinities for diverse ligands and selective ER modulators (Gruber et al, 2002; Rehman & Masson, 2005).

ERα and ERβ are products of different genes and show tissue- and cell-type specific expression (Pettersson & Gustafsson, 2001). Both ERs are widely distributed throughout the body (Rehman & Masson, 2005) and have also been localized in several cerebral areas, such as the cortex, amygdala, HF, basal forebrain, cerebellum, locus coeruleus, rafe, and central grey matter, confirming an involvement of estrogen in controlling cognitive functions in both physiological and pathological conditions (Sherwin, 1997; Sherwin & Henry, 2008).

The cerebral distribution of ERα has been quite well established by steroid autoradiography, immunocytochemistry, and in situ hybridization (Pfaff, 1980) and many studies have shown nuclear and extranuclear ERβ immunoreactivity in several brain regions, especially the hippocampus (Milner et al, 2005; Mitra et al, 2003). The ERα mRNA expression prevail in the hypothalamus and amygdaloid complex, suggesting that the α-subtype could modulate neuronal populations involved in autonomic and reproductive neuroendocrine functions, as well as emotional processes. On the contrary, in the thalamus, HF, entorhinal cortex, and neocortex there is a prevalence of ERβ, indicating a putative role for ERβ in cognition, non-emotional memory and motor functions (Osterlund & Hurd, 2001) The co-localization of ERβ mRNA with cell nuclear ERβ immunoreactivity was revealed in the cerebral cortex, paraventricular nuclei, and preoptic area of hypothalamus, in the rat (Shughrue & Merchenthaler, 2001) It is important to note that the use of I^{125} estrogen, which labels ERs with a higher specific radioactivity compared to ^{3}H estradiol, allowed the detection of label in pyramidal cells of ventral hippocampal CAl and CA3 fields (Shughrue & Merchenthaler, 2000), which are involved in memory processes. Besides its influence on both direct genomic actions, estrogen can also act in the CNS via nonnuclear receptors that implicate interactions of ERs with second messenger systems (Lee & McEwen, 2001; Sherwin & Henry, 2008)

Concerning the subcellular localization of ER, in addition to the nuclear ERs, there is a predominant localization of ERs in proximity to the plasmatic membrane of neuritis, soma, dendritic spines, and axon terminals (Clarke et al, 2000; McEwen et al, 2001). These results also imply that classical ERs may have an intracellular dynamic action and suggest that ERs can be found in different subcellular structures. This is supported by findings showing that estrogen binds and interacts with proteins in the mitochondrial membranes and that ERs are associated with pre-synaptic structures, thus controlling synaptic transmission (Genazzani et al, 2007; Ledoux & Woolley, 2005). In conclusion, estrogen effects on the brain include complex cellular mechanisms ranging from classical nuclear to non-classical membrane-mediated actions. Both forms of cell signaling could be activated separately, even though there is evidence that they are intertwined at several cellular instances and can influence each other reciprocally, yielding synergic effects (Genazzani et al, 2007).

Due to the widespread presence of the ERs in their different forms throughout the brain, estrogen actions are also widespread and affect many neurotransmitter systems including the cholinergic, catecholaminergic, serotonergic, and GABAergic systems (McEwen, 2002). The influence of estrogen on cerebral structures and functions offer possible explanations for the mechanisms of action by which this steroid hormone could affect cognitive functions in women. For example, it was reported that one of the effects of estrogen is to enhance the density of dendritic spine on CAl hippocampal neurons within 24–72 h after its acute administration (Woolley et al, 1990). Moreover, estrogens increase the concentration of choline acetyltransferase (ChAT), critically involved in memory functions and whose levels are markedly decreased in Alzheimer's disease (AD) (Gibbs & Aggarwal, 1998). The neuroprotective action of estrogen could also be exerted through a modulator effect on molecules involved in apoptosis (Pike, 1999) and its antioxidant action. The potential for the numerous mechanisms of action of estrogen to affect the structure and function of cerebral areas that subserve several cognitive functions provides biological plausibility for the hypothesis that estrogen could protect cognitive functions in aging women.

3. Estrogen and cognition

The term cognition indicates the totality of human information processing, including psychomotor skills, pattern recognition, attention, language, learning and memory, problem solving, abstract reasoning or higher-order intellectual functioning.

In female mammals, including rodents and non-human primates, estrogen effects on non-reproductive behaviors include, besides anxiety and depressive-like behaviors, cognitive behaviors (Spencer et al, 2008; Walf & Frye, 2006) When administered to ovariectomized (OVX) rats, estradiol decreases anxiety and depressant behavior in laboratory tests (Walf & Frye, 2006). The effects of estrogen on cognition depend on the type of task performed and on the brain regions involved. For instance, while estradiol impairs performance on striatum-dependent tasks in female rats (Davis et al, 2005; Korol, 2004) it improves performance on prefrontal cortical-dependent learning in female rats (Luine, 2008) rhesus monkeys (Hao et al, 2007; Rapp et al, 2003) and both young adult and post-menopausal women (Berman, 1997) . It also enhances performance on HF-dependent tasks in female mice (Li et al, 2004; Xu & Zhang, 2006) , rats (Daniel et al, 1997; Sandstrom & Williams, 2004) and rhesus monkeys (Lacreuse et al, 2002; Rapp et al, 2003). Findings showing improved performance after estradiol infusion directly into the HF, but not other cerebral areas (Zurkovsky et al, 2006), provides behavioral evidence that the estradiol enhancement of HF-dependent tasks indeed represents a specific effect on HF function. However, estrogen's roles on cognitive function may result from the sum of interacting influences on numerous cerebral regions, including striatum, HF, basal forebrain, and prefrontal cortex (PFC).

3.1 Estrogen in learning and memory

Signaling pathways and gene expression regulated by estrogen include activation of CREB, GABA-A receptors, NMDA receptors, glutamic acid decarboxylase (GAD), ChAT, and synaptic and spine-associated proteins (Frick et al, 2002; McEwen et al, 2001; Rudick & Woolley , 2003).

Studies in knockout mice using the selective estrogen receptor modulators suggest that ERα and ERβ contribute differently to memory mechanisms (Rhodes & Frye, 2006; Rissman et al, 2002). Several studies have shown estrogen regulation of ERα (Hart et al, 2001; 2007) Moreover, it was reported that selective ERβ agonists increased levels of key synaptic proteins in vivo in the HF, and these effects were absent in ERβ knockout mice or after treatment with an ERα agonist. ERβ agonists also induced morphological changes in HF neurons, such as an enhanced density of mushroom-type spines. Most importantly, estrogen or ERβ agonists improved performance in some HF-dependent memory tasks (Liu et al, 2008). Therefore, these results confirm the role of ERβ in memory, but cross-talk between ERα and ERβ receptors cannot be excluded.

It was also evidenced that rapid improvements in cognition could be mediated by membrane associated estrogen receptors activating mitogen-activated protein kinase

(MAPK) signalling pathways in specific neural sites (Bryant et al, 2006). For example, estrogen enhances performance in tasks such as inhibitory avoidance (IA), object recognition and placement within 4h of treatment; a post-training paradigm evidenced that these effects are due to the facilitatory action of estrogen on memory (Frye et al, 2007; Luine, 2008; Rhodes & Frye, 2006; Walf & Frye, 2006). Previous memory studies hypothesized that newly-acquired informations are transferred to long-term memory over time, and seminal work by McGaugh and co-workers has shown that consolidation takes place within 1-2 h post-training (McGaugh, 2000). In addition, the impairment or improvement of the consolidation process due to drugs or hormones can occur if they are given within this time, but not later. Estrogen-related enhancement of consolidation utilizing post-training paradigms have been shown in some memory tasks, such as Morris water maze (MWM), IA, object recognition and object placement (Frye et al, 2007; Luine et al, 2008; Rhodes & Frye, 2006; Walf & Frye, 2006). Administration of the powerful estrogen agonist, diethylstilbestrol, either immediately before or immediately after the presentation of objects, increased discrimination between previously viewed and never viewed items in the recognition trial. Therefore, temporal relations between hormonal application and performance enhancements are in agreement with memory improvement.

Estrogen not only modulates memory formation and maintenance processes in some contexts, but also biases the learning strategy utilized to solve a task, thus changing what and how information is learned, and therefore not only how much is learned, i.e., the strength of the memory (Gasbarri et al, 2009, Pompili et al, 2010).

Rats with high estrogen levels utilize place or allocentric strategies rather successfully, outperforming hormone-deprived rats on tasks requiring the configuration and use of extramaze cues for successful completion. On the contrary, rats with low estrogen levels tend to use response or egocentric strategies on tasks where the use of a directional turn, e.g., left or right, is required for acquisition (Korol, 2004). Taking into account the actions of estrogen across a large range of neural systems, its modulation on cognition could be exerted by altering the relative involvement of specific memory systems, acting much like a conductor, orchestrating the dynamics, timing and coordination of multiple cognitive strategies during learning (McGaugh, 2000) . Influences on neurotransmitters, such as acetylcholine (ACh), regulating other processes, like inhibitory tone and excitability, reflect one of the mechanisms by which estrogen may orchestrate learning and memory. In fact, the ACh system is also activated by estrogen in cerebral areas that are important for memory, such as the basal forebrain and its ACh-containing projections to the HF and frontal cortex (Gibbs et al, 2004; Luine, 2008).

Even though gonadal hormones influence cognition, these hormone-induced changes are not large (Luine, 2008), and they are reported especially when function is compromised by aging or lesions (Gulinello et al, 2006; Scharfman et al, 2007) however, they do not improve all the different aspects of cognition such as, for example, acquisition during memory processes (Dohanich, 2002; Luine, 2007).

Rodents have been evaluated in different tasks, utilizing several kinds of mazes, and they rely on diverse reinforcements or contingencies (positive food rewards or aversive electric shocks) for the learning phase, and the tasks measure different kinds of memory, such as spatial memory, which requires the establishment of relationships between distant cues in the environment and the reinforcement site (Gasbarri et al, 2009). Other tasks use visual memory, based on visual associations. Nonetheless, many studies show positive effects of estradiol on cognition (Dohanich, 2002) . Spatial memory, which is dependent on the HF, has been extensively evaluated using the radial arm maze (RM) and MWM; studies conducted in OVX subjects show enhancements in performance during the acquisition (Dohanich, 2002; Luine et al. 1998) but, after learning how to solve the task (reference memory), estradiol no longer enhances performance (Fader et al, 1999; Luine et al. 1998) and could even impair spatial memory, although the data are not conclusive (Dohanichn 2002). Consistent estrogen-related improvements are reported in studies utilizing spatial tasks for the evaluation of working memory (WM) (Daniel & Dohanich, 2001; Luine, 2008; Sandstrom & Williams, 2001, 2004; Scharfman et al, 2007) defined as the ability to retain information in the face of potentially interfering distraction, in order to guide behavior and make a response (Baddeley, 1992, 1998).

Results of studies, assessing hormonal effects on learning and memory, evidence the importance that context and / or experience can have on performance, and these considerations may account, at least in part, for some inconsistency in the literature. Therefore, it is hypothesized that stress experienced during task performance may interfere with estrogen enhancements of some spatial tasks (Englemann et al, 2006; Frick et al, 2004). In addition, extensive handling, housing conditions, or environmental enrichment can also mitigate hormonal effects on other spatial tasks (Gresack et al, 2007; Rubinow, et al 2004) Taking into account that cognition represents a complex, multidimensional set of higher-order functions that are sub-served by specific, yet inter-related, cerebral areas, the intervention of other stimuli on the effects of estrogen is not unexpected. It is interesting to note that more recent research, evidencing consistent estrogen-related improvements of memory, use tasks evaluating working or short-term memory, tap into higher order memory or executive function, and also rely on cortical integration with HF fields (Ennaceur, et al 1997; Mumby et al, 2002). In addition, subjects are not exposed to stressful circumstances or negative reinforcers during the task. Therefore, recognition memory tests, where subjects have to discriminate between familiar and unfamiliar objects or objects in familiar or unfamiliar locations, appear to be quite consistently improved by estrogen and its agonists in OVX rats (Luine, 2008) or mice (Fernandez & Frick, 2004; Li et al, 2004).

In agreement with OVX models, pro-estrous rats evidenced better recognition memory compared to rats in a different phase of the estrous cycle (Frye et al 2007; Walf & Frye, 2006) and mice show better spatial memory in pro-estrous (Frick et al, 2001). However, rats in pro-estrous phase are often impaired during acquisition (Bowman et al, 2001; Frye, 1995; Warren & Juraska, 1997). Other researchers did not show modifications over the cycle (Berry et al, 1997; Stackman et al, 1997) this inconsistency could be explaining taking into account that they evaluated reference memory, which seems to be insensitive to hormones after acquisition.

3.1.1 Estrogen and working memory

As evidenced by research assessing performances across the estrous and menstrual cycles, ovarian hormones affect cognition and neural substrates subserving learning and memory, including WM, in both rodents (Craig &Murphy , 2007; Daniel, 2006; Warren & Juraska, 1997) and humans (Bimonte & Denenberg, 1999; Janowski et al, 2000). The decrease of estrogen following ovariectomy or menopause enhances the risk of diseases, such as osteoporosis and vasomotor dysfunction (Timins, 2004; Warren & Halpert, 2004), but could also be involved in the development of cognitive impairments (Markou, 2007; Sherwin,

2003). ERT relieves several menopausal symptoms, but whether its benefits include protection of cognitive functions is still controversial (LeBlanc et al, 2007; Tivis et al, 2001).

In recent years, considerable progress has been made towards specifying the neural mechanisms underlying WM in humans (Baddeley, 1998; Repovs & Baddeley , 2006).

Data from OVX rats treated with estrogen, compared to OVX untreated controls, showed improvements in performance of some tasks, including those require spatial WM, such as the RM (Daniel et al, 1997; Fader et al, 1999) and a 2-choice WM task (O'Neal et al, 1996) and impairments in spatial reference memory tests, such as the MWM (Warren & Juraska, 1997). Estrogen replacement therapy (ERT) enhances spatial WM performance both on MWM and RM (Bimonte & Denenberg, 1999; Fader et al, 1999), confirming previous evidence that estrogen selectively improves performance on tasks depending on WM (Daniel et al, 1997; O'Neal et al, 1996). In fact, estrogen treatment improved WM performance during maze acquisition, without affecting reference memory performance; scopolamine treatment impaired WM, but not reference memory, while estrogen prevented the impairment of WM by scopolamine. A recent paper reported substantial sex differences in the effects of gonadectomy and hormone replacement on spatial working and reference memory in male and female rats (Gibbs & Jognson, 2008). An interesting direction of this field is the idea that estrogens may influence learning strategy, independent from memory.

Furthermore, ERT in both physiologically low and moderate doses improved the capability of ovariectomized rats to handle increasing amounts of WM information, when the demand on an animal's WM system was restricted to one to four elements of information (Bimonte & Denenberg, 1999). However, when the demand on the WM system was increased to six elements of information, ERT in physiologically moderate doses provided the maximum benefit, even beyond that of intact females.

Moreover, it was reported that estrogen can prevent deficits in spatial WM induced by neurotoxin treatments aimed to mimic the pathology of early AD (Hruska & Dohanich, 2007).

Cholinergic and HF systems are closely related to learning and memory processes (Hasselmo, 2006), and it can be predicted that estrogen has its most profound effect on HF-dependent cognitive functions such as learning and memory. In fact, estrogen enhances ACh function and the synthesis of ACh in basal forebrain and the Ach neurons projecting to the HF and cortex (Hasselmo, 2006), (Singh et al, 1994), and mediates dendritic spine density in the hippocampal CA1 region (Li et al, 2004; Wallace et al, 2007). The HF and adjacent anatomically related cortex play a crucial role in the explicit encoding and consolidation of verbal and nonverbal information into short-term memory, in humans (Squire, 2004). It has been speculated that estrogen activity in HF might underlie the effects of ERT on memory in postmenopausal women (Maki & Resnick, 2000; Maki, 2005). Estrogen receptors, as well as estradiol-concentrating neurons, were detected in the HF and entorhinal cortex of rodents (Prange-Kiel & Rune, 2006). Circulating estrogens have quantifiable effects on neurotransmitter activities in HF where, for example, a low estrogen state increases serotonin (5-HT) transporter activity in the HF, despite an apparent reduction in 5-HT transporter density (Bertrand, 2005); moreover, a regulation of NMDA and GABA receptors has also been reported (Jelks, 2007; Rudick & Woolley, 2001) Estradiol administration in OVX rats produces increased ChAT activity and high-affinity choline uptake in CA1 field (Singh et al, 1994). Even though research has mainly focused on the medial temporal lobe areas, they do not represent the only neuroanatomical regions involved in human memory. In fact, the PFC mediates a number of cognitive processes contributing to memory function, particularly WM which is strongly related to the PFC in both humans and nonhuman primates. In humans, WM represents the basis for many cognitive functions, including reasoning, reading comprehension, and mental calculations (Baddeley, 1998). Both non verbal (Owen et al, 1996) and verbal (Petrides et al, 1993); stimuli were utilized in experimental tasks with a relevant WM component. The important role of the PFC in WM was demonstrated after lesion and electrophysiological techniques in monkeys (Funahashi et al, 1993; Petrides, 1995) functional neuroimaging techniques in healthy human volunteers (Jonides et al, 1993; Owen et al, 1996); and localized cortical excisions in human neurological patients (Owen et al, 1995). Taking into consideration that, by definition, WM tasks intrinsically involve both temporary retention of verbal or visual information and its active manipulation, some research have clarified that the requirement for active manipulation during WM tasks specifically recruits activity in dorsolateral PFC (Owen et al, 1995; Petrides, 1995; Postle et al, 1999). By contrast, passive storage processes seem to depend on more posterior brain areas, as evidenced by deficits in the immediate span for spatial or verbal information, in patients with lesion of parietal or perisylvian cortex (Milner, 1971) and by changes in functional cerebral activity in parietal and temporal regions of healthy volunteers, during performance of neuroimaging tasks that emphasize passive storage of information (Postle et al, 1999). Therefore, the dorsolateral PFC, as part of the WM system, plays a critical role in mediating the control processes required for the active manipulation, or selective utilization of items contained in WM.

Several lines of research raised the possibility of estrogen's modulating effect on the PFC (Joffe et al, 2006). In particular, analysis of human brain specimens has revealed that in PFC estradiol concentrations was approximately 2 times higher than in temporal cortex or 7 times higher than in HF, showing that the PFC is a principal target for estrogen in the adult female brain (Bixo et al, 1995). Animal studies reported that estrogen influences the activity of several neurotransmitter systems in the PFC. For example, a 56% reduction in ChAT and a 24% reduction in high affinity choline uptake in the frontal cortex of female rats at 28 weeks post-OVX were found; this effect was prevented or reversed in rats treated with ERT (Singh et al, 1994) Estrogen may also regulate neurotransmission in the PFC of nonhuman primates. Remarkable increases in axons immunoreaction for dopamine β-hydroxylase and 5-HT and reductions in the density of axons immunoreactive for ChAT and tyrosine hydroxylase were observed in the dorsolateral PFC of adult rhesus monkeys, following OVX (Kritzer & Kohama, 1998, 1999) In OVX monkeys treated with estrogen, the density of labeling was similar to hormonally intact controls, suggesting that estrogen plays a role in maintaining cholinergic, noradrenergic, serotonergic, and dopaminergic activity in the PFC. In addition, in humans, neuroimaging studies using positron emission tomography (PET) (Berman et al, 1997) or functional magnetic resonance imaging (fMRI) (Shaywitz et al, 1999) have evidenced systematic differences in patterns of task-induced brain activation in PFC, connected to differences in women's estrogen status (Roberts et al, 1997). A behavioral study conducted on rhesus monkeys showed that menopausal and postmenopausal females, compared to age-matched but premenopausal females, exhibited an impairment of performance on the WM delayed response task, which is commonly used to assess PFC dysfunction in nonhuman primates. Taken together, the neuroendocrine and behavioral data supply evidence to suggest that estrogen is active in the PFC. In such a case, estrogen could modulate cognitive functions mediated by the PFC in women.

Taking into account that the dorsolateral PFC is one of the areas of the frontal cortex where estrogen activity was demonstrated (Maki, 2005), this steroid hormone might contribute to WM function by modulating information processing in the PFC (Duff & Hampson, 2000). In order to verify the hypothesis that the WM system is responsive to estrogen in women, Maki et al. (Maki, 2005) designed a study evaluating, in a group of postmenopausal women, two measures, one verbal and one spatial, which strongly recruit the WM system (Digit Ordering, Spatial WM task). Their findings confirmed the hypothesis that estrogen is active within PFC and it can influence functions dependent on this region, like WM.

In agreement with the above findings, evidence exists showing the activation of PFC during the performance of WM tasks (Badre D, Wagner, 2007; Petrides et al, 1993) and decrease of WM with increasing age (Grady & Craik, 2000) . The integrity of both the PFC and its complex neural circuitry, which consolidates input from various modalities via cortical, subcortical, and limbic connections, are critical to intact executive functions, an amalgamation of cognitive processes that includes WM, besides directed attention, response inhibition, dual task coordination, cognitive set switching, and behavioral monitoring. Dopaminergic and serotonergic brain stem afferents to PFC (Jakob & Goldman-Rakic, 1998) modulate the excitability of prefrontal pyramidal neurons. Experimental reduction of prefrontal dopamine in rhesus monkeys and naturally occurring loss of dopaminergic neurons in Parkinson's disease are associated with deficits in WM (Gotham et al, 1988). The dopaminergic D2 receptor agonist bromocriptine improves WM (Luciana et al, 1991) while D2 antagonist raclopride had a minor inhibitory effect (Williams & Goldman-Rakic, 1995). Ovarian steroids are powerful modulators of the dopaminergic neurotransmission. In monkeys ovariectomy reduces, while subsequent estrogen and progesterone replacement restores, the density of axons immunoreactive for tyrosine hydroxylase in the dorsolateral PFC (Kritzer & Kohama, 1998) . Ovariectomy also decreases the density of axons immunoreactive for ChAT and increases the density of fibers immunoreactive for dopamine β–hydroxylase. ERT alone attenuates these effects (Kritzer & Kohama, 1999) estradiol also decreases monoamine oxidase (MAO), involved in the degradation of dopamine (McEwen, 2002).

3.1.1.1 Working memory for emotional facial expressions across the menstrual cycle in young women.

Facial expressions represent non-verbal communicative displays that are critical in social cognition, allowing quick transmission of valence information to cospecifics concerning objects or environments (Blair et al, 1999). In particular, humans and non-human primates use facial expressions to communicate their emotional state. This communication can be reflexive, as situations may induce emotions that are spontaneously expressed on the face. In other cases, particularly in humans, facial expressions may consist in volitional signals with the aim of communicating, and not reflecting, the real emotional state of the subject (Ekman, 1993) . Six basic emotions - happiness, sadness, anger, fear, disgust and surprise - and their corresponding facial expressions are recognized across different cultures (Ekman & Friesen, 1971). Imaging studies showed that different cerebral areas are activated during the processing of different, distinct emotions (Blair et al, 1999). It was also reported that not only subcortical areas, such as amygdala or basal ganglia, but also cortical areas, mainly PFC, cingulate cortex, and temporal cortices, are essential in emotion processing (Blair et al, 1999; Northoff et al, 2000). Many studies on emotion perception in faces have been focused on the identification of the cerebral regions, whose damage causes emotion perception deficits (Adolphs, 2002) . This facial emotion recognition deficit appears to be, at least in part, related to a more general problem in cognitive functions including the categorisation, discrimination and identification of facial stimuli, as well as deficits in other cognitive processes, such as WM, which are impaired in the psychiatric and neurological damages (Addington & Addington, 1998; Kee et al, 1998).

Physiological fluctuations in ovarian hormones across the menstrual cycle allow for non-invasive studies of the effects of estrogen on cognition in young women and underlie a reliable pattern of cognitive change across the menstrual cycle (Maki et al, 2002).

The cognitive performance in a WM task for emotional facial expressions, using the six basic emotions (Ekman &Friesen, 1971) as stimuli in the DMTS, was evaluated in young women in the different phases of the menstrual cycle, in order to point out possible differences related to the physiological hormonal fluctuations (Gasbarri et al, 2008, 2009). Our findings suggest that high levels of estradiol in the follicular phase could have a negative effect on delayed matching-to-sample WM task, using stimuli with emotional valence. Moreover, in the follicular phase, compared to the menstrual phase, the percent of errors was significantly higher for the emotional facial expressions of sadness and disgust (Gasbarri et al, 2008, 2009) The evaluation of the response times (time employed to answer) for each facial expression with emotional valence showed a significant difference between follicular and luteal in reference to the emotional facial expression of sadness (Gasbarri et al, 2008, 2009). Our results show that high levels of estradiol in the follicular phase could impair the performance of WM. However, this effect is specific to selective facial expressions suggesting that, across the phases of the menstrual cycle, in which conception risk is high, women could give less importance to the recognition of the emotional facial expressions of sadness and disgust. This study is in agreement with research conducted on non-human primates, showing that fluctuations of ovarian hormones across the menstrual cycle influence a variety of social and cognitive behaviors. For example, female rhesus monkeys exhibit heightened interest for males and enhanced agonistic interactions with other females during periods of high estrogen level (Lacreuse et al, 2007).

Moreover, our data could also represent a useful tool for investigating emotional disturbances linked to menstrual cycle phases and menopause in women.

3.1.1.2 Working memory for emotional facial expressions in capuchin monkeys

Non-human primates represent important and relevant models for the study of emotional face processing, because they share several cognitive and physiological characteristics with humans. The behavioral evidence includes similarities in innate action patterns such as body movements and communication signals, as well as highly flexible behavioral tactics and clever problem-solving strategies (Preuschoft, 2000) . The capuchin monkey (*Cebus apella*) has been the focus of various researches due to its behavioral similarities with apes. Moreover, capuchins exhibit a rich repertoire of facial expressions and body postures, which convey an array of messages to co-specifics about their internal state (Fragaszy et al, 2004); furthermore, they display tool-using capacities, and can readily solve the WM tasks, such as DNMS and concurrent discrimination learning task (Resende et al, 2003; Tavares & Tomaz, 2002).

Capuchin monkeys have well-developed facial musculature mobility, which allows considerable expressive variability, and they also have excellent visual acuity for discerning signals by others. However, most of the visual signals of capuchin monkeys are accompanied by vocalizations and associated context. In general, movement and body expression are important to understand emotional valence.

In a previous study we developed a pool of 384 pictures of capuchin monkey (*Cebus apella*) faces, classified according to emotional valence (positive/ pleasant, negative/unpleasant and neutral/indifferent), to examine whether WM can benefit from the emotional content of visual stimuli in a delayed non-matching to sample task (DNMTS) (Abreu et al, 2006).

Seven adult capuchin monkeys were tested with a computer system and touch screen. Geometric figures (control) and the co-specific faces pictures were used as stimuli. The subjects obtained a similar performance to positive, negative and neutral pictures. However, the monkeys performed above the upper confidence limits around chance to all kinds of stimulus showing that they are able to learn the tests using emotional faces. Furthermore, the capuchin monkeys had much better performance when using geometric figures compared with the co-specific pictures.

On a whole, our results show that capuchin monkeys were able to perform this new WM task, thus indicating the possible usefulness of applying the paradigm utilized in this study to investigate emotional memory in non-human primates (Abreu et al, 2006).

4. Estrogen and the aging brain

One of the most interesting research fields in women's health of the last decade includes the growing appreciation that estrogen plays relevant neurotrophic and neuroprotective roles during adulthood. This amplifies the relevance of the potential impact of the prolonged post-menopausal hypoestrogenic state on learning and memory processes and the potential increased vulnerability of ageing women to brain injury and neurodegenerative diseases. The longer female life expectancy has implied that nowadays women live one-third of their lives beyond ending of their ovarian function, increasing the need for new therapeutic strategies to facilitate successful aging (defined as low probability of disease), high cognitive and physical abilities, and active engagement in life. Taking into account that changes in the ageing nervous system are subtle, they could be reversed and cognitive performance may be improved by pharmacological treatments.

The ematic concentration of estrogens decreases with age and the post-menopause low values of estrogens are often followed by an acceleration of the age effects on cognition. Cognitive decline during aging affect memory abilities, attention, and speed of information processing (Sherwin & Henry, 2008).

Even though several cognitive functions seem to be unaltered in normal aging, age-related impairments are mainly evident in tasks implying free or cued recall or WM (Small et al, 1999). Although verbal memory has been reported to be the cognitive function most deeply affected with increasing age (Marquis et al, 2002; Rabbitt & Lowe, 2000) other cognitive domains such as attention (Stankov, 1988) visual perception, and verbal fluency (Ashman, 1999) are also influenced. Thus, the attempt to delay or prevent the cognitive impairment occurring with normal aging is an important goal to protect the quality of life for women during the latter one third of their lifespan. Because ERs are present in both the HF and frontal lobes which subserve verbal memory, WM and retrieval, we can hypothesize that estrogen might play an important protective role against the decline in these cognitive functions, occurring with normal aging. Therefore, researchers have tried to verify if the estrogen administration to women at the beginning or during menopause would protect against cognitive impairments that normally take place with increasing age.

During the past few decades, data from basic neuroscience and from animal and human studies have suggested that ERT given to postmenopausal women might protect against specific cognitive declines occurring with normal aging. On the other hand, the numerous inconsistencies in this body of evidence point to the possibility that there are contingencies which modify the supposed neuroprotective effects of ERT on cognitive aging (Sherwin & Henry, 2008).

Even though an extensive literature on the putative neuroprotective effects of estrogen on cognitive functions in postmenopausal women is available, many discrepancies still exist. The critical period hypothesis, introduced many years ago, attempts to account for the inconsistencies in this literature by positing that ERT can have a protective effect on some aspects of cognition in older women, only when it is initiated soon after the menopause. Indeed, data from basic neuroscience and from the animal and human studies provides compelling support for the critical period hypothesis (Sherwin & Henry, 2008). Although it is not completely clarified why estrogen does not protect cognitive functions and may even cause harm when administered to women over the age of 65 years, it is possible that the typical modifications of brain aging, such as a reduction of brain volume, neuronal size, number of dendritic spines, and alterations in neurotransmitter systems form an adverse background preventing the neuroprotective effects of exogenous estrogen. Other factors that have likely contributed to the inconsistencies of the estrogen–cognition literature include differences in the estrogen agonist utilized, their route of administration, cyclic versus continuous regimens, and the concomitant administration of progestins. In conclusion, there is considerable evidence supporting the use of estrogen during the menopause and postmenopausal periods for the prevention and treatment of AD and other neurologic disorders. Nevertheless, the efficacy of estrogen requires that we take into account the most recent data on hormone neurobiology, in order to administer the hormone at the right time, with the right formulation, and to the appropriate population of women (Gleason, 2005; Simpkins & Meharvan, 2008).

5. Conclusions

Besides the mechanisms concerning the neuroprotective role of estrogen in dependence of the age of its administration, further studies are necessary to completely clarify the relative efficacy of cyclic versus continuous hormone regimens, the accessibility to the brain of various estrogen compounds, and their different routes of administration. Moreover, there are no dose response results related to estrogen and cognitive functioning in women, in spite of the increasing clinical trend for administering low doses of estrogen to postmenopausal women. The finding of a prominent dose-dependent effect of estradiol on the density of hippocampal CA1 pyramidal spine synapse in OVX rats (MacLusky et al, 2005) emphasizes the relevance of obtaining such data for women. When the optimal neurobiological and pharmacological parameters of the estrogen–cognition relationship are known, these data could be used clinically to attenuate or to prevent cognitive decline in older women, which represent the fastest growing section of the population in industrialized countries.

6. References

[1] Abreu CT, Tavares MC, Marchetti A, d'Onofrio A, Gasbarri A, Tomaz C. A novel working memory test using capuchin monkey (Cebus apella) emotional faces. Neurobiologia. 2006; 69: 267-274.

[2] Addington J, Addington D. Facial affect recognition and information processing in schizophrenia and bipolar disorder. Schizophr. Res. 1998; 32(3): 171-81.

[3] Adolphs R. Neural systems for recognizing emotion. Curr. Opin. Neurobiol. 2002; 12: 169-177.

[4] Amin Z, Mason GF, Cavus I, Krystal JH, Rothman DL, Epperson CN. The interaction of neuroactive steroids and GABA in the development of neuropsychiatric disorders in women. Pharmacol. Biochem. Behav. 2006; 84: 635-643.
[5] Ashman TA, Mohs RC, Harvey PD. Cognition and aging. In: Principles of geriatric medicine and gerontology (4th edition). Hazzard WR, Blass JP, Ettinger WH, Hatter JB, Ouslander JG (Eds), New York: McGraw-Hill, 1999; 1219–1228.
[6] Baddeley A. Working memory. C. R. Acad. Sci. III. 1998; 321: 167-173.
[7] Baddeley A. Working memory. Science. 1992; 255:556-559.
[8] Badre D, Wagner AD. Left ventrolateral prefrontal cortex and the cognitive control of memory. Neuropsychologia. 2007; 45 (13): 2883-901.
[9] Berman KF et al. Modulation of cognition-specific cortical activity by gonadal steroids: a positron-emission tomography study in women, Proc. Natl. Acad. Sci. USA. 1997; 94: 8836–8841.
[10] Berry B, McMahan R, Gallagher M. Spatial learning and memory at defined points of the estrous cycle: effects on performance of a hippocampal-dependent task. Behav. Neurosci. 1997; 11: 267–274.
[11] Bertrand PP, Paranavitane UT, Chavez C, Gogos A, Jones M, van den Buuse M. The effect of low estrogen state on serotonin transporter function in mouse hippocampus: A behavioral and electrochemical study. Brain Res. 2005; 1064: 10-20.
[12] Bimonte HA, Denenberg VH. Estradiol facilitates performance as working memory load increases. Psychoneuroendocrinology. 1999; 24: 161-173.
[13] Bixo M, Bäckström T, Winblad B, Andersson, A. Estradiol and testosterone in specific regions of the human female brain in different endocrine states. J. Steroid Biochem. Mol. Biol. 1995; 55: 297–303.
[14] Blair RJ, Morris JS, Frith CD, Perrett DI, Dolan RJ. Dissociable neural responses to facial expressions of sadness and anger. Brain. 1999; 122: 883–893.
[15] Bowman RE, Zrull MC, Luine VN. Chronic restraint stress enhances radial arm maze performance in female rats. Brain Res. 2001; 904: 279–289.
[16] Bryant DN, Sheldahl LC, Marriott LK, Shapiro RA, Dorsa DM. Multiple pathways transmit neuroprotective effects of gonadal steroids. Endocrinology. 2006; 29: 199–207.
[17] Carr, B.R. Disorders of the ovaries and female reproductive tract. In: Wilson, J.D; Foster, D.W; Kronenberg, H.M; Larsen, P.R. (Eds.). Williams Textbook of Endocrinology, W.B. Saunders, Philadelphia, 1998; 751–773.
[18] Clark, JH; Schrader, WT; O'Malley, BW; Mechanisms of action of steroid hormones, In: Wilson, J., Foster, D.W. (Eds.), Textbook of Endocrinology. W.B. Saunders, Philadelphia, 1992; 35–90.
[19] Clarke CH, Norfleet AM, Clarke MSF, Watson CS, Cunningham KA, Thomas ML Perimembrane localization of the estrogen receptor alpha protein in neuronal processes of cultured hippocampal neurons. Neuroendocrinology. 2000; 71: 34–42.
[20] Craig MC, Murphy DG. Estrogen: effects on normal brain function and neur neuropsychiatric disorders. Climateric. 2007; 10 (Suppl 2): 97–104.
[21] Daniel JM, Dohanich GP. Acetylcholine mediates the estrogen induced in crease in NMDA receptor binding in CA1 of the hippocampus and the associated improvement in working memory. J. Neurosci. 2001; 21: 6949–6956.
[22] Daniel JM, Fader AJ, Spencer AL, Dohanich GP. Estrogen enhances performance of female rats during acquisition of a radial arm maze. Horm. Behav. 1997; 32:217–225.
[23] Daniel JM. Effects of oestrogen on cognition: what have we learned from basic research? J Neuroendocrinol. 2006; 18: 787-795.

[24] Davis DM, Jacobson TK, Aliakbari S, Mizumori SJ. Differential effects of estrogen on hippocampal- and striatal-dependent learning. Neurobiol. Learn. Mem. 2005; 84: 132–137.

[25] Dohanich GP. Gonadal steroids, learning and memory. In: Hormones, Brain and Behavior. Pfaff DW, Arnold AP, Etgen AM, Fahrbach SE, Rubin RI (Eds), San Diego, CA: Academic Press. 2002; 265–327.

[26] Duff SJ, Hampson E. A beneficial effect of estrogen on working memory in ostmenopausal women taking hormone replacement therapy. Horm. Behav. 2000; 38: 262-276.

[27] Dumas J, Hancur-Bucci C, Naylor M, Sites C, Newhouse P. Estrogen treatment effects on anticholinergic-induced cognitive dysfunction in normal postmenopausal women. Neuropsychopharmacology. 2006; 31: 2065–2078.

[28] Ekman P, Friesen WV. Constants across cultures in the face and emotion. J. Pers. Soc. Psychol. 1971; 17: 124-129.

[29] Ekman P. Facial expression and emotion. Am. Psychol. 1993; 48 (4): 384-92.

[30] Englemann M, Ebner K, Landgraf R, Wotjak CT. Effects of Morris water maze testing on the neuroendocrine stress response and intra hypothalamic release of vasopressin and oxytocin in the rat. Horm. Behav. 2006; 50: 496–501.

[31] Ennaceur A, Neave N, Aggleton JP. Spontaneous object recognition and object location memory in rats: the effects of lesions in the cingulated cortices, the medial prefrontal cortex, the cingulum bundle and the fornix. Exp. Brain. Res. 1997; 113: 509–519.

[32] Fader AJ, Johnson PE, Dohanich GP. Estrogen improves working but not reference memory and prevents amnestic effects of scopolamine of a radial-arm maze. Pharmacol. Biochem. Behav. 1999; 62: 711–717.

[33] Farhat, MY; Lavigne, MC; Ramwell, PW. The vascular protective effects of estrogen. Faseb J. 1996; 10: 615–624.

[34] Fernandez SM, Frick KM. Chronic oral estrogen affects memory and neurochemistry in middle-aged female mice. Behav. Neurosci. 2004; 118: 1340–1351.

[35] Fragaszy DM, Visalberghi E, Fedigan LM. The Complete Capuchin: The Biology of the genus Cebus. Cambridge: Cambridge University Press. 2004.

[36] Frick KM, Berger-Sweeney J. Spatial reference memory and neocortical neurochemistry vary with the estrous cycle in C57Bl/6 mice. Behav. Neurosci. 2001; 115: 229–237.

[37] Frick KM, Fernandez SM, Bennett JC, Prange-Kiel J, Maclusky NJ, Leranth CS. Behavioral training interferes with the ability of gonadal hormones to increase CA1 spine synapse density in ovariectomized female rats. Eur. J. Neurosci. 2004; 19: 1–7.

[38] Frick KM, Fernandez SM, Bulinski SC. Estrogen replacement improves spatial reference memory and increases hippocampal synaptophysin in aged female mice. Neuroscience. 2002; 115: 547–558.

[39] Frye CA, Duffy CA, Walf AA. Estrogens and progestins enhance spatial learning of intact and ovariectomized rats in the object placement task. Neurobiol. Learn. Mem. 2007; 88: 208–216.

[40] Frye CA. Estrus-associated decrements in a water maze task are limited to acquisition. Physiol. Behav. 1995; 57: 5–14.

[41] Funahashi S, Chafee MV, Goldman-Rakic PS. Prefrontal neuronal activity in rhesus monkeys performing a delayed anti-saccade task. Nature. 1993; 365: 753–756.

[42] Gasbarri A, Pompili A, d'Onofrio A, Cifariello A, Tavares MC, Tomaz C. Working memory for emotional facial expressions: role of the estrogen in young women. Psychoneuroendocrinology . 2008; 33 (7): 964-72.

[43] Gasbarri A., Pompili A., Tavares M.C, Tomaz, C. Estrogen and cognitive functions. Expert review of endocrinology & metabolism. 2009; 4: 507-520.

[44] Genazzani AR, Monteleone P, Gambacciani M. Hormonal influence on the central nervous system. Maturitas.2002; 43 (Suppl. 1): S11–S17.

[45] Genazzani AR, Pluchino N, Luisi S, Luisi M. Estrogen, cognition and female ageing. Hum. Reprod. Update. 2007; 13: 175-87.

[46] Gibbs RB, Aggarwal P. Estrogen and basal forebrain cholinergic neurons: Implications for brain aging and Alzheimer's disease-related cognitive decline. Horm. Behav. 1998; 34: 98-111.

[47] Gibbs RB, Gabor R, Cox T, Johnson DA. Effects of raloxifene and estradiol on hippocampal acetylcholine release and spatial learning in the rat. Psychoneuroendocrinology 2004; 29: 741-748.

[48] Gibbs RB, Jognson DA. Sex-specific effects of gonadectomy and hormone treatment on acquisition of 12-arm radial maze task by Sprague Dawley rats. Endocrinology. 2008; 149 (6): 3176-83.

[49] Gleason CE, Carlsson CM, Johnson S, Atwood C, Asthana S. Clinical pharmacology and differential cognitive efficacy of estrogen preparations. Ann N Y Acad Sci. 2005; 1052: 93-115.

[50] Gotham AM, Brown RG, Marsden CP. "Frontal" cognitive function in patients with Parkinson's disease "on" and "off" levodopa. Brain. 1988; 111: 299–321.

[51] Grady CL, Craik FIM. Changes in memory processing with age. Curr. Opin. Neurobiol. 2000; 10: 224–231.

[52] Gresack JE, Kerr KM, Frick KM. Short-term environmental enrichment decreases the mnemonic response to estrogen in young, but not aged female mice. Brain Res. 2007; 1160: 91–101.

[53] Gruber CJ, Tschugguel W, Schneeberger C and Huber JC Production and actions of estrogens. N. Engl. J. Med. 2002; 346: 340–352.

[54] Gulinello M, Lebesgue D, Jover-Mengual T, Zukin RS, Etgen AM. Acute and chronic estradiol treatments reduce memory deficits induced by transient global ischemia in female rats. Horm. Behav. 2006; 49: 246–260.

[55] Hao J, Rapp PR, Janssen WG et al. Interactive effects of age and estrogen on cognition and pyramidal neurons in monkey prefrontal cortex. Proc. Natl. Acad. Sci. U. S. A. 2007; 104: 11465-11470.

[56] Hart SA, Patton JD, Woolley CS. Quantitative analysis of ER alpha and GAD colocalization in the hippocampus of the adult female rat. J. Comp. Neurol. 2001; 440 (2): 144-155.

[57] Hart SA, Snyder MA, Smejkalova T, Woolley CS. Estrogen mobilizes a subset of estrogen receptor-alpha-immunoreactive vesicles in inhibitory presynaptic boutons in hippocampal CA1. J. Neurosci. 2007; 27: 2102-2111.

[58] Hasselmo ME. The role of acetylcholine in learning and memory. Curr. Opin. Neurobiol. 2006; 16: 710-5.

[59] Henderson, V W. Aging, Estrogens, and Episodic Memory in Women. Cogn Behav Neurol., 2009; 22 (4): 205–214.

[60] Henderson, V W. Action of estrogens in the aging brain: Dementia and cognitive aging. Biochimica et Biophysica Acta, 2010; 1800: 1077–1083.

[61] Henderson, V.W. Gonadal hormones and cognitive aging: a midlife perspective. Womens Health (Lond Engl), 2011; Jan 7(1): 81-93.

[62] Hruska Z, Dohanich GP. The effects of chronic estradiol treatment on working memory deficits induced by combined infusion of beta-amyloid (1-42) and ibotenic acid. Horm. Behav. 2007; 52 (3): 297-306.

[63] Jakob RL, Goldman-Rakic PS. 5-hydroxytryptamine2a serotonin receptors in the primate cerebral cortex: possible site of action of hallucinogenic and antipsychotic drugs in pyramidal cell apical dendrites. Proc. Natl. Acad. Sci. USA. 1998; 95: 735–740.

[64] Janowski JS, Chavez B, Orwoll E. Sex steroids modify working memory. J. Cogn. Neurosci. 2000; 12: 407-414.

[65] Jelks KB, Wylie R, Floyd CL, McAllister AK, Wise P. Estradiol targets synaptic proteins to induce glutamatergic synapse formation in cultured hippocampal neurons: critical role of estrogen receptor-alpha. J. Neurosci. 2007; 27: 6903-6913.

[66] Joffe H, Hall JE, Gruber S et al. Estrogen therapy selectively enhances prefrontal cognitive processes: a randomized, double-blind, placebo-controlled study with functional magnetic resonance imaging in perimenopausal and recently postmenopausal women. Menopause. 2006; 13: 411-422.

[67] Jonides J, Smith EE, Koeppe RA, Awh E, Minoshima S, Mintun MA. Spatial working memory in humans as revealed by PET. Nature. 1993; 363: 623–625.

[68] Kee KS, Kern RS, Marshall BD Jr, Green MF. Risperidone versus haloperidol for perception of emotion in treatment-resistant schizophrenia: preliminary findings. Schizophr. Res. 1998; 31 (2-3): 159-65.

[69] Korol DL. Role of estrogen in balancing contributions from multiple memory systems. Neurobiol. Learn. Mem. 2004; 82: 309–323.

[70] Kritzer MF, Kohama SG. Ovarian hormones differentially influence immuno-reactivity for dopamine β-hydroxylase, choline acetyltransferase, and serotonin in the dorsolateral prefrontal cortex of adult rhesus monkeys. J. Comp. Neurol. 1999; 409: 438–451.

[71] Kritzer MF, Kohama SG. Ovarian hormones influence the morphology, distribution, and density of tyrosine hydroxylase immunoreactive axons in the dorsolateral prefrontal cortex of adult rhesus monkeys. J. Comp. Neurol. 1998; 395 :1–17.

[72] Lacreuse A, Wilson ME, Herndon JG. Estradiol, but not raloxifene, improves aspects of spatial working memory in aged ovariectomized rhesus monkeys. Neurobiol. Aging. 2002; 23: 589–600.

[73] Lacreuse, A. Effects of ovarian hormones on cognitive function in nonhuman primates. Neuroscience, 2006; 138(3): 859-67.

[74] Lacreuse J, Martin-Malivel HS, Herndon JG, Effects of the menstrual cycle on looking preferences for faces in female rhesus monkeys. Anim. Cogn. 2007; 105–115.

[75] LeBlanc ES, Neiss MB, Carello PE, Samuels MH, Janowsky JS. Hot flashes and estrogen therapy do not influence cognition in early menopausal women. Menopause. 2007; 14: 191-202.

[76] Ledoux VA, Woolley CS. Evidence that disinhibition is associated with a decrease in number of vesicles available for release at inhibitory synapses. J. Neurosci. 2005; 25: 971-976.

[77] Lee SJ, McEwen BS. Neurotrophic and neuroprotective actions of estrogens and their therapeutic implications. Annu. Rev. Pharmacol. Toxicol. 2001; 41: 569–591.

[78] Li C et al. Estrogen alters hippocampal dendritic spine shape and enhances synaptic protein immunoreactivity and spatial memory in female mice. Proc. Natl. Acad. Sci. USA. 2004; 101: 2185–2190.

[79] Liu F, Day M, Muniz LC et al. Activation of estrogen receptor beta regulates hippocampal synaptic plasticity and improves memory. Nat. Neurosci. 2008; 11:334–343.

[80] Luciana M, Depue RA, Arbisi P, Leon A. Facilitation of working memory in humans by a D2 dopamine receptor agonist. J. Cogn. Neurosci. 1991; 4:58–68.

[81] Luine V, Richards ST, Wu VY, Beck K. Estradiol enhances learning and memory in a spatial memory task and effects levels of monoaminergic neurotransmitters. Horm. Behav. 1998; 34: 149–162.

[82] Luine VN. The prefrontal cortex, gonadal hormones and memory. Horm. Behav. 2007; 51: 181-182.

[83] Luine, VN. Sex steroids and cognitive function. J. Neuroendocrinol., 2008; 20: 866-872.

[84] MacLusky NJ, Luine VN, Hajszan T, Leranth C. The 17 a and b isomers of estradiol both induce rapid spine synapse formation in the CA1 hippocampal subfield of ovariectomized female rats. Endocrinology. 2005; 146:287–293.

[85] Maki PM, Resnick SM. Longitudinal effects of estrogen replacement therapy on PET cerebral blood flow and cognition. Neurobiol. Aging. 2000; 21 (2): 373-83.

[86] Maki PM, Rich JB, Rosenbaum RS. Implicit memory varies across the menstrual cycle: estrogen effects in young women. Neuropsychologia. 2002; 40: 518-529.

[87] Maki PM. Estrogen effects on the hippocampus and frontal lobes. Int. J. Fertil. Womens Med. 2005; 50: 67-71.

[88] Markou A, Duka T, Prelevic GM. Estrogens and brain function. Hormones (Athens). 2007; 4: 9-17.

[89] Marquis S, Moore MM, Howieson DB et al. Independent predictors of cognitive decline in healthy elderly persons. Arch. Neurol. 2002; 59: 601–606.

[90] McEwen B, Akama K, Alves S et al. Tracking the estrogen receptor in neurons: Implications for estrogen-induced synapse formation. PNAS. 2001; 13: 7093–7100.

[91] McEwen, BS; Alves, SH. Estrogen actions in the central nervous system. Endocr Rev, 1999; 20:279–307.

[92] McEwen, B; Akama, K; Alves, S; et al. Tracking the estrogen receptor in neurons: Implications for estrogen-induced synapse formation. PNAS, 2001; 13: 7093–7100.

[93] McEwen B. Estrogen actions throughout the brain. Recent Prog. Horm. Res. 2002; 57: 357-384.

[94] McEwen, BS. Stress, sex, and neural adaptation to a changing environment: mechanisms of neuronal remodeling. Ann N Y Acad Sci., 2010; 1204 Suppl E: 38-59.

[95] McGaugh JL. Memory – A Century of Consolidation. Science. 2000; 287: 248–251.

[96] Micevych PE, Mermelstein PG. Membrane estrogen receptors acting through metabotropic glutamate receptors: an emerging mechanism of estrogen action in the brain. Mol. Neurobiol. 2008; 38 (1): 66-77.

[97] Milner B. Interhemispheric differences in the localization of psychological processes in man. Br. Med. Bull. 1971; 27: 272–277.

[98] Milner TA, Ayoola K, Drake CT et al. Ultrastructural localization of estrogen receptor beta immunoreactivity in the rat hippocampal formation. J. Comp Neurol. 2005; 491:81-95.

[99] Mitra SW, Hoskin E, Yudkovitz J et al. Immunolocalization of estrogen receptor beta in the mouse brain: comparison with estrogen receptor alpha. Endocrinology. 2003; 144: 2055-2067.

[100] Mumby DG, Gaskin S, Glenn MJ, Schramek TE, Lehmann H. Hippocampal damage and exploratory preferences in rats: memory for objects, places, and contexts. Learn. Mem. 2002; 9: 49–57.

[101] Northoff G, Richter A, Gessner M et al. Functional dissociation between medial and lateral prefrontal cortical spatiotemporal activation in negative and positive emotions: a combined fMRI/MEG study. Cereb. Cortex. 2000; 10 (1): 93-107.

[102] O'Neal M, Means L, Poole M, Hamm R. Estrogen affects performance of ovariectomized rats in a two-choice water escape working memory task. Psychoneuroendocrinology. 1996; 21: 51–65.

[103] Osterlund MK, Hurd YL. Estrogen receptors in the human forebrain and the relation to neuropsychiatric disorders. Prog. Neurobiol. 2001; 64: 251–267.

[104] Owen AM, Doyon J, Petrides M, Evans AC. Planning and spatial working memory: A positron emission tomography study in humans. Eur. J. Neurosci. 1996; 8: 353–364.

[105] Owen AM, Sahakian BJ, Semple J, Polkey CE, Robbins TW. Visuo-spatial short-term recognition memory and learning after temporal lobe excisions, frontal lobe excisions or amygdalo-hippocampectomy in man. Neuropsychologia. 1995; 33: 1–24.

[106] Petrides M, Alivisatos B, Evans AC, Meyer E. Dissociation of human mid-dorsolateral from posterior dorsolateral frontal cortex in memory processing. Proc. Natl. Acad. Sci. USA. 1993; 90: 873–877.

[107] Petrides M, Alivisatos B, Meyer E. Functional activation of the human frontal cortex during the performance of verbal working memory tasks. Proc. Natl. Acad. Aci. USA. 1993; 90: 878–882.

[108] Petrides M. Impairments on nonspatial self-ordered and externally ordered working memory tasks after lesions of the mid-dorsal part of the lateral frontal cortex in the monkey. J. Neurosci. 1995; 15: 359–375.

[109] Pettersson K, Gustafsson JA. Role of estrogen receptor beta in estrogen action. Annu. Rev. Physiol. 2001; 63:165-192.

[110] Pfaff DW. Estrogen and Brain Function. Springer-Verlag (Ed.), New York. 1980.

[111] Pike C, Estrogen modulates neuronal Bcl-xL expression and beta-amyloid-induced apoptosis: relevance to Alzheimer's disease. J. Neurochem. 1999; 72: 1552–1563.

[112] Pompili A, Tomaz C, Arnone B, Tavares MC, Gasbarri A. Working and reference memory across the estrous cycle of rat: a long term study in gonadally intact females. Behav. Brain Res. 2010; 213: 10-18."

[113] Postle BR, Berger JS, D'Esposito M. Functional neuroanatomical double dissociation of mnemonic and executive control processes contributing to working memory performance. Proc. Natl. Acad. Sci USA. 1999; 96: 12959–12964.

[114] Prange-Kiel J, Rune GM Direct and indirect effects of estrogen on rat hippocampus. Neuroscience. 2006; 138: 765-772.

[115] Preuschoft S. Primate faces and facial expressions. Soc. Res. 2000; 67: 245-271.

[116] Rabbitt P, Lowe C. Patterns of cognitive aging. Psychol. Res. 2000; 63: 308–316.

[117] Rapp PR, Morrison JH, Roberts JA. Cyclic estrogen replacement improves cognitive function in aged ovariectomized rhesus monkeys. J. Neurosci. 2003; 23: 5708–5714.

[118] Rehman HU, Masson EA. Neuroendocrinology of Female Aging. Gend. Med. 2005; 1: 41-56.

[119] Repovs G, Baddeley A. The multi-component model of working memory: explorations in experimental cognitive psychology. Neuroscience. 2006; 139: 5-21.
[120] Resende MC, Tavares MCH, Tomaz C. Ontogenetic dissociation between habit learning and recognition memory in capuchin monkeys (Cebus apella). Neurobiol. Learn. Mem. 2003; 79: 19-24.
[121] Rhodes ME, Frye CA. ERbeta-selective SERMs produce mnemonic enhancing effects in the inhibitory avoidance and water maze tasks. Neurobiol. Learn. Mem. 2006; 85: 183–191.
[122] Rissman EF, Heck AL, Leonard JE, Shupnik MA, Gustafsson JA. Disruption of estrogen receptor b gene impairs spatial learning in female mice. Proc. Natl. Acad. Sci. USA. 2002; 99: 3996–4001.
[123] Roberts JA, Gilardi KV, Lasley B, Rapp PR. Reproductive senescence predicts cognitive decline in aged female monkeys. Neuroreport. 1997; 8: 2047–2051.
[124] Rubinow MJ, Arseneau LM, Beverly JL, Juraska JM. Effect of the estrous cycle on water maze acquisition depends on the temperature of the water. Behav. Neurosci. 2004; 118: 863–868.
[125] Rudick CN, Woolley CS. Estrogen regulates functional inhibition of hippocampal CA1 pyramidal cells in the adult female rat. J. Neurosci. 2001; 21: 6532- 6543.
[126] Rudick CN, Woolley CS. Selective estrogen receptor modulators regulate phasic activation of hippocampal CA1 pyramidal cells by estrogen. Endocrinology. 2003; 144: 179–187.
[127] Sandstrom NJ, Rowan MH. Acute pretreatment with estradiol protects against CA1 cell loss and spatial learning impairments resulting from transient global ischemia. Horm. Behav. 2007; 51: 335–345.
[128] Sandstrom NJ, Williams CL. Memory retention is modulated by acute estradiol and progesterone replacement. Behav. Neurosci. 2001; 115: 384–393.
[129] Sandstrom NJ, Williams CL. Spatial memory retention is enhanced by acute and continuous estradiol replacement. Horm. Behav. 2004; 45: 128–135.
[130] Scharfman HE, Hintz TM, Gomez J et al. Changes in hippocampal function of ovariectomized rats after sequential low doses of estradiol to simulate the preovulatory estrogen surge. Eur. J. Neurosci. 2007; 26: 2595–2612.
[131] Shaywitz SE, Shaywitz BA, Pugh KR et al. Effect of estrogen on brain activation patterns in postmenopausal women during working memory tasks. JAMA. 1999; 281: 1197–1202.
[132] Sherwin BB, Henry JF. Brain aging modulates the neuroprotective effects of estrogen on selective aspects of cognition in women: A critical review. Front. Neuroendocrinol. 2008; 29: 88–113.
[133] Sherwin BB. Estrogen and cognitive function in women. Endocr. Rev. 2003; 24: 133–151.
[134] Sherwin BB. Estrogen effects on cognition in menopausal women. Neurology. 1997; 48: S21–S26.
[135] Shughrue PJ, Merchenthaler I. Distribution of estrogen receptor β immunoreactivity in the rat central nervous system. J. Comp. Neurol. 2001; 436: 64–81.
[136] Shughrue PJ, Merchenthaler I. Estrogen is more than just in "sex hormones": novel sites for estrogen action in the hippocampus and cerebral cortex. Front. Neuroendocrinol. 2000; 21: 95-101.

[137] Shughrue PJ, Scrimo PJ, Merchenthaler I. Estrogen binding and estrogen receptor characterization (ERα and ERβ) in the cholingergic neurons of the rat basal forebrain. Neuroscience. 2000; 96: 41–49.

[138] Simpkins JW, Meharvan S. More than a decade of estrogen neuroprotection. Alzheimer & dementia. 2008; S131-S136.

[139] Singh M, Meyer EM, Millard WJ, Simpkins JW. Ovarian steroid deprivation results in a reversible learning impairment and compromised cholinergic function in female Sprague–Dawley rats. Brain Res. 1994; 644: 305–312.

[140] Small SA, Perera GM, DeLa Paz R, Mayeux R, Stern Y. Differential regional sfunction of the hippocampal formation among elderly with memory decline and Alzheimer's disease. Ann. Neurol. 1999; 45: 466–472.

[141] Spencer JL, Waters EM, Romeo RD, Wood GE, Milner TA, McEwen BS. Uncovering the mechanisms of estrogen effects on hippocampal function. Front. Neuroendocrinol. 2008; 29: 219–237.

[142] Squire LR, Stark CE, Clark RE. The medial temporal lobe. Annu. Rev. Neurosci., 2004; 27: 279–306.

[143] Stackman WR, Blasberg ME, Langan CJ, Clark AS. Stability of spatial working memory across the estrous cycle of Long-Evens rats. Neurobiol. Learn. Mem. 1997; 67: 167–171.

[144] Stankov L. Aging, attention, and intelligence. Psychol. Aging.1988; 3(1): 59-74.

[145] Tavares MCH, Tomaz C. Working memory in capuchin monkeys (Cebus apella). Behav. Brain Res 2002; 131: 131-137.

[146] Timins JK. Current issues in hormone replacement therapy. N. J. Med. 2004; 101: 21-27.

[147] Tivis LJ, Nixon SJ, Green MD. Estrogen replacement therapy: a perspective on cognitive impact. Assessment. 2001; 8 (4): 403-16.

[148] Turner, RT; Riggs, BL; Spelsberg, TC. Skeletal effects of estrogen. Endocrine Rev, 1994; 15: 275–296.

[149] Walf AA, Frye CA. A review and update of mechanisms of estrogen in the hippocampus and amygdala for anxiety and depression behavior. Neuropsychopharmacology. 2006; 31: 1097–1111.

[150] Wallace M, Frankfurt M, Arellanos A, Inagaki T, Luine V. Impaired recognition memory and decreased prefrontal cortex spine density in aged female rats. Ann. NY Acad. Sci. 2007; 1097: 54-57.

[151] Warren MP, Halpert S. Hormone replacement therapy: controversies, pros and cons. Best Pract. Res. Clin. Endocrinol. Metab. 2004; 18: 317-332.

[152] Warren SG, Juraska JM. Spatial and nonspatial learning across the rat estrous cycle. Behav. Neurosci. 1997; 111: 259–266.

[153] Williams G, Goldman-Rakic PS. Modulation of memory fields by dopamine D1 receptors in prefrontal cortex. Nature. 1995; 376: 572–575.

[154] Woolley CS, Gould E, Frankfurt M, McEwen BS. Naturally occurring fluctuation in dendritic spine density on adult hippocampal pyramidal neurons. J. Neurosci. 1990; 10: 4035–4039.

[155] Xu X, Zhang Z. Effects of estradiol benzoate on learning-memory behavior and synaptic structure in ovariectomized mice. Life Sci. 2006; 79: 1553–1560.

[156] Ziegler, DR; Gallagher, M. Spatial memory in middle-aged female rats: Assessment of estrogen replacement after ovariectomy. Brain Research, 2005; 1052: 163 - 173.

[157] Zurkovsky L, Brown SL, Korol DL. Estrogen modulates place learning through estrogen receptors in the hippocampus. Neurobiol. Learn. Mem. 2006; 86: 336–343.

9

An Integrative Review of Estradiol Effects on Dendritic Spines and Memory over the Lifespan

Victoria Luine[1] and Maya Frankfurt[2]
[1]*Department of Psychology, Hunter College of CUNY, New York,*
[2]*Department of Science Education, Hofstra North Shore-LIJ School of Medicine, 500 Hofstra University, Hempstead, USA*

1. Introduction

Estradiol enhances some aspects of learning and memory in both humans and animal models. These enhancements are present throughout the adult lifespan (Luine, 2008) and extend into old age (Frick, 2008). While many neurochemicals and neurotrophins have been shown to be regulated by estrogen, the mechanism(s) responsible for estrogen's positive effects on cognition remain elusive. It has, however, been demonstrated that gonadal hormones, both estrogens and progestins, influence neural morphology in areas important for cognitive function such as the hippocampus and medial prefrontal cortex (PFC). Spines, which are located on the dendrites of pyramidal neurons in both of these areas, have been shown to contribute to cognitive function (Morgado-Bernal, 2011). Therefore, we will review estradiol's effects on dendritic spine density in the hippocampus and PFC in relation to cognitive function. Moreover, we also consider whether changes in spine density are important for estrogen's role in the maintenance of memory. The studies are primarily from our own laboratories, but, when available, data from other labs are compared. In our studies, spine density has been investigated by Golgi impregnation, and memory has been evaluated using the spatial memory tasks of radial arm maze and object placement, and non-spatial memory has been assessed by object recognition. In most of the studies to be discussed, both morphology and cognitive function were assessed in the subjects. This current research provides substantial data suggesting a relationship between hormones, spines and cognitive function, but we point out the need for further research to establish causal relationships between these variables and to identify how spines promote memory consolidation and are integrated into memory networks.

2. Dendritic spines and memory

Neuron to neuron communication occurs mainly when axons synapse on dendrites. Dendritic spines are small protrusions of the dendrite which receive the majority of synaptic input. Although dendritic spines are present on many neurons, they are extremely numerous on pyramidal cells of both the hippocampus and the PFC (See Figure 1, schematic of pyramidal neuron). Most excitatory synapses occur on dendritic spines where there is a concentration of neurotransmitter receptors.

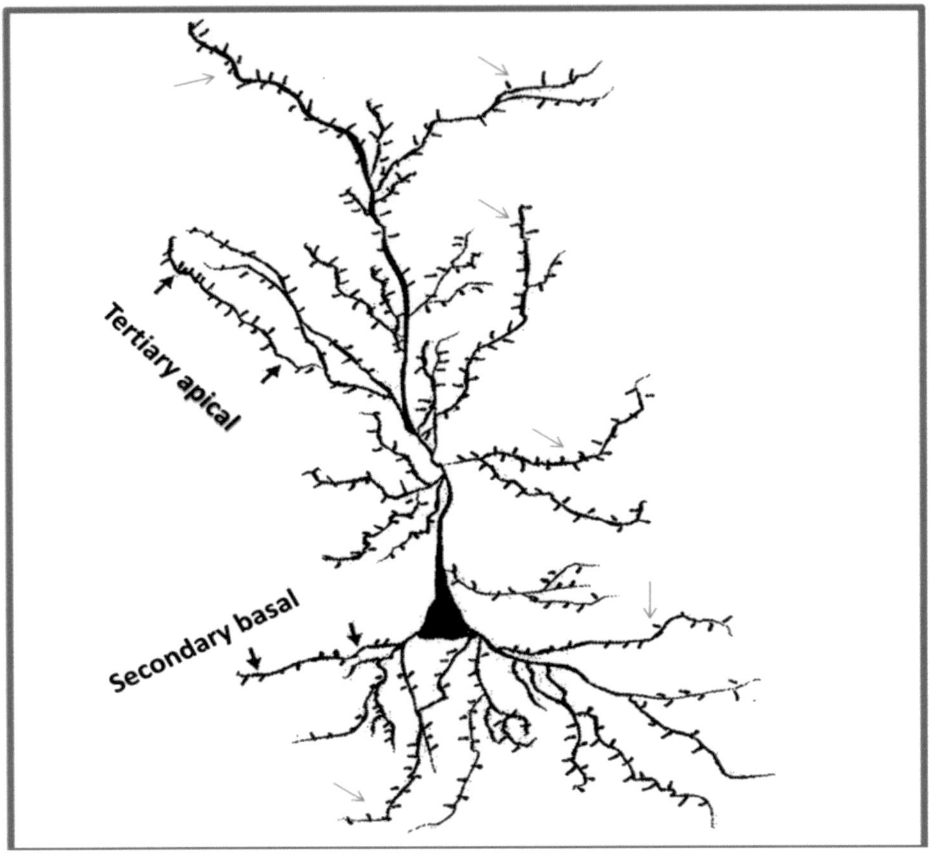

Shown are the parts of the apical and basal trees that are used for Golgi analysis in our studies. Blue arrows denote dendritic spines. Drawn by Landry McMeans.

Fig. 1. Schematic of a pyramidal cell.

Several subtypes of dendritic spines are recognized. The classification varies depending on the author but generally dendritic spines consist of a protrusion and either have a bulbous termination (mushroom spines) or not. One may also distinguish between thin spines with a smaller head and stubby spines that lack any terminal enlargement (reviewed by Bourne and Harris 2008). Golgi impregnation is used to study spine density because it labels the cell body and the adjacent dendritic structures completely (See Figure 2, photomicrograph of a pyramidal neuron). Using this technique it has been clearly demonstrated that dendritic spine density and the type of dendritic spines observed actually change with many conditions such as hormone state (Gould et al., 1990; Kinsley, 2008; Li et al., 2004; Woolley et al., 1990), stress (Radley et al. 2008) and drug administration (Robinson et al., 2001; Robinson and Kolb, 2004; Frankfurt, et al., 2011).

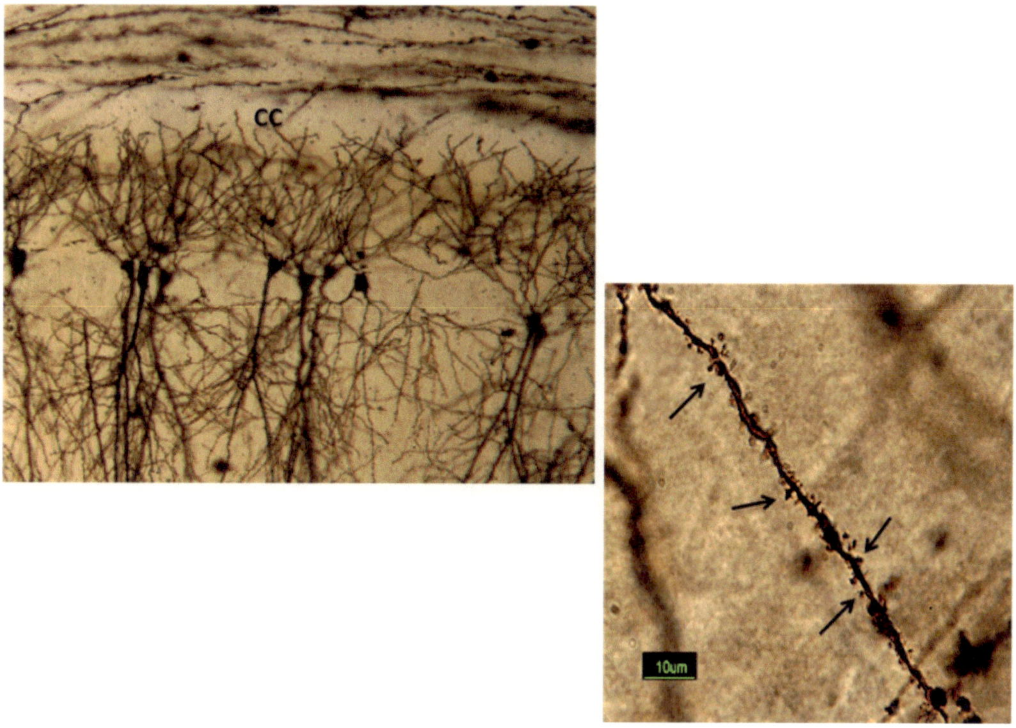

Left: CA1 region of the adult rat hippocampus. CC = corpus callosum. 10x magnification. Right: Photomicrograph of golgi-impregnated dendrites taken under oil (100x). Arrows denote spines. Frankfurt, Unpublished.

Fig. 2. Examples of Golgi impregnation.

3. Use of golgi impregnation techniques to study spines

There is increasing evidence that the processes underlying learning and memory involve neural plasticity, which includes neurogenesis and dendritic remodeling. Ultimately memory seems to require dendritic remodeling which leads to an increase in LTP and synaptic strength (See Figure 3, schematic of a spine). This idea that memory requires alterations in dendritic spines is supported by the demonstration that the acquisition of new memories is associated with changes in dendritic spine density in the CA1 hippocampal region in adult male rats (Leuner et al, 2003; Jedlicka et al, 2008; Beltran-Campos, 2011). In addition, there is increasing evidence that existing spines undergo structural alterations that result in LTP (Jedlicka et al, 2008; Morgado-Bernal, 2011). Spine assembly involves a complex sequence of events and many proteins which have been demonstrated to be altered following memory tasks (Hotulainen and Hoogenraad, 2010; Morgado-Bernal, 2011). For example the polymerization of actin, which is highly concentrated in dendritic spines, appears to be required for the induction of LTP (reviewed by Fortin et. al, 2011).

4. Estrogens and spines

The hippocampal region not only contains a high density of spines, but these spines are plastic, i.e. their numbers fluctuate depending upon the state of the host. A dramatic 30%

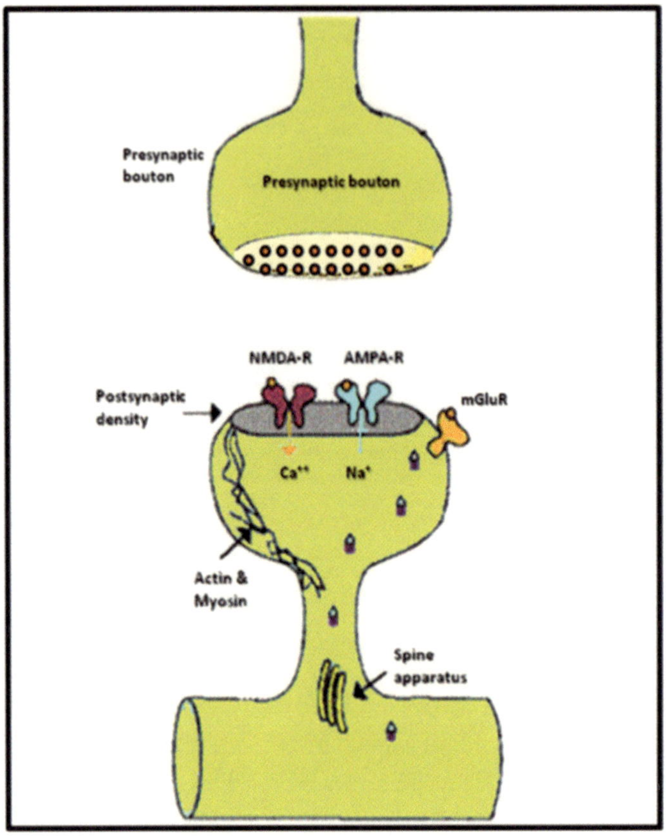

The axon terminal contains vesicles which release their contents , then bind to the post synaptic receptor and then initiate a series of events that induce structural changes in the dendritic spine. Drawn by Dr. A. Bornstein

Fig. 3. Schematic representation of the events that occur at the axo-spinous synapse.

change in spine density has been shown in the hippocampus during the 4-5 day estrus cycle of the female rat in concert with the changes in estradiol and progesterone (Woolley, et al, 1990). These changes occur in the CA1, but not the CA3 or dentate gyrus region of the hippocampus and allow for changes in neural traffic through frontal cortex and the hippocampus itself. Ovariectomy (Ovx) is associated with decreased spine density in CA1 (Gould et al. 1990, Wallace et al, 2006), and it has been recently demonstrated that the PFC also undergoes spine (Wallace et al, 2006) and spine synapse (Leranth et al, 2003) loss following gonadectomy. Since memory function undergoes similar changes with alterations in gonadal hormones (see Estrogens and memory below), dendritic spines in CA1 and the medial PFC may be important in mediating gonadal hormone influences on cognitive function in females.

5. Estrogens and memory

A substantial literature has demonstrated that gonadal hormones, mainly estradiol, influence cognition function during development, at adulthood and during aging (Luine,

2008; Frick, 2008); however, the changes are often small in magnitude. Nonetheless, estradiol administration to Ovx rats or mice has been shown to enhance performance of radial arm maze, T-maze, Morris water maze, and object recognition/placement tasks (see Dohanich, 2002 for review). A critical consideration is that hormones do not usually enhance all aspects of cognition. For example, learning to play a card game like Bridge (*acquisition* of the extensive rules of play) is different from playing the game and remembering which cards have been played (*short-term/working memory*). Thus, acquisition/learning is different than memory, and it appears that estradiol may not enhance both (Luine, 2008). In understanding memory in animal models, it should be noted that the rats face the same issues when they learn a task and then use memory to solve or complete the task. Thus, it is important to consider both learning and memory when examining the influence of gonadal hormones on cognitive function. In this review, we focus on the role of hormone-dependent changes in spines in mediating memory function. Thus, we have applied tasks which utilize memory to female rats, but there are also different types of memory. Spatial memory is the most widely assessed form of memory in rodents, and a variety of tasks have been developed for its measurement, for example, radial arm maze, Morris water maze and object placement. These strongly hippocampal-dependent tasks rely on the innate ability of rodents to know and defend a territory by utilization of salient environmental landmarks to establish a cognitive map which resides within hippocampal neurons or networks. Thus, if the hippocampus is ablated, the rats can no longer perform spatial tasks (Broadbent et al, 2004). We have applied the object placement task because this task, unlike other tasks, requires minimal learning and it also does not entail use of positive (food) or negative (drowning) rewards which might inadvertently influence performance through stress or other influences. Object placement relies on the observation that rats seek novelty and readily explore their environment. When a delay is interspersed between presentation of objects in a new as compared to an old location, then memory can be assessed by determining whether the subjects spend more time exploring the object in the new location than in the old location (Ennaceur et al, 1997). The task is conducted as depicted in Figure 4. Rats spend three minutes exploring two identical objects on an open field in the sample trial (T1). After inter-trial delays of 1 to 4 h, the subject is returned to the field where one object has been moved to a different location (retention trial or T2). The time spent exploring the object in the old and in the new location is noted. Spending significantly more time exploring at the new vs. the old location indicates that the rat remembers the old location and hence explores at the novel location, i.e. significantly discriminates between locations. Object placement memory can also be reported using the exploration ratio (time exploring new place/time exploring old + time exploring new place) where ratios of 0.5 indicate chance performance (poor memory) and ratios higher than 0.5 indicate that subjects remember the old location and significantly discriminate between the locations. This task can also be configured as a visual memory task which relies on visual associations by the prefrontal cortex as well as integration of the PFC with hippocampal memory circuits (Broadbent et al, 2004; Ennaceur et al, 1997). See Figure 5. The sample trial is the same as in object placement, but in the retention trial, a new object is switched for one of the two identical objects. Scoring in the retention trial is as in object placement. Estradiol, given to Ovx rats or mice, has been shown to enhance memory in these tasks by a number of laboratories (Luine et al, 2003; Li et al, 2004; Walf et al, 2006, 2007; Frye et al, 2007; Scharfman et al, 2007; Jacome et al, 2010).

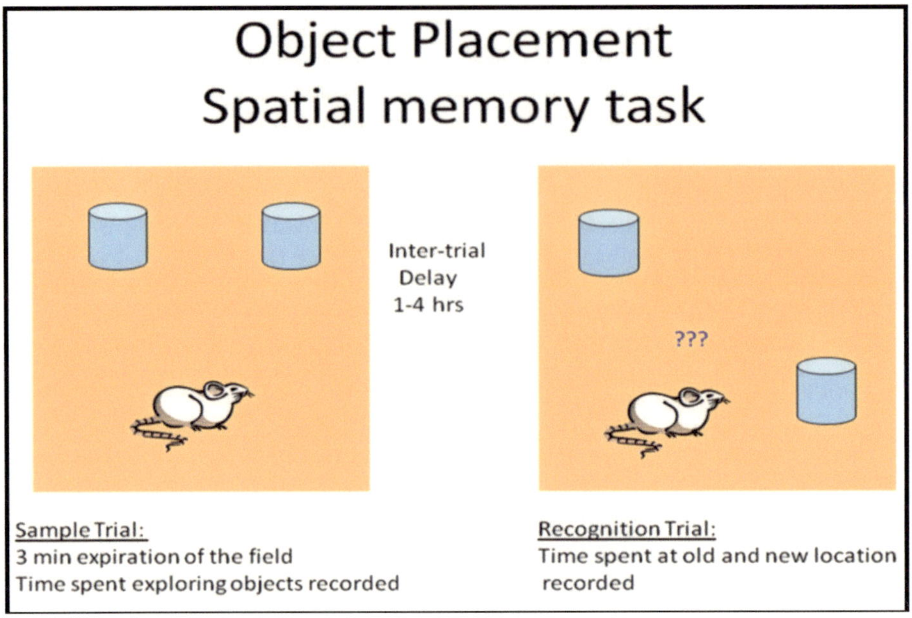

The rat is shown on an open field with objects to be explored.

Fig. 4. Depiction of the object placement memory task.

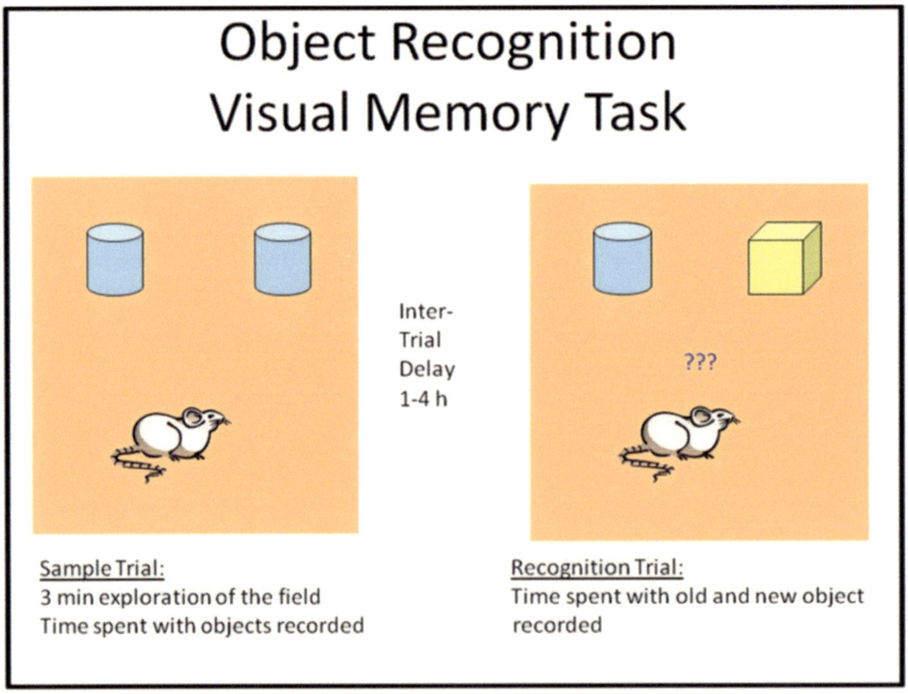

The rat is shown on an open field with objects to be explored.

Fig. 5. Depiction of the object recognition memory task.

6. Estrogens, memory and spines

6.1 Declines in estrogen following Ovx

As indicated earlier, some cognitive functions appear optimal in the presence of circulating gonadal hormones, but whether maintenance of dendritic spines at critical levels contributes to gonadal hormone influences on cognition has not received extensive investigation; however, we assessed the effects of gonadectomy on recognition memory (object recognition) and spatial memory (object placement) and spine density in the medial prefrontal cortex (PFC) and in hippocampal sub-regions (Wallace et al, 2006). Prior to Ovx, rats could significantly discriminate between old and new objects and between objects in new and old locations when tested 4 hours after first viewing the objects. One week following surgery, Ovx females showed impaired object recognition memory because they could not discriminate between old and new objects (ratio less than 50%) while gonadally intact females still discriminated in the task (Wallace et al, 2006). At this time interval post Ovx, place memory showed different results because both gonadally intact and Ovx rats could significantly discriminate between objects in new and old locations (ratios of approximately 0.65), however by four weeks post-Ovx, rats could not significantly discriminate locations (See Figure 6). These results suggest that gonadal hormones contribute to the performance of the memory tasks. Moreover,

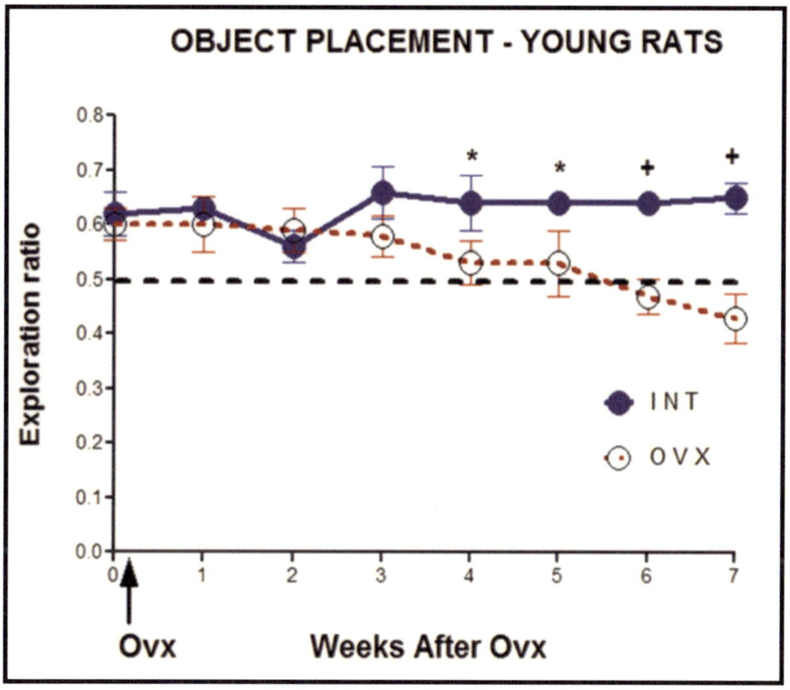

The exploration ratio ± SEM is shown for gonadally intact, sham (solid circles) and Ovx (open circles) rats before Ovx (0 week) and weeks 1-7 post Ovx. Dashed line at 0.5 indicates chance performance of task (same amount of time spent exploring the object at the old and new locations). Two way ANOVA (group x week) of ratios showed no significant main effects but a significant group x week interaction ($F(1,16)=2.22$, $p<0.047$). Post hoc testing by t-tests showed significant differences between groups at weeks 4, 5, 6 and 7, by at least $p < 0.02$. Adapted from Wallace et al. (2006)

Fig. 6. The effect of ovariectomy on object placement memory task.

recognition memory may be more sensitive to ovarian steroids than spatial memory since performance of object recognition was lost faster after Ovx. However, it is important to consider the possible effects of stress on the results because stressing female rats has been shown to enhance object placement (Bowman et al, 2003). Since corticosterone, released during stress, acts within the hippocampus, it is possible that anesthesia-induced stress in this study may have masked any early effects of Ovx on object placement.

The Ovx and gonadally intact subjects were sacrificed 7 weeks post Ovx and brain morphology was analyzed following Golgi impregnation. Spines were counted on tertiary apical and secondary basal dendrites of pyramidal neurons in layer II/III of the medial prefrontal cortex (PFC) and in CA1 and CA3 of the hippocampus (See Figure 1). In the PFC and CA1 (but not CA3), Ovx females had lower spine density in both apical and basal dendrites than intact rats, ranging from 17% decreases in apical CA1 to 53% decreases in apical PFC. Thus, poorer memory in the Ovx subjects was associated with lower spine densities in the hippocampus and PFC. Unfortunately, behavior could not be directly correlated with spine density as the subjects were not sacrificed immediately following behavior testing. Similar results have been reported recently by Beltran-Campos et al (2011) who found that CA1 apical dendrite spines were 55% lower in Ovx as compared to intact rats. Moreover, the Ovx rats were impaired in acquisition of the platform location in the Morris Water Maze spatial memory task.

6.2 Declines in estrogens with aging

Given that gonadal hormones decrease with age, aged rats also provide interesting subjects for assessing relationships between spines and memory. It is well known that aged rats, as well as aged humans, show declines in both learning and memory as compared to young subjects (Frick, 2008). We examined memory function, brain spine densities and estradiol levels in young (four months old) and aged (21 months old) Fischer 344 rats (Wallace et al, 2007; Luine et al, 2011). Fischer 344 rats are maintained by the National Institute for Aging of the National Institutes of Health as a standard model for studies on the physiological and neural aspects of aging. Consistent with many previous studies on spatial memory using tasks like the radial arm maze (Luine and Hearns, 1990) and its water version (Bimonte et al, 2003), Y and T mazes (Aggleton et al, 1980), Barnes maze (Barrett et al, 2009) and the most widely applied spatial memory task, the Morris water maze (Markowska et al, 1999, Veng et al, 2003) the aged females showed poorer object placement performance; they were unable to discriminate between old and new location with 1.5 h inter-trial delay while young rats could discriminate (Luine et al, 2011). Likewise, aged rats are also impaired in visual memory; they could not discriminate between old and new objects at a one hr inter-trial delay (Wallace et al, 2007). Examination of spine densities in the PFC and hippocampus (Table 1) showed that aged rats had 16% decreases, as compared to young rats, in apical dendrites of the PFC and CA1, but no changes in CA3. This decline in densities with aging was smaller than the decline following Ovx. Moreover, the whole pyramidal neuron was affected following Ovx; both apical and basal dendrites were decreased by Ovx, but only apical dendrites were affected with aging. It is notable that the Fischer 344, aged rats (Luine et al, 2011) still had appreciable circulating estradiol levels, 7.9 $\pm$ 1 pg/ml serum, a level which is comparable to a young rat at diestrus. With further aging, estradiol levels become negligible, but spine densities have not been examined in this age group so it is not known whether spine densities would further decline with aging to levels seen in young Ovx females.

Group	PFC Apical	PFC Basal	CA1 Apical	CA1 Basal	CA3 Apical	CA3 Basal
Young	8.13 ± 0.40	7.80 ± 0.41	7.87 ± 0.58	5.37 ± 0.21	5.42 ± 0.36	5.52 ± 0.29
Aged	6.86 ± 0.52*	7.19 ± 0.31	6.59 ± 0.39*	5.96 ± 0.15	6.30 ± 0.39	4.79 ± 0.36

Entries are mean number of spines/10μm ± S.E.M. for 6-8 rats/group. Young is 4 months and aged is 21 months old. * $p < .05$ by Student's T-test. Data from Wallace et al, 2007 and Luine et al, 2011.

Table 1. Spine density in young vs aged Fischer 344 rats

Von Bohlen et al (2006) also reported decreased CA1 spine density in a group of aged rats of both sexes that had impaired Morris water maze performance. However, our data is different from the only other published study in females. Markham et al. (2005), who applied Golgi techniques, reported no changes in CA1 spine density in rats of a similar age as ours (19-22 mo.) but of a different strain, Long Evans. Nonetheless, it is notable that Markham and Juraska (2002) reported decreased spine density in the PFC of their aged females. In neither of these studies was memory assessed. An important variable which may have contributed to our demonstration of decreased hippocampal spine density with aging is the reproductive history of the females utilized. The Fischer 344 female rats supplied to us by N.I.A. were virgins. In the other studies (Markham and Juraska, 2002; Juraska et al, 2005) retired Long-Evans breeding dams were used. As discussed in detail below, rats that have been pregnant and reared pups (multiparous) generally have better memory abilities than female rats that have never experienced motherhood (virgin or nulliparous; see Macbeth and Luine, 2010 for review). For example, middle-aged rats (12 months old) that have had 4-5 pregnancies and births demonstrated better object placement performance and other memory tasks than age-matched, virgin rats (Macbeth et al., 2008). Reproductive experience also apparently imparts long lasting effects on memory processes because multiparous females show better spatial memory than age-matched virgins at 24 months of age (Kinsley, 2008; Macbeth and Luine, 2010). Moreover, pregnant or lactating females have greater spine density in CA1 than females at all stages of the estrus cycle (Kinsley, et al, 2006; Kinsley 2008). Whether pregnancy-related spine changes are as enduring as the memory changes is, however, unknown, and needs to be investigated. Thus, the reproductive history of female rats may be an important variable when investigating neural and behavioral function.

Overall, our studies indicate that aging in females is accompanied by losses in memory abilities, neural spines and lower estradiol levels. Whether there is a causal relationship among the variables needs further investigation.

7. Increases in estrogens

7.1 Pregnancy

During pregnancy levels of gonadal hormones are elevated so pregnant dams provide an interesting model for further assessing relationships between memory function and dendritic spines. We found that pregnant females on days 7 and 16 of gestation showed better place memory than virgin females (Macbeth et al, 2008). While spine density was not measured in these subjects, there are several reports of alterations in spine density on pyramidal neurons in CA1 and the PFC with pregnancy. Leuner and Gould (2010) demonstrated that pregnant rats had increased dendritic spine density in both apical and basal branches of neurons in CA1 and the medial PFC as well as enhanced cognitive function 20 days after birth when compared to virgin females. However, the effects of pregnancy on spine density in CA1 have been determined in several studies with variable results. In a recent study, we found that dendritic spine density was decreased on the apical branch of CA1 neurons on the day of birth in dams when compared with the virgin females (Frankfurt et al, 2011) whereas Kinsley et al. (2006) demonstrated that dendritic spine density on the apical branch of CA1 neurons was greatest in late pregnancy and during lactation (day 5) when compared with virgin rats in different stages of estrous. Brusco et al. (2008) demonstrated that, starting at day four postpartum, there were no differences in either spine density or spine type in CA1 between postpartum and virgin Wistar rats. The differences between these studies may be attributed to the fact that the animals were examined at different postpartum times and therefore the gonadal hormone levels also differ.

7.2 Replacement of Estradiol to Ovx rats

As indicated earlier, Estradiol Benzoate (EB) treatment for two days increases CA1 apical spine density (Gould et al, 1990,), and estrogens and other gonadal hormones regulate the density of synapses on these CA1 spines (Parducz et al, 2006; MacLusky et al, 2005); however, neither learning nor memory was assessed in these studies. Conrad and colleagues (McLaughlin et al, 2008) examined the of effects two doses of EB, 5 and 10 ug, given twice to Ovx rats on object placement and other cognitive tasks as well as spine densities. The higher doses resulted in significant discriminations in object placement and a doubling of spine density in the apical dendrites of CA1 (but not in the basal dendrites). Interestingly, if rats were Ovx for ten weeks without any hormonal replacement, then estradiol did not alter spine density (memory was not assessed).

We have reported that Ovx females chronically fed regular rat chow (Purina LabDiet), which contains high levels of a variety of phytoestrogens, have better memory function and greater dendritic spine density in some brain areas than Ovx rats fed chow low in phytoestrogens (Teklad 2016) (Luine et al, 2006). Phytoestrogens are plant derived estrogens which have a much lower affinity for the estrogen receptor than estradiol but nonetheless exert some estrogenic effects. Following 7 weeks on the diets, the high phytoestrogen diet group significantly discriminated between objects at old and new locations while the Ovx rats fed the low phytoestrogen diet could not. Interestingly, Ovx rats fed either diet could not significantly discriminate between old and new objects after 6, 8 or 9 weeks on the diets. Thus, phytoestrogens were insufficient to enhance object recognition memory which again suggests that behaviors mediated by the medial prefrontal cortex maybe very sensitive to losses in circulating estrogens. Apical spine density was assessed in pyramidal cells in CA1 and the PFC, areas where we previously saw differences between Ovx and gonadally intact rats. Spine density of the low phytoestrogen diet group was 32% lower in CA1 and 21% lower in the PFC than the high phytoestrogen group. Comparison of the two experiments utilizing Ovx rats (Ovx vs. intact rats; low vs. high phytoestrogen diet in Ovx rats) suggests that a reduction of 20-30% in CA1 apical spines is sufficient to impact spatial memory function but that larger declines are necessary in PFC in order to affect recognition memory. However, the relationship between spine density and memory may not be direct since spines were decreased in the low phytoestrogen diet group but object recognition memory was not.

Working with groups at Rockefeller University (Li et al, 2003), we found a somewhat different pattern of estrogen treatment in mice vs. rats. Ovx mice received 1 ug of EB daily for 5 days and then received object placement testing. EB treatment enhanced object placement, but the density of spines in apical CA1 was not increased. Interestingly, the density of mushroom spines was increased by 38%. Combined with other ICC data, it was suggested that estradiol may be facilitating the spine-maturation process. While this could be a species difference, the longer treatment time compared with McLaughlin et al (2008) is consistent with the notion that estradiol, in general, may facilitate the spine maturation process.

8. Conclusions

The data presented here show that estrogen effects on memory are associated with dendritic remodeling in the hippocampus and PFC. It is impossible, at present, to state conclusively which dendritic spines are involved in mediating a given function because most of the studies done to date include confounding variables. For example, some evidence suggests that learning (Beltran-Campos, 2011) or forming associative memories (Leuner and Shors 2003) increases spine density in CA1, but Beltran-Campos, in the same study, found that spines were not increased by training in Ovx rats, only in gonadally intact rats. Moreover, Frick et al (2004) reported that behavioral training in the water maze interfered with the ability of estradiol to increase CA1 spine synapse density in Ovx rats. While an influence of the stress of swimming cannot be discounted, the above studies indicate a complex interaction between hormones, memory and spines. Since there is some evidence of different hormonal or learning effects on different spines, counting of mushroom, thin and filapodial spines might be informative for future studies. Also critical is the comparison of behaviorally tested vs. non-behaviorally tested subjects and how long the subjects have been without circulating estrogens as well as how long after behavioral testing spine density is analyzed. Nonetheless, estrogenic facilitations of memory functions regulated by the hippocampus and prefrontal cortex provide a rich context in which to examine the mechanisms underlying memory consolidation and retrieval. Using estradiol as a physiological probe, it should be possible to identify the intracellular signals whereby spines are generated, strengthened or shed, and how newly generated spines promote memory consolidation and may be ultimately integrated into memory networks.

9. Acknowledgments

We thank many students who have assisted with these studies: Luis Jacome, Claris Gautreaux, Tomoko Inagaki, Govini Mohan, Sara Attala, Ana Costa and Leo Arellanos. Experiments were supported by NIH grants GM60654 and RR03037 with supplement from NIA.

10. References

Aggleton JP, Blindt HS, Candy JM (1989) Working memory in aged rats. Behav Neurosci 103: 975-983.

Barrett, GL, Bennie A, Trieu J, Ping S, Tsafoulis C (2009). The chronology of age-related spatial learning impairment in two rat strains, as tested by the Barnes maze. 123: 533-8.

Beltran-Campos, RA Pado-Alcala, U. Leon-Jacinto, A. Aguilar-Vazquez, GL Quirarte, V Ramirez-Amaya, S Diaz-Cintra (2011) Increase of mushroom spine density in CA1 apical dendrites produced by water maze training is prevented by ovariectomy. Brain Research 1369: 119-130.

Bimonte HA, Nelson ME, Granholm AE (2003). Age-related deficits as working memory load increases: relationships with growth factors. Neurobiol Aging 24, 37-48.

Bowman, RE, Beck, KD and Luine, VN (2003) Chronic stress effects on memory: Sex differences in performance and monoamines. Hormones and Behavior 43: 48-59.

Bourne JN, Harris KM (2008) Balancing structure and function at hippocampal dendritic spines. Annu Rev Neurosci. 31:47-67.

Broadbent, N, Squire, L and Clark, R (2004). Spatial memory, recognition memory, and the hippocampus. PNAS 101 (40), 14515-14520.

Brusco J, Wittmann R, de Azevedo MS, Lucion AB, Franci CR, Giovenardi M, Rasia-Filho AA. (2008). Plasma hormonal profiles and dendritic spine density and morphology in the hippocampal CA1 stratum radiatum, evidenced by light microscopy, of virgin and postpartum female rats. Neurosci Lett 438(3):346-50.

Dohanich, GP (2002) Gonadal Steroids, learning and memory In: Pfaff DW, Arnold AP, Etgen AM, Fahrbach SE, Rubin RI, eds. Hormones, Brain and Behavior. San Diego, CA: Academic Press, 2002: 265-327.

Ennaceur, A, Neave, N and Aggleton, J (1997). Spontaneous object recognition and object location memory in rats: the effects of lesions in the cingulate cortices, the medial prefrontal cortex, the cingulum bundle and the fornix. Exp. Brain Research 113, 509-519.

Fortin DA, Srivastava T, Soderling TR (2011) Structural Modulation of Dendritic Spines during Synaptic Plasticity. Neuroscientist. 2011 Jun 13. [Epub ahead of print]

Frankfurt, M, Salas-Ramirez, K., Friedman, E. and Luine, VN (2011). Cocaine alters dendritic spine density in cortical and subcortical regions of the postpartum and virgin female rat. Synapse 65: 955-61. .

Frick, KM, Fernandez, SM, Bennett JC, Prange-Kiel J, MacLusky NJ and Leranth C (2004) Behavioral training interferes with the ability of gonadal hormones to increase CA1 spine synapse density in ovariectomized female rats. European J. Neuroscience 19: 3026-32.

Frick KM (2008) Estrogens and age-related memory decline in rodents: what have we learned and where do we go from here? Horm Behav. 55 2-23.Frye, CA, Duffy, CK, Walf, AA (2007). Estrogens and progestins enhance spatial learning of intact and ovariectomized rats in the object placement task. Neurobiol. Learn Mem.88, 208-16.

Gould E, Woolley CS, Frankfurt, M, McEwen, BS. (1990). Gonadal steroids regulate dendritic spine density in hippocampal pyramidal cells in adulthood. J Neurosci 10:1286–1291.

Hotulainen P and Hoogenraad, CC (2010) Actin in dendritic spines: connecting dynamics to function J Cell Biol. 189(4):619-29.

Jacome, LF, Gautreaux, C, Inagaki, T, Mohan, G, Arellanos, A., MacLusky, N., Alves, S., Lubbers, L and Luine, VN. (2010). ERβ Agonists Enhance Recognition Memory and Alter Monoamines in Ovariectomized Rats. Neurobiology of Learning and Memory 94: 488-98 PMC 2975833.

Jedlicka P, Vlachos A, Schwarzacher SW, Deller T (2008) A role for the spine apparatus in LTP and spatial learning. Behav Brain Res. 192(1):12-9.

Kinsley, CH (2008). The neuroplastic maternal brain. Horm Behav. 55, 1-4.

Kinsley CH, Trainer R, Stafisso-Sandoz G, Quadros P, Marcus LK, Hearon C, Meyer EA, Hester N, Morgan M, Kozub FJ, Lambert KG. 2006. Motherhood and the hormones of pregnancy modify concentrations of hippocampal neuronal dendritic spines. Horm Behav 49(2):131-42.

Leranth C, Petnehazy O, MacLusky NJ. (2003). Gonadal hormones affect spine synaptic density in the CA1 hippocampal subfield of male rats. J Neurosci. 23: 1588-92.

Leuner B, Falduto J, Shors TJ. (2003) Associative memory formation increases the observation of dendritic spines in the hippocampus. J Neurosci. 23(2):659-65.

Leuner B, Gould E. (2010) Dendritic growth in medial prefrontal cortex and cognitive flexibility are enhanced during the postpartum period. J Neurosci. 2010 30:13499-503.

Li, C, Brake, WG, Romeo, RD, Dunlop, J.C., Gordon, M, Buzescu, R, Magarinos, A, Allen, P, Greengard, P. Luine, V, and McEwen, BS. (2004).Estrogen alters hippocampal dendritic spine shape and enhances synaptic protein immunoreactivity and spatial memory tasks in female mice Proc. Nat'l Acad. Science 101: 2185-2190.

Luine, V.N., Wallace, M. Frankfurt, M. (2011). Age-related deficits in spatial memory and hippocampal spines in virgin, female, Fischer-344 rats. Current Gerontology and Geriatric Research. 2011:316386. Epub 2011 Aug 18.

Luine, V and Hearns, M Spatial memory deficits in aged rats: Contributions of the cholinergic system assessed by ChAT. Brain Research 523: 321-324 (1990).

Luine, V, Attalla, S, Mohan, G, Costa, A and Frankfurt, M (2006). Dietary phytoestrogens enhance spatial memory and spine density in the hippocampus and prefrontal cortex of ovariectomized rats. Brain Research 1126: 183-187.

Luine, VN. (2008). Sex steroids and cognitive function. J. Neuroendocrinology 20: 866-72.

Luine, VN, Jacome, L F and MacLusky, NJ., (2003). Rapid enhancements of visual and place memory by estrogens in rats. Endocrinology 144 (7), 2836-2844.

Macbeth AH, Luine VN (2010) Changes in anxiety and cognition due to reproductive experience: a review of data from rodent and human mothers. Neuroscience & Biobehavioral Reviews. 34, 452-467.

Macbeth AH, Scharfman HE, MacLusky NJ, Gautreaux C, Luine VN (2008) Effects of multiparity on recognition memory, monoaminergic neurotransmitters, and brain-derived neurotrophic factor (BDNF). Hormones & Behavior 54 7-17.

Macbeth, AH, Gautreaux, C and Luine, VN (2008). Pregnant rats show enhanced spatial memory, decreased anxiety, and altered levels of monoaminergic neurotransmitters. Brain Research 1241:136-47.

MacLusky, NJ, Luine, VN, Hajszan, T, Prange-Kiel and Leranth C. (2005). The 17 α and βisomers of estradiol both induce rapid spine synapse formation in the CA1 hippocampal subfield of ovariectomized female rats. Endocrinology 146: 287-293.

Markham JA, Juraska JM. (2002) Aging and sex influence the anatomy of the rat anterior cingulated cortex. Neurobiol Aging 23, 579-588.

Markham, JA, McKian, KP, Stroup, TS, Juraska, JM (2005) Sexually dimorphic aging of dendritic morphology in CA1 of hippocampus. Hippocampus 15, 97-103.

Markowska, AL (1999) Sex dimorphisms in the rate of age-related decline in spatial memory: relevance to alterations in the estrous cycle. J. Neurosci. 19, 8122-8133.

McLaughlin, KJ, H Bimonte-Nelson, JL Neisewander, CD Conrad (2008). Assessment of estradiol influence on spatial tasks and hippocampal CA1 spines: Evidence that the duration of hormone deprivation after ovariectomy compromises 17β-effectiveness in altering CA1 spines. Hormones & Behavior 54: 386-395.

Morgado-Bernal I. (2011) Learning and memory consolidation: Linking molecular and behavioral data. *Neuroscience* 176:12–19.

Parducz A, Hajszan T, Maclusky NJ, Hoyk Z, Csakvari E, Kurunczi A, Prange-Kiel J, Leranth C.(2006) Synaptic remodeling induced by gonadal hormones: neuronal plasticity as a mediator of neuroendocrine and behavioral responses to steroids. Neuroscience. 138: 977-85.

Radley JJ, Rocher AB, Rodriguez A, Ehlenberger DB, Dammann M, McEwen BS, Morrison JH, Wearne SL, Hof PR (2008) Repeated stress alters dendritic spine morphology in the rat medial prefrontal cortex. J Comp Neurol. 507:1141-50.

Robinson TG, Gorny G, Mitton E, Kolb B. 2001. Cocaine self administration alters the morphology of dendrites and dendritic spines in the nucleus accumbens and neocortex. Synapse 39: 257–266.

Robinson TE, Kolb B, 2004. Structural plasticity associated with exposure to drugs of abuse. Neuropharmacology. 2004;47 Suppl 1:33-46.

Scharfman, HE, Hintz, TM, Gomez, J, Stormes, KA., Barouk, S, Malthankar-Phatak, DH, McLoskey, DP, Luine, VN and MacLusky, NJ (2007). Changes in hippocampal function of ovariectomized rats after sequential low doses of estradiol to simulate the preovulatory estrogen surge. European J. Neuroscience 26: 2595-2612.

Son J, Song. S, Lee , S, C hang, S and Kim, M (2011) Morphological change tracking of dendritic spines based on structural features. J. of Microscopy, Vol. 241, pp. 261–272.

Veng LM, Granholm A-C, Rose GM (2003) Age-related sex differences in spatial learning and basal forebrain cholinergic neurons in F344 rats. Physiology & Behavior 80, 27-36.

Von Bohlen und Halbach O, Zacher C, Gass P, Unsicker K (2006) Age-related alterations in hippocampal spines and deficiencies in spatial memory in mice. J Neurosci Res. 83, 525-31.

Walf, AA, Koonce, CJ, Frye, CA. (2008). Estradiol or diarylpropionitrile administration to wild type, but not estrogen receptor beta knockout, mice enhances performance in the object recognition and object placement tasks. Neurobiol Learn. Mem. 89, 513-21.

Walf, AA, Rhodes, E, Frye, CA (2006). Ovarian steroids enhance object recognition in naturally cycling and ovariectomized, hormone-primed rats. Neurobiol. Learn. Mem. 86, 35-46.

Wallace, M, Luine, V, Arellanos, A and Frankfurt, M (2006). Ovariectomized rats show decreased recognition memory and spine density in hippocampus and prefrontal cortex. Brain Research 1126: 176-182.

Wallace, M, Frankfurt, M, Arellanos, A, Inagaki, T and Luine, V (2007). Impaired recognition memory and decreased frontal cortex spine density in aged rats. Imaging and the Aging Brain Annals NYAS 1097: 54-57.

Woolley CS, Gould E, Frankfurt M, McEwen BS (1990) Naturally occurring fluctuation in dendritic spine density on adult hippocampal pyramidal neurons. J Neurosci. 12: 4035-9.

Part 3

Sex Steroids and the Immune Response

10

Sex Steroids Modulate Fish Immune Response

Elena Chaves-Pozo[1], Isabel Cabas[2] and Alfonsa García-Ayala[2]
[1]*Centro Oceanográfico de Murcia, Instituto Español de Oceanografía (IEO), Carretera de la Azohía s/n. Puerto de Mazarrón, Murcia*
[2]*Department of Cell Biology and Histology, Faculty of Biology, University of Murcia, Murcia*
Spain

1. Introduction

For some time behavioural and ecological studies have suggested that sex steroid hormones regulate several immune processes in fish. For example, the immunocompetence handicap hypothesis relates the heritability of parasite resistance with secondary sexual ornaments, which are determined and maintained by androgens. Such ornaments are probably a good indicator to potential mates of genetic resistance to infections (Dijkstra et al., 2007; Roberts et al., 2004). Among vertebrates, the prevalence and intensity of parasitic infections is higher in males than females (Klein, 2004). Some fish species show altered sex steroid hormones levels upon parasite infection. The main alterations recorded upon infection are decreases in androgen, estrogen and vitelogenin serum levels (Hecker & Karbe, 2005). For example, during an infective period of vibriosis, silver seabream showed gradually increasing testosterone serum levels, whereas serum estradiol levels significantly decreased at an early stage of infection and remained low until death. This process coincided with increasing macrophages phagocytic activity (Deane et al., 2001). Such field studies prompted immunologists to try to establish how sex steroid hormones are able to alter the functions of the circulating leukocytes. In fish, most existing information on reproductive-immune interactions deals with the modulation of immune responses by circulating hormones, including cortisol, growth hormone, prolactin and reproductive hormones and some proopiomelanocortin-derived peptides (Engelsma et al., 2002; Harris & Bird, 2000). Although the exact effect of these endocrine mediators depends on the species, in general, they are known to modulate immune responses by integrating the activities of all the systems. In this way they help to adapt the organism to its environment (Lutton & Callard, 2006).
From a reproductive biology point of view, the leukocytes located in mammalian gonads orchestrate important reproductive physiology processes, including gametogenesis and steroidogenesis. A long time has passed since leukocytes were first described in the gonad of teleosts. Since them, several types of leukocytes have been described in the testis of different teleost species using light and electron microscopy. Moreover, differences in the number and localization of leukocytes within the testis have also been observed during the different stages of the reproductive cycle (Besseau & Faliex, 1994; Billard, 1983; Beruslé-Sicard & Fourcault, 1997; Lo Nostro, 2004; Scott & Sumpter, 1989). Thus, in the gametogenic activity and spawning stages some macrophages have been described in the interstitial tissue of the rainbow trout testis (Loir et al., 1995), whereas in the post-spawning stage a

high population of phagocyte cells has been described in several teleost fish (Henderson, 1962; Loir et al., 1995; Scott & Sumpter, 1989; Shrestha & Khanna, 1976). Although macrophages, granulocytes and lymphocytes have been described in the testis of some sparid fish, only macrophages have been shown to be phagocytic cells (Besseau & Faliex, 1994; Puslé-Sicard & Fourcault, 1997; Micale et al., 1987).

The gilthead seabream (*Sparus aurata* L.) is a protandrous hermaphrodite seasonal breeding teleost with a bisexual gonad (Figure 1) that offers an interesting model for studying immune-reproductive interactions. This is because the remodelling events of the gonad, especially during the post-spawning and testicular involution stages, compromise the immune system. The specimens undergo sex change during the second or third year of life, depending on the natural environment of the populations studied (Lasserre, 1972). Our previous studies performed in the western Mediterranean area demonstrated that gilthead seabream are males during the first and second reproductive cycles although their gonads possess a non-developed ovarian area separated from the testicular area by connective tissue (Chaves-Pozo et al., 2005a; Liarte et al., 2007). The reproductive cycle of males is divided into four gonad stages: gametogenic activity, spawning, post-spawning and resting. Resting is replaced by a testicular involution stage when the fish are ready to undergo sex change (Chaves-Pozo et al., 2005a; Liarte et al., 2007).

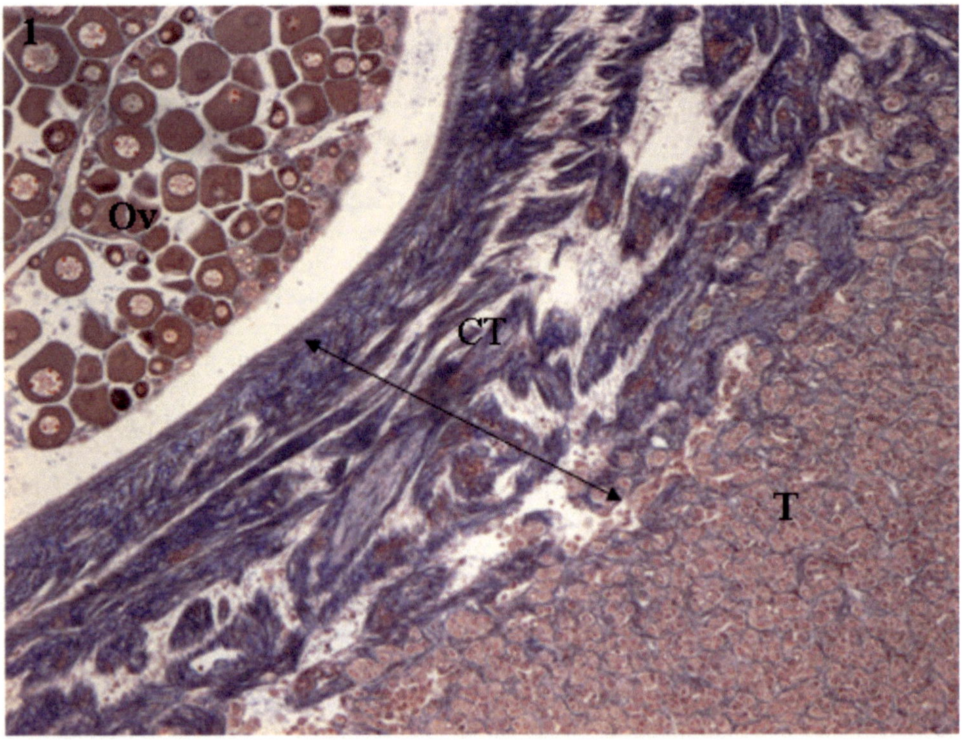

Fig. 1. Section of the gonad of gilthead seabream (*Sparus aurata* L.) during the male phase. The bisexual gonad is formed of a testis and an ovary separated by a thin layer of connective tissue. The testis is constituted by seminiferous tubules which are in the initial stage of spermatogenesis and the ovary is occupied with pre-vitellogenic ovocytes. T, testis; Ov, ovary; CT, connective tissue. (Mallory trichromic) Magnification x 10.

During the first reproductive cycle, 11-ketotestosterone and testosterone, the main androgens in fish, play different and specific roles in the testicular physiology as they peak at different stages of the reproductive cycle. Moreover, the profiles of testosterone serum levels during the second reproductive cycle demonstrated that this androgen is not essential to the testicular regression process that occurs during this cycle. In contrast, changes in 17β-estradiol serum levels suggest that this hormone orchestrates the testicular regression process during both reproductive cycles. Moreover, the data suggest that there is a threshold level of 17β-estradiol that determines the initiation of ovarian development during the second reproductive cycle without promoting complete feminization (Chaves-Pozo et al., 2008a).

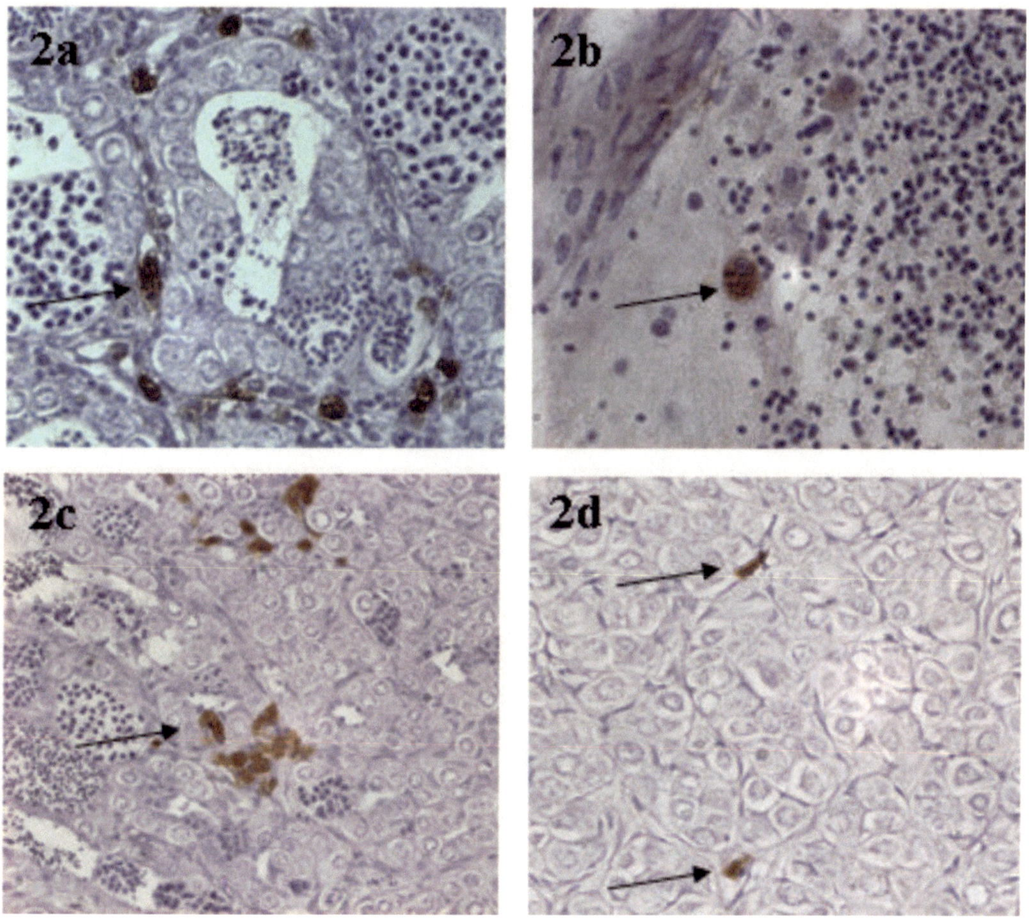

Fig. 2. Sections of the testis of gilthead seabream in the spermatogenesis (a), spawning (b), post-spawning (c) and resting (d) stages immunostained with a monoclonal antibody specific to gilthead seabream acidophilic granulocytes (Sepulcre et al., 2002). Acidophilic granulocytes (arrows) are seen in the blood vessels (a) during spermatogenesis, in the lumen of the tubules between the spermatozoa (b) and in the seminal epithelium in contact with germ cells (c) during spawning and post-spawning and in the interstitial tissue (d) during resting. Magnification x 400.

Few studies have dealt with the presence of leukocytes in the gonad of teleosts, their functions and the molecular pathways that regulate them. However, our studies in recent years have suggested that sex hormones might be key regulators of leukocyte functions in the gonad. For example, a massive infiltration of leukocytes, mainly acidophilic granulocytes (Figure 2), is orchestrated by gonadal factors including sex steroid hormones during post-spawning and testicular involution stages (Chaves-Pozo et al., 2003, 2005a, 2005b, 2007). The immune cells are produced in the head-kidney, the main haematopoietic organ in fish. However, when the acidophilic granulocytes infiltrate the testis, they show heavily impaired reactive oxygen intermediate production and phagocytic activity (hardly 1% of the testicular acidophilic granulocytes are able to phagocytise) (Figure 3) while the production of interleukin-1β (IL-1β) is sharply induced (Chaves-Pozo et al., 2003, 2005b, 2008a).

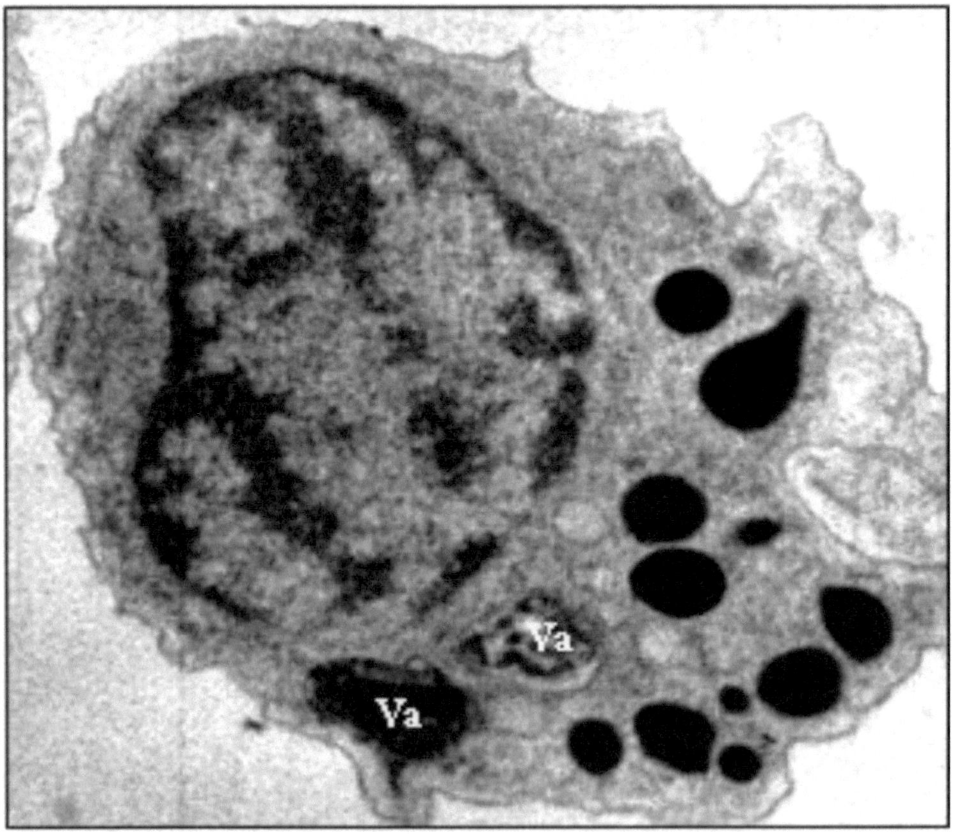

Fig. 3. An electron micrograph showing a testicular acidophilic granulocyte with the typical ultrastructure of acidophilic granulocytes and two phagosomes containing *Vibro anguillarum* cells (Va). Magnification x 5000.

Interestingly, it is the gonad itself which actively regulates the presence of these immune cells in the testis by stimulating their extravasation from the blood (Chaves-Pozo et al., 2005b). Moreover, 17β-estradiol and testosterone seem to be related with the infiltration of acidophilic granulocytes and probably with the magnitude of the infiltration since both hormones peak when the infiltration of these cells into the gonad occurred (Chaves-Pozo et al., 2008a). Moreover, the infiltration of acidophilic granulocytes was correlated with an increase in the expression of gonadal aromatase, the enzyme that transforms testosterone to 17β-estradiol. Such expression was seen to remain high during the period that acidophilic granulocytes are present in the gonad (Chaves-Pozo et al., 2005a, 2008b; Liarte et al., 2007). Moreover, experimentally induced increases of 17β-estradiol serum levels in spermatogenically active males triggered the migration of acidophilic granulocytes to the gonad in a way that resembles an inflammatory process (Chaves-Pozo et al., 2007). In the adult gilthead seabream gonad, macrophages and lymphocytes have also been observed in the interstitial tissue (Chaves-Pozo et al., 2008a; Liarte et al., 2007). However, the number of testicular macrophages remains steady throughout the reproductive cycle when the specimens are males, while no data related to lymphocytes are available (Chaves-Pozo et al., 2008a). Acidophilic granulocytes and B lymphocytes (Figure 4) also infiltrated the gonad and were located in the interstitial tissue and among the spermatozoa when fish were treated with an estrogenic endocrine disruptor, 17α-ethynilestradiol. This pharmaceutical compound, used for oral contraceptives and hormone replacement therapy, has a widespread presence in the aquatic environment (Ternes et al., 1999) and may reach concentrations of 0.5 to 62 ng/l in European seawage and surface waters (Hinteman et al., 2006; Johnson et al., 2005; Kuch and Ballschmiter, 2000).

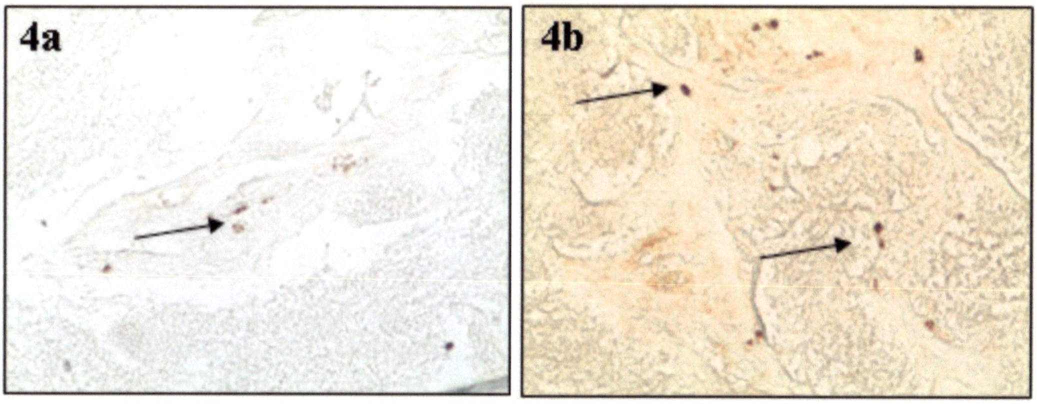

Fig. 4. Sections of the gilthead seabream testis in the spermatogenesis stage of specimens control (a) and specimens treated with 5 μg of 17α-ethynilestradiol/g food (b) immunostained with a specific anti-gilthead seabream IgM serum. B lymphocytes can be seen in the interstitial tissue of the testis, the numbers slightly increasing after 17α-ethynilestradiol treatment. Magnification x 200.

Testosterone administration *in vivo* modulates particular components of the physiological response of professional phagocytes such as respiratory burst, but does not alter their phagocytic activity. Testosterone is also able to regulate the gene expression profile of immune related molecules in head-kidney and other immune competent organs. This effect is characterized by a strong pro-inflammatory activation in the first week, after which it changes into an anti-inflammatory response (Águila et al., 2010).

These observations which, taken together, suggest that the presence of immune cells and cytokines in the gonad guarantees and modulates the reproductive functions (Figure 5), prompted us to investigate the role of 17β-estradiol and testosterone in immune cell functions and in the regulation of the inflammatory response.

In this context, we studied the effects of estrogens and androgens on the immune system responses, bringing together the views of both immunologists and reproductive biologists. An *in vitro* approach was used to determine which types of leukocytes are able to respond to sex steroid hormones.

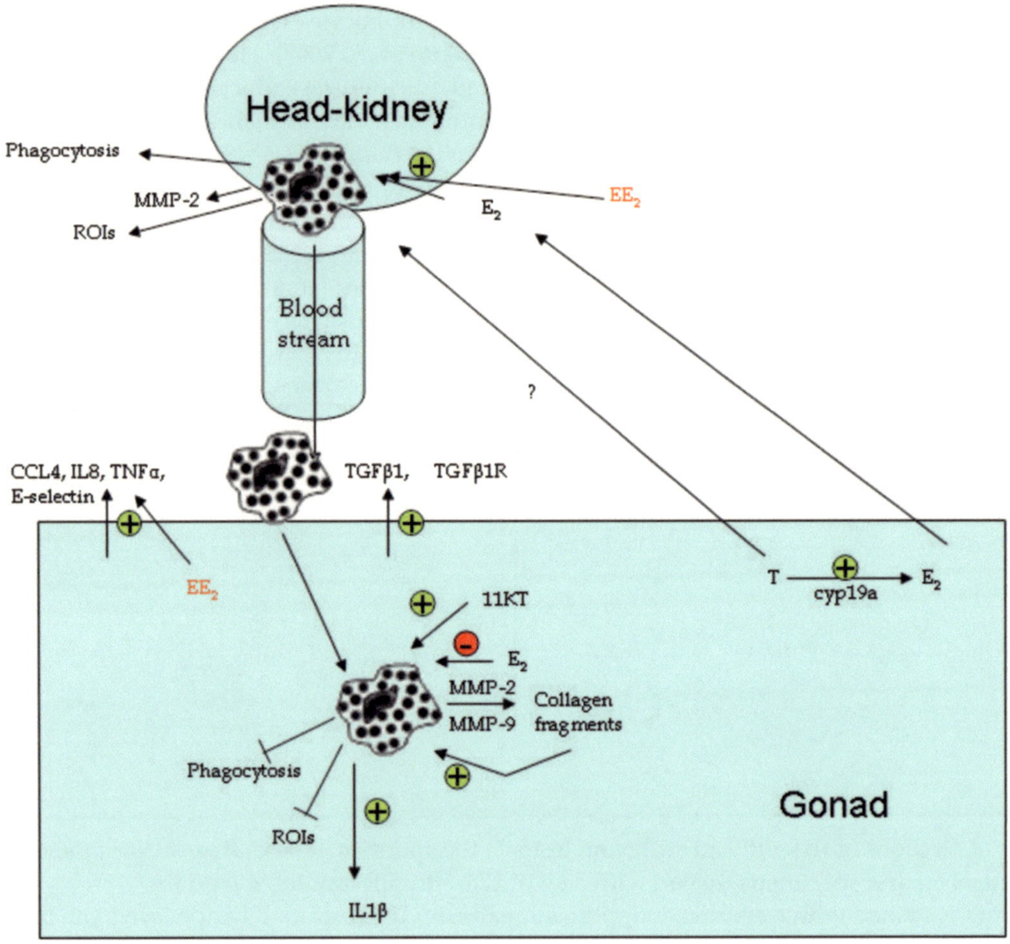

Fig. 5. Molecules involved in the mobilisation of acidophilic granulocytes from the head-kidney to the testis, as deduced from our *in vivo* and *in vitro* data (Chaves-Pozo et al., 2003, 2005 a,b, 2007, 2008a,b,c; Cabas et al., 2010). Although further studies are needed, the data clearly identify estrogens (17β-estradiol and 17α-ethynilestradiol) as key modulators of this process. MMP, matrix metalloproteinase; ROIs, reactive oxygen intermediates; E_2, 17β-estradiol; EE_2, 17α-ethynilestradiol; CCL4, CC chemokine-like 4 ; IL, interleukin; TNFα, tumour necrosis factor α; E-selectin, leukocyte adhesion molecule E-selectin; TGFβ1, transforming growth factor β1; TGFβ1R, transforming growth factor β1 receptor; 11KT, 11-ketotestosterone; cyp19a, P450 aromatase.

2. Sex steroid hormones as regulators of the immune response

In mammals, androgens and estrogens exert their main long-term effects on cell growth, cell differentiation and cell functions through intracellular androgen receptors (AR) and estrogen receptors (ER), ERα and ERβ, respectively, all of which belong to the nuclear receptor superfamily (Evans & Bergeron, 1988). These AR and ER are ligand-inducible transcription factors that cause the activation or repression of genes (Beato & Klug, 2000; Kumar & Tindall, 1998). In different mammalian models, the preponderance of ERα gene over the ERβ gene is accepted as being one of the mechanism that control the effects of 17β-estradiol on the immune system (Straub, 2007). The main effect of estrogens on the immune response involve enhancing the immune/inflammatory response by activating the nuclear factor κB (NFkB) signalling pathway (Cutolo et al., 2004) and stimulating the secretion of tumor necrosis factor (TNF) (Janele et al., 2006). Furthermore, using ER knock-out mice, researchers have shown that ER participates in the stimulation of interleukin (IL)-10 and immunoglobulin (Ig) M production. In accordance with these roles, a number of epidemiological studies have highlighted the relationship between plasma estrogen levels, IL production, and autoimmune disorders linked to some diseases (Cutolo et al., 2006). However, 17β-estradiol also has an inhibitory effect on bone resorption and the suppression of inflammation in several animal models of chronic inflammatory diseases (Straub, 2007). Unlike estrogens, androgens are thought to be exclusively immunosuppressive in mammals. For example, androgens have a negative effect on the expression of inflammatory cytokines, increase apoptosis in human monocytes/macrophages, and inhibit lymphocyte proliferation (Cutolo & Straub, 2009; Cutolo et al., 2005; Lehmann et al., 1988).

In teleosts, the large number of different species and the genome duplications that have occurred during their phylogeny make it very difficult to assess the number of AR and ER existing in each specie. Depending on the species studied, three or four different ER genes have been described. Thus, in some species (gilthead seabream, atlantic croaker, zebrafish, goldfish) one ERα and two ERβ have been cloned, while in others (rainbow trout and *Spinibarbus denticulatus*) two ERα and two ERβ were found (Iwanowicz & Ottinger, 2009; Nagler et al., 2007). In order to determine whether immune tissues are potential targets for estrogens, several studies have looked at the expression of ER in immune tissues. In immature and mature male and female channel catfish, for example, ERα is expressed in spleen, blood and head-kidney, while ERβ is only expressed in spleen (Xia et al., 2000). ERβ is expressed in the spleen and head-kidney of male and female common solea (Caviola et al., 2007). In the gilthead seabream, *in vitro* long term treatment of head-kidney leukocytes with 17β-estradiol revealed a suppressive effect on the production of reactive oxygen intermediates and the *Vibrio anguillarum* DNA (VaDNA)-stimulated production of IL-1β (Chaves-Pozo et al., 2003). However, short term treatment with higher concentrations of 17β-estradiol inhibited the phagocytic capability, while the percentage of phagocytic cells and the VaDNA-stimulated production of reactive oxygen intermediates and cell migration activity remained steady (Liarte et al., 2011b). In the case of AR, most vertebrates are believed to have one active form of nuclear AR with high specificity for the androgen 5α-dihydrotestosterone, whereas there appear to be two subtypes of AR in some teleosts, ARα and ARβ. These are differentially expressed in tissues and show high affinity for both testosterone and 11β-hidroxytestosterone (review in Rempel & Schlenk, 2008). However, little is known about the expression of these AR in fish immune tissues, although in mammalian models AR are present in liver, spleen and thymus (Butts et al., 2011).

There is increasing evidence supporting the transcription-independent non-genomic actions of steroid hormones, including testosterone and 17β-estradiol (Christ et al., 1997; Falkenstein et al., 2000). For example, mammalian mast cells, T and B cells and macrophages shows membrane AR and membrane ER (Benten et al., 1998, 2001, 2002; Zaitsu et al., 2007). A membrane ER (Pang et al., 2008) and a membrane AR (review in Thomas et al., 2006) have recently been cloned and characterized in atlantic croaker, although nothing is known about membrane AR in fish immune tissues. The complexity of the way in which sex steroid hormones act in fish through membrane and intracellular receptors, as well as the complexity of the systemic and gonadal immune responses and the several cell types involved, prompted researchers to characterize sex steroid hormone receptors and the effects of their ligands in purified immune cells and cell lines. However, since each cell type has its own response pattern these issues will be dealt with separately.

2.1 Macrophages

Macrophages are ubiquitous cells that play a central role in the innate immune response through the secretion of inflammatory cytokines, such as IL-1β and TNFα, the production of cytotoxic reactive oxygen intermediates, and the secretion of leukostatic factors and other regulatory molecules. They are also important accessory cells for many other immune responses. In addition, during development, these cells are thought to have a trophic role through their remodelling capabilities and ability to produce cytokines. Interestingly, whereas a similar pattern of functioning has been demonstrated for macrophages in different tissues (Guillemin & Brew, 2004; Laskin et al., 2001; Stout & Suttles, 2004), testicular macrophages and their functions are largely determined by the local environment (Hedger, 1997, 2002), including not only cytokines and chemokines, but also steroid hormones. In mammals, it has been known for many years that ER are expressed in monocytes (Cunningham & Gilkeson). However, their response to estrogens and the predominance of ERα or ERβ expression appear to be dependent on their stage of differentiation. For example, Mor et al. (2003) demonstrated that monocytes express more ERβ and macrophages express more ERα. The behaviour of 17β-estradiol functions in mammalian macrophages has been described as double-edge-sword (depending on 17β-estradiol concentration). Thus, lower 17β-estradiol concentrations stimulated IL-1β production, whereas higher concentrations inhibited lipopolysaccharide (LPS)-induced TNFα production. This dichotomous effect of 17β-estradiol on IL-1β and TNFα at high and low concentrations is most probably due to inhibition of NF-κB at high concentrations (review in Straub, 2007).

Gilthead seabream macrophages constitutively express only the ERα gene, although stimulation with VaDNA drastically up-regulates the expression of ERα, ERβ1 and ERβ2 genes, suggesting that the immune system is able to increase its sensitivity to 17β-estradiol during development of the immune response (Liarte et al., 2011b). In long-term leukocyte cell lines of monocytes/macrophages from channel catfish, the expression of both ERα and ERβ has been described (Iwanowicz & Ottinger, 2009). Although evidence conclusively demonstrates that fish leukocytes express ER genes, the literature in this respect does not deal with the possible differential roles of the two ERβ genes (ERβ1 and ERβ2) present in fish. Our data in the gilthead seabream demonstrate for the first time that ERβ1 and ERβ2 are differentially regulated in macrophages. Thus, ERβ1 gene expression is only induced by VaDNA and its VaDNA-induced expression is slightly increased by 17β-estradiol, in contrast to ERβ2 gene whose expression is induced by both stimuli, which, moreover, have a synergic effect on ERβ2 gene expression (Liarte et al., 2011b).

The biological effect of 17β-estradiol on fish head-kidney macrophages is mainly anti-inflammatory, although controversial data were observed depending on whether the studies were *in vivo* or *in vitro*. Intra-peritoneal injections of 17β-estradiol in common carp inhibit phagocytosis and the production of reactive oxygen intermediates and reactive nitrogen intermediates by head-kidney macrophages in a dose-dependent manner (Watanuki et al., 2002). However, upon *in vitro* treatment, these head-kidney macrophages only showed impaired phagocytic capability (Yamaguchi et al., 2001) and, in goldfish macrophages, 17β-estradiol inhibited the percentage of phagocytic cells (Wang & Belosevic, 1995). In the European flounder, microarray studies have revealed that 17β-estradiol suppresses immune system-related transcripts in liver (Williams et al., 2007). In rainbow trout, 17β-estradiol repressed the acute phase immune response genes (Tilton et al., 2006), as occurs in mammalian macrophages (Kramer & Wray, 2002). However, in gilthead seabream macrophages, 17β-estradiol up-regulates some genes coding for key immune molecules, including inflammatory and anti-inflammatory molecules, innate immune receptors, molecules related to leukocyte infiltration, matrix metalloproteinases (MMP) and the anti-viral molecule *Myxovirus* (*influenza*) resistance protein (Mx). Moreover, the soluble factors produced by those 17β-estradiol-stimulated macrophages modify the immune functions of head-kidney leukocytes (Liarte et al., 2011b), suggesting that the soluble factors produced by testicular macrophages in response to 17β-estradiol contribute by blocking the phagocytic activity of testicular acidophilic granulocytes (Chaves-Pozo et al., 2005b). A suppression subtractive library was constructed to isolate and identify mRNA species up-regulated by a supra-physiological dose of 17β-estradiol (50 ng/ml) to macrophages. Interestingly, this showed that 4% of up-regulated genes are related with the immune response, 6% with the stimulus response and 0.5% with physiological interactions between different organism categories, all of them probably involved in the interaction of immune cells with the immune stimulus. Although the number of identified genes within these categories was relatively low, other well-represented subcategories such as these related with biological regulation could contain genes whose functions may influence the behaviour of macrophages and thus affect their ability to respond to an immunological challenge upon exposure to estrogens (Liarte et al., 2011a; Xia & Yue, 2010).

Although less data are available for AR than for ER in mammalian species, several studies have demonstrated that testosterone alters macrophage functions in a complex manner, since it has both pro-inflammatory and anti-inflammatory effects. For example, wound healing is impaired in males, especially the elderly, which has been directly linked to a pro-inflammatory action of testosterone on tissue macrophages in the skin (Ashcroft & Mills, 2002). Moreover, castration increased macrophage-mediated damage at sites of injury in the skin, suggesting an anti-inflammatory role for testosterone (Ashcroft & Mills, 2002). Testosterone also inhibits inducible nitric oxide synthase and nitric oxide production in a mouse macrophage cell line (Friedl et al., 2000). The expression of AR in microglia, the brain macrophage, increases after injury and indicates that the innate immune cells of the brain may be modulated by androgens (García-Ovejero et al., 2002). Other data indicate that 5α-dihydrotestosterone acts as an anti-inflammatory agent and depresses both nitric oxide and TNFα production in a dose-dependent fashion. However, testosterone treatment of microglia and peritoneal macrophages increased supernatant nitrite levels, suggesting a pro-inflammatory effect (Brown & Angel, 2005).

In fish, the data obtained show that androgens are also able to modulate the immune system responses. In common carp, intraperitoneal injections of 11-ketotestosterone inhibit phagocytosis and the production of reactive oxygen intermediates and reactive nitrogen intermediates by head-kidney macrophages in a dose-dependent manner (Watanuki et al., 2002). However, *in vitro* studies with head-kidney macrophages have demonstrated that this hormone inhibits phagocytosis and the production of reactive nitrogen intermediates and has no effect on the production of reactive oxygen intermediates (Yamaguchi et al., 2001). Interestingly, although gilthead seabream macrophages do not express the AR at a level detectable by real time polymerase chain reaction, both testosterone and 11-ketotestosterone up-regulated different immune genes, such as immune receptors and pro-inflammatory cytokines, and down-regulated the anti-inflammatory cytokine, transforming growth factor (TGF) β (Águila et al., 2011). Taking into account the complexity of sex steroid hormone signalling through intracellular and membrane receptors and sex steroid hormone conversion through transformation in other derivatives (such as reduced derivatives or even 17β-estradiol) and bearing in mind that both testosterone and 11-ketotestosterone alter the macrophage gene expression and functions analyzed, it can not be discounted that macrophages convert testosterone into 11-ketotestosterone or another molecule capable of signalling through other receptors in this cell type. In this sense, mammalian macrophages lack AR but are able to respond to androgens through a membrane AR that triggers a Ca^{2+} influx (Benten et al., 2004). Moreover, mammalian testicular macrophages have a steroidogenic capability as they are able to produce and secrete 25-hydroxycholesterol, which affects Leydig cell steroidogenesis (Hales, 2002). In light of the above, further studies are needed to complete our understanding of the effect of androgens on fish innate immunity and macrophages.

2.2 Acidophilic granulocytes

The acidoplilic granulocytes of gilthead seabream display some functions similar to human neutrophils despite their opposite staining pattern. In brief, they are the most abundant circulating granulocytes and are recruited from the head-kidney to the site of inflammation (Chaves-Pozo et al., 2004, 2005c), where they attach themselves to, internalize and kill bacteria through the production of reactive oxygen intermediates (Chaves-Pozo et al., 2004, 2005c; Meseguer et al., 1994; Sepulcre et al., 2002). However, they also show a monocyte/macrophage-like behaviour as they are able to specifically target a tissue and respond to physiological stimuli by displaying modified functions, as do the monocytes/macrophages of mammals (Chaves-Pozo et al., 2005c; Stout & Suttles, 2004). In fact, gilthead seabream acidophilic granulocytes infiltrate the testis in a way that resembles an inflammatory process triggered by physiological stimuli, and their main activities are strongly inhibited by the testicular microenvironment in order to preserve reproductive functions (Chaves-Pozo et al., 2005b). Previous data showed that 17β-estradiol is related *in vivo* with the mobilization of acidophilic granulocytes from the head-kidney to the gonad and probably with the degree of this infiltration (Chaves-Pozo et al., 2007, 2008a). Interestingly, neither testicular nor head-kidney acidophilic granulocytes express any of the ER known in the gilthead seabream (Pinto et al., 2006; Liarte et al., 2011b). However, studies performed with conditioned medium from 17β-estradiol-treated macrophages suggest that some, but not all, the acidophilic granulocyte functions modified by the testicular microenvironment might be regulated by the factors produced by 17β-estradiol-treated macrophages (Liarte et al., 2011b). In this sense, there is evidence that suggests a pro-inflammatory role for 17β-estradiol in the gilthead seabream, since it is able to stimulate *in vivo* specific leukocyte migration and promote acidophilic granulocytes infiltration into the gonad (Chaves-Pozo et al., 2007). However, *in vitro,* 17β-estradiol failed to promote chemiotaxis in purified acidophilic granulocytes, although it is produced a positive migration of leukocytes when head-kidney suspensions were exposed to 17β-estradiol (Liarte et al., 2011b).

In so far as androgens are concerned, acidophilic granulocytes constitutively express AR, the expression of which is modified by 11-ketotestosterone and testosterone, but only when the cells are co-stimulated with VaDNA (Águila et al., 2011). The effects of 11-ketotestosterone and testosterone on acidophilic granulocytes differ: while testosterone increased, 11-ketotestosterone decreased the expression of IL-1β and toll-like receptors (TLRs), although both up-regulated the VaDNA-induced expression of IL-1β (Águila et al., 2010).

2.3 Lymphocytes

T and B lymphocytes are the acknowledged cellular pillars of adaptative immunity. T cells are primarily responsible for cell-mediated immunity, while B lymphocytes are responsible for humoral immunity, but, in conjunction with other cell types, both mediate effective adaptive immunity (Pancer & Cooper, 2006). Recently, in long-term leukocyte cell lines of T-cells and B-cells from channel catfish, the differential expression of ERα and ERβ was described. Thus, ERα is expressed in both cell types, while only T-cells express ERβ2 (Iwanowicz & Ottinger, 2009). In the gilthead seabream, lymphocytes only express the ERα gene (Liarte et al., 2011b). In mammals, however, B lymphocytes express both ERα and ERβ genes, while there is debate as to whether or not T cells contain classical nuclear ER (Benten et al., 1998; Harkonen & Vaananen, 2006). *In vitro* functional assays demonstrated that 17β-estradiol stimulates lymphocyte proliferation (Cook et al., 1994).

To determine whether fish lymphocytes respond to androgens, the classical chemical characterization of AR was performed in salmonid lymphocytes (Slater et al., 1995). In these species, 11-ketotestosterone inhibits lymphocyte proliferation, while testosterone reduces the number of antibody-producing cells and acts with cortisol to produce a greater inhibitory effect (Cook et al., 1994; Slater & Schreck, 1993).

2.4 Endothelial cells

Leukocyte recruitment is an early and pivotal event in any inflammatory response. Since gilthead seabream acidophilic granulocytes are recruited from the blood stream into the testis in a process that might be orchestrated by 17β-estradiol (Chaves-Pozo et al., 2005b, 2007, 2008a), we investigated the role of the endothelium in this process. Leukocyte-endothelial interactions are a special case of cell sorting, in which the endothelium discriminates between circulating leukocytes in order to select cells for transmigration into surrounding tissue (Ebnet et al., 1996a). Endothelial cells play a singular role in this process, receiving information from the underlying tissue and transforming it into information that can be read rapidly by the passing leukocytes (Ebnet et al., 1996b). Accumulated evidence on mammalian models of cardiovascular disease points to the prominent role of estrogens in the ability of endothelial cells to trigger inflammation and participate in the leukocyte infiltration process (Nilsson, 2007; Straub, 2007). In mammals, endothelial cells constitutively express both ERα and ERβ, although ERα plays a prominent role in the vascular physiology (Ihionkhan et al., 2002; Straub, 2007). Gilthead seabream endothelial cells constitutively express ERα and ERβ1 but not ERβ2 (Liarte et al., 2011c). However, few studies have been carried out into the effect of 17β-estradiol on endothelial cell physiology in fish. In the Japanese eel, 17β-estradiol stimulated the production of vascular endothelial cell growth factor in endothelial cells (Huang et al., 2006). In the gilthead seabream endothelial cell cultures, 17β-estradiol induced the expression of genes coding for chemokines, adhesion molecules and MMPs, which agrees with previous studies that demonstrated that 17β-estradiol promotes acidophilic granulocyte infiltration into the testis (Chaves-Pozo et al., 2007). These effects contrast with that which occurs in mammals, where 17β-estradiol inhibits *in vivo* the migration of leukocytes into inflamed areas and exerts tissue-protective activities through the down-regulation of adhesion molecules and the proforms of MMPs (Straub, 2007). On the other hand, 17β-estradiol did not affect the expression in endothelial cells of the genes encoding major pro-inflammatory cytokines, such as IL-1β, IL-6 and TNFα, which may prevent the detrimental effects of 17β-estradiol-induced inflammation through leukocyte recruitment (Liarte et al., 2011c).

Little is known about androgens and their receptors in fish endothelial cells. There are very recent studies that suggest that androgens influence fish endothelial cell physiology, although further effort is needed to really understand how androgens affect endothelial cells and their molecular pathways. Trout testicular endothelial cells possess AR, as located by immunocytochemistry (Galas et al., 2009). In the gilthead seabream, recent studies determined that testosterone up-regulated TNFα, cyclooxigenase 2 (Cox2) and IL-1β, and down-regulated TGFβ and aromatase (the enzyme that transforms testosterone into 17β-estradiol) gene expression (Águila et al., 2011).

3. Effects of endocrine disruptors on the immune response

In several species, the affinity for ER of several agonists, including natural estrogens like 17β-estradiol, estrone or estriol, and estrogenic disruptor compounds, like 17α-ethynilestradiol or diethylstilbestrol, has been tested. The different types of ER show differential binding preferences for ligands and their expression patterns are tissue-dependant (Iwanowicz & Ottinger, 2009). Taking into account that ER and AR are widely distributed in immune tissues, including the spleen, liver and anterior kidney (Lynn et al., 2008; Shved et al., 2009; Slater et al., 1995; Todo et al., 1999), the study of endocrine disruptor compounds as potential aquatic pollutants has taken on some importance for fish immunologists. Several anatomical and morphological changes were observed in lymphoid tissues following exposure to xenoestrogens and xenoandrogens. Spleno-somatic and hepato-somatic indices and thymus volume are affected by exposure to sex-steroids (androgens and estrogens) or to their related endocrine disruptor compounds (Grinwis et al., 2009; Kurtz et al., 2007; Tellez-Banuelos et al., 2009; van Ginneken et al., 2009). In the gilthead seabream the dietary intake of 17α-ethynilestradiol promotes the up-regulation of several genes related with leukocyte recruitment (e.g. E-selectin (sele), the CC chemokine-like 4 (CCL4), TNFα and IL-8). Moreover, the heavy chain of IgM and IgT genes has also been seen to be up-regulated (Cabas et al., 2011). An increase in the spleno-somatic index was also recorded.

Surprisingly, *in vitro* 17α-ethynilestradiol treatment of gilthead seabream endothelial cells dramatically reduces the expression of chemokines, adhesion molecules and MMPs in

VaDNA-activated endothelial cells unlike in 17β-estradiol-treated endothelial cells (see point 2.4). Although, the differential expression profile in stimulated 17α-ethynilestradiol-treated endothelial cells, compared with 17β-estradiol-treated endothelial cells, indicates that this compound would be able to impair the recruitment and activation of fish leukocytes, other molecular pathways might promote an inflammatory process in the gonad *in vivo,* as described by Cabas et al. (2011). These data show the complex effect of endocrine disruptor compounds on immune functions and the need to deepen our knowledge of their molecular action mechanism. As also occurs in mammals, 17β-estradiol, but not 17α-ethynilestradiol, significantly enhances nitric oxide production in gilthead seabream endothelial cells, indicating that some estrogens regulate nitric oxide production by endothelial cells from fish to mammals (Arnal et al., 1996; Liarte et al., 2011c; Nilsson, 2007). As far as we know, most studies on this topic have dealt with the effects of estrogenic and anti-androgenic disruptor compounds on reproductive functions. It is known that these disruptor compounds mainly affect several enzymes in the steroidogenic pathway, such as 20β-hydroxysteroid deshydrogenase, 17β- hydroxysteroid deshydrogenase and 11β-hydroxysteroid deshydrogenase, aromatase and 5α-reductase (Rempel & Schlenk, 2008). Further studies are needed into androgenic disruptor compounds as well as into estrogenic, anti-androgenic and androgenic disruptor compound mixtures to better understand how chemically and pharmaceutically polluted water might affect the reproductive and immune function of fish. Future studies and analyses along these times are being undertaken in our laboratory.

4. Conclusion

It is known that both estrogens and androgens modulate the fish immune response, although the molecular mechanisms by which they act are not completely understood. *In vivo* and *in vitro* analyses have demonstrated that gilthead seabream leukocyte (macrophages, acidophilic granulocytes and lymphocytes) express intracellular AR and/or ER, whose expression pattern upon stimulation depend on the cell type and the stimuli in question. Estrogens and androgens compromise the immune response, affecting cell types other than leukocytes. Thus, endothelial cells are involved in the leukocyte trafficking that occurs during the inflammatory process and their activities are also modulated by sex steroids. A wide variety of chemicals discharged from industrial and municipal sources has been reported to disrupt the endocrine system of animals via the food chain and contaminated water. Some of these contaminants have a widespread presence in the aquatic environment. Although, current knowledge concerning the sensitivity of marine fish to estrogenic and androgenic chemical in the environment is limited, we have seen that the most widespread (estrogenic) disruptor compound drastically affects leukocyte trafficking and recruitment into tissues. The short time of exposure (3 hours) used in our *in vitro* experiments suggests that, together with ER and AR activation, some transcription-independent non-genomic actions might be acting on sex steroid hormones-stimulated leukocytes. Taking all this into account, further effort will focus on the cloning and characterization of membrane AR and ER, their expression pattern in immune cells and the molecular characterization of the way of which estrogenic and androgenic compounds disrupt the molecular signalling pathways of intracellular and membrane androgen and estrogen receptors.

5. Acknowledgments

This work was supported by the Fundación Séneca, Coordination Center for Research, CARM (proyect 04538/GERM/06 to A.G.A and grant to I.C.), the Spanish Ministry of Science and Innovation (contract RYC-2009-05451 to E.C.P., project AGL2008-04575-C02-01 to A.G.A.). We thank the "Servicio de Apoyo a la Investigación" of the University of Murcia for their assistance with cell culture and gene expression analysis and the "Centro Oceanográfico de Murcia, Instituto Español de Oceanografía" for their assistance with fish care.

6. References

Águila S.; Castillo-Briceño P.; Mulero V.; Meseguer J. & García-Ayala A. (2010). Testosterone modulates the immune response in vivo of the teleost fish gilthead seabream. First symposium of the European Organisation of Fish Immunology (EOFFI). Viterbo, Italy.

Águila S.; Sánchez M.; Castillo Briceño P.; García Alcázar A.; Meseguer J.; Mulero V. & García Ayala A. (2011). Androgens modulate *in vitro* the activation of professional phagocytes from the bony fish gilthead seabream. GIA 2011. Heraklion, Crete, Greece.

Arnal J. F.; Tack I.; Besombes J. P.; Pipy B. & Negre-Salvayre A. (1996). Nitric oxide and superoxide anion production during endothelial cell proliferation. American Journal of Physiology, Vol.271, No.5, (November 1996), pp. 1521-1526, ISSN 0002-9513.

Ashcroft G. S. & Mills S. J. (2002). Androgen receptor-mediated inhibition of cutaneous wound healing. Journal of Clinical Investigation, Vol.110, No.5, (September 2002), pp. 615-624, ISSN 0021-9738.

Beato M. & Klug J. (2000). Steroid hormone receptors: an update. Human Reproduction Update, Vol.6, No.3, (May-June 2000), pp. 225-236, ISSN 1355-4786.

Benten W. P.; Guo Z.; Krucken J. & Wunderlich F. (2004). Rapid effects of androgens in macrophages. Steroids, Vol.69, No.8-9, (August 2004), pp. 585-590, ISSN 0039-128X.

Benten W. P.; Lieberherr M.; Giese G. & Wunderlich F. (1998). Estradiol binding to cell surface raises cytosolic free calcium in T cells. FEBS Letters, Vol.422, No.3, (February 1998), pp. 349-53, ISSN 0014-5793.

Benten W. P.: Stephan C.; Lieberherr M. & Wunderlich F. (2001). Estradiol signaling via sequestrable surface receptors. Endocrinology, Vol.142, No.4, (April 2001), pp. 1669-1677, ISSN 0013-7227.

Benten W. P.; Stephan C. & Wunderlich F. (2002). B cells express intracellular but not surface receptors for testosterone and estradiol. Steroids, Vol.67, No.7, (June 2002), pp. 647-654, ISSN 0039-128X.

Besseau L. & Faliex E. (1994). Resorption of unemitted gametes in *Lithognathus mormyrus* (Sparidae, Teleostei): a possible synergic action of somatic and immune cells. Cell and Tissue Research, Vol.276, No.1, (April 1994), pp. 123-132, ISSN 0302-766X.

Billar R. (1983). A quantitative analysis of spermatogenesis in the trout, *Salmo trutta fario*. Cell and Tissue Research, Vol, 230, No.3, (April 1983), pp. 495-502, ISSN 0302-766X.

Brown P. A. & Angel J. B. (2005). Granulocyte-macrophage colony-stimulating factor as an immune-based therapy in HIV infection. Journal of Immune Based Therapies and Vaccines, Vol.3, No.1, (May 2005), pp. 3-10, ISSN 1476-8518.

Truslé-Sicard S. & Fourcault B. (1997). Recognition of sex-inverting protandric *Sparus aurata*: ultrastructural aspects. Journal of Fish Biology, Vol.50, (December 1997), pp. 1094-1103, ISSN 0022-1112.

Butts C. L.; Jones Y. L.; Lim J. K.; Salter C. E.; Belyavskaya E. & Sternberg E. M. (2011). Tissue expression of steroid hormone receptors is associated with differential immune responsiveness. Brain, Behaviour and Immunity, Vol.25, No.5, (July 2001), pp. 1000-1007, ISSN 1090-2139.

Cabas I.; Liarte S.; Meseguer J.; Mulero V. & García-Ayala A. (2010). 17α-ethynylestradiol *in vivo* treatment alters inflammatory gene expression profile in the gilthead seabream (*Sparus aurata* L.). 9th International Congress on the Biology of Fish. Barcelona, Spain.

Cabas I.; Chaves-Pozo E.; García-Alcazar A.; Meseguer J.; Mulero V. & García-Ayala A. (2011). Dietary intake of 17 alpha-ethinylestradiol promotes leukocytes infiltration in the gonad of the hermaphrodite gilthead seabream. Molecular Immunology. ISSN 0161-5890. DOI:10.1016/j.molimm.2011.05.019.

Caviola E.; Dalla Valle L.; Belvedere P. & Colombo L. (2007). Characterisation of three variants of estrogen receptor beta mRNA in the common sole, *Solea solea* L. (Teleostei). General and Comparative Endocrinology, Vol.153, No.1-3, (August-September 2007), pp. 31-39, ISSN 0016-6480.

Cook G. A.; Elliott D.; Metwali A.; Blum A. M.; Sandor M.; Lynch R. & Weinstock J. V. (1994). Molecular evidence that granuloma T lymphocytes in murine schistosomiasis mansoni express an authentic substance P (NK-1) receptor. Journal of Immunology, Vol.152, No. 4, (February 1994), pp. 1830-1835, ISSN 0022-1767.

Cunningham M. & Gilkeson G. (2011). Estrogen receptors in immunity and autoimmunity. Clinical Reviews in Allergy and Immunology, Vol.40, No.1, (February 2011), pp. 66-73, ISSN 1559-0267.

Cutolo M.; Capellino S.; Montagna P.; Ghiorzo P.; Sulli A. & Villaggio B. (2005). Sex hormone modulation of cell growth and apoptosis of the human monocytic/macrophage cell line. Arthritis Research and Therapy, Vol.7, No.5, (July 2005), pp. 1124-1132, ISSN 1478-6362.

Cutolo M.; Montecucco C. M.; Cavagna L.; Caporali R.; Capellino S.; Montagna P.; Fazzuoli L.; Villaggio B.; Seriolo B. & Sulli A. (2006). Serum cytokines and steroidal hormones in polymyalgia rheumatica and elderly-onset rheumatoid arthritis. Annals of the Rheumatic Diseases, Vol.65, No.11, (November 2006), pp. 1438-1443, ISSN 0003-4967.

Cutolo M. & Straub R. H. (2009). Insights into endocrine-immunological disturbances in autoimmunity and their impact on treatment. Arthritis Research and Therapy, Vol.11, No.2, (April 2009), pp. 218-225, ISSN 1478-6362.

Cutolo M.; Sulli A.; Capellino S.; Villaggio B.; Montagna P.; Seriolo B. & Straub R. H. (2004). Sex hormones influence on the immune system: basic and clinical aspects in autoimmunity. Lupus, Vol.13, No.9, (September, 2004) pp. 635-638, ISSN 0961-2033.

Chaves-Pozo, E., Liarte, S., Fernández-Alacid, L., Abellán, E., Meseguer, J., Mulero, V. & García-Ayala, A. (2008a). Pattern of expression of immune-relevant genes in the gonad of a teleost, the gilthead seabream (*Sparus aurata* L.). Molecular Immunology, Vol.45, No.10, (May 2008), pp.2998-3011, ISSN 0161-5890.

Chaves-Pozo E.; Arjona F. J.; García-López A.; García-Alcázar A.; Meseguer J. & García-Ayala A. (2008b). Sex steroids and metabolic parameter levels in a seasonal breeding fish (*Sparus aurata* L.). General and Comparative Endocrinology, Vol.156, No.3, (May 2008), pp. 531-536, ISSN 0016-6480.

Chaves-Pozo E.; Castillo-Briceño P.; García-Alcázar A.; Meseguer J.; Mulero V. & García-Ayala A. (2008c). A role for matrix metalloproteinases in granulocyte infiltration and testicular remodelation in a seasonal breeding teleost. Molecular Immunology, Vol.45, No.10, (May 2008), pp. 2820-2830, ISSN 0161-5890.

Chaves-Pozo E.; Liarte S.; Vargas-Chacoff L.; García-López A.; Mulero V.; Meseguer J.; Mancera J. M. & García-Ayala A. (2007). 17Beta-estradiol triggers postspawning in spermatogenically active gilthead seabream (*Sparus aurata* L.) males. Biolology of Reproduction, Vol.76, No.1, (January 2007), pp. 142-148, ISSN 0006-3363.

Chaves-Pozo E.; Mulero V.; Meseguer J. & García-Ayala A. (2005a). An overview of cell renewal in the testis throughout the reproductive cycle of a seasonal breeding teleost, the gilthead seabream (*Sparus aurata* L). Biology of Reproduction, Vol.72, No.3, (March 2005), pp. 593-601, ISSN 0006-3363.

Chaves-Pozo E.; Mulero V.; Meseguer J. & García-Ayala A. (2005b). Professional phagocytic granulocytes of the bony fish gilthead seabream display functional adaptation to testicular microenvironment. Journal of Leukocyte Biology, Vol.78, No.2, (August 2005), pp. 345-351, ISSN 0741-5400.

Chaves-Pozo E.; Muñoz P.; López-Muñoz A.; Pelegrín P.; García-Ayala A.; Mulero V. & Meseguer J. (2005c). Early innate immune response and redistribution of inflammatory cells in the bony fish gilthead seabream experimentally infected with *Vibrio anguillarum*. Cell and Tissue Research, Vol.320, No.1, (April 2005), pp. 61-68, ISSN 0302-766X.

Chaves-Pozo E.; Pelegrín P.; García-Castillo J.; García-Ayala A.; Mulero V. & Meseguer J. (2004). Acidophilic granulocytes of the marine fish gilthead seabream (*Sparus aurata* L.) produce interleukin-1beta following infection with *Vibrio anguillarum*. Cell and Tissue Research, Vol.316, No.2, (May 2004), pp. 189-195, ISSN 0302-766X.

Chaves-Pozo E.; Pelegrín P.; Mulero V.; Meseguer J. & García-Ayala A. (2003). A role for acidophilic granulocytes in the testis of the gilthead seabream (*Sparus aurata* L., Teleostei). Journal of Endocrinology, Vol.179, No.2, (November 2003), pp. 165-174, ISSN 0022-0795.

Christ M.; Haseroth K.; Falkenstein E. & Wehling M. (1997). Nongenomic steroid actions: fact or fantasy? Vitamines and Hormones, Vol.57, pp. 325-373, ISSN 0083-6729.

Deane E. E.; Li J. & Woo N. Y. (2001). Hormonal status and phagocytic activity in sea bream infected with vibriosis. Comparative Biochemistry and Physiology. Part B, Biochemistry and Molecular Biology, Vol.129, No.2-3, (June 2001), pp. 687-693, ISSN 1096-4959.

Dijkstra P. D.; Hekman R.; Schulz R. W. & Groothuis T. G. G. (2007). Social stimulation, nuptial colouration, androgens and immunocompetence in a sexual dimorphic cichlid fish. Behavioural Ecology and Sociobiology, Vol.61, No.2, (February 2007), pp. 599-609, ISSN 0340-5443.

Ebnet K.; Kaldjian E. P.; Anderson A. O. & Shaw S. (1996a). Orchestrated information transfer underlying leukocyte endothelial interactions. Annual Review of Immunology, Vol.14, (April 1996), pp. 155-177, ISSN 0732-0582.

Ebnet K.; Simon M. M. & Shaw S. (1996b). Regulation of chemokine gene expression in human endothelial cells by proinflammatory cytokines and Borrelia burgdorferi. Annals of the New York Academy of Sciences, Vol.797, (October 1996), pp. 107-117, ISSN 0077-8923.

Engelsma M. Y.; Huising M. O.; van Muiswinkel W. B.; Flik G.; Kwang J.; Savelkoul H. F. & Verburg-van Kemenade B. M. (2002). Neuroendocrine-immune interactions in fish: a role for interleukin-1. Veterinary Immunology, Vol.87, No.3-4, (September 2002), pp. 467-479, ISSN 0165-2427.

Evans W. H. & Bergeron J. J. (1988). Nuclear receptors: a re-evaluation. Trends in Biochemical Sciences, Vol.13, No.1, (January 1988), pp. 7-8, ISSN 0968-0004.

Falkenstein E.; Tillmann H. C.; Christ M.; Feuring M. & Wehling M. (2000). Multiple actions of steroid hormones, a focus on rapid, nongenomic effects. Pharmacologycal Reviews, Vol.52, No.4, (December 2000), pp. 513-556, ISSN 0031-6997.

Friedl R.; Brunner M.; Moeslinger T. & Spieckermann P. G. (2000). Testosterone inhibits expression of inducible nitric oxide synthase in murine macrophages. Life Sciences, Vol.68, No.4, (Decemver 2000), pp. 417-429, ISSN 0024-3205.

Galas J. F.; Hejmej A.; Glogowski J. & Bilinska B. (2009). Morphological and functional alterations in testes and efferent ducts of homogametic rainbow trout *Oncorhynchus mykiss* Walbaum. Annals of the New York Academy of Sciences, Vol.1163, (April 2009), pp. 398-401, ISSN 1749-6632.

García-Ovejero D.; Veiga S.; García-Segura L. M. & Doncarlos L. L. (2002). Glial expression of estrogen and androgen receptors after rat brain injury. The Journal of Comparative Neurology, Vol.450, No.3, (August 2002), pp. 256-271, ISSN 0021-9967.

Grinwis G. C.; Wester P. W. & Vethaak A. D. (2009). Histopathological effects of chronic aqueous exposure to bis(tri-n-butyltin)oxide (TBTO) to environmentally relevant concentrations reveal thymus atrophy in European flounder (*Platichthys flesus*). Environmental Pollution, Vol.157, No.10, (October 2009), pp. 2587-2593, ISSN 1873-6424.

Guillemin G. J. & Brew B. J. (2004). Microglia, macrophages, perivascular macrophages, and pericytes: a review of function and identification. Journal of Leukocyte Biology, Vol.75, No.3, (March 2004), pp. 388-397, ISSN 0741-5400.

Hales D. B. (2002). Testicular macrophage modulation of Leydig cell steroidogenesis. Journal of Reproductive Immunology, Vol.57, No.1-2, (October-November 2002), pp. 3-18, ISSN 0165-0378.

Harkonen P. L. & Vaananen H. K. (2006). Monocyte-macrophage system as a target for estrogen and selective estrogen receptor modulators. Annals of New York Academy of Sciences, Vol.1089, (November 2006), pp. 218-227, ISSN 0077-8923.

Harris J. & Bird D. J. (2000). Modulation of the fish immune system by hormones. Veterinary Immunology and Immunopathology, Vol.77, No.3-4, (December 2000), pp. 163-176, ISSN 0165-2427.

Hecker M. & Karbe L. (2005). Parasitism in fish: an endocrine modulator of ecological relevance? Aquatic Toxicology, Vol.72, No.3, (April 2005), pp. 195-207, ISSN 0166-445X.

Hedger M. P. (1997). Testicular leukocytes: what are they doing? Review of Reproduction, Vol.2, No.1, (January 1997), pp. 38-47, ISSN 1359-6004.

Hedger M. P. (2002). Macrophages and the immune responsiveness of the testis. Journal of Reproductive Immunology, Vol.57, No.1-2, (October-November 2002), pp. 19-34, ISSN 0165-0378.

Henderson N. E. (1962). The annual cycle in the testis of eastern brook trout *Salvelinus fontinalis* (Mitchell). Canadian Journal of Zoology, Vol.40, No. 4, pp. 631-641, ISSN 0008-4301.

Hinteman T.; Schneider C.; Scholer H. F. & Schneider R. J. (2006). Field study using two immunoassays for the determination of estradiol and ethinylestradiol in the aquatic environment. Water Research, Vol.40, No.12, (July 2006), pp. 2287-2294, ISSN 0043-1354.

Huang Y. S.; Huang W. L.; Lin W. F.; Chen M. C. & Jeng S. R. (2006). An endothelial-cell-enriched primary culture system to study vascular endothelial growth factor (VEGF A) expression in a teleost, the Japanese eel (*Anguilla japonica*). Comparative Biochemistry and Physiology. Part A, Molecular and Integrative Physiology, Vol.145, No.1, (September 2006), pp. 33-46, ISSN 1095-6433.

Ihionkhan C. E.; Chambliss K. L.; Gibson L. L.; Hahner L. D.; Mendelsohn M. E. & Shaul P. W. (2002). Estrogen causes dynamic alterations in endothelial estrogen receptor expression. Circulation Research, Vol.91, No.9, (November 2002), pp. 814-820, ISSN 1524-4571.

Iwanowicz L. R. & Ottinger C. A. (2009). Estrogens, estrogen receptors and their role as immunoregulators in fish, In: Fish Defenses, G. Zaccone; J. Meseguer; A. García-Ayala and B. G. Kapoor, (Eds), Vol. 1 Immunology, pp. 277-322, Science publisher, ISBN 978-1 -57 808 -327 -5, Enfield.

Janele D.; Lang T.; Capellino S.; Cutolo M.; Da Silva J. A. & Straub R. H. (2006). Effects of testosterone, 17beta-estradiol, and downstream estrogens on cytokine secretion from human leukocytes in the presence and absence of cortisol. Annals of New York Academy of Sciences, Vol.1069, (June 2006), pp. 168-182, ISSN 0077-8923.

Johnson A. C.; Aerni H. R.; Gerritsen A.; Gibert M.; Giger W.; Hylland K.; Jurgens M.; Nakari T.; Pickering A.; Suter M. J.; Svenson A. & Wettstein F. E. (2005). Comparing steroid estrogen, and nonylphenol content across a range of European sewage plants with different treatment and management practices. Water Research, Vol.39, No.1, (January, 2005), pp. 47-58, ISSN 0043-1354.

Klein S. L. (2004). Hormonal and immunological mechanisms mediating sex differences in parasite infection. Parasite Immunology, Vol.26, No.6-7, (June-July 2004), pp. 247-264, ISSN 0141-9838.

Kramer P. R. & Wray S. (2002). 17-Beta-estradiol regulates expression of genes that function in macrophage activation and cholesterol homeostasis. The Journal of Steroid Biochemistry and Molecular Biology, Vol.81, No.3, (July 2002), pp. 203-216, ISSN 0960-0760.

Kuch H. M. & Ballschmiter K. (2000). Determination of endogenous and exogenous estrogens in effluents from sewage treatment plants at the ng/L-level. Fresenius Journal of Analytical Chemistry, Vol.366, pp. 392-395, ISSN 1061-9348.

Kumar M. V. & Tindall D. J. (1998). Transcriptional regulation of the steroid receptor genes. Progress in Nucleic Acid Research and Molecular Biology, Vol.59, pp. 289-306, ISSN 0079-6603.

Kurtz J.; Kalbe M.; Langefors A.; Mayer I.; Milinski M. & Hasselquist D. (2007). An experimental test of the immunocompetence handicap hypothesis in a teleost fish: 11-ketotestosterone suppresses innate immunity in three-spined sticklebacks. The American Naturalist, Vol.170, No.4, (October 2007), pp. 509-519, ISSN 1537-5323.

Lasserre G. (1972). Le coefficient de condition chez la daurade *Sparus auratus* L. 1758 de la région de Sète en 1971-1972. Travaux du Laboratoire de Biologie Halieutique, Université de Rennes 6, 141–150.

Laskin D. L.; Weinberger B. & Laskin J. D. (2001). Functional heterogeneity in liver and lung macrophages. Journal of Leukocyte Biolology, Vol.70, No.2, (August 2001), pp. 163-170, ISSN 0741-5400.

Lehmann D.; Siebold K.; Emmons L. R. & Muller H. (1988). Androgens inhibit proliferation of human peripheral blood lymphocytes in vitro. Clinical Immunology and Immunopathology, Vol.46, No.1, (January 1988), pp. 122-128, ISSN 0090-1229.

Liarte S.; Chaves-Pozo E.; Abellán E.; Meseguer J.; Mulero V.; Canario A. V. & García -Ayala A. (2011a). Estrogen-responsive genes in macrophages of the bony fish gilthead seabream: A transcriptomic approach. Developmental and Comparative Immunology, Vol.35, No.8 (March 2011), pp. 840-849, ISSN 1879-0089.

Liarte S.; Chaves-Pozo E.; Abellán E.; Meseguer J.; Mulero V. & García-Ayala A. (2011b). 17beta-Estradiol regulates gilthead seabream professional phagocyte responses through macrophage activation. Developmental and Comparative Immunology, Vol.35, No.1(January 2011), pp. 19-27, ISSN 1879-0089.

Liarte S.; Cabas I.; Chaves-Pozo E.; Arizcun M.; Meseguer J.; Mulero V. & García-Ayala A. (2011c). Natural and synthetic estrogens modulate the inflammatory response in the gilthead seabream (*Sparus aurata* L.) through the activation of endothelial cells. Molecular Immunology, ISSN 0161-5890. DOI:10.1016/j.molimm.2011.05.019.

Liarte S.; Chaves-Pozo E.; García-Alcázar A.; Mulero V.; Meseguer J. & García-Ayala A. (2007). Testicular involution prior to sex change in gilthead seabream is characterized by a decrease in DMRT1 gene expression and by massive leukocyte infiltration. Reproductive Biology and Endocrinology, Vol.5, (June 2007), pp. 20-35, ISSN 1477-7827.

Lo Nostro F. L.; Antoneli F. N.; Quagio-Grassiotto I. & Guerrero G. A. (2004). Testicular interstitial cells, and steroidogenic detection in the protogynous fish, *Synbranchus marmoratus* (Teleostei, Synbranchidae). Tissue and Cell, Vol.36, No.4, (August, 2004), pp. 221-231, ISSN 0040-8166.

Loir M.; Sourdaine P.; Mendis-Handagama S. M. & Jegou B. (1995). Cell-cell interactions in the testis of teleosts and elasmobranchs. Microscopy Research and Technique, Vol.32, No. 6, (December 1995), pp. 533-552, ISSN 1059-910X.

Lutton B. & Callard I. (2006). Evolution of reproductive-immune interactions. Integrative and Comparative Biology, Vol.46, No.6, (December 2006), pp. 1060-1071, ISSN 1540-7063.

Lynn S. G.; Birge W. J. & Shepherd B. S. (2008). Molecular characterization and sex-specific tissue expression of estrogen receptor alpha (esr1), estrogen receptor beta a (esr2a) and ovarian aromatase (cyp19a1a) in yellow perch (*Perca flavescens*). Comparative Biochemistry and Physiology. Part B, Biochemistry and Molecular Biology, Vol.149, No.1, (January 2008), pp. 126-147, ISSN 1096-4959.

Meseguer J.; Esteban M. A.; Lopez-Ruiz A. & Bielek E. (1994). Ultrastructure of nonspecific cytotoxic cells in teleosts. I. Effector-target cell binding in a marine and a freshwater species (seabream: *Sparus aurata* L., and carp: *Cyprinus carpio* L.). The Anatomical Record, Vol.239, No.4, (August 1994), pp. 468-474, ISSN 0003-276X.

Micale V.; Perdichizzi F. & Santangelo G. (1987). The gonadal cycle of captive white bream, *Diplodus sargus* (L.). Journal of Fish Biology, Vol.31, (May 1987), pp. 435-440, ISSN 002-1112.

Mor G.; Sapi E.; Abrahams V. M.; Rutherford T.; Song J.; Hao X. Y.; Muzaffar S. & Kohen F. (2003). Interaction of the estrogen receptors with the Fas ligand promoter in human monocytes. Journal of Immunology, Vol.170, No.1, (January 2003), pp. 114-122, ISSN 0022-1767.

Nagler J. J.; Cavileer T.; Sullivan J.; Cyr D. G. & Rexroad III C., 3rd. (2007). The complete nuclear estrogen receptor family in the rainbow trout: discovery of the novel ERα2 and both ERβ isoforms. Gene, Vol.392, No.1-2, (May 2007), pp. 164-173, ISSN 0378-1119.

Nilsson B. O. (2007). Modulation of the inflammatory response by estrogens with focus on the endothelium and its interactions with leukocytes. Inflammation Research, Vol.56, No.7, (July 2007), pp. 269-273, ISSN 1023-3830.

Pancer Z. & Cooper M. D. (2006). The evolution of adaptive immunity. Annual Review of Immunology, Vol.24, (April 2006), pp. 497-518, ISSN 0732-0582.

Pang Y.; Dong J. & Thomas P. (2008). Estrogen signaling characteristics of Atlantic croaker G protein-coupled receptor 30 (GPR30) and evidence it is involved in maintenance of oocyte meiotic arrest. Endocrinology, Vol.149, No.7, (July 2008), pp. 3410-3426, ISSN 0013-7227.

Pinto P. I.; Passos A. L.; Martins R. S.; Power D. M. & Canário A. V. (2006). Characterization of estrogen receptor betab in sea bream (*Sparus auratus*): phylogeny, ligand-binding, and comparative analysis of expression. General and Comparative Endocrinology, Vol.145, No.2, (January, 2006), pp. 197-207, ISSN 0016-6480.

Rempel M. A. & Schlenk D. (2008). Effects of environmental estrogens and antiandrogens on endocrine function, gene regulation, and health in fish. International Review of Cell and Molecular Biology, Vol.267, (June 2008), pp. 207-252, ISSN 1937-6448.

Roberts M. L.; Buchanan K. L. & Evans M. R. (2004). Testing the immunocompetence handicap hypothesis: a review of the evidence. Animal Behaviour, Vol.68, No. 2, (August 2004), pp. 227-239, ISSN 0003-3472.

Scott A. P. & Sumpter J. P. (1989). Seasonal variations in testicular germ cell stages and in plasma concentrations of sex steroids in male rainbow trout (*Salmo gairdneri*) maturing at 2 years old. General and Comparative Endocrinology, Vol.73, No.1, (January 1989), pp. 46-58, ISSN 0016-6480.

Sepulcre M. P.; Pelegrín P.; Mulero V. & Meseguer J. (2002). Characterisation of gilthead seabream acidophilic granulocytes by a monoclonal antibody unequivocally points to their involvement in fish phagocytic response. Cell and Tissue Research, Vol.308, No.1, (April 2002), pp. 97-102, ISSN 0302-766X.

Shrestha T. K. & Khanna S. S. (1976). Histology and seasonal changes in the testes of a hill-stream fish Schizothorax plagiostomus. Zeitschrift für Mikroskopisch-Anatomische Forschung, Vol.90, No.4, pp. 749-761, ISSN 0044-3107.

Shved N.; Berishvili G.; Hausermann E.; D'Cotta H.; Baroiller J. F. & Eppler E. (2009). Challenge with 17alpha-ethinylestradiol (EE2) during early development persistently impairs growth, differentiation, and local expression of IGF-I and IGF-II in immune organs of tilapia. Fish and Shellfish Immunology, Vol.26, No.3, (March 2009), pp. 524-530, ISSN 1095-9947.

Slater C. H.; Fitzpatrick M. S. & Schreck C. B. (1995). Characterization of an androgen receptor in salmonid lymphocytes: possible link to androgen-induced immunosuppression. General and Comparative Endocrinology, Vol.100, No.2, (November 1995), pp. 218-225, ISSN 0016-6480.

Slater C. H. & Schreck C. B. (1993). Testosterone alters the immune response of chinook salmon, *Oncorhynchus tshawytscha*. General and Comparative Endocrinology, Vol.89, No.2, (February 1993), pp. 291-298, ISSN 0016-6480.

Stout R. D. & Suttles J. (2004). Functional plasticity of macrophages: reversible adaptation to changing microenvironments. Journal of Leukocyte Biology, Vol.76, No.3, (September 2004), pp. 509-513, ISSN 0741-5400.

Straub R. H. (2007). The complex role of estrogens in inflammation. Endocrine Reviews, Vol.28, No.5, (August 2007), pp. 521-574, ISSN 0163-769X.

Tellez-Bañuelos M. C.; Santerre A.; Casas-Solis J.; Bravo-Cuellar A. & Zaitseva G. (2009). Oxidative stress in macrophages from spleen of Nile tilapia (*Oreochromis niloticus*) exposed to sublethal concentration of endosulfan. Fish and Shellfish Immunology, Vol.27, No.2, (August 2009), pp. 105-111, ISSN 1095-9947.

Ternes T. A.; Stumpf M.; Mueller J.; Haberer K.; Wilken R. D. & Servos M. (1999). Behavior and occurrence of estrogens in municipal sewage treatment plants--I. Investigations in Germany, Canada and Brazil. The Science of the Total Environment, Vol,225, No.1-2, (January, 1999), pp. 81-90, ISSN 0048-9697.

Thomas P.; Dressing G.; Pang Y.; Berg H.; Tubbs C.; Benninghoff A. & Doughty K. (2006). Progestin, estrogen and androgen G-protein coupled receptors in fish gonads. Steroids, Vol.71, No.4, (April 2006), pp. 310-316, ISSN 0039-128X.

Tilton S. C.; Givan S. A.; Pereira C. B.; Bailey G. S. & Williams D. E. (2006). Toxicogenomic profiling of the hepatic tumor promoters indole-3-carbinol, 17beta-estradiol and beta-naphthoflavone in rainbow trout. Toxicological Scieces, Vol.90, No.1, (March 2006), pp. 61-72, ISSN 1096-6080.

Todo T.; Ikeuchi T.; Kobayashi T. & Nagahama Y. (1999). Fish androgen receptor: cDNA cloning, steroid activation of transcription in transfected mammalian cells, and tissue mRNA levels. Biochemical and Biophysical Research Communications, Vol.254, No.2, (January 1999), pp. 378-383, ISSN 0006-291X.

van Ginneken V.; Palstra A.; Leonards P.; Nieveen M.; van den Berg H.; Flik G.; Spanings T.; Niemantsverdriet P.; van den Thillart G. & Murk A. (2009). PCBs and the energy cost of migration in the European eel (*Anguilla anguilla* L.). Aquatic Toxicology, Vol.92, No.4, (May 2009), pp. 213-220, ISSN 1879-1514.

Wang R. & Belosevic M. (1995). The in vitro effects of estradiol and cortisol on the function of a long-term goldfish macrophage cell line. Developmental and Comparative Immunology, Vol.19, No.4, (July-August 1995), pp. 327-336, ISSN 0145-305X.

Watanuki H.; Yamaguchi T. & Sakai M. (2002). Suppression in function of phagocytic cells in common carp *Cyprinus carpio* L. injected with estradiol, progesterone or 11-ketotestosterone. Comparative Biochemistry and Physiology. Part C, Pharmacology, Toxicology and Endocrinology, Vol.132, No.4, (August 2002), pp. 407-413, ISSN 1532-0456.

Williams T. D.; Diab A. M.; George S. G.; Sabine V. & Chipman J. K. (2007). Gene expression responses of European flounder (*Platichthys flesus*) to 17-beta estradiol. Toxicology Letters, Vol.168, No.3, (February 2007), pp. 236-248, ISSN 0378-4274.

Xia J. H. & Yue G. H. (2010). Identification and analysis of immune-related transcriptome in Asian seabass *Lates calcarifer*. BMC Genomics, Vol.11, (June 2010), pp. 356-368, ISSN 1471-2164.

Xia Z.; Gale W. L.; Chang X.; Langenau D.; Patino R.; Maule A. G. & Densmore L. D. (2000). Phylogenetic sequence analysis, recombinant expression, and tissue distribution of a channel catfish estrogen receptor beta. General and Comparative Endocrinology, Vol.118, No.1, (April 2000), pp. 139-149, ISSN 0016-6480.

Yamaguchi T.; Watanuki H. & Sakai M. (2001). Effects of estradiol, progesterone and testosterone on the function of carp, *Cyprinus carpio*, phagocytes in vitro. Comparative Biochemistry and Physiology. Part C, Pharmacology, Toxicology & Endocrinology, Vol.129, No.1, (May 2001), pp. 49-55, ISSN 1532-0456.

Zaitsu M.; Narita S.; Lambert K. C.; Grady J. J.; Estes D. M.; Curran E. M.; Brooks E. G.; Watson C. S.; Goldblum R. M. & Midoro-Horiuti T. (2007). Estradiol activates mast cells via a non-genomic estrogen receptor-alpha and calcium influx. Molecular Immunology, Vol.44, No.8, (March 2007), pp. 1977-1985, ISSN 0161-5890.

11

Interactions Between Reproductive and Immune Systems During Ontogeny: Roles of GnRH, Sex Steroids, and Immunomediators

Liudmila A. Zakharova and Marina S. Izvolskaia
Institute of Developmental Biology/Russian Academy of Sciences
Russian Federation

1. Introduction

Reproduction is an essential function of every animal species, and its realization depends on a complex of interrelated neural, endocrine, immune, and behavioral reactions. It is now accepted that the neuroendocrine system (including its reproductive component) and the immune system have a reciprocal regulatory influence development and functioning during pre- and postnatal ontogeny (Watanobe & Hayakawa, 2003; Zakharova et al., 2005; Carreras et al., 2008; Li et al., 2007; Chapman et al., 2009; Wu et al., 2011). The functions of these systems change during ontogeny. In the perinatal period, they are involved not only in regulatory but also in morphogenetic processes, unlike in the postnatal period. The tight bilateral connection between these systems is of special significance during the early, critical period of ontogeny, when the functions necessary for postnatal life of newborns are being established. The key role in the interaction of the reproductive and immune systems is played by the hypothalamic neuropeptide gonadotropin-releasing hormone (GnRH) and sex hormones. During the perinatal period, they regulate the growth and differentiation of various fetal tissues, including the lymphoid tissue. In postnatal life, the dynamics of endocrine processes related to reproduction are regulated by the level of GnRH secretion into the hypothalamo-pituitary portal circulation. GnRH regulates secretion of pituitary gonadotropins, which regulate secretion of sex hormones. GnRH is also involved in regulation of sexual behavior, transmission of olfactory signals, and control of humoral and cell-mediated immunity. Sex hormones, in turn, regulate GnRH production in the hypothalamus (and, therefore, secretion of pituitary gonadotropins) and also its production in the thymus and spleen (Azad et al, 1998; Hrabovszky et al., 2000). On the other hand, immune system mediators such as thymic peptides and proinflammatory cytokines have a role in controlling the development and functioning of the reproductive system.

Interactions of the reproductive and immune systems during early ontogeny are prerequisite to their normal functioning in adult life. Changes in the normal levels of GnRH and sex steroids in the developing fetus or newborn and their exposure to adverse environmental factors cause disturbances in long-term programming of the regulatory mechanisms of both reproductive and immune systems (Jacobson et al., 2000; Razia et al., 2006; Cameron et al., 2008; Champagne & Curley, 2008). The brain is especially sensitive to perinatal programming by sex steroids, which not only contribute to the patterning of brain structures during early ontogeny but also activate sexual behavior in prepubertal and pubertal males and females. Thus, the brain retains its plasticity for programming at later stages of ontogeny, being most responsive to sex steroids in adolescence as well as in the perinatal period (Shulz et al., 2009). The formation of individual structural–functional elements of the reproductive and immune systems and the establishment of relationships between them are not strictly genetically controlled. These processes are characterized by high functional lability and sensitivity to various regulatory factors, which provides the possibility of correcting disturbances in the reproductive process.

2. Effect of the reproductive system on the immune system: Roles of GnRH and sex steroids

Distinctive features of GnRH-producing neurons include their small population size (800–2000 cells), diffuse distribution in the septo-preoptic hypothalamic region, and extracerebral origin during ontogeny. Most these neurons have axons terminating in the median eminence, where GnRH is released in the portal circulation and regulates the synthesis and secretion of the luteinizing hormone (LH) and follicle-stimulating hormone (FSH) by gonadotrope cells. GnRH isolated from the mammalian brain was initially regarded only as the hormone controlling the reproductive function, but subsequent studies have demonstrated that GnRH occurs in a variety of functionally different forms. To date, 23 such forms have been identified in vertebrates. Three of them—GnRH1, GnRH2, and GnRH3—are the most frequent, being expressed in groups of neurons differing in origin, location, and functional role. In adult animals, GnRH1 is expressed mainly in the hypothalamus; GnRH2, in the midbrain and tectum; and GnRH3, in the rostral regions of the forebrain. The population of hypothalamic neurons expressing GnRH1 is usually referred to as the GnRH1 system, and its basic function is to regulate the release of gonadotropins. GnRH2 and GnRH3 supposedly function as neuromodulators, the former being involved in the regulation of sexual behavior and the latter, in the integration of olfactory signals and other processes related to reproduction. Extracerebral synthesis is characteristic mainly of GnRH2, which has been revealed in the thymus, spleen, ovaries, testes, prostate, mammary gland, and placenta (Jacobson et al., 2000; Zakharova et al., 2005). Along with hypothalamic GnRH, extracerebral GnRH2 plays a role in the development and functioning of the immune system at different stages of ontogeny (Morale et al., 1991; Zakharova et al., 2005). According to Marchetti et al. (1998), GnRH is one of the most important signal molecules involved in the neuroendocrine–immune interaction.

Sex steroids, in turn, control the development and functioning of the hypothalamo-pituitary and immune systems. In particular, they account for the programming of sexual dimorphism in the structure and functions of the hypothalamo-pituitary system of vertebrates and regulate GnRH production in the hypothalamus and expression of GnRH receptors in the pituitary, thereby modulating the response of gonadotrope cells to this hormone. Sex steroids also modulate the molecular processing of GnRH in the thymus and its concentrations in the thymus and spleen (Azad et al, 1998).

The effects of these hormones on the immune and endocrine systems apparently differ depending on the period of ontogeny, as is the case with many other factors. During the early period, they cause long-lasting or irreversible changes in the structure and functions of the above systems, whereas their effects in adult animals are short-term and reversible.

2.1 Role of GnRH in immune system development and functioning at different stages of ontogeny

The involvement of GnRH in the differentiation of lymphocytes and regulation of immune response is lifelong. Its neonatal administration in normal mice accelerates the development of immune reactions (Marchetti et al., 1989). In rats and monkeys, central or peripheral blockade of the GnRH receptor antagonists in the neonatal period leads to reduction of mature T- and B-lymphocyte counts in the thymus, spleen, and circulating blood and suppression of antibody production and mitogen-induced proliferative response of T cells, with the immune reactions returning to the norm only by the age of 3 months in rats and 5 years in monkeys (Morale et al., 1991). Thymic and splenic lymphocytes differ in sensitivity to GnRH. Neonatal administration of a GnRH antagonist in rats results in complete block of the mitogen-induced proliferative response of thymocytes, whereas this response of splenocytes is blocked only partially. GnRH and its agonists prevent age-related involution of the thymus and normalize the suppressed functional activity of thymocytes (Marchetti et al., 1989). In pregnancy, the functional activity of GnRH in controlling the numbers of thymocytes is suppressed due to the intensified synthesis of prohibitin, an antiproliferative protein; as a consequence, the maternal thymus undergoes involution. The suppression of T-lymphocyte development in pregnancy is an adaptation against allogeneic fetal rejection. Administration of an GnRH agonist results in normalization of thymocyte count (Dixit et al., 2003).

There is evidence that GnRH exacerbates progression of autoimmune diseases. In particular, this follows (by contradiction) from the data by Jacobson et al. (2000) that administration of an GnRH antagonist to New Zealand mice with systemic lupus erythematosus leads to a drop in the levels of both total IgG and anti-DNA antibodies, relief of disease symptoms, and extension of life span, with these effects being observed in both intact and castrated animals of both sexes. It should be noted that the diseases progresses more severely in females than males, which the authors attribute to sex-related differences in the expression of GnRH receptors or G protein (Jacobson et al., 2000). Although the available data on the involvement of GnRH in immune response modulation and exacerbation of autoimmune diseases in adults are fairly abundant, its role in these processes is not yet completely clear. However, since the functions of many hormones in postnatal life are aimed at the maintenance of immune system homeostasis in response to changes in ambient conditions (Dorshkind & Horseman, 2000), such a function cannot be excluded for GnRH.

According to our data (Zakharova et al., 2000), GnRH becomes involved in the regulation of T-cell immunity as early as during prenatal ontogeny. Surgical ablation of the hypothalamus (encephalectomy) *in utero* in 18-day rat fetuses results in 30–40% suppression of concanavalin A (Con A)-induced response in thymocytes isolated on day 22, but intraperitoneal injection of GnRH (0.2 μg per fetus) immediately after surgery restores this response to the norm. No such effect has been observed in experiments with sham-operated fetuses. Moreover, GnRH (10^{-9} and 10^{-7} M) added to a culture of thymocytes from encephalectomized fetuses has proved to enhance their Con A-induced proliferative response in a dose-dependent manner. The involvement of GnRH at early stages of immune system development is also confirmed by the results of experiments on central or peripheral blockade of the synthesis of GnRH or its receptors in rat fetuses (Zakharova et al., 2005). On day 20 of pregnancy, fetuses in one uterine horn were intraperitoneally injected with either the selective GnRH antagonist D-pGlu-D-Phe-D-Trp-Ser-Tyr-D-Trp-Leu-Arg-Pro-Gly-NH_2 or anti-GnRH antibodies, and fetuses in the other horn, with 0.9% NaCl solution or nonimmune rabbit serum. The GnRH antagonist (2 μg per fetus) caused 40–50%

suppression of Con A-induced proliferative response of thymocyte on day 22, compared to that in fetuses injected with saline (0.9% NaCl). It should be noted that this response did not differ between male and female fetuses, either in the norm or after the antagonist injection. When thymocytes from 22-day fetuses were cultured in the presence of the GnRH antagonist (10^{-5} or 10^{-6} M), no such decrease in the proliferative response was observed. In the case of injection with anti-GnRH antibodies, Con A-induced proliferative response of thymocytes was suppressed fivefold, compared to that in fetuses injected with either saline or nonimmune serum.

On the other hand, the injection of a long-acting GnRH agonist to prepubertal female mice has been found to suppress T- and B-cell maturation in the primary lymphoid organs. It appears that GnRH acts on lymphocyte precursors so that changes in its initial concentration lead to suppression of their differentiation in the central organs of the immune system (the thymus and bone marrow), which, in turn, accounts for the decreased numbers of differentiated T and B cells in spleen, a secondary lymphoid organ (Rao et al., 1995).

The synthesis of GnRH and its receptors in the thymus and spleen of adult animals has been confirmed experimentally. As shown by Azad et al. (1997), the *Jurkat* human leukemia T-cell line (phenotypically similar to normal human T lymphocytes) expresses GnRH mRNA and secretes this hormone and its precursor into the culture medium. The proliferative activity of these cells increases under the effect of either endogenous or exogenous GnRH, whereas its antagonist suppresses their proliferation. According to the same authors (Azad et al., 1998), the concentration of GnRH in the thymus significantly increases in castrated rats, but this increase is prevented by testosterone injection. It is considered that sex steroids modulate molecular processing of the GnRH precursor, with its processing in the thymus differing from that in the hypothalamus.

The results of our experiments exhibit that GnRH is also synthesized in the fetal thymus (Zakharova et al., 2005). Immunocytochemical analysis for GnRH in the thymus of 21-day rat fetuses revealed the presence of GnRH-positive cells morphologically identical to thymocytes. Quantitative assessment of GnRH in the thymus exhibited that its content was minimal in 18-day fetuses, increased by a factor of about 1.5 in 21-day fetuses, and further increased by postnatal day 3 (by 65 and 40%, compared to intrauterine days 18 and 21), reaching the level characteristic of the hypothalamus. The GnRH contents in the thymus were similar in males and females. A considerable GnRH level was also detected in the blood serum of rat fetuses. It reached a peak in 18-day fetuses and decreased by half in 21-day fetuses, remaining fairly high relative to those in the thymus and hypothalamus. After surgical ablation of the hypothalamus (encephalectomy) on intrauterine day 18, the concentrations of GnRH in the thymus and peripheral blood of 21-day fetuses, either male or female, was half as low as in sham-operated fetuses. The origin of circulating GnRH is as yet unclear. Since its level drops after encephalectomy, it appears that at least half its amount is of brain origin and, therefore, the level of this hormone at the periphery is controlled by the hypothalamus. It cannot be excluded, however, that GnRH found in the circulating blood of fetuses comes from other sources (e.g., the placenta).

All the above data suggest that GnRH can control the development and functioning of the immune system via the hypothalamo-pituitary axis and is involved in an autocrine or paracrine regulation of the immune response during postnatal life. There are several possible mechanisms of GnRH action on the immune system: it can interact with specific receptors on thymic epithelial cells that synthesize peptides participating in T-cell maturation, as well as directly interact with such receptors on lymphocytes. In addition, GnRH can induce both the expression of interleukin (IL)-2 receptors on lymphocytes and the synthesis of gamma-interferon (IFNγ), which, in turn, induces IL-2 production by T cells, thereby regulating their numbers (Grasso et al., 1998).

2.2 Role of sex steroids in the development of immune and endocrine systems

During early ontogeny, sex hormones (along with other hormones) participate in the development of the hypothalamo-pituitary and immune systems. It is known that exposure of the fetus to adverse factors can affect the structural and functional programming of these systems, with consequent disease susceptibility in adulthood (Langley-Evans, 2006). Alterations in a certain developing system usually entail alterations in other systems. External factors such as stress, treatment with pharmaceuticals, and mother's inadequate diet and behavior during pregnancy and breast feeding place the fetus (newborn) at risk for autoimmune, allergic, metabolic, nervous, and mental disorders in later life (Fowden & Forhead, 2004; Wang et al., 2009; Wu et al., 2011).

A strong stimulus changing homeostasis of the fetus is exerted by sex steroids. The mechanisms of sexual differentiation of the brain were addressed even in the first studies on prenatal programming of the GnRH system. It has been shown long ago that the development of the brain in male mammals initially follows the female pattern, but specific brain regions in a certain period of ontogeny are influenced by testosterone aromatized into estradiol, which leads to masculinization of the brain and its subsequent development according to the male scenario. This period is critical for organization of the GnRH system, and its timing varies between species. In rodents, brain masculinization takes place during the late intrauterine–early postnatal period; in guinea pigs, during midpregnancy; in rhesus monkeys and humans, this process is accomplished by the second trimester of pregnancy; whereas in sheep it continues from days 30--37 to 147 of intrauterine development.

An increase in the concentration of androgens in mice between intrauterine day 18 and postnatal day 14 causes changes in the development of the hypothalamo-pituitary system. Male transgenic hCGαβ+ mice overproducing human chorionic gonadotropin are characterized by an elevated GnRH level in the hypothalamus, a reduced FSH level in the pituitary and circulating blood, and inhibited expression of the mRNA of receptors for GnRH and estrogens in the pituitary (Gonzalez et al., 2011). The sexual behavior of a pregnant female has an effect on the functioning of the endocrine system in its offspring, which is mediated by epigenetic modifications at the promoter for oestrogen receptor alpha (ERα) and subsequent effects on gene expression (Cameron et al., 2008). Estradiol and testosterone injected to female mice during the neonatal period induce the development of infertility, whereas their injection on postnatal day 7 causes no disturbances in the reproductive system. Hydrocortisone injected together with estradiol prevents the development of infertility (Chapman et al., 2009).

Sex hormones also modulate the development of lymphoid organs, the thymus being their main target in the immune system. The drop in the level of sex hormones in male mice after pre- or postpubertal castration causes thymic hypertrophy (with increase in thymocyte count) and enhancement of graft rejection reaction. The phenomenon of twofold increase in thymus weight in castrated males was discovered more than a century ago, but its mechanism has not yet been elucidated in detail. Injection of androgens to castrated animals results in a rapid decrease in thymus weight, with signs of active apoptosis being observed in the organ. The effects of androgens are realized via traditional receptor-mediated mechanisms (Olsen et al., 1996). Receptors for estrogens and androgens in the thymus are expressed as early as during embryonic development, with their level increasing by birth (Staples et al., 1999). Thymocytes carry the same numbers of functional androgen receptors as do target cells for these hormones in the reproductive system, with the least mature thymocyte subpopulations being the richest in such receptors. The thymic stroma also expresses androgen receptors. Estrogen receptors are expressed on mature peripheral T and B lymphocytes, which mediate the immunomodulatory effects of sex hormones (Tanriverdi et al., 2003.

Injection of testosterone, estrogen, or their derivatives to chick or quail embryos results in atrophy of the bursa of Fabricius, degeneration of lymphoid tissue in follicles and its substitution by fibrous tissue, and disturbances in the development of thymic stromal elements creating the microenvironment for lymphocyte maturation (Razia et al., 2006). In addition, excess sex steroids cause disturbances in mammal immune system. In particular, they suppress differentiation of regulatory and cytotoxic T cells in the thymus, with consequent increase in the numbers of immature lymphocytes in the circulation, and cause an impairment of negative selection mechanisms, which results in the formation of self-reactive T cells (Chapman et al., 2009). Estrogens also stimulate an increase in the numbers of self-reactive B lymphocytes and the level of circulating autoantibodies (Olsen & Kovacs, 1996; Tanriverdi et al., 2003). These data are in agreement with the observation that females, especially when pregnant, are more vulnerable to autoimmune diseases, compared to males. On the other hand, it has been noted that the level of testosterone in male mice genetically resistant to infectious diseases is maintained high after infection with bacterial (Salmonella enteritis) endotoxin, whereas this level in sensitive males dropped significantly on day 14 after infection (Zala et al., 2008).

Female mice kept at high density in the presence of only one male in the cage become aggressive, unresponsive to mating attempts and do not copulate. The aggressive behavior of females correlates with elevated levels of testosterone, corticosterone, and progesterone. Compared to female mice kept under standard conditions, the weight of their ovaries and adrenals is greater, while that of the thymus and uterus is smaller, and the lysis of corpora lutea in the ovaries is prolonged and incomplete. Supposedly, high corticosterone suppresses the activity of T lymphocytes normally involved in this process (Chapman et al., 2000).

Despite general similarity in the effects of male and female sex hormones on the thymus, the resultant changes in the composition of cell subpopulations in this organ are different: estrogens cause a decrease in the number of cortical T lymphocytes and an increase in the contents of more mature cell forms, whereas androgens have an opposite effect (Olsen and Kovacs, 1996).

Sex hormones also regulate the development of bone tissue and bone marrow and have an immunomodulatory effect on B lymphocytes in adults. Estrogens control differentiation of osteoclasts, mesenchymal stem cells, and myelopoiesis in the bone marrow (Carreras et al., 2008). Interacting with receptors on bone marrow stromal cells, sex hormones modulate B-cell differentiation. In either males or females, castration results in the increased numbers of pre-B cells in the bone marrow and mature B cells in peripheral organs, with the spleen growing in size (Olsen et al., 1996). In pregnancy, at a high estrogen background, the relative numbers of B lymphocytes in the bone marrow are decreased at almost all stages of differentiation (Tanriverdi et al., 2003).

Estrogens have a protective effect on the progression of autoimmune diseases, in particular, multiple sclerosis and autoimmune encephalomyelitis as its model. In pregnant women with multiple sclerosis, clinical remission is observed during the last trimester, at a high level of estrogens and progesterone; after delivery, this level drops, and the disease is exacerbated. Exogenous estrogens at physiological concentrations suppress the progression of experimental encephalomyelitis, supposedly by inhibiting the synthesis of proinflammatory cytokines (Van den Broek et al., 2005). The protective effect of sex steroids is dependent on a number of factors, including their dose and the age, sex, and metabolic pattern of animals. Thus, in NZB/NZW mice, which spontaneously develop lethal glomerulonephritis by the age of 8–14 months, castration of 14-day-old females accompanied by testosterone injection significantly prolongs their life span. On the other hand, castration and estradiol injection in males has an opposite effect. Moreover, males castrated at the age of 14 days die of this disease earlier than do males castrated at the age of 5 weeks, while castration of 14- to 15-week-old males has no effect on their life span.

It is noteworthy that the patterning of sexual behavior by sex steroids takes place not only during early ontogeny. As noted above, the brain retains its plasticity at later stages, and its responsiveness to sex steroids in males reaches a second peak during adolescence. Such a peak during the late postnatal period is also characteristic of females, but its exact timing has not yet been determined for them (Shulz et al., 2009).

2.3 Effect of immune system on the development of reproductive system: Role of cytokines and thymic peptides

Numerous data are available on the effect of the neuroendocrine system, including its reproductive component, on the establishment and functioning of the immune system. The immune system, in turn, is not only the target for hormones but is itself involved in the regulation of neuroendocrine system functioning. Mediators produced by the immune system have a role in programming the development of reproductive system in the fetus (Igaz et al., 2006; Li et al., 2007; Goya et al., 2004). The thymus is the central organ of the immune system, and its absence in homozygous athymic or neonatally thymectomized mice leads to severe disturbances in immune–neuroendocrine regulation. These disturbances manifest themselves not only in the inhibited functions of the immune system but also in the impaired synthesis and secretion of neuropeptides and hormones of the hypothalamus, pituitary, and peripheral endocrine glands (Goya et al, 2004; Chapman et al., 2009; Zakharova, 2009). The impaired neuroendocrine functions can be modulated by thymic peptides (Goya et al., 2007). There is evidence that bacterial endotoxins and proinflammatory cytokines have influence on the GnRH system of newborns (Li et al., 2007). In particular, neonatal activation of the immune system by these factors results in long-term sensitization of the adult GnRH system to the inhibitory effect of stress.

2.3.1 Regulation of the GnRH system in adult mammals

As noted above, GnRH has a modulatory effect on the development and functions of the neuroendocrine and immune systems, which, in turn, control the functioning of the GnRH system. It is through GnRH neurons that various neurotransmitters and neuropeptides (monoamines, gamma-aminobutyric acid, neuropeptide Y, opioids, tec.) and also cytokines convey signals from external stimuli influencing the state of the reproductive system (Karsch et al., 2002; Ciechanowska et al., 2007; Pereira A et al., 2010). Sex steroids are the most powerful regulators of the GnRH system. During the estrous cycle, for example, the GnRH level in the anterior pituitary varies in antiphase to the level of plasma estrogens, with estradiol having been shown to reduce the content of GnRH mRNA in this pituitary region. On the other hand, estradiol increases the level of GnRH in the hypothalamus immediately before ovulation. It has long been considered that sex steroid exert their effect through steroid-sensitive sites of the brain, because no specific receptors have been found on GnRH neurons. However, this concept was questioned after identification of estrogen-sensitive regions in the promoter of human GnRH gene and estrogen receptors ERα and ERβ on cells of mouse GnRH neuronal cell line GT1-7 expressing the rat GnRH gene. Using improved techniques of in situ hybridization and binding of a radioactive estrogen analog, it has been shown that at least part of GnRH neurons in rats contain ERβ-receptor mRNA and can bind the radioactive estradiol analog (Hrabovszky et al., 2000). Estradiol and progesterone regulate the expression of receptors for GnRH on gonadotrope cells. Progesterone also regulates GnRH secretion depending on the physiological body state. Before ovulation, it activates GnRH neurons and stimulates its secretion. After ovulation, in the luteal phase of the estrous cycle, corpus luteum enhances progesterone synthesis in preparation for probable zygote implantation; under such conditions, progesterone inhibits the pulse secretion of GnRH.

Long-term studies on the complex pathways of sex steroid action on GnRH neurons have shown that they involve various neurotransmitter systems operating in different brain regions of adult mammals. In rodents, the main steroid-sensitive brain region is the preoptic area (anterior hypothalamus), including anteroventral periventricular, arcuate, and medial preoptic nuclei.

A major role in regulating the functional activity of GnRH neurons is played by catecholamines, primarily by dopamine and noradrenaline delivered by afferent fibers from the hypothalamic periventricular nucleus and brain stem. A long known fact is that noradrenaline coming from the brain stem is a "releasing factor" for the preovulatory GnRH surge. As shown in sheep, the noradrenergic neurons A1 and A2 projecting to the bed nucleus of stria terminalis carry receptors for estradiol and can directly or indirectly influence GnRH secretion (Pereira et al., 2010). It is also known that the seasonal inhibition of GnRH synthesis in the sheep hypothalamus is directly correlated with activation of dopaminergic neurons A15. The synthesis of dopamine by neurons of this group is intensified under the effect of gamma-aminobutyric acid (GABA)- and glutamatergic neurons of the ventromedial preoptic area and ventromedial and arcuate nuclei containing receptors for estradiol (Goldman et al., 2010). The majority of studies on the innervation of GnRH neurons by catecholaminergic terminals have been performed on rats and sheep Tillet et al, 1993). Using electron microscopy and stereotactic surgery, their authors have not only revealed the fact of such innervation but also made attempts to identify the origin of these catecholaminergic terminals. In rats, the noradrenergic system appears to innervate mainly the bodies of GnRH neurons in the septo-preoptic region, while the dopaminergic system innervates both the bodies of these neurons and their terminals in the organum vasculesum of lamina terminalis (OVLT) and median eminence. In sheep, unlike in rats, the bodies of GnRH neurons in the septo-preoptic region are innervated mainly by noradrenergic fibers from the locus coeruleus and brain stem, whereas their terminals in the median eminence are innervated by the dopaminergic system of the hypothalamus. Catecholamines exert their effect through receptors expressed on the surface of GnRH neurons (Hosny & Jennes, 1998).

As noted above, various neurotransmitters and neuropeptides (monoamines, neuropeptide Y, opioids, etc.) are involved in the transmission of signals from external stimuli that have an effect on the state of the reproductive system. Thus, long-term stress induced by electric shock results in the inhibition of GnRH expression in the hypothalamus, and this effect is jointly mediated by the opioidergic, noradrenergic, and serotonergic systems (Ciechanowska et al., 2007). It has been shown that steroid-dependent control of GnRH neurons is also accounted for by other factors, including GABA, somatostatin and kisspeptin (Pillon et al., 2004; Oakley et al., 2009).

Stimulation of the immune system by inflammatory bacterial endotoxins also inhibits the activity of the GnRH system in adult animals (Karsch et al., 2002). In the course of inflammation, immune system cells produce various pro- and antiinflammatory cytokines that activate the cascade of hormone secretion in the hypothalamo-pituitary system, thereby inducing the hormonal stress response. Bacterial endotoxins are often used in laboratory experiments as activators of the immune system. In particular, this concerns the lipopolysaccharide (LPS) from the outer membrane of Gram-negative bacteria, which is known as a factor stimulating the synthesis and secretion of pro- and antiinflammatory cytokines not only at the periphery but also in the CNS. Endothelial cells forming the hematoencephalic barrier have binding sites for LPS and its complex with accessory proteins (Singh & Jiang, 2004). Under the effect of LPS, these cells, along with cells of the immune system, can synthesize proinflammatory cytokines such as IL-1α, IL-1β, and IL-6; tumor necrosis factor alpha (TNFα); regulatory cytokine IL-10; and granulocyte/macrophage colony-stimulating factor (GM-CSF). Bacterial inflammation is also accompanied by an increase of another proinflammatory cytokine, the leukemia inhibitory factor (LIF) in the blood level, which penetrates the hematoencephalic barrier via a special transport system (Pan et al., 2008). Thus, bacterial inflammation stimulates signal transmission through vascular endothelium and cytokine transport through the hematoencephalic barrier. These cytokines act upon the GnRH system either directly or by inducing the synthesis or secretion of prostaglandins, neuropeptides, and catecholamines (Karsch et al., 2002).

Among cytokines mediating the effect of LPS on the GnRH system, the main role is played by IL-1β and TNFα. During bacterial inflammation, both these cytokines are almost equally effective in inhibiting the secretion of GnRH and, therefore, of the luteinizing hormone (Watanobe & Hayakawa, 2003). Injection of IL-1β into the rat brain ventricles markedly reduces both the synthesis of GnRH in the septo-preoptic region and the secretion of this hormone, which leads to disturbances of the estrous cycle (Kang et al., 2000). Moreover, IL-1β inhibits the expression of the c-fos protein in the nuclei of GnRH neurons, thereby altering GnRH synthesis during proestrus in rats. The role of IL-6 in GnRH secretion is as yet unclear. According to some publications, IL-6 inhibits the secretion of this hormone by neurons, whereas others conclude that IL-6 has no such effect even at high concentrations. However, it was shown, that LPS also stimulates the secretion of IL-6 in the preoptic area, which is followed by a drop in GnRH level within 30 min (Watanobe & Hayakawa, 2003). GM-CSF can also inhibit GnRH secretion in the mediobasal hypothalamic region by stimulation of GM-CSF receptors expressed on GABAergic neurons. Activation of these receptors leads to increased production of GABA, which influence on specific receptors on GnRH terminals and thereby inhibits NO synthase activity; as a result, the level of GnRH decreases (Kimura et al., 1997).

The direct involvement of proinflammatory cytokines in the regulation of GnRH secretion has been demonstrated on the model of the immortalized GnRH-expressing neuronal cell line Gnv-4 derived from the rat hypothalamus. These cells have been shown to carry receptors for IL-1β and the accessory protein necessary for its activation as well as for the α chain of IL-6 and the β chain of oncostatin M, a functional analog of LIF participating in inflammatory processes (Igaz et al., 2006). Numerous data are also available on indirect effects of LPS and interleukins on GnRH secretion. In particular, it has been shown that IL-1β blocks nitric oxide (NO)-induced GnRH secretion in the mediobasal region of the hypothalamus, which, in turn, blocks the pulse secretion of the luteinizing hormone into circulation; as a result, the sexual behavior regulated by GnRH is suppressed (McCann et al., 2000). Similar to GM-CSF, IL-1β blocks GnRH release from the axons of GnRH by inhibiting NO synthase activity (Rettori et al., 1994). It also inhibits GnRH secretion induced by noradrenaline. Thus, in experiments with perfused fragments of the mediobasal hypothalamic region, the level of GnRH secretion proved to decrease when IL-1β was added to the incubation medium together with noradrenaline (Rettori et al., 1994). The suppression of GnRH secretion by LPS can also be mediated by opioids (He et al., 2003). Therefore, activation of the immune system in response to bacterial infection entails a complex of reactions in the neuroendocrine system that result in the suppression of female reproductive function.

2.3.2 Neuroendocrine and immune regulatory mechanisms in the development of GnRH system

During early embryonic development, GnRH neurons originate in the olfactory placodes, wherefrom they migrate rostrocaudally, toward the forebrain, along terminal, vomeronasal, and olfactory nerves. Entering the brain, these neurons reach their definitive location and begin to form axonal connections with circumventricular organs. The process of their migration to the brain can be divided into three stages: intramesenchymal migration from the olfactory placodes to the cribriform plate of the ethmoid bone, penetration through this plate into the brain, and intracerebral migration to the septo-preoptic hypothalamic region.

The general pattern of development of the GnRH system is common to most mammals, although the timing of formation and migration of its neurons varies between species depending on the duration of pregnancy and the degree of maturity at birth. In particular, GnRH neurons in mice are formed on day 11, and in rats, on days 12–14 of intrauterine development.

In the past two decades, many attempts have been made to reveal factors influencing the migration and differentiation of GnRH neurons. The main factors identified to date are the neural cell adhesion molecule (NCAM), which forms a substrate for migrating GnRH neurons, and peripherin, a member of the intermediate filament protein family (Fueshko & Wray, 1994). Disturbances of GnRH neuron migration caused by the absence of NCAM are responsible for the Kallmann syndrome in humans, which involves hypogonadism and anosmia. Other factors influencing the development of the GnRH system include chemoattractants and chemorepellents such as netrin, ephrin, and semaphorin 4D (Schwarting et al., 2007; Giacobini et al., 2008); neurotransmitters produced by the microenvironment of migrating GnRH neurons (GABA, serotonin, and catecholamines), which regulate the rate of their migration (Bless et al., 2000; Izvolskaia et al., 2009); and growth factors, including the fibroblast growth factor (FGF), brain-derived neurotrophic factor (BDNF), hepatocyte growth factor/scatter factor (HGF/SF), and LIF (Cronin et al., 2004; Chung et al., 2008).

The migration of GnRH neurons in the nasal region of rats is confined to the bundles of nerve fibers expressing polysialylated forms of NCAM (PSA-NCAM). Experiments on the removal of NCAM from this migration route (by gene knockout, enzyme treatment, or anti-NCAM antibodies) have shown that such disturbances entail significant reduction in the number of migrating neurons but do not completely block their migration. On this basis, it has been concluded that NCAM does not play the key role in the migration of GnRH neurons, although is involved in the formation of their migration route. Moreover, nerve fibers on the migration route of rat GnRH neurons in the nasal region also express other cell adhesion proteins, TAG-1 and CC-2. In mice, their migration in this region is connected with the bundles of nerve fibers expressing peripherin (Fueshko & Wray, 1994).

The development of the olfactory system proceeds with the involvement of numerous guiding molecules, in particular, chemoattractants, chemorepellents, and chemotrophic factors. The last group includes proteins such as Slit, semaphorins, and netrins, which provide directional and positional cues for growing axons of olfactory nerves and, supposedly, for GnRH neurons migrating in the nasal region and forebrain. The latter apparently pertains to netrins, a small family of secreted proteins involved in the formation of many nerve bundles in the brain. The receptor protein for netrins, DCC, has been identified and shown to be expressed in parallel to GnRH in normal mice and rats and also in mice with the DCC gene knockout. The DCC protein is present in peripherin-expressing nerve fibers guiding the migration of GnRH neurons in the nasal region, and its mRNA can also be detected in some GnRH neurons located in the nasal region but disappears after they enter the brain. Their migration in the nasal region is also guided by one more chemoattractant protein, HGF/SF, with its receptor protein (c-Met) being expressed in the immediate vicinity of migrating GnRH neurons (Giacobini et al., 2002).

The migration rate of GnRH neurons is regulated by neurotransmitters. Many neurotransmitters controlling the functions of the GnRH system in adults can also provide spatiotemporal cues to migrating GnRH neurons during development. In particular, penetration of these neurons to the forebrain is guided by GABA. GABAergic neurons found in the nasal region of mouse, rat, and human fetuses are derived from the epithelium of olfactory placodes, as are GnRH neurons. Their axons extend to the cribriform plate of the ethmoid bone, where they can interact with GnRH neurons located there. Injection of GABA receptor antagonists in pregnant mice retards the migration GnRH neurons (Bless et al., 2000). In chick embryos, a natural decrease in the rate of their migration in the zone of cribriform plate has been observed. The role of this phenomenon is unclear. It may be that the delay in migration is necessary for maturation of GnRH neurons or reorganization of their migration behavior prior to entering the forebrain. The migration of GnRH neurons in the forebrain is also guided by GABA. Injection of pregnant females with bicuculline, a GABA receptor antagonist, results in deviation of these neurons from the caudal segments of their migration route formed by peripherin-expressing fibers, with consequent disturbances in the pattern of their distribution in the forebrain (Bless et al., 2000).

Glutamate is another neurotransmitter producing an effect on the migration of GnRH neurons. Mechanisms of this effect in the nasal region and forebrain appear to be different. Blockade of AMPA glutamate receptors in mice retards penetration of GnRH neurons to the forebrain (Simonian & Herbison, 2001), but no such receptors have been found on these neurons in the nasal region. In the forebrain, the effect of glutamate is apparently mediated by a different type of receptors. This follows from the fact that GnRH neurons of mouse fetuses have been found to contain NMDAR1 glutamate receptors and that prenatal blockade of these receptors accelerates the migration of GnRH neurons in the forebrain (Simonian & Herbison, 2001). The question as to the mechanisms of glutamate action on these neurons remains open.

The migration of GnRH-neurons to the definitive location in the septo-preoptic region is stimulated also by monoamines. Data on the distribution of GnRH neurons and the level of GnRH in the rostral brain region and hypothalamus of 21-day rat with chronic serotonin deficiency provide a basis for the conclusion that the migration of GnRH neurons is stimulated by serotonin (Pronina et al., 2001). The stimulating effect of serotonin is potentiated by testosterone, since it is better manifested in males than in females.

During the "preneurotransmitter" period of brain development, catecholamines function as highly effective morphogenetic factors influencing differentiation and migration of target cells. In mice, dopamine appears on day 10, and noradrenaline and adrenaline, on day 11 of embryonic development. In rats, the first neurons expressing tyrosine hydroxylase (TH) and catecholamines have been found on embryonic day 13 both in the midbrain and sympathetic ganglia. The migration of GnRH neurons to the forebrain in rats on embryonic days 16–18 coincides with the arrival of growing catecholaminergic afferent fibers to their target neurons in this brain region, i.e., with the appearance of an additional, local source of catecholamines. There is evidence that embryonic GnRH neurons and other topographically close neurons transiently expressing TH may also be involved in local metabolism of catecholamines.

According to our data, suppression of catecholamine synthesis in rat embryos by alpha-methyl-p-tyrosine (αMPT, a competitive TH inhibitor) beginning from day 11 of development leads to an increase in the number of GnRH neurons in the rostral segments of their migration route by day 17 and their accumulation in the zone of their entry into the forebrain by days 18–21 (Izvolskaia et al., 2009).

Experiments with double immunohistochemical labeling allowed us to determine the regions of interaction of the catecholaminergic brain systems with migrating and differentiating GnRH neurons. The close topographic location of GnRH-immunoreactive neurons and TH-immunoreactive nerve fibers was observed in the nucleus accumbens on days 17 and 20 and in the median eminence on day 20.

A quantitative radioimmunoassay for GnRH in the caudal regions of the GnRH neuron migration route in 21-day rat fetuses showed that injection of αMPT resulted in a drop of GnRH level in the anterior hypothalamus of female fetuses (Izvolskaia et al., 2009). This is additional evidence that catecholamines contribute to the regulation of development of GnRH neurons during prenatal ontogeny.

Probable mechanisms of the stimulating effect of catecholamines on the migration of differentiating GnRH neurons may involve regulation of the exchange of calcium ions, since the rate of their migration depends on the intracellular concentration of these ions. In mice, retardation of GnRH neuron migration at the cribriform plate of the ethmoid bone takes place against the background of sharp increase in intracellular calcium under the effect of tonic depolarization of GABAergic neurons (Bless et al., 2000). In the case of differentiating GnRH neurons, noradrenaline is apparently a signal molecule that reduces the level of GnRH secretion and probably causes cell membrane hyperpolarization. This neurotransmitter can serve as a functional antagonist of GABA and, acting upon previously depolarized GnRH neurons entering the brain through the cribriform plate, contribute to the maintenance of intracellular calcium level, thereby stimulating the migration of GnRH

neurons. It is also possible that catecholamines exert an indirect effect on the migration of these neurons by acting on their immediate cellular environment, in particular, on GABAergic neurons and cells synthesizing cell adhesion molecules. However, there is no evidence that GABAergic neurons migrating together with GnRH neurons are innervated by catecholaminergic nerve fibers and express catecholamine receptors. It is also less probable that the effect of catecholamines is mediated via regulation of the metabolism of cell adhesion molecules. Indeed, neither catecholamines themselves nor their antagonists (e.g., 6-hydroxydopamine) have influence on the synthesis of cell adhesion molecules in the nervous system of fetuses or adult animals (Messenger et al., 1999). On the other hand, some data indicate that noradrenaline partially inhibits the synthesis of β-tubulin, a cytoskeletal protein, which may results in the reduced rate of neuron migration (Messenger et al., 1999).
Sex-related differences in the distribution of GnRH neurons along their migration route manifest themselves only against the background of catecholamine deficiency.
Special attention has been recently devoted to the influence of cytokines on differentiation of GnRH neurons, but relevant published data are as yet scarce. One of such cytokines is HGF/SF, which has mitogenic, motogenic (stimulating cell motility), and chemoattractant properties with respect to nerve and other cells. HGF/SF appears in the nasal mesenchyme of embryos on day 12 of development, with its concentration increasing toward the brain and its c-Met receptor being expressed on GnRH neurons. The migration of GnRH neurons and the growth of their axonal cones become retarded if the HGF/SF concentration gradient is disturbed (Giacobini et al, 2007).
Another cytokine, LIF, exhibits a pleiotropic action during ontogeny, producing an effect on proliferation of primordial germ cells, differentiation of spermatocytes, blastocyst implantation, and the development of the pituitary and olfactory system . Experiments with the immature GnRH neuronal cell line GN11 have shown that LIF can induce hemokinesis of these cells. Both LIF and its receptor (LIFβ) are expressed in the nasal region of mouse embryos on day 13 of development, indicating a role for this cytokine in the migration of GnRH neurons.
The macrophage chemotactic protein-1 (MCP-1) is a powerful chemoattractant for many immune and nonimmune cells. Its main function is to guide the migration of leukocytes from hematopoietic organs to inflammation foci. As found recently, MCP-1 also stimulates migration of nervous stem cells in rats. Experiments with immortalized neuronal cell lines GT1-7 and GN11 and in vivo studies have shown that GnRH neurons themselves produce MCP-1 and express receptors for his factor, while MCP-1 has a stimulating effect on their migration in culture (Chattopadhyay et al, 2006).
The above facts suggest that the development of GnRH neurons and the hypothalamo-pituitary-gonadal system as a whole is apparently subject to dramatic changes upon activation of the mother's immune system during pregnancy. This assumption is confirmed by recent data on the effect of LPS on fetal brain development. It has been shown that LPS induces the synthesis of the vascular endothelial growth factor, nerve growth factor (NGF), antiapoptotic protein YB-1, neuronal differentiation factor (necdin), and BDNF in the fetal rat brain cortex (Liverman et al., 2006). On day 18 of embryonic development in mice, LPS suppresses the expression of factors involved in neuron migration and axonal cone growth, namely, of semaphorin 5b and chromatin-associated Groucho protein (Liverman et al., 2006). In addition, LPS increases the content of glial fibrillary acidic protein (GFAP), an intermediate filament protein, in hippocampal and cortical astrocytes and reduces the

content of myelin and immunoreactivity of the microglia in the offspring of LPS-injected rats during postnatal development. Intrauterine infection of LPS in rats results in an elevated level of GFAP in the brain white matter and hippocampus on postnatal day 7 and in the brain cortex and corpus callosum on postnatal day 14 (Yu et al., 2004). Chronic endotoxin-induced inflammation processes in the brain cause lesions in the white matter of pups examined on postnatal days 1 and 7, with these pups also showing a high level of GFAP expression on postnatal days 1 and 3 followed by active proliferation and differentiation of astrocytes (astrogliosis), on day 7 (Rousset et al., 2006).

Prenatal activation of the immune system by endotoxins modifies the stress response of the hypothalamo-pituitary system, the expression of proinflammatory cytokines in the brain, and the functioning of dopamin- and serotonergic systems (Wang et al., 2009). All these changes affect brain development, increasing the risk for neurological and mental disorders in remote periods. Induction of mother's immune response by LPS leads to changes in the levels of cytokines in different organs of the fetus. Proinflammatory cytokines are regarded as a connecting link between intrauterine infection during pregnancy and subsequent disturbances of brain functions in the fetus. Injection of LPS to pregnant mice induces increased expression of TNFα, IL-1β, and MCP-1 in fetuses (Liverman et al., 2006). In rats, the expression of TNFα is observed as early as 1 h after LPS injection and its level remaining unchanged for 24 h, while the level of IL-1β gradually decreases. The highest level of TNFα and IL-1β expression is observed during the first postnatal days. During intrauterine infection, cytokines TNFα и IL-1β appear to affect mainly the white matter of the fetal brain, which entails the development of cerebral palsy in newborn pups and characteristic symptoms of schizophrenia in remote periods (Yu et al., 2004).

Prenatal infection also affects the dopaminergic system of the fetus. In pregnant rats injected with LPS on day 11 of pregnancy, postnatal offspring are characterized by reduced numbers of dopaminergic neurons, increased activity of microglia, and a high level of proinflammatory cytokines, especially TNFα, in the substantia nigra. It is considered that, что LPS suppresses the secretion of glutathione (an antioxidant) in glial cells, which leads to the death of dopaminergic neurons and the development of Parkinson's disease. As shown recently, prenatal LPS infection in rats results in the attrition of dopaminergic neurons in the substantia nigra and serotoninergic neurons in the locus coeruleus, with consequent decrease in the contents of dopamine and serotonin in postnatal offspring (Wang et al., 2009). Such infection of pregnant rats can probably affect differentiation of monoaminergic neurons not only in the brain stem but also in other regions of the fetal brain, including the hypothalamus.

Initial data are also available on the effect of LPS on the GnRH system of newborn rat pups (Li et al., 2007). Stimulation of their immune system on the first postnatal days results in long-term sensitization of the GnRH system and its vulnerability to the inhibitory effect of stress in adult age. This effect is mediated by corticotropin-releasing hormone and its receptors in the median preoptic region.

According to our data, a single LPS injection to pregnant rats on day 12 of pregnancy suppresses the migration of GnRH neurons, whereas such an injection on day 15 has no effect on their distribution along the migration route (Fig. 3). After the injection on day 12 (but not on day 15), the total number of GnRH-immunoreactive neurons in the fetus was decreased on day 17 but returned to the normal (control) level by day 19. The effect observed on day 17 can be explained either by a general reduction of GnRH synthesis in these neurons or by a delay in the onset of their differentiation. In rats, GnRH neurons begin to synthesize this hormone on day 15, i.e., one or two days after their formation, and the levels of LPS-induced cytokines in mother's blood and fetal tissues remain high only during 24 h after injection and then return to the baseline (Liverman et al., 2006). Therefore, the decrease in the numbers of fetal GnRH neurons observed on day 5 after LPS injection is unlikely to result from the direct influence of proinflammatory cytokines on GnRH synthesis in these cells. However, their indirect influence cannot be excluded, IL-1α and GM-CSF in adult animals block the release of GnRH from the axons of GnRH neurons by inhibiting the activity of NO synthase (Rettori et al., 1994). In view of these and our data, the most probable explanation is that LPS delays the onset of differentiation of GnRH neuron precursors. It should be noted that the total number of GnRH neurons returns to the norm by birth, but this does not exclude the occurrence of disturbances in the GnRH system functions during later periods of postnatal ontogeny.

Stimulation of the immune system in pregnant females by LPS on day 12 results to the suppression of not only differentiation but also migration of fetal GnRH neurons, which manifests itself in the increased numbers of these cells accumulating in the rostral brain regions, compared to the control (Fig. 1). On the other hand, LPS injection on day 15 does not lead to redistribution of GnRH-immunoreactive cells along their migration route by day 17 or 19. Thus, as GnRH cell differentiation is delayed, the start of migration of GnRH neurons shifts to later dates, and the rate of their intramesenchymal (intranasal) migration is retarded. On the other hand, LPS has no effect on the rate of their migration at later stages, when GnRH neurons pass through the cribriform plate of the ethmoid bone to the forebrain.

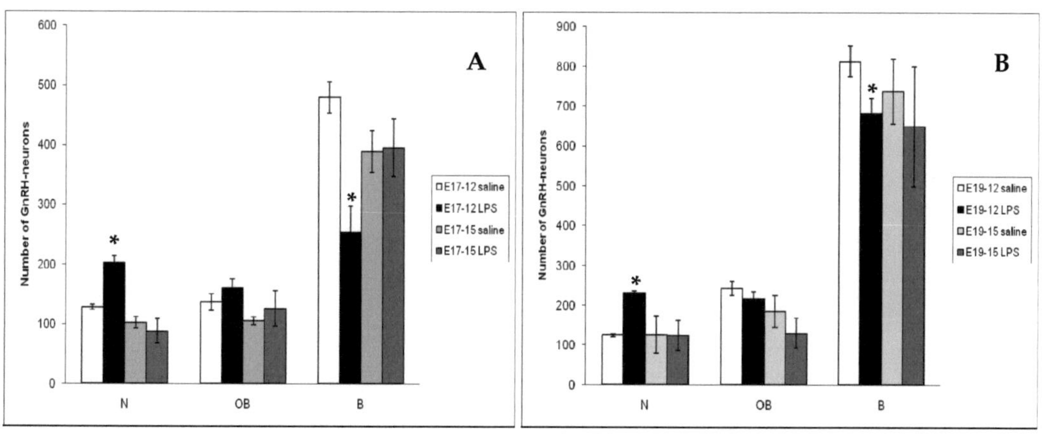

Fig. 1. Distribution of GnRH neurons in different areas of their migration in (A) 17-day and (B) 19-day rat fetuses injected with saline (control) or LPS on embryonic days (E) 12 and 15, $m \pm SD$ (E12: saline, n=6; LPS, n=6; E15: saline, n=3; LPS, n=3): N, nasal region; OB, olfactory bulbs; (B) brain. (*) Differences between the indicated values are significant at $p < 0.05$.

It is during the intramesenchymal migration that GnRH neurons express receptors for cytokines, primarily for IL-6 and LIF (Dozio et al., 2009), while their migration within the brain is apparently regulated by a different mechanism.

In the experiments described above, the migration of GnRH neurons within the nasal region appeared to be regulated via LPS-induced activation of the synthesis of proinflammatory cytokines. Therefore, we decided to analyze the effect of LPS at low doses (causing no more than 25–30% fetal mortality) on the levels of cytokines IL-6, TNFα, LIF, and MCP-1 in pregnant mice and fetuses. Pregnant females were intraperitoneally injected with LPS (45 μg/kg body weight), and cytokines in the blood sera of females and fetuses and in fetal cerebrospinal and amniotic fluids were determined by means of flow cytometry and ELISA. The results showed that the blood levels of antiinflammatory cytokines in LPS-injected females were increased drastically, compared to the control: the increase was 38-fold for LIF, 28-fold for IL-6, 23-fold for MCP-1, and 20-fold for TNFα (Fig. 2). In fetuses, MCP-1 and IL-6 in tissues were increased by factors of two and seven, respectively, and LIF in the amniotic fluid was increased threefold. Thus, activation of the immune system by LPS in pregnant females has proved to result in elevated levels of proinflammatory cytokines in their peripheral blood and then in fetuses, with consequent disturbances in the migration and differentiation of GnRH neurons. The strongest effect on the migration of these neurons is apparently characteristic of IL-6, LIF and MCP-1.

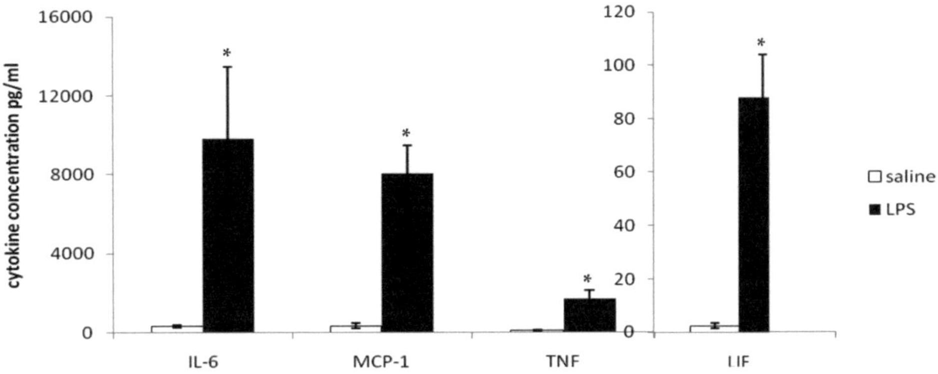

Fig. 2. Serum concentrations of proinflammatory cytokines in 12-day mouse fetuses 1.5 in 12-day mouse 1.5 hours after injection of saline (control) or LPS to the mother, $m \pm SD$ (saline, $n = 6$; LPS, $n = 5$). Abbreviations: IL-6, interleukin 6; LIF, leukemia inhibitory factor; MCP-1, macrophage chemotactic protein-1; TNF, tumor necrosis factor alpha. (*) Differences from the control are significant at $p < 0.05$.

2.3.3 Role of thymic peptides in reproductive system development and functioning

The thymus, being the primary organ of the immune system, can also be regarded as an endocrine organ. Moreover, it contains cells of neural origin that synthesize neuropeptides, which is evidence for its obvious relation to the nervous system. The thymus is the lymphoepitelian organ formed at the earliest stages of ontogeny. Its development begins on embryonic day 10 in rodents and embryonic week 4 in humans. Embryonic T-cell precursors migrate into thymus from the yolk sac, para-aortic splanchnopleura, and embryonic liver; in the postnatal period, the source of precursor cells is the bone marrow. Several systems of humoral regulatory factors operate in the thymus, including thymic peptides, hormones, neuropeptides, and cytokines. Their basic role is to provide for and regulate the development and functioning of T lymphocytes and thymic stroma and to control processes in the peripheral compartments of the immune and, probably, neuroendocrine systems (Goya et al, 2004).

A special place in thymus endocrinology belongs to thymic peptides, or hormones, which are relatively specific for this organ. These hormones, synthesized by epithelial cells of the thymus and released into the circulation, are distinguished into a separate group for the reason of their local synthesis (in the thymus) and sphere of action confined to the immune system. However, there is evidence for the synthesis of these peptides (except for thymulin) beyond the thymus and, in particular, in the nervous system (Hannappel et al., 2007). Thymic peptides appear to be cofactors in processes related to differentiation of thymocytes as well as to regulate the production of other hormones, neuropeptides, and cytokines in the thymus, hypothalamus, and pituitary. They are also involved in T-cell differentiation in the secondary lymphoid organs and in interactions with the hypothalamo-pituitary-adrenal and reproductive systems (Goya et al, 2004).

The thymus has a significant role in the functioning of the reproductive system (Fig.3). Thymic peptides, primarily α- and β-thymosins and thymulin, stimulate GnRH secretion in the mediobasal hypothalamus and gonadotropin secretion in the pituitary of female rats (Garcia et al., 2005). In male rats, prepubertal thymectomy is followed after 45 days by a drop of FSH and a rise of luteinizing hormone and testosterone levels in the peripheral blood.

In perinatal ontogeny, the thymus is indispensable for the formation of the pituitary-gonadal axis. Prenatal thymectomy in primates and neonatal thymectomy in rats or mice result in suppressed oogenesis, reduced weights of the ovaries and adrenals, and decreased levels of gonadotropins in the pituitary and circulating blood during postnatal life (Farookhi, 1988). Disturbances in the immune system manifest themselves 25–30 days after thymectomy. In particular, thymectomy on postnatal day 3 leads to the paucity of regulatory T cells, loss of peripheral tolerance, and development of organ-specific autoimmune disease in adult mice. Moreover, it induces production of auto-oocyte antibodies detectable in the circulation, with consequent development of autoimmune ovarian dysgenesis. Importantly, day 3 thymectomy does not necessarily lead to autoimmune disease in all mouse strains, indicating that processes responsible for the disease development are genetically controlled (Roper et al., 2002).

Neonatal thymectomy also affects the male reproductive system, but its consequences manifest themselves relatively late. A drop in the levels of luteinizing hormone and prolactin takes place on days 60–90 after thymectomy, and symptoms observed on days 13-170 include testicular atrophy, hypertrophy of pituitary β-cells, and lymphoid infiltration of the pituitary, thyroid, and prostate (Farookhi, 1988). It should be noted that thymectomy on postnatal day 10 also results in retarded sexual development (with reduced numbers of follicles, low levels of blood estrogens, etc.), as does neonatal thymectomy. Thymulin corrects these disturbances, while in normal mice it has no effect on estrogen secretion (Goya et al, 2004; García et al., 2005).

In mutant nude (athymic) mice, disturbances are observed not only in the immune system but also in the neuroendocrine and reproductive systems. Embryonic development of the thymus in these mice is controlled by gene *Foxn1* located on chromosome 11. It proceeds normally until embryonic day 11, when the complex architecture of the thymus becomes distorted, which interferes with differentiation of thymic epithelial cells and colonization of the organ by lymphoid precursor cells. Changes in the reproductive system of athymic mutants are similar to those in neonatally thymectomized mice.

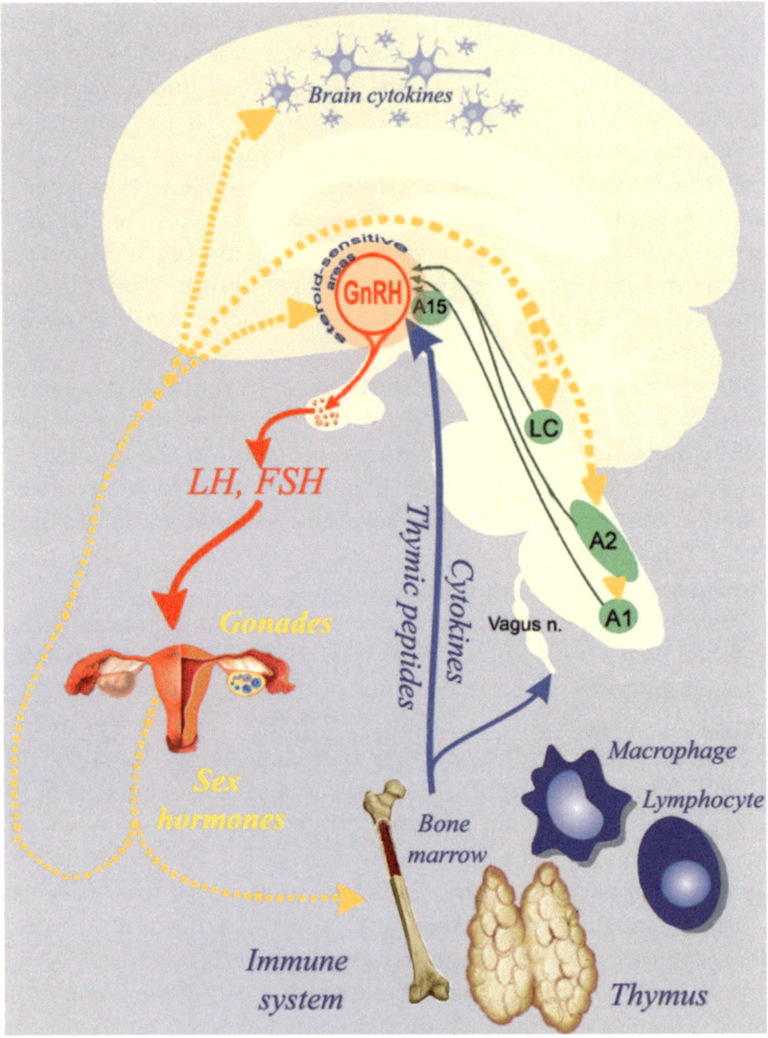

Fig. 3. Interactions of the GnRH system with the hypothalamo-pituitary-gonadal axis and immune system. Abbreviations: GnRH, gonadotropin releasing hormone-producing neurons; LH, luteinizing hormone; FSH, follicle stimulating hormone; LC, locus coeruleus; A1, A2, and A15, catecholamine-producing (tyrosine hydroxylase-immunoreactive) cell groups in the brain.

Acidophilic and basophilic pituitary cells in the mutants are smaller than normal, and the synthesis of the growth hormone, prolactin, FSH, and luteinizing hormone is reduced (Goya et al, 2004). Thymic peptides, thymulin in particular, correct these disturbances (García et al., 2005). Neonatal thymulin gene therapy in nude mice results in normalization of blood thymulin and gonadotropin levels at maturity (Goya et al., 2007). Thus, the hormonal hypofunction of the thymus during early ontogeny entails long-term or irreversible disturbances in the structure and functions of both immune and reproductive systems.

The sum of available data suggests the following scheme of interactions between the hypothalamo-pituitary reproductive system and the thymus (Fig. 3). Hypothalamic GnRH interacts with specific receptors on epithelial cells of the thymus, thereby inducing the synthesis of thymic peptides by these cells and differentiation of T lymphocytes, the latter process involving participation of thymic GnRH and sex hormones. Thymic peptides, in turn, stimulate the secretion and functional activity of hypothalamic GnRH, which induces the secretion of gonadotropins and thereby modulates steroidogenesis.

3. Conclusion

The data considered in this review demonstrate that interactions of the hypothalamo–pituitary-gonadal and immune systems are a lifelong phenomenon that begins during embryonic development. The pattern of establishment and development of their interactions during early ontogeny is a major factor in programming the health of an individual. Changes in these systems upon perinatal exposure to various adverse factors upset the normal homeostatic balance of the body, causing disturbances in their functioning throughout the subsequent life span. The plasticity of physiological systems during early ontogeny provides for effective adaptation of the developing organism to variable ambient conditions; on the other hand, it is responsible for long-term or even permanent alteration of general response to environmental factors. Thus, thymic peptide deficiency in neonatally thymectomized or nude mice or increased levels of proinflammatory cytokines resulting from bacterial infection in a pregnant female cause disturbances in the formation of various brain systems, thereby affecting differentiation of GnRH neurons and, therefore, the establishment of the reproductive function. Since high concentrations of sex steroids can significantly intrude on the formation of the neuroendocrine–immune axis, caution should be taken in prescribing sex steroids and their synthetic analogs. In particular, this concerns prenatal treatment with estriol recommended by some specialists. Special attention should also be given to the children whose mothers suffered an infectious disease during pregnancy. On the other hand, experimental and clinical data accumulated to date provide evidence for a favorable effect of estrogens on patients with autoimmune diseases, e.g., multiple sclerosis.

The patterning of sexual behavior of sex steroids takes place not only during early development: these hormones can alter the prenatal programming of relevant systems at later stages of ontogeny, with adolescence being most responsive to their influence. The effects of GnRH and sex hormones on the immune system during adult life are apparently nonspecific and serve to maintain its homeostasis in response to changes in ambient conditions or to stress-induced immunosuppression. Indeed, thymocyte deficiency resulting from age-related thymus involution or stress can be reversed by treatment with hormones, including GnRH and its agonists.

4. Acknowledgments

This study was supported by the Russian Foundation for Basic Research (projects №10-04-01101).

5. References

Azad, N., LaPaglia, N., Kirsteins, L., Uddin, S., Steiner, J., Williams, D.W., Lawrence, A.M., & Emanuele, N.V. (1997). Jurkat cell proliferative activity is increased by luteinizing hormone-releasing hormone. *J. Endocrinol.* Vol.153. No.2. (May 1997), pp. 241-249. ISSN: 0022-0795.

Azad, N., LaPaglia, N., Agrawal, L., Steiner, J., Uddin, S., Williams, D.W., Lawrence, A.M. & Emanuele, N.V. (1998). The role of gonadectomy and testosterone replacement on thymic luteinizing hormone-releasing hormone production. *J. Endocrinol.* Vol.158. No.2. (August 1998), pp. 229–235. ISSN: 0022-0795.

Bless E.P., Westaway W.A., Schwarting G.A. & Tobet S.A. (2000). Effects of gamma-aminobutyric acid (A) receptor manipulation on migrating gonadotropin-releasing hormone neurons through the entire migratory route in vivo and in vitro. *Endocrinology*. Vol.141. No.3. (March 2000), 1254-1262. ISSN: 0013-7227.

Shahrokh, D., Del Corpo, A., Dhir S.K., Szyf, M., Champagne, F.A. & Meaney, M.J. (2008). Epigenetic programming of phenotypic variations in reproductive strategies in the rat through maternal care. *J. Neuroendocrinol.* Vol.20. No.6. (June 2008), pp. 795-801. ISSN: 0953-8194.

Carreras, E., Turner, S., Paharkova-Vatchkova, V., Mao, A., Dascher, C. & Kovats S. (2008). Estradiol acts directly on bone marrow myeloid progenitors to differentially regulate GM-CSF or Flt3 ligand-mediated dendritic cell differentiation. *J. Immunol.* Vol.180. No.2. (January 2008), pp. 727–738. ISSN: 0022-1767.

Champagne, F.A. & Curley, J.P. (2008). Maternal regulation of estrogen receptor alpha methylation. *Curr. Opin. Pharmacol.* Vol.8. No. 6. (December 2008), pp. 735-739. ISSN: 0271-0137.

Chapman, J.C., Christian, J.J., Pawlikowski, M.A., Yasukawa, N., & Michael, S.D. (2000). Female house mice develop a unique ovarian lesion in colonies that are at maximum population density. *Proc. Soc. Exp. Biol .Med.* Vol.225. No.1. (October 2000), pp. 80-90. ISSN: 0037-9727.

Chapman, J.C., Min, S.H., Freeh, S.M. & Michael, S.D. (2009). The estrogen-injected female mouse: new insight into the etiology of PCOS. *Reprod. Biol. Endocrinol.* Vol.18. (May 2009), pp. 7-47. ISSN: 1477-7827.

Chattopadhyay, N., Jeong, K.H., Yano, S., Huang, S., Pang, J.L., Ren, X., Terwilliger, E., Kaiser, U.B., Vassilev, P.M., Pollak, M R. & Brown, E.M. (2007). Calcium receptor stimulates chemotaxis and secretion of MCP-1 in GnRH neurons in vitro: potential impact on reduced GnRH neuron population in CaR-null mice. *Am J Physiol Endocrinol Metab.* Vol.292. No.2. (February 2007), pp. E523-32. ISSN: 0193-1849.

Chung W.C., Moyle S.S., Tsai P.S. Fibroblast growth factor 8 signaling through fibroblast growth factor receptor 1 is required for the emergence of gonadotropin-releasing hormone neurons. *Endocrinology*. Vol.149. No.10/ (October 2008), pp. 4997–5003. ISSN: 0013-7227.

Ciechanowska, M., Lapot, M., Malewski, T., Misztal, T., Mateusiak, K. & Przekop F. (2007). Effect of stress on the expression of GnRH and GnRH receptor (GnRH-R) genes in the preoptic area-hypothalamus and GnRH-R gene in the stalk/median eminence and anterior pituitary gland in ewes during follicular phase of the estrous cycle. *Acta Neurobiol Exp (Wars)*. Vol.67. No.1. (2007), pp. 1-12. ISSN 0065-1400.

Cronin, A.S, Horan, T.L., Spergel, D.J., Brooks, A.N., Hastings, M.H. & Ebling, F.J. (2004). Neurotrophic effects of BDNF on embryonic gonadotropin-releasing hormone

(GnRH) neurons. *Eur. J. Neurosci.* Vol.20. No.2. (July 2004), pp. 338–344. ISSN: 1460-9568.

Dixit, V.D., Sridaran, R., Edmonsond, M.A., Taub, D. & Thompson W.E. (2003). Gonadotropin-releasing hormone attenuates pregnancy-assotiated thymic involution and modulates the expression of antiproliferative gene product prohibitin. *Endocrinology.* Vol.144. No.4. pp. (July 2003), ISSN: 0013-7227.

Dorshkind, K., & Horseman N.D. (2000). The roles of prolactin, growth hormone, insulin-like growth factor-I, and thyroid hormones in lymphocyte development and function: insights from genetic models of hormone and hormone receptor deficiency. *Endocr. Rev.* Vol.21. No3. (June 2000), pp. 292–312. ISSN: 0163-769X.

Dozio, E., Ruscica, M., Galliera, E., Corsi, M.M. & Magni, P. (2009). Leptin, ciliary neurotrophic factor, leukemia inhibitory factor and interleukin-6: class-I cytokines involved in the neuroendocrine regulation of the reproductive function. *Curr Protein Pept Sci.* Vol.10. No. 6. (December 2009), pp. 577-84. ISSN: 1389-2037.

Farookhi, R., Wesolowski, E., Trasler, J.M. & Robaire, B. (1988). Modulation by neonatal thymectomy of the reproductive axis in male and female rats during development. *Biol. Reprod.* Vol.38. No.1. (February 1988), pp. 91–99. ISSN: 0006-3363.

Fowden, A.L., & Forhead, A.J. (2004). Endocrine mechanisms of intrauterine programming. *Reproduction.* Vol.127. No.5. (May 2004), pp. 515–526. ISSN: 1470-1626.

Fueshko, S. & Wray S. (1994). LHRH cells migrate on periferin fibers in embryonic olfactory explant cultures: an in vitro model for neurotrophic migration. *Dev. Biol.* Vol.166. No.1. (November 1994), pp. 331-348. ISSN: 0012-1606.

García, L., Hinojosa, L., Domínguez, R., Chavira, R. & Rosas, P. (2005). Effects of injecting thymulin into the anterior or medial hypothalamus or the pituitary on induced ovulation in prepubertal mice. *Neuroimmunomodulation.* Vol.12. No.5. (May 2005), pp. 314-320. ISSN:1021-7401.

Giacobini, P., Messina, A., Morello, F., Ferraris, N., Corso, S., Penachioni, J., Giordano, S., Tamagnone, L. & Fasolo, A. (2008). Semaphorin 4D regulates gonadotropin hormone-releasing hormone-1 neuronal migration through PlexinB1-Met complex . *J. Cell Biol.* V. 183. No. 3. (November 2008), pp 555–566. ISSN: 0021-9525.

Giacobini, P., Messina, A., Wray, S., Giampietro, C., Crepaldi, T., Carmeliet, P. & Fasolo, A. (2007). Hepatocyte growth factor acts as a motogen and guidance signal for gonadotropin hormone-releasing hormone-1 neuronal migration. *J. Neurosci.* Vol. 27. No.2. (January 2007), pp. 431-45. ISSN: 0270-6474.

Gonzalez, B., Ratner, L.D., Di Giorgio, N.P., Poutanen, M., Huhtaniemi, I.T., Calandra, R.S., Lux-Lantos, V.A. & Rulli, S.B. (2011). Endogenously elevated androgens alter the developmental programming of the hypothalamic-pituitary axis in male mice. *Mol. Cell. Endocrinol.* Vol.332. No.1-2. (Januare 2011), pp. 78-87. ISSN: 0303-7207.

Goodman, R.L., Jansen, H.T., Billings, H.J., Coolen, L.M. & Lehman, M.N. (2010). Neural systems mediating seasonal breeding in the ewe. *J. Neuroendocrinol.* Vol22. No.7. (July 2010), pp. 674-81. ISSN: 0953-8194.

Goya, R.G., Brown, O.A., Pléau, J.M. & Dardenne, M. (2004). Thymulin and the neuroendocrine system. *Peptides.* Vol.25. No.1. (January), pp. 139-142. ISSN: 0196-9781.

Goya, R.G., Reggiani, P.C., Vesenbeckh, S.M., Pléau, J.M., Sosa, Y.E., Cónsole, G.M., Schade, R., Henklein, P. & Dardenne M. (2007) Thymulin gene therapy prevents the reduction in circulating gonadotropins induced by thymulin deficiency in mice. *Am. J. Physiol. Endocrinol. Metab.* Vol.293. No.1. (July 2007), pp. E182–187. ISSN: 0193-1849.

Grasso, G., Massai, L., De Leo, V., & Muscettola, M. (1998). The effect of LHRH and TRH on human interferon-gamma production in vivo and in vitro. *Life Sci.* Vol.62. No.22. (April 1998), pp. 2005-2014. ISSN: 0024-3205.

Hannappel, E. (2007). beta-Thymosins. *Ann. N. Y. Acad. Sci.* (September 2007). Vol.1112, pp. 21-37. ISSN 0077-8923.

He, D., Sato, I., Kimura, F. & Akema, T.(2003). Lipopolysaccharide inhibits luteinizing hormone release through interaction with opioid and excitatory amino acid inputs to gonadotropin-releasing hormone neurones in female rats: possible evidence for a common mechanism involved in infection and immobilization stress. *Neuroendocrinol.* Vol. 15. No.5. (June 2003), pp. 559-563. ISSN 0028-3835.

Herbison, A.E. (1997). Noradrenergic regulation of cyclic GnRH secretion. Rev Reprod. Vol.2. No.1.(January 1997), pp.1-6. ISSN: 1470-1626.

Hosny, S., Jennes, L. (1998). Identefication of a1B adrenergic receptors in gonadotropin releasing hormone neurons of the female rat. *J. Neuroendocrinol.* Vol. 10. No9. (September 1998), pp. 687-692. ISSN: 0953-8194.

Hrabovszky, E., Shughrue, P.J., Merchenthaler, I., Hajszán, T., Carpenter, C.D., Liposits, Z., Petersen, S.L. (2000). Detection of estrogen receptor-beta messenger ribonucleic acid and 125I-estrogen binding sites in luteinizing hormone-releasing hormone neurons of the rat brain. *Endocrinology.* Vol. 141. No.9. (September 2000), pp. 3506-3509. ISSN: 0013-7227.

Igaz, P., Salvi, R., Rey, J.P., Glauser, M., Pralong, F.P. & Gaillard, R.C. (2006). Effects of cytokines on gonadotropin-releasing hormone (GnRH) gene expression in primary hypothalamic neurons and in GnRH neurons immortalized conditionally. *Endocrinology.* Vol. 147. No.2. (February 2006), pp. 1037-1043. ISSN: 0013-7227.

Izvolskaia, M., Duittoz, A.H., Tillet, Y. & Ugrumov, M.V. (2009). The influence of catecholamine on the migration of gonadotropin-releasing hormone-producing neurons in the rat foetuses. *Brain Struct Funct.* Vol.213. No. 3. (February 2009), pp. 289-300. ISSN: 1863-2653.

Jacobson, J.D. (2000). Gonadotropin-releasing hormone and G proteins: potential roles in autoimmunity. *Ann. N. Y. Acad. Sci.* Vol.917. (January 2000), pp. 809-818. ISSN: 0077-8923.

Kang, S.S., Kim, S.R., Leonhardt, S., Jarry, H., Wuttke, W. & Kim K. (200). Effect of interleukin-1beta on gonadotropin-releasing hormone (GnRH) and GnRH receptor gene expression in castrated male rats. *J Neuroendocrinol.* Vol.12. No.5.(May 2000), pp. 421-429. ISSN: 0953-8194.

Karsch, F.J., Battaglia, D.F., Breen, K.M., Debus, N. & Harris, T.G. (2002). Mechanisms for ovarian cycle disruption by immune/inflammatory stress. Stress. Vol. 5. No.2 (June 2002), pp. 101-112. ISSN: 1025-3890.

Kimura, M., Yu, W.H., Rettori, V. & McCann SM. (1997). Granulocyte-macrophage colony stimulating factor suppresses LHRH release by inhibition of nitric oxide synthase and stimulation of gamma-aminobutyric acid release // *Neuroimmunomodulation*. Vol. 4. No.5-6. (September-December 1997), pp. 237-43. ISSN:1021-7401.

Langley-Evans, S.C. (2006). Developmental programming of health and disease. *Proc. Nutr. Soc.* Vol.65. No.1. (February 2006), pp. 97–105. ISSN: 0029-6651.

Li, X.F., Kinsey-Jones, J.S., Knox, A.M., Wu, X.Q., Tahsinsoy, D., Brain, S.D., Lightman, S.L. & O'Byrne, K.T. (2007). Neonatal lipopolysaccharide exposure exacerbates stress-induced suppression of luteinizing hormone pulse frequency in adulthood. *Endocrinology*. Vol.148. No.12. (December 2007), pp.5984-90. ISSN: 0013-7227.

Liverman, C.S., Kaftan, H.A., Cui, L., Hersperger, S.G., Taboada, E., Klein, R.M. & Berman, N.E.(2006). Altered expression of pro-inflammatory and developmental genes in the fetal brain in a mouse model of maternal infection. *Neurosci Lett.* Vol.399. No.3. (May 2006), pp.220-225. ISSN: 0304-3940.

Magni, P., Dozio, E., Ruscica, M., Watanobe, H., Cariboni, A., Zaninetti, R., Motta, M. & Maggi, R. Leukemia inhibitory factor induces the chemomigration of immortalized gonadotropin-releasing hormone neurons through the independent activation of the Janus kinase/signal transducer and activator of transcription 3, mitogen-activated protein kinase/extracellularly regulated kinase 1/2, and phosphatidylinositol 3-kinase/Akt signaling pathways. *Mol. Endocrinol.* 2007. Vol.21. No.5, (May 2007), pp. 1163–1174. ISSN: 0888-8809.

Marchetti, B., Gallo, F., Farinella, Z., Tirolo, C., Testa, N., Romeo, C. & Morale, M.C. (1998). Luteinizing hormone-releasing hormone is a primary signaling molecule in the neuroimmune network. *Ann. N.Y. Acad. Sci.* Vol.840. (May 1998), pp. 205–248. ISSN: 0077-8923.

Messenger, N.J., Rowe S.J. & Warner A.E. (1999). The neurotransmitter noradrenaline drives noggin-expressing ectoderm cells to activate N-tubulin and become neurons. *Dev. Biol.* Vol.205.No.2. (January 1999), pp. 224-232. ISSN: 0012-1606.

Morale, M.C., Batticane, N., Bartoloni, G., Guarcello, V., Farinella, Z., Galasso, M.G., & Marchetti, B. (1991). Blocade of central and peripheral luteinizing hormone-releasing hormone (LHRH) receptors in neonatal rats with a potent LHRH-antagonist inhibits the morphofunctional development of the thymus and maturation of the cell-mediated and humoral immune responses. *Endocrinology*. Vol.128. No.2. (February 1991), pp. 1073–1085. ISSN: 0013-7227.

Oakley, A.E., Clifton, D.K. & Steiner, R.A. (2009). Kisspeptin signaling in the brain. *Endocr Rev.* Vol.30. No.6. (October 2009), pp. 713-43. ISSN: 1945-7189.

Olsen, N.J. & Kovacs, W.J. (1996). Gonadal Steroids and Immunity. *Endocr. Rev.* Vol.17. No.4 (August 1996), pp. 369-384. ISSN: 1945-7189.

Pan, W., Yu, C., Hsuchou, H., Zhang, Y. & Kastin, A.J. (2008). Neuroinflammation facilitates LIF entry into brain: role of TNF. *Am J Physiol Cell Physiol.* Vol. No.6. (June 2008), pp.1436-1442. ISSN: 0363-6143.

Pereira, A., Rawson, J., Jakubowska, A. & Clarke, I.J. (2010). Estradiol-17beta-responsive A1 and A2 noradrenergic cells of the brain stem project to the bed nucleus of the stria terminalis in the ewe brain: a possible route for regulation of gonadotropin releasing hormone cells. *Neuroscience*. Vol.165. No3. (Februry 2010), pp. 758-73. ISSN: 03064522.

Pillon, D., Caraty, A., Fabre-Nys, C., Lomet, D., Cateau, M. & Bruneau, G. (2004). Regulation by estradiol of hypothalamic somatostatin gene expression: possible involvement of somatostatin in the control of luteinizing hormone secretion in the ewe. *Biol Reprod.* Vol.71. No.1. (July 2004), pp.38-44. ISSN: 0006-3363.

Pronina, T., Ugrumov, M., Adamskaya, E., Kuznetsova, T., Shishkina, I., Babichev, V., Calas, A., Tramu, G., Mailly, P. & Makarenko, I. (2003). Influence of serotonin on the development and migration of gonadotropin-releasing hormone neurones in rat fetuses. *J. Neuroendocrinol.* Vol.15. No.6. (June 2003), pp. 549–558. ISSN: 0953-8194.

Rao, L.V. Cleveland, R.P., Kimmel, R.J. & Ataya, K.M. (1995). Hematopoietic stem cell antigen-1 (Sca-1) expression in different lymphoid tissues of female mice treated with GnRH agonist. *Am. J. Reprod. Immunol.* Vol.34. No.4. (October 1995), pp. 257–266. ISSN: 8755-8920.

Razia, S., Maegawa, Y., Tamotsu, S. & Oishi, T. (2006). Histological changes in immune and endocrine organs of quail embryos: exposure to estrogen and nonylphenol. *Ecotoxicol. Environ. Saf.* Vol.65. No.3. (November 2006), pp. 364-371. ISSN: 0147-6513.

Rettori, V., Dees, W.L., Hiney, J.K., Lyson, K. & McCann, S.M. (1994). An interleukin-1-alpha-like neuronal system in the preoptic-hypothalamic region and its induction by bacterial lipopolysaccharide in concentrations which alter pituitary hormone release. *Neuroimmunomodulation.* Vol. 1. No. 4. (July-Augest 1994), pp.251-258. ISSN:1021-7401.

Rivest, S. & Rivier, C. (1993). Centrally injected interleukin-1 beta inhibits the hypothalamic LHRH secretion and circulating LH levels via prostaglandins in rats. *J Neuroendocrinol.* Vol.5. No.4. (Augest 1993), pp. 445-50. ISSN: 0953-8194.

Roper, R.J., Ma, R.Z., Biggins, J.E., Butterfield, R.J., Michael, S.D., Tung, K.S., Doerge, R.W. & Teuscher, C. (2002). Interacting quantitative trait loci control loss of peripheral tolerance and susceptibility to autoimmune ovarian dysgenesis after day 3 thymectomy in mice. *J. Immunol.* Vol.169. No.3. (August 2002), pp. 1640-1646. ISSN: 0022-1767.

Rousset, C.I., Chalon, S., Cantagrel, S., Bodard, S., Andres, C., Gressens, P. & Saliba, E. (2006). Maternal exposure to LPS induces hypomyelination in the internal capsule and programmed cell death in the deep gray matter in newborn rats. *Pediatr Res.* Vol.59. No.3. (March 2006), pp. 428-33. ISSN: 0031-3998.

Schwarting, G.A., Kostek, C., Bless, E.P., Ahmad, N. & Tobet S.A. (2001). Deleted in colorectal cancer (DCC) regulates the migration of luteinezing hormone-releasing hormone neurons to the basal forebrain. *J. Neurosci.* Vol.21. No3. (February 2001), pp.911-919. ISSN: 0270-6474.

Shulz, K.M., Molenda-Figueira, H.A. & Sisk, C.L. (2009). Back to the future: the organizational-activational hypothesis adapted to puberty and adolescence. *Horm Behav.* Vol.55. No.5. (May 2009), pp. 597–604. ISSN: 0018-506X.

Simonian S.X, Herbison A.E. Differing, spatially restricted roles of ionotropic glutamate receptors in regulating the migration of GnRH neurons during embryogenesis. J. Neurosci. Vol.21. No.3. (February 2001), pp.934-943. ISSN: 0270-6474.

Singh, A.K. & Jiang, Y. (2004). How does peripheral lipopolysaccharide induce gene expression in the brain of rats? *Toxicology*. V. 201. No1-3. (September 2004), pp. 197-207. ISSN: 0300-483X.

Staples, J.E., Gasiewicz, T.A. & Fiore, N.C (1999). Estrogen receptor alpha is necessary in thymic development and estradiol-induced thymic alterations. *J. Immunol.* Vol.163. No.8. (October 1999), pp. 4168–4174. ISSN: 0022-1767.

Tanriverdi, F., Silveira, L.F.G., MacColl, G.S. & Bouloux, P.M.G. (2003).The hypothalamic-pituitary-gonadal axis: immune function and autoimmunity. *J. Endocrinol.* Vol.176. No.3. (March 2003), pp. 293–304. ISSN: 0022-0795.

van den Broek, H.H., Damoiseaux, J .G., De Baets, M.H. & Hupperts, R.M. (2005). The influence of sex hormones on cytokines in multiple sclerosis and experimental autoimmune encephalomyelitis: a review. *Mult. Scler.* Vol.11. No.3. (June 2005), pp. 349-359. ISSN: 1352-4585.

Verma, S., Nakaoke, R., Dohgu, S. & Banks, W.A.(2006). Release of cytokines by brain endothelial cells: A polarized response to lipopolysaccharide. *Brain. Behav. Immun.* Vol. 20. No.5 (September 2006), pp. 449-455. ISSN: 0889-1591.

Wang, S., Yan, J.Y., Lo, Y.K., Carvey, P.M. & Ling, Z. (2009). Dopaminergic and serotoninergic deficiencies in young adult rats prenatally exposed to the bacterial lipopolysaccharide. *Brain Res.* Vol.10. No. 1265. (April 2009), pp. 196-204. ISSN: 0006-8993.

Watanobe, H. & Hayakawa, Y. (2003) Hypothalamic Interleukin-1 and Tumor Necrosis Factor, But Not Interleukin-6, Mediate the Endotoxin- Induced Suppression of the Reproductive Axis in Rats. *Endocrinology*. Vol. 144. No.11. (November 2003), pp. 4868-4875. ISSN: 0013-7227.

Wu, X.Q., Li, X.F., Ye, B., Popat, N., Milligan, S.R., Lightman, S.L. & O'Byrne, K.T. (2011). Neonatal programming by immunological challenge: effects on ovarian function in the adult rat. *Reproduction*. Vol. 41. No.2. (February 2011), pp. 241-248. ISSN: 1470-1626.

Yoshida, K., Rutishauser, U., Crandall, J.E. & Schwarting, G.A. (1999). Polysialic acid facilitates migration of luteinizing hormone-releasing hormone neurons on vomeronasal axons. *J. Neurosci.* Vol.19. No.2. (January 1999), pp. 794–801. ISSN: 0270-6474.

Yu, H.M., Yuan, T.M., Gu, W.Z. & Li, J.P. (2004). Expression of glial fibrillary acidic protein in developing rat brain after intrauterine infection. *Neuropathology*. Vol. 24. No.2. (June 2004), pp. 136-43. ISSN 0919-6544.

Zakharova, L.A., Ermilova, I.Y., Melnikova, V.I., Malyukova, I.V. & Adamskaya, E.I. (2005). Hypothalamic control of the cell-mediated immunity and of the Luteinizing Hormone-Releasing Hormone level in thymus and peripheral blood of rat fetuses. *Neuroimmunomodulation*. Vol.12. No.2. (October 2005), pp. 85–91. ISSN:1021-7401.

Zakharova, L.A. (2009). Plasticity of neuroendocrine-immune interactions during ontogeny: role of perinatal programming in pathogenesis of inflammation and stress-related diseases in adults. *Recent Patents on Endocrine, Metabolic & Immune Drug Discovery.* Vol.3. No.1. (July 2009), pp. 11-27. ISSN: 1872-2148.

Zakharova, L.A., Malyukova, I.V., Proshlyakova, E.V., Potapova, A.A., Sapronova, A.Y., Ershov, P.V., Ugrumov, M.V. (2000). Hypothalamo-pituitary control of the cell-mediated immunity in rat embryos: role of LHRH in regulation of lymphocyte proliferation. *J. Reprod. Immunol.* Vol.47. No.1. (May 2000), pp. 17–32. ISSN: 0165-0378.

Zala, S.M., Chan, B.K., Bilbo, S.D., Potts, W.K., Nelson, R.J. & Penn, D.J. (2008). Genetic resistance to infection influences a male's sexual attractiveness and modulation of testosterone. *Brain Behav. Immun.* Vol.22. No.3. (March 2008), pp. 381-387. ISSN: 0889-1591.

12

Modulation of Immune Senescence by Menopause and Hormone Therapy

Flora Engelmann[1], Mark Asquith[1] and Ilhem Messaoudi[1,2,3]
[1]*Vaccine and Gene Therapy Institute,*
Oregon Health and Science University, Portland, OR
[2] *Division of Pathobiology and Immunology,*
Oregon National Primate Research Center, Beaverton, OR
[3]*Molecular Microbiology and Immunology,*
Oregon Health and Science University, Portland, OR
USA

1. Introduction

The immune system must overcome daily challenges from pathogens to protect the body from infection. The success of the immune response to infection relies on the ability to sense and evaluate microbial threats and coordinate their elimination - all the while limiting damage to host tissues. This delicate balance is achieved through coordinated action of innate and adaptive arms of the immune system. The main distinguishing characteristic of these two branches of the immune response is the way they recognize antigens. Whereas innate immunity relies on germline-encoded receptors to sense the presence of pathogens, adaptive immunity employs a highly diverse set of receptors generated through somatic mutation and recombination that are tailored to specific pathogens. The second major defining characteristic of the adaptive immune system is the development of immunological memory that manifests with increased functionality and frequency of responding cells upon re-exposure to the same antigen.

Several immune cell subsets play a critical role in mediating innate immune responses. These include neutrophils, natural killer (NK) cells, dendritic cells (DC), and macrophages. These cells are alerted to the presence of pathogens via recognition of microbial non-self, missing self, or altered self (Medzhitov and Janeway 2002). Recognition of microbial entities relies on the detection of conserved molecular patterns referred to as pathogen-associated molecular patterns (PAMPs) by pattern recognition receptors (PRRs) of the innate immune system. The three best-characterized families of PRRs are the toll-like receptors (TLR), the NOD-Like Receptors (NLR) and the retinoic acid-inducible gene (RIG-I)-like RNA helicases (RLHs). Following PAMP encounter, these receptors initiate signaling cascades that drive production of several anti-microbial molecules that ultimately limit pathogen replication and spread. Furthermore innate immune cells activate the adaptive arm of the immune system through the action of soluble mediators and antigen processing and presentation (Kabelitz and Medzhitov 2007; Medzhitov 2007).

DCs can be divided into myeloid (mDC) also known as conventional DCs and plasmacytoid DCs (pDCs) (Sallusto and Lanzavecchia 1994; Olweus, BitMansour et al.

1997). Myeloid DCs detect pathogens via TLR-3, -4, -7, and -8 and respond to infection by upregulating surface expression of CD40 and CD86 and producing IL-12 (Ketloy, Engering et al. 2008). Their main function is to process and present pathogen-derived peptides to naïve T cells (Siegal, Kadowaki et al. 1999). On the other hand, pDCs recognize viral DNA and RNA via TLR-7 and TLR-9 and produce vast amounts of type I interferons, which are potent antiviral cytokines, such as interferon α (IFNα) in response to viral infection (Cella, Jarrossay et al. 1999; Teleshova, Kenney et al. 2004; Chung, Amrute et al. 2005; Ketloy, Engering et al. 2008).

NK cells mediate the recognition of missing and altered self through the expression of inhibitory and activation receptors (Christopher E. Andoniou 2008). These receptors are member of either the immunoglobulin-like superfamily (IgSF) or the C-type lectin-like receptor (CTLR) superfamily (Radaev and Sun 2003). Recognition of MHC class I molecules is mediated by killer inhibitory receptors (KIR) such as CD94/NKG2 heterodimers/complexes, which deliver an inhibitory signal to NK cells (Biron, Nguyen et al. 1999; Biassoni 2008). Some viruses down-regulate MHC class I molecules to evade detection by CD8 T cells (discussed later). However, NK cells that do not receive a signal through inhibitory receptors receive an activation signal and can eliminate the infected cells (Biassoni 2008). Cell damage and some additional viral infections can also result in the upregulation of stress-induced molecules such as MIC-A, MIC-B, and ULBPs (Radaev and Sun 2003). These altered self-molecules function as ligands for NK cell activating receptors such as NKG2D (Radaev and Sun 2003; Biassoni 2008). NK cells can be subdivided based on the expression of CD16 (Lanier 2008). The majority of blood and spleen resident NK cells are $CD16^{pos}$ (85-90%); they are highly cytotoxic and secrete moderate amounts of inflammatory cytokines (Werner Held 2008). The $CD16^{neg}$ NK cells cannot kill target cells but they secrete large amounts of inflammatory cytokines.

Neutrophils and macrophages play a critical role in the elimination of pathogens via phagocytosis. Neutrophils are short-lived cells that are recruited by a chemotactic gradient into infected/inflamed tissues where they then phagocytose bacteria (Svanborg, Godaly et al. 1999). Neutrophils can also kill bacteria by respiratory burst, the release of reactive oxygen species (Dahlgren and Karlsson 1999), or the release of antimicrobials (Medzhitov 2003). Neutrophils are required for the clearance of bacteria from mucosal sites (Svanborg, Godaly et al. 1999). Macrophages also play a critical role in elimination of pathogens via phagocytosis, pinocytosis, or receptor-mediated endocytosis (Aderem and Underhill 1999). As described for DCs, macrophages express several PRRs, notably TLR 4 (Aderem and Underhill 1999). Activation of PRRs on macrophages activates the release of intracellular antimicrobial molecules (Linehan, Martinez-Pomares et al. 2000) as well as inflammatory cytokines such as IL-6, IL-8, and TNFα (Larsson, Larsson et al. 1999; Beutler 2000). Like DCs, macrophages can also stimulate lymphocytes and initiate the development of the adaptive immune response (Beutler 2000).

The adaptive immune branch is composed of B and T lymphocytes, which unlike cells of the innate immune system can generate a response tailored specifically to each pathogen. This specificity is acquired through the expression of diverse, clonally distributed antigen receptors on T and B cells. The initial diversity is produced in primary lymphoid organs (the thymus in the case of T cells and the bone marrow in the case of B cells) through a series of gene recombination events; further diversification occurs by somatic hypermutation of the B-cell receptor (BCR, antibody) and by functional diversification of effector T cells.

T cells are broadly divided into αβ CD4 and CD8 T cells (90%) as well as γδ T cells (10%). T cells recognize antigens in the form of small peptides bound to major histocompatibility (MHC) class I or class II molecules. CD8 T cells, commonly known as cytotoxic T cells, recognize foreign peptide bound to MHC-I molecules and have evolved to monitor for and eliminate tumor cells and cells harboring intracellular pathogens. CD4 T cells, or helper T cells, recognize foreign peptides bound to MHC-II and secrete a broad range of cytokines, which play a crucial role in the maturation of the B cell response as well as the development and establishment of the CD8 T cell response. Once activated, CD4 T cells can differentiate into four major lineages, Th1, Th2, Th17, and regulatory (Treg) cells. These subsets can be distinguished by their unique cytokine production profiles and their functions: Th1 cells predominantly produce IFNγ and mediate responses to intracellular viral and bacterial pathogens; Th2 cells produce IL-4, IL-5, IL-9, IL-13, and IL-25 and are critical for expelling extracellular parasites such as helminths; Th17 cells are responsible for controlling extracellular bacteria and fungi through their production of IL-17a, IL-17f, and IL-22; Treg cells are important in maintaining immune tolerance, as well as in regulating lymphocyte homeostasis, activation and function and produce regulatory cytokines TGFβ and IL-10 (Zhu and Paul 2010).

The maintenance of a structurally and functionally diverse T cell repertoire is a dynamic process governed by thymic output and the exposure to antigen and cytokines, which modulate T cell survival, proliferation and death. A rigorous analysis developed over several years has demonstrated that human CD4 and CD8 T cells can be subdivided into naïve, central memory (CM) and effector memory (EM) in addition to several transitional subsets (Lanzavecchia and Sallusto 2005). Studies have identified IL-7 and IL-15 as key players in T cell homeostasis (Surh and Sprent 2008). IL-7 and MHC contact are critical for the survival of naïve T cells (Jared F. Purton 2007). These signals do not induce differentiation but rather a low level of homeostatic proliferation and promote the survival of these cells. Memory T cells on the other hand, do not require MHC contact for survival (Boyman, Purton et al. 2007), but do require both IL-7 and IL-15 (Purton, Tan et al. 2007).

Upon antigen encounter, naïve antigen-specific B cells quickly differentiate into short-lived plasma cells that can immediately produce antibodies while others travel to germinal centers to undergo the longer process of becoming memory cells and long-lived plasma cells (Tangye and Tarlinton 2009). B cells within the germinal centers undergo vigorous proliferation, isotype class switching (from IgM to IgG, IgA or IgE) and somatic hypermutation thereby differentiating into memory and plasma cells that produce high affinity antibodies (Tarlinton 1998). Naïve B cells express IgM and IgD and are induced to class switch by T cell produced cytokines (Chaplin 2010). For example, IL-10 and possibly IFN-γ induces switching to IgG, while IL-4 and IL-13 induce switching to IgE, and TGF-β to IgA (Chaplin 2010). Different antibody classes target different pathogens as a result of the activation of different T_H types. IgA are produced in response to infection of mucosal surfaces (Tiwari, Agrawal et al. 2010), IgE are important for allergic responses (Johansson) and IgG are critical for the anti-viral immune response. Long lived plasma cells continue to secrete antibodies well after antigen clearance while memory B can rapidly proliferate and differentiate into plasma cells upon antigen re-exposure (Tangye and Tarlinton 2009). B cells are also capable of T cell independent activation by polymeric antigens with a repeating structure such as LPS. However somatic mutation does not usually occur in this process and immune response tends to be weak (Chaplin 2010).

2. Gender and the immune response to infection/vaccination

The incidence and severity of several viral diseases is higher in men than women (Klein 2010). For instance, coxsackie virus associated myocarditis occurs more often in men than women (Woodruff 1980). These gender differences were recapitulated by a murine infection model, where pro-inflammatory cytokines TNFα and IL-1β are induced more strongly in male mice, resulting in the increased recruitment and accumulation of macrophages in the heart and the subsequent development of myocarditis (Huber and Pfaeffle 1994; Huber, Kupperman et al. 1999; Huber 2005). Adult women also generate a more robust cell mediated response following cytomegalovirus (CMV) infection with higher IFNγ and IL-2 production (Villacres, Longmate et al. 2004), a stronger humoral response to Epstein Barr virus (EBV) (Wagner, Hornef et al. 1994), and a better immune response to herpes simplex virus (HSV)-1 and 2 than men (Han, Lundberg et al. 2001). During human immune deficiency virus (HIV) infection pre-menopausal women have higher CD4 lymphocyte counts throughout infection and lower viral loads early during infection than men (van Benthem, Vernazza et al. 2002). Moreover, HIV+ women have higher levels of CD8+ T cell activation than men with equivalent viral loads (Meier, Chang et al. 2009). Similarly, female mice generate more robust immune responses and are better protected following infection with vesicular stomatitis virus and picornavirus (Curiel, Miller et al. 1993; Barna, Komatsu et al. 1996)

It is now well recognized that men experience greater morbidity and mortality due to bacterial infection and sepsis after trauma than women (reviewed by Marriott et al. (Marriott and Huet-Hudson 2006)). Moreover, more men develop severe septic shock than women (Schroder, Kahlke et al. 1998; Schroder, Kahlke et al. 2000; Wichmann, Inthorn et al. 2000). Similarly, male gender is a risk factor for major infections after surgery (Offner, Moore et al. 1999). The notion that males are more vulnerable to bacterial infections than females is supported by animal studies. *Mycobacterium marinum* infection in male mice results in higher bacterial burden and worse disease outcome than females (Yamamoto, Saito et al. 1991). Male rats also experience higher mortality than females following intravenous injection of LPS (Merkel, Alexander et al. 2001). Similar findings were reported in mice models of sepsis (Zellweger, Wichmann et al. 1997; Diodato, Knoferl et al. 2001). This gender difference in survival is most likely mediated by a difference in cytokine production. Whereas male patients produced higher levels of the inflammatory cytokines TNFα and IL-6 during sepsis, females produced higher levels of the regulatory cytokine IL-10 (Schroder, Kahlke et al. 1998; Offner, Moore et al. 1999).

Parasitic infections also show a strong sex bias with higher prevalence of infection and disease severity in men compared to women (Klein 2004). This increased resistance seems to be mediated by a gender difference in T cell polorization. Female mice generate a Th1 response following infection with *Plasmodium brasiliensis* whereas males produce a Th2 response (Pinzan, Ruas et al. 2010). Moreover, when castrated male mice are treated with 17ß estradiol (E2), their spleen cells produced higher levels of IFNγ and lower levels of IL-10 following stimulation with *P. brasiliensis* compared to control males (Pinzan, Ruas et al. 2010). Similarly, ovariectomized (OVX) mice treated with E2 produced higher levels of IFNγ and IL-10 (associated with a protective response) as well as higher antibody responses after *Plasmodium chabaudi* infection compared to OVX mice treated with placebo (Klein, Easterbrook et al. 2008). OVX mice receiving E2 also experienced less weight and hematocrit loss, as well as less hypothermia following malaria infection than OVX mice receiving placebo (Klein, Easterbrook et al. 2008). Finally, E2 treatment induces resistance to *Toxoplasma gondii* infection in both female and male mice (Klein 2004). These data are consistent with the hypothesis that estrogen promotes a protective Th1 response following parasitic infections.

As described for infections, women also generate a more robust response to most vaccines as evidenced by higher rates of seroconversion and lower rates of disease after vaccination than men (Cook 2008; Klein, Jedlicka et al. 2010) as well as higher plasma levels of immunoglobulins than men (Ansar Ahmed, Penhale et al. 1985). In an influenza vaccine trial, participants aged 18-49 were given either a full or half dose of vaccine. Women who received a half dose developed an equivalent antibody response as men who received the full dose of vaccine (Engler, Nelson et al. 2008). Similarly, vaccines against HSV-2 also show sex differences in immunogenicity and efficacy. Early vaccine formulations showed some protection in women (26%) and no protection in men (4%) (Corey, Langenberg et al. 1999). More recent subunit vaccines expressing glycoprotein D resulted in 73 to 74% protection in HSV negative women while protection in men remained negligible (11%) (Stanberry, Spruance et al. 2002; Bernstein, Aoki et al. 2005).

2.1 Mechanisms of action of female sex hormomes

The mechanisms by which ovarian steroids modulate the immune response are beginning to emerge. Several lines of evidence suggest that E2 enhances the immune response whereas progesterone dampens it. For instance, prolonged exposure to progesterone in the form of the contraceptive Depo-Provera (Depo) increases susceptibility of female mice to HSV-2 genital infection (Gillgrass, Ashkar et al. 2003) and of female nonhuman primates to *Chlamydia trachomatis* (Kaushic, Murdin et al. 1998), SIV (Marx, Spira et al. 1996) and SHIV (Trunova, Tsai et al. 2006). Clinical studies also found associations between Depo use and increased chlamydia, HSV-2, HIV and HPV incidence in adult women (Marx, Spira et al. 1996; Baeten, Nyange et al. 2001; Brabin 2002; Morrison, Richardson et al. 2007). In contrast to Depo treatment, E2 administration to ovariectomized (OVX) female mice protected them from HSV-2 infection (Gillgrass, Fernandez et al. 2005). Similarly, female rhesus macaques treated with estrogen were protected from SIV transmission (Smith, Baskin et al. 2000). Interestingly, vaccination studies in humans indicate that vaginal immunizations might be more effective for induction of genital tract antibodies if performed during the mid-follicular phase of the menstrual cycle when estrogen levels are highest (Kozlowski, Williams et al. 2002).

Estrogen and progesterone can directly modulate T and B cell function or indirectly impact their function by modifying the function of innate immune cells such as DCs, or a combination of both. There are two types of nuclear estrogen receptors (ER): α and β, which form homo and heterodimers (Kovats and Agrawal 2010). The expression of ERα has been reported on lymphocytes, DCs, macrophages, monocytes, NK cells, and mast cells (Suenaga, Evans et al. 1998; Komi and Lassila 2000; Curran, Berghaus et al. 2001; Grimaldi, Cleary et al. 2002; Mor, Sapi et al. 2003; Paharkova-Vatchkova, Maldonado et al. 2004; Phiel, Henderson et al. 2005; Harkonen and Vaananen 2006). The level of expression differs between immune cell types. For instance, CD4 T cells express higher amounts of ERα than ERβ while the inverse expression profile is observed in B cells (Phiel, Henderson et al. 2005). CD8 T cells and monocytes express only low amounts of both receptor types (Phiel, Henderson et al. 2005). This difference in ER expression levels is likely to result in differential modulation of the of these immune cells by estradiol.

Progesterone receptors (PR) are not as ubiquitous as ERs and no nuclear PR have been detected in peripheral blood mononuclear cells (PBMC) (Kovats and Agrawal 2010). T cells do however express membrane bound progesterone receptors α and β (Dosiou, Hamilton et al. 2008). The expression of PRα is also upregulated on CD8+ T cells during the luteal phase of the menstrual cycle (Dosiou, Hamilton et al. 2008). Adding to the complexity of the effects of sex steroids, PR are primarily induced by estrogen via ER, thus creating an intricate interaction between these two hormones (Kovats and Agrawal 2010). NK cells and monocytes are the only other immune cell types known to express PRs (Kovats and Agrawal 2010). Both ER and PR function as transcription factors by binding to estrogen and progesterone responsive elements upon ligation or by binding to other transcription factors (Kovats and Agrawal 2010).

Estrogen treatment of B cells increases the expression of the anti-apoptotic molecule Bcl-2 thereby potentially increasing the resistance of auto-reactive B cells to apoptosis (Evans, MacLaughlin et al. 1997; Verthelyi and Ahmed 1998; Rider, Jones et al. 2001). Estrogen also enhances B cell activation (Paavonen, Andersson et al. 1981), IgG production (Kanda and Tamaki 1999), and upregulates activation-induced deaminase (AID), thereby enhancing somatic hypermutation frequency and class-switch recombination, resulting in greater antibody affinity-maturation (Karpuzoglu and Zouali 2011). In vitro studies examining the effect of E2 on T cell proliferation and cytokine production have often yielded contradictory results when using PBMC (Bouman, Heineman et al. 2005) although some observations do suggest a potential bias towards Th2, Th17 (Polanczyk, Hopke et al. 2006) and Treg polarization in E2 treated T cell cultures (Khan, Dai et al. 2010).

Several studies have demonstrated the modulation of innate immunity by estrogen. E2 regulates TLR2 expression on lipopolysaccharide (LPS) stimulated microglial cells *in vivo* after both intracerebral and systemic LPS injection (Soucy, Boivin et al. 2005). A recent study showed that presence of estrogen related receptor ERRα on macrophages was required for IFNγ production and efficient clearance of *Listeria monocytogenes* (Sonoda, Laganiere et al. 2007). Moreover, E2 administration significantly increases mRNA for the inflammatory cytokines IL-1β, IL-6, and TNFα as well as inducible NO synthase in thioglycate-elicited macrophages from OVX mice(Calippe, Douin-Echinard et al. 2010). This mechanism was ERα dependant (Calippe, Douin-Echinard et al. 2010). Human dendritic cells matured in the presence of E2 and TNFα, but not TNFα alone, promote the differentiation of naïve CD4 T cells into Th2 cells (Uemura, Liu et al. 2008). However, E2 treatment may limit the capacity of mature DC to stimulate T cell proliferation (Segerer, Muller et al. 2009). Mouse pDCs stimulated with CpG in the presence of E2 have higher expression of the co-stimulatory molecules CD40 and CD86 as well as higher IFN-α production (Li, Xu et al. 2009). When co-cultured with B cells, these E2 treated pDCs increase B cell viability, but as described for T cells above, not proliferative capacity (Li, Xu et al. 2009). Similarly, in vitro stimulation of PBMC with HIV-1 antigens which stimulate pDC via binding to TLR-7 resulted in higher IFNα production by women than by men (Meier, Chang et al. 2009). In contrast to these data, progesterone treatment reduces the ability of dendritic cells to take up antigenic peptides, stimulate T cell responses (Butts, Shukair et al. 2007), and secrete the potent antiviral cytokine IFNα (Hughes, Thomas et al. 2008).

3. Immune senescence

Increasing age results in a gradual erosion of immune function that is commonly referred as "immune senescence" (Larbi, Franceschi et al. 2008). This age-related loss of immune fitness is believed to result in greater morbidity and mortality from infection in this age group.

Immuno-senescent changes have been described for both innate and adaptive immunity. Specifically, circulating monocyte numbers are increased in the elderly, although circulating neutrophil numbers remain unaltered (Chatta, Andrews et al. 1993; Born, Uthgenannt et al. 1995; Lord, Butcher et al. 2001; Della Bella, Bierti et al. 2007). This may reflect the skewing of bone marrow hematopoietic stem cell (HSC) progenitors in the elderly towards the myeloid lineage (Beerman, Bhattacharya et al. 2010). Nonetheless, age-related decreases in circulating mDC numbers have been reported (Della Bella, Bierti et al. 2007). In addition, aged myeloid cells exhibit hyporesponsiveness to several innate stimuli, which may reflect reduced expression of PRR and their downstream signaling mediators, or increased negative regulation of these pathways (Dunston and Griffiths 2010; Shaw, Joshi et al. 2010). Furthermore, innate immune function may be compromised by diminished phagocytic activity in the elderly (Wenisch, Patruta et al. 2000; Lloberas and Celada 2002), compounded by reduced superoxide production and intracellular killing ability in the case of Gram-positive bacteria (Lord, Butcher et al. 2001). Some reports have suggested that although NK cell numbers are conserved with age (Tarazona 2009), there is a decrease in proliferation and cytokine production (Mocchegiani and Malavolta 2004; Murasko and Jiang 2005; Zhang, Wallace et al. 2007). Changes in NK cytotoxicity with age are somewhat controversial with some studies showing a decrease while others show no change (Tarazona 2009). Preserved NK cytotoxicity is associated with lower infection and mortality rates and better vaccine response in the elderly (Ogata, Yokose et al. 1997; Mysliwska, Trzonkowski et al. 2004). Moreover, aging is associated with an increase in $CD56^{dim}$ NK cells which are cytotoxic and a decrease in $CD56^{bright}$ cells which are immuno-regulatory (Borrego, Alonso et al. 1999). Age-related changes in frequency and function of innate immune cells impact the protective immune response by decreasing anti-bacterial function as well as by impacting antigen presentation and the generation of adaptive immunity in the elderly.

Although, it is clear that aging affects innate immune function, accumulating evidence indicate that the adaptive arm of the immune system, and more specifically in the T cell compartment, exhibits more profound and consistent changes than the innate arm (Pawelec, Larbi et al. 2009). The hallmarks of T cell senescence include: 1) loss of naïve T cells and accumulation of memory T cells; 2) reduced CD4:CD8 T cell ratio; 3) increased T cell production of inflammatory cytokines; and 4) reduced T cell proliferative ability. Several phenomena are believed to contribute to these changes. Decreased production of hematopoietic stem cells in the bone marrow leads to decreased migration of early T cell progenitors to the thymus, which in turn leads to thymic atrophy and a decline in naïve T cell production (Chen 2004). Other factors that contribute to naïve T cell loss include accelerated conversion of naïve T cells into memory T cells due to increased turnover (Naylor, Li et al. 2005), and a life-long exposure to chronic/persistent viruses, notably CMV (Pawelec, Derhovanessian et al. 2009). The loss of naïve T cells is accompanied by a concomitant increase in memory T cell number/frequency, especially terminally differentiated T cells. These cells preferentially accumulate within the CD8 T cell subset where they can reach significant proportions in the aged (Vallejo 2005; Sansoni, Vescovini et al. 2008) and can often be oligoclonal (expressing a single T cell receptor) (Schwab, Szabo et al. 1997). These T cell clonal expansions (TCE) are often CMV-specific and may play a role in controlling CMV viral burden (Derhovanessian, Larbi et al. 2009), but high frequencies of terminally differentiated T cells have also been associated with the poor responses to influenza vaccines (Saurwein-Teissl, Lung et al. 2002; Trzonkowski, Mysliwska et al. 2003) and increased inflammation (Vallejo, Weyand et al. 2004).

Both quantitative and qualitative changes in the B cell compartment have been reported with age. The frequency of B cells decreases with age (Huppert, Solomou et al. 1998; Colonna-Romano, Bulati et al. 2003). More importantly, there is a consistent reduction in the antibody response to infection and vaccination. For instance, 25% of persons over the age of 65 fail to develop a neutralizing antibody response following influenza vaccination, whereas 90% of adults aged 25 to 45 successfully do so (Beyer, Palache et al. 1989). This decline was also reported in response to other vaccines such as hepatitis B (Cook, Gualde et al. 1987) and A (D'Acremont, Herzog et al. 2006; Genton, D'Acremont et al. 2006). It was initially proposed that reduced B cell function is due to diminished CD4 T cell help. However, accumulating evidence points to the fact that there are intrinsic defects within the B cell compartment independent of the CD4 helper function. One of the possible intrinsic B cell deficiencies is that isotype class switching and/affinity maturation is compromised in the elderly (Aydar, Balogh et al. 2004; Frasca, Riley et al. 2004; Cancro, Hao et al. 2009). Another contributing factor to the decreased B cell response in the elderly is the reduction in the B cell repertoire. As described for T cells, B cell clonal expansions are detected with greater frequency in the elderly and could potentially interfere in the development of a protective immune response by constricting the proliferative burst, establishment of new memory B cell population or reducing naïve B cell output (LeMaoult, Delassus et al. 1997; LeMaoult, Szabo et al. 1997; LeMaoult, Manavalan et al. 1999; Weksler and Szabo 2000; Szabo, Li et al. 2004).

Last but not least, immune senescence is associated with the upregulation of circulating pro-inflammatory cytokines, notably IL-6 and TNFα and to a lesser extent IL-1β (De Martinis, Franceschi et al. 2005; Wikby, Nilsson et al. 2006). Increased production of chemokines such as RANTES, MIP-1a,α IL-8 and MCP-1 was also reported (Gerli, Monti et al. 2000; Pulsatelli, Meliconi et al. 2000; Mariani, Pulsatelli et al. 2002). This chronic inflammatory state has been correlated with overall mortality rate and is believed to significantly contribute to the development of age-related diseases such as Alzheimer's, atherosclerosis, sarcopenia, diabetes, rheumatoid arthritis and certain types of cancer (Vasto, Candore et al. 2007).

4. Menopause and hormone therapy regimens

In women, aging is accompanied by a dramatic loss in ovarian function and subsequent menopause around the age of 51. Thus, with the average life span of ~80 years, women can expect to spend a significant portion of their lives in a post-menopausal state (Hall 2004). The endocrine changes associated with entry into menopause appear to be driven by the age-related depletion of follicular reserve, which leads to a failure to produce the hormonal support necessary to maintain levels of inhibin B. The decrease in inhibin B production results in deregulated production of follicular stimulating hormone (FSH), which in turn results in altered estrogen production and eventually a decrease in the levels of circulating estrogen (Wu, Zelinski et al. 2005; Burger, Hale et al. 2008). This diminished responsiveness results in a cycle that culminates in menopause.

Menopause not only affects women's fertility, but also exacerbates several age-related diseases such as osteoporosis, cardiovascular disease, loss of cognitive abilities and the incidence of some cancers (Prior 1998; Grady 2006). Interestingly, some of these diseases, notably osteoporosis and atherosclerosis correlate with increased inflammatory cytokine production (Ginaldi, Di Benedetto et al. 2005), thereby establishing a complex interaction between immune senescence and menopause. However, few studies have investigated the impact of menopause and hormone therapy on immune senescence.

There are three basic forms of hormone replacement therapy (HRT): 1) unopposed estrogen therapy; 2) sequentially combined HRT (scHRT) where estrogens are taken daily and; 3) progesterone or progestins are taken intermittently, and continuous combined HRT (ccHRT) where both hormones are taken daily. Estrogen administration can be accomplished orally via tablets, or transdermally through a variety of vehicles including patches, creams, and vaginal inserts. Estrogen is most commonly prescribed as conjugated equine estrogens (CEE) in the U.S. (Nelson HD 2007), but other forms such as synthetic conjugated estrogens, estradiol estropipate, esterified estrogen, and ethinylestradiol are gaining in popularity. The method of delivery is often determined by the target symptoms and patient preference. Progesterones can be prescribed as progesterone or as a wide array of synthetic congeners or progestins.

Treatment of postmenopausal symptoms with estrogen began in the 1940's (Nelson HD 2007). In the 1970's progesterone was added to regimens when a link was made between unopposed estrogen treatment and endometrial cancer (Smith, Prentice et al. 1975; Ziel and Finkle 1975). In the 1980's estrogen began to be prescribed as a prophylactic against osteoporosis when it was shown to reduce fractures (Weiss, Ure et al. 1980; Kiel, Felson et al. 1987) and was thought to be potentially beneficial against other chronic illnesses such as heart disease and dementia (Bluming and Tavris 2009). A sharp decline in prescription of HRT occurred after the termination of the combination estrogen-progestin therapy arm of the Women's Health Initiative (WHI) in 2002 (Hing and Brett 2006). Since 2002 the WHI has made a number of updated reports warning of the dangers of HRT, however careful review of the data reveals these dangers are largely unfounded in most women (Bluming and Tavris 2009). The only conclusive danger is that of an increased cardiac risk in women over the age 60 taking HRT for the first time, and only for the first year (Bluming and Tavris 2009). There is no conclusive evidence that exogenous estrogens increase the risk of breast cancer (Bluming and Tavris 2009).

5. Impact of menopause on immune cell function

In contrast to the plethora of studies examining the effect of hormone therapy on cardiovascular disease, bone metabolism and breast cancer, very few studies have examined the effects of menopause and HRT on immunological parameters. Given that female sex hormones modulate immune response to infection in young women and animal models, it has been hypothesized that that the loss of ovarian steroids during menopause could exacerbate immune senescence (Gameiro and Romao 2010; Gameiro, Romao et al. 2010; Rehman and Masson 2005). This hypothesis is supported by the observation that rhinovirus infection induces a higher IFNγ and IL-13 response in women than men, however this sex difference is no longer detected after the age of 50 (Carroll, Yerkovich et al. 2010). Similarly, hepatitis vaccines induce higher antibody titers and seroconversion rates in adult women, but this gender difference is no longer evident in vaccinees over the age of 60 (Klein, Jedlicka et al. 2010). The incidence of herpes zoster is also higher in women 50 years of age and older compared to males (Chapman, Cross et al. 2003; Fleming, Cross et al. 2004).

The mechanisms underlying these observations are being examined in rodent and nonhuman primate models where menopause was induced surgically via bilateral removal of the ovaries (ovariectomy). This approach allows the investigation of the impact of menopause without the confounding factor of age. In adult female rats, ovariectomy resulted in decreased chemotaxis (migration in response to chemokine gradients) and LPS-induced proliferation by leukocytes as well as decreased NK cell lysis, suggestive of premature immunosenescence (Baeza, De Castro et al. 2011). More recently, studies from the same group showed that ovariectomy results in increased oxidative damage and inflammatory cytokine production by peritoneal macrophages (Baeza, De Castro et al. 2011).

Similarly, in a mouse model of HSV-2 challenge, ovariectomy resulted in a reduced response to HSV vaccine and ovariectomized female mice experienced the same rate of vaginal infection as unvaccinated controls following challenge (Pennock, Stegall et al. 2009). E2 treatment of control or OVX mice enhanced protection and decreased disease severity (Pennock, Stegall et al. 2009). Interestingly, antibody titers in E2 treated mice were not significantly higher than those observed in untreated mice, but the neutralization potential was significantly improved (Pennock, Stegall et al. 2009).

We have also recently shown that ovariectomy results in several changes in T cell homeostasis in the female rhesus macaque and that these changes were in part modulated by the age at which ovariectomy was perfomed (Engelmann, Barron et al. 2010). Young adult OVX rhesus macaques had a higher frequency of CD4 naïve T cells, whereas OVX aged female rhesus macaques had an increased frequency of terminally differentiated CD4 memory T cells. Moreover, in contrast to young adult females, OVX aged female rhesus macaques showed increased inflammatory cytokine production by T cells compared to intact aged animals. These data suggest that ovariectomy may accelerate some aspects of immune senescence in aged but not young female rhesus macaques. More importantly, both adult and aged OVX animals generated a reduced T and B cell response to vaccination compared to ovary-intact females. Specifically, T and B cell proliferative bursts were delayed and reduced in magnitude in OVX animals. Consequently IgG titers and frequency of IFNγ+ T cells were significantly reduced in OVX animals (Engelmann, Barron et al. 2010). Thus, as described in rodent models, loss of ovarian steroids results in diminished T cell responses to vaccination/infection in nonhuman primates but the mechanisms underlying this reduced immune response remain unclear. The exacerbation of immune senescence by menopause is likely mediated by changes in immune cell frequencies as well as functions discussed in the sections below.

6. Impact of menopause and hormone therapy on immune cell frequency

As reviewed earlier, aging leads to several perturbations in the frequency of several immune cell subsets. However, the contribution of menopause to those changes is not entirely clear. Some studies have reported a significant decline in total lymphocyte numbers (Giglio, Imro et al. 1994), while others report no change (Kamada, Irahara et al. 2000). Women receiving HRT were reported to have higher lymphocyte numbers than post-menopausal women not using HRT within one to six months following treatment (Kamada, Irahara et al. 2000). Peripheral blood monocytes increase after menopause (Ben-Hur, Mor et al. 1995) but the number of tissue specific macrophages in the ovary diminish (Best, Pudney et al. 1996; Katabuchi, Suenaga et al. 1997). HRT can restore the levels of circulating monocytes to levels seen in cycling women (Ben-Hur, Mor et al. 1995).

One of the most conserved age-related changes is the decrease in the percentage of naïve T cells and the accumulation of memory T cells. There is a significant decrease in naïve T cells and an increase in memory and activated T cells between early and late menopause and the use of HRT has no effect on these changes (Fahlman, Boardley et al. 2000; Kamada, Irahara et al. 2000; Yang, Chen et al. 2000), suggesting that chronological age has a more significant impact on the loss of naïve T cells than menopause. Another hallmark of T cell senescence is a reduced CD4/CD8 ratio (Larbi, Franceschi et al. 2008). Data from a few studies suggest that menopause decreases the CD4/CD8 ratio by reducing the frequency of CD4 T cells (Gameiro and Romao 2010; Giglio, Imro et al. 1994). Since women of reproductive age have more CD4 T cells and respond more vigorously to infection/vaccination than men (Tollerud, Clark et al. 1989; Maini, Gilson et al. 1996), menopause-associated loss of CD4 T cells could be one of the mechanisms by which ovarian senescence contributes to immune senescence.

Total B cell numbers also decline with age and with menopause (Giglio, Imro et al. 1994). B cells can be broadly divided into B1 and B2 cells and their frequency is altered with increasing age (Weksler and Szabo 2000). B1 cells produce predominantly non-specific binding IgM whereas B2 cells, or conventional B cells are involved in the adaptive humoral immune response. The reduction in B cell numbers through menopause appears to be isolated to the B2 cells, which are significantly lower in late menopause compared to early and perimenopause (Kamada, Irahara et al. 2001). Furthermore, B2 cells are significantly higher in HT users than non-users (Kamada, Irahara et al. 2001). These studies suggest that menopause leads to a reduced humoral response and this change can potentially explain the disappearance of sex differences in antibody responses following infection and vaccination (Carroll, Yerkovich et al. 2010; Engler, Nelson et al. 2008; Klein, Jedlicka et al. 2010).

Similarly, oopherectomy results in a decrease in circulating B cells, CD4/CD8 ratio, and an increase in the percentage of NK cells in adult women (Kumru, Godekmerdan et al. 2004). Similarly, surgical menopause leads to increased NK cell frequencies (Giglio, Imro et al. 1994). All these changes are hallmarks of immune senescence and suggest that loss of ovarian steroids exacerbates aging of the immune system. Estrogen therapy reverses the decrease in CD4 and B cells and the increase in NK cells that is seen in patients who have undergone a hysterectomy (Giglio, Imro et al. 1994; Kumru, Godekmerdan et al. 2004). Similarly, combined hormone therapy reverses the age-related decrease in number of circulating B cells and T cell proliferative potential in post-menopausal women (Porter, Greendale et al. 2001) and leads to an increase in B2 B cells (Kamada, Irahara et al. 2001). Furthermore, estrogen has been shown to decrease the number of CD8 T cells in post-menopausal women thereby increasing the CD4/CD8 ratio (Holl, Donat et al. 2001).

7. Inflammation and menopause

It is well accepted that aging is accompanied by the establishment of a chronic proinflammatory state, notably via increased levels of IL-6 and TNFα (Krabbe, Pedersen et al. 2004; Vasto, Candore et al. 2007; Vasto, Carruba et al. 2009). This process is often referred to as inflamm-aging (Franceschi, Bonafe et al. 2000), and is associated with the development of several chronic diseases such as sarcopenia, Alzheimer's, osteoporosis and certain types of cancer (Kim, Chae et al. 2011; Giuliani, Sansoni et al. 2001; Yasui, Maegawa et al. 2007). The age related increase in IL-6 levels could in part be explained by the decline in sex hormones. Both IL-6 and soluble IL-6 receptor are significantly higher in postmenopausal than premenopausal women (Giuliani, Sansoni et al. 2001). Similarly, IL-6 production after *in vitro* stimulation also increases with age. More specifically, in vitro stimulation of PBMC with LPS results in higher production of IL-6 ,TNFα and IL-1β in women aged 52 to 63 compared to young adult women (Kim, Chae et al. 2011). Interestingly, IL-6 production by LPS stimulated PBMC is higher in women taking combined hormone therapy compared to nonusers, but not in post-menopausal women receiving unopposed estrogen (Brooks-Asplund, Tupper et al. 2002). Similarly, women receiving transdermal estrogen experienced a significant decrease in IL-6 serum levels three months after treatment compared to post-menopausal women who did not receive estradiol (Saucedo, Rico et al. 2002). Indeed, serum IL-6 levels show a negative correlation with serum estrogen levels in users (Saucedo, Rico et al. 2002) and in women spanning the transitional stages of menopause aged 40 to 65 years (Yasui, Maegawa et al. 2007).

A trend toward an increase in serum IFNγ levels is seen during early menopause (< 5 years post menopause) followed by a slight decrease in late menopause (Yasui, Maegawa et al. 2007). Similarly, IFNγ production in whole blood or PBMC in response to either PHA or LPS stimulation *in vitro*, begins to increase at around the age of 40 and peaks during early to mid menopause before again decreasing during late menopause (Deguchi, Kamada et al. 2001; Kamada, Irahara et al. 2001; Stopinska-Gluszak, Waligora et al. 2006). Previous *in vitro* studies have shown that estrogen has a biphasic effect on IFNγ production by LPS stimulated whole blood samples, with low estrogen levels stimulating and high levels inhibiting IFNγ production (Matalka 2003). Therefore, it is possible that the initial decrease in estrogen levels during early menopause stimulates an increase in IFNγ production, but during late menopause, estrogen levels become too low to have an effect (Goetzl, Huang et al. 2010). In support of this hypothesis, IFNγ serum levels decreased in women who have had a bilateral oopherectomy and increase once estrogen treatment is initiated (Kumru, Godekmerdan et al. 2004). On the other hand, combined hormone therapy is associated with lower IFNγ production possibly due to the opposing effect of progesterone (Deguchi, Kamada et al. 2001; Stopinska-Gluszak, Waligora et al. 2006)

A transient increase in serum IL-2 was described in women within the first five years of menopause and the data suggest a weak negative correlation with serum estrogen levels (Yasui, Maegawa et al. 2007). Similarly, IL-2 production following LPS stimulation of whole blood cultures increases with age, peaking during early menopause before declining (Deguchi, Kamada et al. 2001). HRT reduces plasma IL-2 levels as well as IL-2 production by T cells following stimulation of purified PBMC with PHA (Stopinska-Gluszak, Waligora et al. 2006). In contrast, transdermal administration of estrogen does not change IL-2 levels, probably because plasma levels achieved via this delivery route are too low to modulate T cell functions (Saucedo, Rico et al. 2002). IL-4 plasma levels were reported to increase after menopause and HT reverses this increase (Vural, Canbaz et al. 2006; Yasui, Maegawa et al. 2007). In PHA stimulated whole blood, IL-4 production increases in mid menopause and then becomes significantly lower in late menopause (Deguchi, Kamada et al. 2001). In contrast, oopherectomy decreases IL-4 levels and unopposed estrogen therapy does not affect this decrease (Kumru, Godekmerdan et al. 2004).

Menopause-induced changes in circulating levels of additional cytokines are controversial. Some studies reported an increase in TNFα and IL-1β after menopause that is reversed by HRT (Kamada, Irahara et al. 2001; Vural, Canbaz et al. 2006), while other studies reported no changes (Yasui, Maegawa et al. 2007). The impact of menopause on IL-10 and IL-12 is equally controversial with some studies reporting an increase (Deguchi, Kamada et al. 2001; Vural, Canbaz et al. 2006), while others report no change (Yasui, Maegawa et al. 2007) or a decrease in these cytokines (Kamada, Irahara et al. 2001). HRT and transdermal estrogen do not seem to have an impact on IL-10 levels (Saucedo, Rico et al. 2002; Vural, Canbaz et al. 2006). A negative correlation of IL-8 with estrogen level was reported in both humans and mice (Yasui, Maegawa et al. 2007; Abu-Taha, Rius et al. 2009).

8. Alternative approaches and their effect on immunity in post menopausal women

Alternative approaches for dealing with menopausal symptoms have gained significant interest in recent years. One of the most popular interventions is nutritional supplementation with estrogen-like substances that might not have the undesirable side effects of hormones. Dietary phyto-estrogens are organic compounds found in soy products, fruits and legumes (Huntley and Ernst 2004). It has been proposed that the beneficial effects of soybean compounds are mediated by isoflavones such as genistein since they show structural similarities to estradiol (Bingham, Atkinson et al. 1998).

Some rodent studies support a beneficial effect of isoflavones on immune function in post-menopausal animals. In mature ovariectomized female rats, nutritional supplementation with soybean or soybean and green tea improved chemotaxis, phagocytic index as well as the production of reactive oxygen species by peritoneal macrophages (Baeza, De Castro et al. 2010). This nutritional supplementation also improved T and B cell proliferative potential and NK cell killing (Baeza, De Castro et al. 2010). Similar results were reported for human (Zhang, Song et al. 1999) and murine (Guo, McCay et al. 2001) NK cells after exposure to another isoflavone, genistein. Genistein treatment of murine splenocytes in vitro increased IL-10 production thereby tilting the cytokine balance towards a Th2 response (Rachon, Rimoldi et al. 2006).

Post-menopausal women receiving a daily dose of 70mg of isoflavones either in the form of soy milk (700ml) or oral supplements for 16 weeks experienced an increase in the frequency of circulating B cells as well as a reduction in plasma concentrations of 8-hydroxy-2-deoxy-guanosine (8-OHdg), an oxidative damage marker (Ryan-Borchers, Park et al. 2006). No changes in the plasma levels of IL-2, IFNγ or TNFα were observed in this and a second study where women consumed comparable amount of soymilk (Beavers, Serra et al. 2009). However in an earlier study where women consumed 1064 ml of soymilk for 16 weeks, a decrease in plasma levels of TNFα and IL-1, but not IL-6, were detected (Huang, Cao et al. 2005). These data suggest that additional studies with a bigger range of doses in different populations of post-menopausal women need to be conducted in order to define dynamic ranges and individuals who stand to benefit the most from such nutritional interventions (Genazzani and Pluchino 2011).

Dehydroepiandrosterone (DHEA) is produced by the adrenal cortex and is the most abundant steroid in humans. Serum levels of DHEA and its sulfated conjugation product, DHEA sulfate (DHEAS), peak in men and women in the third decade and decrease progressively and profoundly with age. In the longitudinal Baltimore study, plasma levels of DHEAS emerged at the most consistent aging biomarker and correlated with longevity. In addition to its role as a precursor for androgens and estrogens, DHEA can exert a direct, physiologically relevant, agonistic effect on ERβ, a lesser antagonistic effect on androgen receptor, and a modest effect on ERα (Chen, Knecht et al. 2005). Therefore, DHEA supplementation has been explored as an alternative to classical hormone therapy. Early studies in aged mice, showed that age-related upregulation of IL-6 production could be effectively prevented and/or reversed by supplementing aging animals with DHEA (Daynes, Araneo et al. 1993). More importantly, either DHEA or DHEA sulfate supplementation promoted enhanced antibody responses against recombinant hepatitis B surface antigen by aged mice when incorporated directly into the vaccine (Araneo, Woods et al. 1993). In contrast to the rodent data, the effect of DHEA on the immune response to influenza vaccine in older humans is controversial. Earlier studies showed one oral dose of DHEAS before influenza vaccination was associated with a demonstrable increase in the number of individuals with a fourfold increase in hemagglutinin inhibition (HI) titers following vaccination (Araneo, Dowell et al. 1995). Similarly, one dose of DHEAS administered at the time of influenza vaccination appeared to enhance the HI titer in a small group of older adults with lower prevaccination titers and lower DHEAS concentrations (Degelau, Guay et al. 1997). In contrast, a 6-day course of DHEA treatment that began 2 days before vaccination did not improve the age-related declined response to immunization against influenza in human subjects (Danenberg, Ben-Yehuda et al. 1997). These results suggest additional detailed immunologic investigations on the role of DHEAS in the aging human immune response are warranted.

9. Conclusions and perspectives

A considerable body of data strongly suggests that sex hormones modulate immune function with estrogen having an immune stimulatory effect whereas progesterone an immune inhibitory effect. Aging results in several changes in both the immune and the endocrine systems. However the interplay between these two organ systems remains poorly understood. While it is clear that some changes (such as increased IL-6 levels) can be strongly attributed to loss of ovarian steroids, other changes such as lymphocyte function are not easily attributable to menopause. Moreover, the effects of hormone therapy on the post-menopausal immune system are controversial. The discrepancies between studies are in large part due to the variety of hormone replacement regimens available (conjugated equine estrogens, 17β estradiol, progestin), but also reflect the lack of consensus over which immune parameters are analyzed. As new safer hormone replacement therapies become available such as transdermal low levels of estradiol, the immune modulatory capacities of these treatments should be characterized. Future studies should also examine how changes in additional sex hormones such as FSH, LH and increased androgen production by the senescent ovary affect the immune system.

10. Acknowledgments

This work was supported by American Heart Association career development grant 0930234N, NIH R01AG037042, NIH P51 RR00163-51, the Center for Gender Based Medicine and the Brookdale Foundation. We would like to thank Kristen Haberthur and Dr. Delphine Malherbe for reviewing and editing this chapter.

11. References

Abu-Taha, M., C. Rius, et al. (2009). "Menopause and ovariectomy cause a low grade of systemic inflammation that may be prevented by chronic treatment with low doses of estrogen or losartan." J Immunol 183(2): 1393-402.

Aderem, A. and D. M. Underhill (1999). "Mechanisms of phagocytosis in macrophages." Annu Rev Immunol 17: 593-623.

Ansar Ahmed, S., W. J. Penhale, et al. (1985). "Sex hormones, immune responses, and autoimmune diseases. Mechanisms of sex hormone action." Am J Pathol 121(3): 531-51.

Araneo, B., T. Dowell, et al. (1995). "DHEAS as an effective vaccine adjuvant in elderly humans. Proof-of-principle studies." Ann N Y Acad Sci 774: 232-48.

Araneo, B. A., M. L. Woods, 2nd, et al. (1993). "Reversal of the immunosenescent phenotype by dehydroepiandrosterone: hormone treatment provides an adjuvant effect on the immunization of aged mice with recombinant hepatitis B surface antigen." J Infect Dis 167(4): 830-40.

Aydar, Y., P. Balogh, et al. (2004). "Follicular dendritic cells in aging, a "bottle-neck" in the humoral immune response." Ageing Res Rev 3(1): 15-29.

Baeten, J. M., P. M. Nyange, et al. (2001). "Hormonal contraception and risk of sexually transmitted disease acquisition: results from a prospective study." Am J Obstet Gynecol 185(2): 380-5.

Baeza, I., N. M. De Castro, et al. (2010). "Soybean and green tea polyphenols improve immune function and redox status in very old ovariectomized mice." Rejuvenation Res 13(6): 665-74.

Baeza, I., N. M. De Castro, et al. (2011). "Ovariectomy causes immunosenescence and oxi-inflamm-ageing in peritoneal leukocytes of aged female mice similar to that in aged males." Biogerontology 12(3): 227-38.

Baeza, I., N. M. De Castro, et al. (2010). "Ovariectomy, a model of menopause in rodents, causes a premature aging of the nervous and immune systems." J Neuroimmunol 219(1-2): 90-9.

Barna, M., T. Komatsu, et al. (1996). "Sex differences in susceptibility to viral infection of the central nervous system." J Neuroimmunol 67(1): 31-9.

Beavers, K. M., M. C. Serra, et al. (2009). "Soymilk supplementation does not alter plasma markers of inflammation and oxidative stress in postmenopausal women." Nutrition research (New York, N.Y.) 29(9): 616-622.

Beerman, I., D. Bhattacharya, et al. (2010). "Functionally distinct hematopoietic stem cells modulate hematopoietic lineage potential during aging by a mechanism of clonal expansion." Proc Natl Acad Sci U S A 107(12): 5465-70.

Ben-Hur, H., G. Mor, et al. (1995). "Menopause is associated with a significant increase in blood monocyte number and a relative decrease in the expression of estrogen receptors in human peripheral monocytes." Am J Reprod Immunol 34(6): 363-9.

Bernstein, D. I., F. Y. Aoki, et al. (2005). "Safety and immunogenicity of glycoprotein D-adjuvant genital herpes vaccine." Clin Infect Dis 40(9): 1271-81.

Best, C. L., J. Pudney, et al. (1996). "Localization and characterization of white blood cell populations within the human ovary throughout the menstrual cycle and menopause." Hum Reprod 11(4): 790-7.

Beutler, B. (2000). "Endotoxin, toll-like receptor 4, and the afferent limb of innate immunity." Curr Opin Microbiol 3(1): 23-8.

Beyer, W. E., A. M. Palache, et al. (1989). "Antibody induction by influenza vaccines in the elderly: a review of the literature." Vaccine 7(5): 385-94.

Biassoni, R. (2008). "Natural killer cell receptors." Adv Exp Med Biol 640: 35-52.

Bingham, S. A., C. Atkinson, et al. (1998). "Phyto-oestrogens: where are we now?" Br J Nutr 79(5): 393-406.

Biron, C. A., K. B. Nguyen, et al. (1999). "Natural killer cells in antiviral defense: function and regulation by innate cytokines." Annu Rev Immunol 17: 189-220.

Bluming, A. Z. and C. Tavris (2009). "Hormone replacement therapy: real concerns and false alarms." Cancer J 15(2): 93-104.

Born, J., D. Uthgenannt, et al. (1995). "Cytokine production and lymphocyte subpopulations in aged humans. An assessment during nocturnal sleep." Mech Ageing Dev 84(2): 113-26.

Borrego, F., M. C. Alonso, et al. (1999). "NK phenotypic markers and IL2 response in NK cells from elderly people." Exp Gerontol 34(2): 253-65.

Bouman, A., M. J. Heineman, et al. (2005). "Sex hormones and the immune response in humans." Hum Reprod Update 11(4): 411-23.

Boyman, O., J. F. Purton, et al. (2007). "Cytokines and T-cell homeostasis." Current Opinion in Immunology 19(3): 320-326.

Brabin, L. (2002). "Interactions of the female hormonal environment, susceptibility to viral infections, and disease progression." AIDS Patient Care STDS 16(5): 211-21.

Brooks-Asplund, E. M., C. E. Tupper, et al. (2002). "Hormonal modulation of interleukin-6, tumor necrosis factor and associated receptor secretion in postmenopausal women." Cytokine 19(4): 193-200.

Burger, H. G., G. E. Hale, et al. (2008). "Cycle and hormone changes during perimenopause: the key role of ovarian function." Menopause 15(4 Pt 1): 603-12.

Butts, C. L., S. A. Shukair, et al. (2007). "Progesterone inhibits mature rat dendritic cells in a receptor-mediated fashion." Int. Immunol. 19(3): 287-296.

Calippe, B., V. Douin-Echinard, et al. (2010). "17{beta}-Estradiol Promotes TLR4-Triggered Proinflammatory Mediator Production through Direct Estrogen Receptor {alpha} Signaling in Macrophages In Vivo." J Immunol 185(2): 1169-1176.

Cancro, M. P., Y. Hao, et al. (2009). "B cells and aging: molecules and mechanisms." Trends Immunol 30(7): 313-8.

Carroll, M. L., S. T. Yerkovich, et al. (2010). "Adaptive immunity to rhinoviruses: sex and age matter." Respir Res 11: 184.

Cella, M., D. Jarrossay, et al. (1999). "Plasmacytoid monocytes migrate to inflamed lymph nodes and produce large amounts of type I interferon [see comments]." Nat Med 5(8): 919-23.

Chaplin, D. D. (2010). "Overview of the immune response." J Allergy Clin Immunol 125(2 Suppl 2): S3-23.

Chapman, R. S., K. W. Cross, et al. (2003). "The incidence of shingles and its implications for vaccination policy." Vaccine 21(19-20): 2541-2547.

Chatta, G. S., R. G. Andrews, et al. (1993). "Hematopoietic progenitors and aging: alterations in granulocytic precursors and responsiveness to recombinant human G-CSF, GM-CSF, and IL-3." J Gerontol 48(5): M207-12.

Chen, F., K. Knecht, et al. (2005). "Direct agonist/antagonist functions of dehydroepiandrosterone." Endocrinology 146(11): 4568-76.

Chen, J. (2004). "Senescence and functional failure in hematopoietic stem cells." Exp Hematol 32(11): 1025-32.

Christopher E. Andoniou, J. D. C., Mariapia A. Degli-Esposti, (2008). "Killers and beyond: NK-cell-mediated control of immune responses." European Journal of Immunology 38(11): 2938-2942.

Chung, E., S. B. Amrute, et al. (2005). "Characterization of virus-responsive plasmacytoid dendritic cells in the rhesus macaque." Clin Diagn Lab Immunol 12(3): 426-35.

Colonna-Romano, G., M. Bulati, et al. (2003). "B cells in the aged: CD27, CD5, and CD40 expression." Mech Ageing Dev 124(4): 389-93.

Cook, I. F. (2008). "Sexual dimorphism of humoral immunity with human vaccines." Vaccine 26(29-30): 3551-5.

Cook, J. M., N. Gualde, et al. (1987). "Alterations in the human immune response to the hepatitis B vaccine among the elderly." Cell Immunol 109(1): 89-96.

Corey, L., A. G. Langenberg, et al. (1999). "Recombinant glycoprotein vaccine for the prevention of genital HSV-2 infection: two randomized controlled trials. Chiron HSV Vaccine Study Group." JAMA 282(4): 331-40.

Curiel, R. E., M. H. Miller, et al. (1993). "Does the gender difference in interferon production seen in picornavirus-infected spleen cell cultures from ICR Swiss mice have any in vivo significance?" J Interferon Res 13(6): 387-95.

Curran, E. M., L. J. Berghaus, et al. (2001). "Natural killer cells express estrogen receptor-alpha and estrogen receptor-beta and can respond to estrogen via a non-estrogen receptor-alpha-mediated pathway." Cell Immunol 214(1): 12-20.

D'Acremont, V., C. Herzog, et al. (2006). "Immunogenicity and safety of a virosomal hepatitis A vaccine (Epaxal) in the elderly." J Travel Med 13(2): 78-83.

Dahlgren, C. and A. Karlsson (1999). "Respiratory burst in human neutrophils." J Immunol Methods 232(1-2): 3-14.

Danenberg, H. D., A. Ben-Yehuda, et al. (1997). "Dehydroepiandrosterone treatment is not beneficial to the immune response to influenza in elderly subjects." J Clin Endocrinol Metab 82(9): 2911-4.

Daynes, R. A., B. A. Araneo, et al. (1993). "Altered regulation of IL-6 production with normal aging. Possible linkage to the age-associated decline in dehydroepiandrosterone and its sulfated derivative." J Immunol 150(12): 5219-30.

De Martinis, M., C. Franceschi, et al. (2005). "Inflamm-ageing and lifelong antigenic load as major determinants of ageing rate and longevity." FEBS Lett 579(10): 2035-9.

Degelau, J., D. Guay, et al. (1997). "The effect of DHEAS on influenza vaccination in aging adults." J Am Geriatr Soc 45(6): 747-51.

Deguchi, K., M. Kamada, et al. (2001). "Postmenopausal changes in production of type 1 and type 2 cytokines and the effects of hormone replacement therapy." Menopause 8(4): 266-73.

Della Bella, S., L. Bierti, et al. (2007). "Peripheral blood dendritic cells and monocytes are differently regulated in the elderly." Clin Immunol 122(2): 220-8.

Delpy, L., V. Douin-Echinard, et al. (2005). "Estrogen enhances susceptibility to experimental autoimmune myasthenia gravis by promoting type 1-polarized immune responses." J Immunol 175(8): 5050-7.

Derhovanessian, E., A. Larbi, et al. (2009). "Biomarkers of human immunosenescence: impact of Cytomegalovirus infection." Curr Opin Immunol 21(4): 440-5.

Diodato, M. D., M. W. Knoferl, et al. (2001). "Gender differences in the inflammatory response and survival following haemorrhage and subsequent sepsis." Cytokine 14(3): 162-9.

Dosiou, C., A. E. Hamilton, et al. (2008). "Expression of membrane progesterone receptors on human T lymphocytes and Jurkat cells and activation of G-proteins by progesterone." J Endocrinol 196(1): 67-77.

Dunston, C. R. and H. R. Griffiths (2010). "The effect of ageing on macrophage Toll-like receptor-mediated responses in the fight against pathogens." Clin Exp Immunol 161(3): 407-16.

Engelmann, F., A. Barron, et al. (2010). "Accelerated immune senescence and reduced response to vaccination in ovariectomized female rhesus macaques." Age (Dordr).

Engler, R. J., M. R. Nelson, et al. (2008). "Half- vs full-dose trivalent inactivated influenza vaccine (2004-2005): age, dose, and sex effects on immune responses." Arch Intern Med 168(22): 2405-14.

Evans, M. J., S. MacLaughlin, et al. (1997). "Estrogen decreases in vitro apoptosis of peripheral blood mononuclear cells from women with normal menstrual cycles and decreases TNF-alpha production in SLE but not in normal cultures." Clin Immunol Immunopathol 82(3): 258-62.

Fahlman, M. M., D. Boardley, et al. (2000). "Effects of hormone replacement therapy on selected indices of immune function in postmenopausal women." Gynecol Obstet Invest 50(3): 189-93.

Fleming, D. M., K. W. Cross, et al. (2004). "Gender difference in the incidence of shingles." Epidemiol Infect 132(1): 1-5.

Franceschi, C., M. Bonafe, et al. (2000). "Inflamm-aging. An evolutionary perspective on immunosenescence." Ann N Y Acad Sci 908: 244-54.

Frasca, D., R. L. Riley, et al. (2004). "Effect of age on the immunoglobulin class switch." Crit Rev Immunol 24(5): 297-320.

Gameiro, C. and F. Romao (2010). "Changes in the immune system during menopause and aging." Front Biosci (Elite Ed) 2: 1299-303.

Gameiro, C. M., F. Romao, et al. (2010). "Menopause and aging: changes in the immune system--a review." Maturitas 67(4): 316-20.

Genazzani, A. R. and N. Pluchino (2010). "DHEA therapy in postmenopausal women: the need to move forward beyond the lack of evidence." Climacteric 13(4): 314-6.

Genton, B., V. D'Acremont, et al. (2006). "Hepatitis A vaccines and the elderly." Travel Med Infect Dis 4(6): 303-12.

Gerli, R., D. Monti, et al. (2000). "Chemokines, sTNF-Rs and sCD30 serum levels in healthy aged people and centenarians." Mech Ageing Dev 121(1-3): 37-46.

Giglio, T., M. A. Imro, et al. (1994). "Immune cell circulating subsets are affected by gonadal function." Life Sci 54(18): 1305-12.

Gillgrass, A. E., A. A. Ashkar, et al. (2003). "Prolonged exposure to progesterone prevents induction of protective mucosal responses following intravaginal immunization with attenuated herpes simplex virus type 2." J Virol 77(18): 9845-51.

Gillgrass, A. E., S. A. Fernandez, et al. (2005). "Estradiol regulates susceptibility following primary exposure to genital herpes simplex virus type 2, while progesterone induces inflammation." J Virol 79(5): 3107-16.

Ginaldi, L., M. C. Di Benedetto, et al. (2005). "Osteoporosis, inflammation and ageing." Immun Ageing 2: 14.

Giuliani, N., P. Sansoni, et al. (2001). "Serum interleukin-6, soluble interleukin-6 receptor and soluble gp130 exhibit different patterns of age- and menopause-related changes." Exp Gerontol 36(3): 547-57.

Goetzl, E. J., M. C. Huang, et al. (2010). "Gender specificity of altered human immune cytokine profiles in aging." FASEB J 24(9): 3580-9.

Grady, D. (2006). "Clinical practice. Management of menopausal symptoms." N Engl J Med 355(22): 2338-47.

Grimaldi, C. M., J. Cleary, et al. (2002). "Estrogen alters thresholds for B cell apoptosis and activation." J Clin Invest 109(12): 1625-33.

Guo, T. L., J. A. McCay, et al. (2001). "Genistein modulates immune responses and increases host resistance to B16F10 tumor in adult female B6C3F1 mice." J Nutr 131(12): 3251-8.

Hall, J. E. (2004). "Neuroendocrine physiology of the early and late menopause." Endocrinol Metab Clin North Am 33(4): 637-59.

Han, X., P. Lundberg, et al. (2001). "Gender influences herpes simplex virus type 1 infection in normal and gamma interferon-mutant mice." J Virol 75(6): 3048-52.

Harkonen, P. L. and H. K. Vaananen (2006). "Monocyte-macrophage system as a target for estrogen and selective estrogen receptor modulators." Ann N Y Acad Sci 1089: 218-27.

Hing, E. and K. M. Brett (2006). "Changes in U.S. prescribing patterns of menopausal hormone therapy, 2001-2003." Obstet Gynecol 108(1): 33-40.

Holl, M., H. Donat, et al. (2001). "[Peripheral blood lymphocyte subpopulations of postmenopausal women with hormone replacement therapy]." Zentralbl Gynakol 123(9): 543-5.

Huang, Y., S. Cao, et al. (2005). "Decreased Circulating Levels of Tumor Necrosis Factor-Œ± in Postmenopausal Women during Consumption of Soy-Containing Isoflavones." Journal of Clinical Endocrinology & Metabolism 90(7): 3956-3962.

Huber, S. A. (2005). "Increased susceptibility of male BALB/c mice to coxsackievirus B3-induced myocarditis: role for CD1d." Med Microbiol Immunol 194(3): 121-7.

Huber, S. A., J. Kupperman, et al. (1999). "Hormonal regulation of CD4(+) T-cell responses in coxsackievirus B3-induced myocarditis in mice." J Virol 73(6): 4689-95.

Huber, S. A. and B. Pfaeffle (1994). "Differential Th1 and Th2 cell responses in male and female BALB/c mice infected with coxsackievirus group B type 3." J Virol 68(8): 5126-32.

Hughes, G. C., S. Thomas, et al. (2008). "Cutting Edge: Progesterone Regulates IFN-{alpha} Production by Plasmacytoid Dendritic Cells." J Immunol 180(4): 2029-2033.

Huntley, A. L. and E. Ernst (2004). "Soy for the treatment of perimenopausal symptoms--a systematic review." Maturitas 47(1): 1-9.

Huppert, F. A., W. Solomou, et al. (1998). "Aging and lymphocyte subpopulations: whole-blood analysis of immune markers in a large population sample of healthy elderly individuals." Exp Gerontol 33(6): 593-600.

Jared F. Purton, J. S., Charles D. Surh, (2007). "Staying alive - naïve CD4(+) T cell homeostasis." European Journal of Immunology 37(9): 2367-2369.

Johansson, S. G. "The History of IgE: From discovery to 2010." Curr Allergy Asthma Rep 11(2): 173-7.

Kabelitz, D. and R. Medzhitov (2007). "Innate immunity--cross-talk with adaptive immunity through pattern recognition receptors and cytokines." Curr Opin Immunol 19(1): 1-3.

Kamada, M., M. Irahara, et al. (2001). "Transient increase in the levels of T-helper 1 cytokines in postmenopausal women and the effects of hormone replacement therapy." Gynecol Obstet Invest 52(2): 82-8.

Kamada, M., M. Irahara, et al. (2001). "Postmenopausal changes in serum cytokine levels and hormone replacement therapy." American Journal of Obstetrics and Gynecology 184(3): 309-314.

Kamada, M., M. Irahara, et al. (2000). "Effect of hormone replacement therapy on post-menopausal changes of lymphocytes and T cell subsets." J Endocrinol Invest 23(6): 376-82.

Kamada, M., M. Irahara, et al. (2001). "B cell subsets in postmenopausal women and the effect of hormone replacement therapy." Maturitas 37(3): 173-179.

Kanda, N. and K. Tamaki (1999). "Estrogen enhances immunoglobulin production by human PBMCs." J Allergy Clin Immunol 103(2 Pt 1): 282-8.

Karpuzoglu, E. and M. Zouali (2011). "The multi-faceted influences of estrogen on lymphocytes: toward novel immuno-interventions strategies for autoimmunity management." Clin Rev Allergy Immunol 40(1): 16-26.

Katabuchi, H., Y. Suenaga, et al. (1997). "Distribution and fine structure of macrophages in the human ovary during the menstrual cycle, pregnancy and menopause." Endocr J 44(6): 785-95.

Kaushic, C., A. D. Murdin, et al. (1998). "Chlamydia trachomatis infection in the female reproductive tract of the rat: influence of progesterone on infectivity and immune response." Infect Immun 66(3): 893-8.

Ketloy, C., A. Engering, et al. (2008). "Expression and function of Toll-like receptors on dendritic cells and other antigen presenting cells from non-human primates." Vet Immunol Immunopathol 125(1-2): 18-30.

Khan, D., R. Dai, et al. (2010). "Estrogen increases, whereas IL-27 and IFN-gamma decrease, splenocyte IL-17 production in WT mice." Eur J Immunol 40(9): 2549-56.

Kiel, D. P., D. T. Felson, et al. (1987). "Hip fracture and the use of estrogens in postmenopausal women. The Framingham Study." N Engl J Med 317(19): 1169-74.

Kim, O. Y., J. S. Chae, et al. (2011). "Effects of aging and menopause on serum interleukin-6 levels and peripheral blood mononuclear cell cytokine production in healthy nonobese women." Age (Dordr).

Klein, P. W., J. D. Easterbrook, et al. (2008). "Estrogen and progesterone affect responses to malaria infection in female C57BL/6 mice." Gend Med 5(4): 423-33.

Klein, S. H., S. (2010). Sex Differences in Susceptibility to Viral Infection. Sex Hormones and Immmunity to Infection. S. R. Klein, C. Berlin/Heidelberg, Springer.

Klein, S. L. (2004). "Hormonal and immunological mechanisms mediating sex differences in parasite infection." Parasite Immunology 26(6-7): 247-264.

Klein, S. L., A. Jedlicka, et al. (2010). "The Xs and Y of immune responses to viral vaccines." Lancet Infect Dis 10(5): 338-49.

Komi, J. and O. Lassila (2000). "Nonsteroidal anti-estrogens inhibit the functional differentiation of human monocyte-derived dendritic cells." Blood 95(9): 2875-82.

Kovats S, E. C., and Hemant Agrawal (2010). Sex Steroid Receptors in Immune Cells. Sex Hormones and Immunity to Infection. R. C. Klein S. Berlin/Heidelberg, Springer.

Kozlowski, P. A., S. B. Williams, et al. (2002). "Differential induction of mucosal and systemic antibody responses in women after nasal, rectal, or vaginal immunization: influence of the menstrual cycle." J Immunol 169(1): 566-74.

Krabbe, K. S., M. Pedersen, et al. (2004). "Inflammatory mediators in the elderly." Exp Gerontol 39(5): 687-99.

Kumru, S., A. Godekmerdan, et al. (2004). "Immune effects of surgical menopause and estrogen replacement therapy in peri-menopausal women." J Reprod Immunol 63(1): 31-8.

Lanier, L. L. (2008). "Up on the tightrope: natural killer cell activation and inhibition." Nat Immunol 9(5): 495-502.

Lanzavecchia, A. and F. Sallusto (2005). "Understanding the generation and function of memory T cell subsets." Curr Opin Immunol 17(3): 326-32.

Larbi, A., C. Franceschi, et al. (2008). "Aging of the Immune System as a Prognostic Factor for Human Longevity." Physiology 23(2): 64-74.

Larsson, B. M., K. Larsson, et al. (1999). "Gram positive bacteria induce IL-6 and IL-8 production in human alveolar macrophages and epithelial cells." Inflammation 23(3): 217-30.

LeMaoult, J., S. Delassus, et al. (1997). "Clonal expansions of B lymphocytes in old mice." J Immunol 159(8): 3866-74.

LeMaoult, J., J. S. Manavalan, et al. (1999). "Cellular basis of B cell clonal populations in old mice." J Immunol 162(11): 6384-91.

LeMaoult, J., P. Szabo, et al. (1997). "Effect of age on humoral immunity, selection of the B-cell repertoire and B-cell development." Immunol Rev 160: 115-26.

Li, X., Y. Xu, et al. (2009). "17beta-estradiol enhances the response of plasmacytoid dendritic cell to CpG." PLoS One 4(12): e8412.

Linehan, S. A., L. Martinez-Pomares, et al. (2000). "Macrophage lectins in host defence." Microbes Infect 2(3): 279-88.

Lloberas, J. and A. Celada (2002). "Effect of aging on macrophage function." Exp Gerontol 37(12): 1325-31.

Lord, J. M., S. Butcher, et al. (2001). "Neutrophil ageing and immunesenescence." Mech Ageing Dev 122(14): 1521-35.

Maini, M. K., R. J. Gilson, et al. (1996). "Reference ranges and sources of variability of CD4 counts in HIV-seronegative women and men." Genitourin Med 72(1): 27-31.

Mariani, E., L. Pulsatelli, et al. (2002). "RANTES and MIP-1alpha production by T lymphocytes, monocytes and NK cells from nonagenarian subjects." Exp Gerontol 37(2-3): 219-26.

Marriott, I. and Y. M. Huet-Hudson (2006). "Sexual dimorphism in innate immune responses to infectious organisms." Immunol Res 34(3): 177-92.

Marx, P. A., A. I. Spira, et al. (1996). "Progesterone implants enhance SIV vaginal transmission and early virus load." Nat Med 2(10): 1084-9.

Matalka, K. Z. (2003). "The effect of estradiol, but not progesterone, on the production of cytokines in stimulated whole blood, is concentration-dependent." Neuro Endocrinol Lett 24(3-4): 185-91.

Medzhitov, R. (2003). The Innate Immune System. Fundamental Immunology. W. Paul, Lippincott Williams & Wilkins: 509.

Medzhitov, R. (2007). "Recognition of microorganisms and activation of the immune response." Nature 449(7164): 819-26.

Medzhitov, R. and C. A. Janeway, Jr. (2002). "Decoding the patterns of self and nonself by the innate immune system." Science 296(5566): 298-300.

Meier, A., J. J. Chang, et al. (2009). "Sex differences in the Toll-like receptor-mediated response of plasmacytoid dendritic cells to HIV-1." Nat Med 15(8): 955-9.

Merkel, S. M., S. Alexander, et al. (2001). "Essential role for estrogen in protection against Vibrio vulnificus-induced endotoxic shock." Infect Immun 69(10): 6119-22.

Mocchegiani, E. and M. Malavolta (2004). "NK and NKT cell functions in immunosenescence." Aging Cell 3(4): 177-84.

Mor, G., E. Sapi, et al. (2003). "Interaction of the estrogen receptors with the Fas ligand promoter in human monocytes." J Immunol 170(1): 114-22.

Morrison, C. S., B. A. Richardson, et al. (2007). "Hormonal contraception and the risk of HIV acquisition." Aids 21(1): 85-95.

Murasko, D. M. and J. Jiang (2005). "Response of aged mice to primary virus infections." Immunol Rev 205: 285-96.

Mysliwska, J., P. Trzonkowski, et al. (2004). "Immunomodulating effect of influenza vaccination in the elderly differing in health status." Exp Gerontol 39(10): 1447-58.

Naylor, K., G. Li, et al. (2005). "The Influence of Age on T Cell Generation and TCR Diversity." J Immunol 174(11): 7446-52.

Nelson HD, N. P., Freeman M, Chan BKS. (2007). "Drug Class Review on Hormone Therapy." from http://www.ohsu.edu/drugeffectiveness/reports/final.cfm.

Offner, P. J., E. E. Moore, et al. (1999). "Male gender is a risk factor for major infections after surgery." Arch Surg 134(9): 935-8; discussion 938-40.

Ogata, K., N. Yokose, et al. (1997). "Natural killer cells in the late decades of human life." Clin Immunol Immunopathol 84(3): 269-75.

Olweus, J., A. BitMansour, et al. (1997). "Dendritic cell ontogeny: a human dendritic cell lineage of myeloid origin." Proc Natl Acad Sci U S A 94(23): 12551-6.

Paavonen, T., L. C. Andersson, et al. (1981). "Sex hormone regulation of in vitro immune response. Estradiol enhances human B cell maturation via inhibition of suppressor T cells in pokeweed mitogen-stimulated cultures." J Exp Med 154(6): 1935-45.

Paharkova-Vatchkova, V., R. Maldonado, et al. (2004). "Estrogen preferentially promotes the differentiation of CD11c+ CD11b(intermediate) dendritic cells from bone marrow precursors." J Immunol 172(3): 1426-36.

Pawelec, G., E. Derhovanessian, et al. (2009). "Cytomegalovirus and human immunosenescence." Rev Med Virol 19(1): 47-56.

Pawelec, G., A. Larbi, et al. (2009). "Senescence of the Human Immune System." J Comp Pathol.

Pennock, J. W., R. Stegall, et al. (2009). "Estradiol improves genital herpes vaccine efficacy in mice." Vaccine 27(42): 5830-6.

Phiel, K. L., R. A. Henderson, et al. (2005). "Differential estrogen receptor gene expression in human peripheral blood mononuclear cell populations." Immunol Lett 97(1): 107-13.

Pinzan, C. F., L. P. Ruas, et al. (2010). "Immunological basis for the gender differences in murine Paracoccidioides brasiliensis infection." PLoS ONE 5(5): e10757.

Polanczyk, M. J., C. Hopke, et al. (2006). "Estrogen-mediated immunomodulation involves reduced activation of effector T cells, potentiation of Treg cells, and enhanced expression of the PD-1 costimulatory pathway." J Neurosci Res 84(2): 370-8.

Porter, V. R., G. A. Greendale, et al. (2001). "Immune effects of hormone replacement therapy in post-menopausal women." Exp Gerontol 36(2): 311-26.

Prior, J. C. (1998). "Perimenopause: the complex endocrinology of the menopausal transition." Endocr Rev 19(4): 397-428.

Pulsatelli, L., R. Meliconi, et al. (2000). "Chemokine production by peripheral blood mononuclear cells in elderly subjects." Mech Ageing Dev 121(1-3): 89-100.

Purton, J. F., J. T. Tan, et al. (2007). "Antiviral CD4+ memory T cells are IL-15 dependent." J. Exp. Med. 204(4): 951-961.
Rachon, D., G. Rimoldi, et al. (2006). "In vitro effects of genistein and resveratrol on the production of interferon-gamma (IFNgamma) and interleukin-10 (IL-10) by stimulated murine splenocytes." Phytomedicine 13(6): 419-24.
Radaev, S. and P. D. Sun (2003). "Structure and function of natural killer cell surface receptors." Annu Rev Biophys Biomol Struct 32: 93-114.
Rehman, H. U. and E. A. Masson (2005). "Neuroendocrinology of female aging." Gender Medicine 2(1): 41-56.
Rider, V., S. Jones, et al. (2001). "Estrogen increases CD40 ligand expression in T cells from women with systemic lupus erythematosus." J Rheumatol 28(12): 2644-9.
Ryan-Borchers, T. A., J. S. Park, et al. (2006). "Soy isoflavones modulate immune function in healthy postmenopausal women." The American Journal of Clinical Nutrition 83(5): 1118-1125.
Sallusto, F. and A. Lanzavecchia (1994). "Efficient presentation of soluble antigen by cultured human dendritic cells is maintained by granulocyte/macrophage colony-stimulating factor plus interleukin 4 and downregulated by tumor necrosis factor alpha." J Exp Med 179(4): 1109-18.
Sansoni, P., R. Vescovini, et al. (2008). "The immune system in extreme longevity." Exp Gerontol 43(2): 61-5.
Saucedo, R., G. Rico, et al. (2002). "Transdermal estradiol in menopausal women depresses interleukin-6 without affecting other markers of immune response." Gynecol Obstet Invest 53(2): 114-7.
Saurwein-Teissl, M., T. L. Lung, et al. (2002). "Lack of antibody production following immunization in old age: association with CD8(+)CD28(-) T cell clonal expansions and an imbalance in the production of Th1 and Th2 cytokines." J Immunol 168(11): 5893-9.
Schroder, J., V. Kahlke, et al. (2000). "Gender differences in sepsis: genetically determined?" Shock 14(3): 307-10; discussion 310-3.
Schroder, J., V. Kahlke, et al. (1998). "Gender differences in human sepsis." Arch Surg 133(11): 1200-5.
Schwab, R., P. Szabo, et al. (1997). "Expanded CD4+ and CD8+ T cell clones in elderly humans." J Immunol 158(9): 4493-9.
Segerer, S. E., N. Muller, et al. (2009). "Impact of female sex hormones on the maturation and function of human dendritic cells." Am J Reprod Immunol 62(3): 165-73.
Shaw, A. C., S. Joshi, et al. (2010). "Aging of the innate immune system." Curr Opin Immunol 22(4): 507-13.
Siegal, F. P., N. Kadowaki, et al. (1999). "The nature of the principal type 1 interferon-producing cells in human blood." Science 284(5421): 1835-7.
Smith, D. C., R. Prentice, et al. (1975). "Association of exogenous estrogen and endometrial carcinoma." N Engl J Med 293(23): 1164-7.
Smith, S. M., G. B. Baskin, et al. (2000). "Estrogen protects against vaginal transmission of simian immunodeficiency virus." J Infect Dis 182(3): 708-15.
Sonoda, J., J. Laganiere, et al. (2007). "Nuclear receptor ERR alpha and coactivator PGC-1 beta are effectors of IFN-gamma-induced host defense." Genes Dev 21(15): 1909-20.

Soucy, G., G. Boivin, et al. (2005). "Estradiol is required for a proper immune response to bacterial and viral pathogens in the female brain." J Immunol 174(10): 6391-8.
Stanberry, L. R., S. L. Spruance, et al. (2002). "Glycoprotein-D-adjuvant vaccine to prevent genital herpes." N Engl J Med 347(21): 1652-61.
Stopinska-Gluszak, U., J. Waligora, et al. (2006). "Effect of estrogen/progesterone hormone replacement therapy on natural killer cell cytotoxicity and immunoregulatory cytokine release by peripheral blood mononuclear cells of postmenopausal women." J Reprod Immunol 69(1): 65-75.
Suenaga, R., M. J. Evans, et al. (1998). "Peripheral blood T cells and monocytes and B cell lines derived from patients with lupus express estrogen receptor transcripts similar to those of normal cells." J Rheumatol 25(7): 1305-12.
Surh, C. D. and J. Sprent (2008). "Homeostasis of Naive and Memory T Cells." Immunity 29(6): 848-862.
Svanborg, C., G. Godaly, et al. (1999). "Cytokine responses during mucosal infections: role in disease pathogenesis and host defence." Curr Opin Microbiol 2(1): 99-105.
Szabo, P., F. Li, et al. (2004). "Evolution of B-cell clonal expansions with age." Cell Immunol 231(1-2): 158-67.
Tangye, S. G. and D. M. Tarlinton (2009). "Memory B cells: effectors of long-lived immune responses." Eur J Immunol 39(8): 2065-75.
Tarazona, R. (2009). NK Cells in Human Aging. Handbook on Immunosenescence, Springer.
Tarlinton, D. (1998). "Germinal centers: form and function." Curr Opin Immunol 10(3): 245-51.
Teleshova, N., J. Kenney, et al. (2004). "CpG-C immunostimulatory oligodeoxyribonucleotide activation of plasmacytoid dendritic cells in rhesus macaques to augment the activation of IFN-gamma-secreting simian immunodeficiency virus-specific T cells." J Immunol 173(3): 1647-57.
Tiwari, S., G. P. Agrawal, et al. (2010). "Molecular basis of the mucosal immune system: from fundamental concepts to advances in liposome-based vaccines." Nanomedicine (Lond) 5(10): 1617-40.
Tollerud, D. J., J. W. Clark, et al. (1989). "The influence of age, race, and gender on peripheral blood mononuclear-cell subsets in healthy nonsmokers." J Clin Immunol 9(3): 214-22.
Trunova, N., L. Tsai, et al. (2006). "Progestin-based contraceptive suppresses cellular immune responses in SHIV-infected rhesus macaques." Virology 352(1): 169-77.
Trzonkowski, P., J. Mysliwska, et al. (2003). "Association between cytomegalovirus infection, enhanced proinflammatory response and low level of anti-hemagglutinins during the anti-influenza vaccination--an impact of immunosenescence." Vaccine 21(25-26): 3826-36.
Uemura, Y., T. Y. Liu, et al. (2008). "17 Beta-estradiol (E2) plus tumor necrosis factor-alpha induces a distorted maturation of human monocyte-derived dendritic cells and promotes their capacity to initiate T-helper 2 responses." Hum Immunol 69(3): 149-57.
Vallejo, A. N. (2005). "CD28 extinction in human T cells: altered functions and the program of T-cell senescence." Immunol Rev 205: 158-69.
Vallejo, A. N., C. M. Weyand, et al. (2004). "T-cell senescence: a culprit of immune abnormalities in chronic inflammation and persistent infection." Trends Mol Med 10(3): 119-24.
van Benthem, B. H., P. Vernazza, et al. (2002). "The impact of pregnancy and menopause on CD4 lymphocyte counts in HIV-infected women." AIDS 16(6): 919-24.

Vasto, S., G. Candore, et al. (2007). "Inflammatory networks in ageing, age-related diseases and longevity." Mech Ageing Dev 128(1): 83-91.

Vasto, S., G. Carruba, et al. (2009). "Inflammation, ageing and cancer." Mech Ageing Dev 130(1-2): 40-5.

Verthelyi, D. (2001). "Sex hormones as immunomodulators in health and disease." Int Immunopharmacol 1(6): 983-93.

Verthelyi, D. I. and S. A. Ahmed (1998). "Estrogen increases the number of plasma cells and enhances their autoantibody production in nonautoimmune C57BL/6 mice." Cell Immunol 189(2): 125-34.

Villacres, M. C., J. Longmate, et al. (2004). "Predominant type 1 CMV-specific memory T-helper response in humans: evidence for gender differences in cytokine secretion." Hum Immunol 65(5): 476-85.

Vural, P., M. Canbaz, et al. (2006). "Effects of menopause and postmenopausal tibolone treatment on plasma TNFalpha, IL-4, IL-10, IL-12 cytokine pattern and some bone turnover markers." Pharmacol Res 53(4): 367-71.

Wagner, H. J., M. Hornef, et al. (1994). "Sex difference in the serostatus of adults to the Epstein-Barr virus." Immunobiology 190(4-5): 424-9.

Weiss, N. S., C. L. Ure, et al. (1980). "Decreased risk of fractures of the hip and lower forearm with postmenopausal use of estrogen." N Engl J Med 303(21): 1195-8.

Weksler, M. E. and P. Szabo (2000). "The effect of age on the B-cell repertoire." J Clin Immunol 20(4): 240-9.

Wenisch, C., S. Patruta, et al. (2000). "Effect of age on human neutrophil function." J Leukoc Biol 67(1): 40-5.

Werner Held (2008). "Tolerance and reactivity of NK cells: Two sides of the same coin?" European Journal of Immunology 38(11): 2930-2933.

Whitacre, C. C., S. C. Reingold, et al. (1999). "A gender gap in autoimmunity." Science 283(5406): 1277-8.

Wichmann, M. W., D. Inthorn, et al. (2000). "Incidence and mortality of severe sepsis in surgical intensive care patients: the influence of patient gender on disease process and outcome." Intensive Care Med 26(2): 167-72.

Wikby, A., B. O. Nilsson, et al. (2006). "The immune risk phenotype is associated with IL-6 in the terminal decline stage: findings from the Swedish NONA immune longitudinal study of very late life functioning." Mech Ageing Dev 127(8): 695-704.

Woodruff, J. F. (1980). "Viral myocarditis. A review." Am J Pathol 101(2): 425-84.

Wu, J. M., M. B. Zelinski, et al. (2005). "Ovarian aging and menopause: current theories, hypotheses, and research models." Exp Biol Med (Maywood) 230(11): 818-28.

Yamamoto, Y., H. Saito, et al. (1991). "Sex differences in host resistance to Mycobacterium marinum infection in mice." Infect Immun 59(11): 4089-96.

Yang, J. H., C. D. Chen, et al. (2000). "Hormone replacement therapy reverses the decrease in natural killer cytotoxicity but does not reverse the decreases in the T-cell subpopulation or interferon-gamma production in postmenopausal women." Fertil Steril 74(2): 261-7.

Yasui, T., M. Maegawa, et al. (2007). "Changes in serum cytokine concentrations during the menopausal transition." Maturitas 56(4): 396-403.

Zellweger, R., M. W. Wichmann, et al. (1997). "Females in proestrus state maintain splenic immune functions and tolerate sepsis better than males." Crit Care Med 25(1): 106-10.

Zhang, Y., T. T. Song, et al. (1999). "Daidzein and genistein glucuronides in vitro are weakly estrogenic and activate human natural killer cells at nutritionally relevant concentrations." J Nutr 129(2): 399-405.

Zhang, Y., D. L. Wallace, et al. (2007). "In vivo kinetics of human natural killer cells: the effects of ageing and acute and chronic viral infection." Immunology 121(2): 258-65.

Zhu, J. and W. E. Paul (2010). "Peripheral CD4+ T-cell differentiation regulated by networks of cytokines and transcription factors." Immunol Rev 238(1): 247-62.

Ziel, H. K. and W. D. Finkle (1975). "Increased risk of endometrial carcinoma among users of conjugated estrogens." N Engl J Med 293(23): 1167-70.

13

The Role of Sex Steroids in the Host-Parasite Interaction

Karen Nava-Castro[1], Romel Hernández-Bello[2], Saé Muñiz-Hernández[3] and Jorge Morales-Montor[2]
[1]*Departamento de Infectología e Inmunología, Instituto Nacional de Perinatología, Secretaria de Salud*
[2]*Departamento de Inmunología, Instituto de Investigaciones Biomédicas, Universidad Nacional Autónoma de México*
[3]*Subdirección de Investigación Básica, Instituto Nacional de Cancerología, Secretaria de Salud*
México

1. Introduction

In this Chapter, we intend to review and discuss the current literature, and the state of the art related to the role that sex steroids play in the complex host-parasite relationship, particularly during *Taenia crassiceps* and *Taenia solium* cysticercosis. It is well known that sex-steroids regulate a variety of cellular and physiological functions of organisms such as growth, reproduction and differentiation. More recently the ability of sex steroids to affect the immunological response directed against pathogenic agents, and importantly the direct effect of these molecules on these organisms, have gained attention. These effects are clearly evident during various parasitic diseases including malaria, schistosomiasis, toxoplasmosis, cysticercosis, trypanosomiasis and leishmaniasis, where strong steroid hormone regulation of the immune response, has been described (Remoué et al., 2001; do Prado et al., 1998; Satoskar & Alexander, 1995; Vargas-Villavicencio et al., 2006; Libonati et al., 2006; Liesenfield et al., 2001). For instance, sex steroids play a significant role in regulating the parasite load in experimental intraperitoneal *Taenia crassiceps* cysticercosis of male and female Balbc/anN mice. Briefly, estrogens increase parasite loads and androgens decrease them (1) by acting directly on the parasite, favoring or hindering its reproduction, respectively, and (2) by biasing the hosts' immune response towards a parasite-permissive Th2 or a parasite-restrictive Th1 response. Recent experimental evidence, suggests that either steroids hormones may exert their effects directly upon the parasite, which may be able to exploit the host hormonal microenvironment for its exclusive benefit. The fact that steroids can directly influence parasites has been described in at least 17 different species of helminths and protozoan with medical and veterinary relevance. Briefly, we detail some of the most important experimental evidence about direct effects of steroid upon parasites. In fact, the hormonal microenvironment inside an immunocompetent host is so important, that experimental evidence suggests that an inadequate hormonal environment may lead to apoptosis of crucial parasite cells, as has been proposed in some parasites (e.g., retinoic acid has been shown to affect female *Litomosoides carinii* and microfilariae of *L. carinii, Brugia malayi, B. pahangi* and *Acanthocheilonema viteae*) (Zahner et al., 1989). In the same sense, *in vitro* experiments have shown that testosterone negatively affects fecundity in *Schistosoma. haematobium* adult worms (Remoué et al., 2002). Interestingly, this hormonal microenvironment also modulates the gene expression of female and male *S. mansoni* adult parasites. This finding may represent an interesting approach, because if we know that sex-steroids can specifically down-regulate genes involved in the fecundity and oviposition of *S. mansoni* and *S. haematobium,* we can propose the use of sex-steroid analogues to modulate this effect (Barrabes et al., 1979). Finally, parasites have developed diverse mechanisms of survival within the host, which facilitate the establishment of infection. These can be grouped into two types: those in which the immune response is evaded by strategies such as antigenic variation and molecular mimicry and those in which the parasite exploits some system of the host to its benefit, and thus obtains an advantage such as establishment, growth or reproduction. Thus *Naeglerai fowleria* is capable of internalizing antigen antibody complexes from their surface with the dual benefit of gaining the amino acids for their own metabolism and preventing the surface bound antibody from interfering with parasite host cell interactions (Shibayama et al., 2003). Other pathogens, including *Chlamydia trachomatis* and *Coxiella burnetii* have developed molecules that directly of interfere with antigen processing and presentation (Brodsky et al., 1999). A striking example of exploitation of host molecules is the ability of a number of parasites to use host-synthesized cytokines as indirect growth factors for the parasite. Recent experimental evidence has led us to suggest a mechanism of host exploitation by the parasite. In this system of 'trans-regulation' the parasite benefits directly from host derived hormones or growth factors, to allow rapid establishment, increased growth and reproduction.

In view of this evidence, it is clear that the endocrine system, particularly sex steroids, not only influences the course of parasitic infection by the modulation of the immune system, but can also be directly exploited by parasites. In this way host hormones, by means of genomic and non-genomic mechanisms, regulate important parasite processes such as growth, differentiation and reproduction, through a mechanism described as trans-regulation. This mechanism allows the parasite to accomplish a more successful infection.

Comprehension of these concepts, as well as the study of sex steroid receptors and of those that regulate the activity of various second messenger cascades in parasites opens interesting research perspectives in the complex host-parasite evolutionary relationship. Reports on nuclear receptors in parasites are extremely scarce and to date have only been described in six parasites. However as more parasite genome projects reach completion, evidence for these receptors in other parasites is likely to grow. The ability of a parasite to differentially affect a female or a male of the same species (sexual dimorphism of an infection) can be due to hormonal regulation of the immune response or direct hormonal affects on the parasite. Understanding the contribution of each of these and characterization of the parasite molecules involved may facilitate the development of drugs that counteract the effects of hormones on the immune system or the parasite.

The relationship between parasites (P), particularly helminthes, and their hosts (H) implies biochemical co-evolution and communication between their complex physiological and metabolic systems among themselves and with the environment, at all levels of biological organization. Hormones are known to regulate a variety of cellular and physiological functions of organisms such as growth, reproduction and differentiation (Verthelyi, 2001).

Hormones and immune actors are prominent in H-P relationships (Klein, 2004). The comparatively sophisticated immune systems of vertebrates add complexity to H-P interactions. Mammals sense and react with their innate and acquired immunological systems to the presence of a parasite and the parasite is also sensitive and reactive to the host's immune systems effectors. Host's hormones are also involved in the modulation of the immune system's protective or pathogenic functions and also on the parasite's metabolism and reproduction (Roberts et al., 2001; Escobedo et al., 2005). Host's adrenal hormones are well known immune modulators (Tait et al., 2008), whilst sex steroids (estradiol, progesterone and testosterone) are progressively being recognized to also significantly affect the immune system's functions (Bouman et al., 2005; Verthelyi, 2001). More recently the ability of hormones to affect, the immunological response directed against pathogenic agents has gained attention (Roberts et al., 2001).

2. Sexual dimorphism of the immune response

As stated above, sex steroids regulate a variety of cellular and physiological functions of organisms such as growth, reproduction and differentiation (Derijk & Berkenbosh, 1991; Grossman et al., 1991). More recently the ability of sex steroids to affect the immunological response directed against pathogenic agents has gained attention (Klein, 2004; Roberts et al., 2001; Escobedo et al., 2005). This is clearly evident during various parasitic diseases including malaria, schistosomiasis, toxoplasmosis, cysticercosis, trypanosomiasis and leishmaniasis where strong hormonal regulation of the immune response has been described (Remoue et al., 2001; do Prado et al., 1998; Satoskar & Alexander, 1995; Vargas-Villavicencio et al., 2006; Libonati et al., 2006; Liesenfield et al., 2001). In many sexually dimorphic species the determination of the sexual genotype upon conception, followed by the organism's physiological and endocrinological development, brings about numerous and complex differences between males and females. Starting in infancy, and thereafter along reproductive life, these differences are based on the production, secretion, and circulating concentrations of estrogens, progesterone and testosterone and caused mainly on the function and development of the hypothalamus-pituitary-gonad axis (HPG) (Angioni et al., 1991). The complex interaction between hormones produced by the HPG axis and other hormones, in addition to sex-independent gene products, determine the male and female phenotypes (Besedovsky & del Rey, 2002).

It may thus be inferred that, in addition to their effects on sexual differentiation and reproduction, sex hormones may also determine the differences between the sexes regarding their immune response to the same antigenic stimulus. These differences include sexual dimorphism of the immune response as well as dimorphism associated to infection parameters (Bouman et al., 2005; Morales-Montor et al., 2002b; Zuk & McKean, 1996).

Besides their effects on sexual differentiation and reproduction, sex steroids (estradiol, progesterone and testosterone) can influence the immune system by affecting differently many of the functions of virtually all-immune cells types (Muñoz-Cruz et al., 2011). In fact, sexual hormones modulate a large variety of phenomena involved in the immune response, including thymocyte maturation and selection, cellular transit, lymphocyte proliferation, expression of class II major histocompatibility complex molecules and receptors, and cytokine production (Bebo et al., 2001; Da Silva, 1999). Furthermore, the presence of sex steroid receptors on immune cells (Muñoz-Cruz et al., 2011) indicates that one mechanism by which sex steroids may exert their biological effects involves interactions with either cytoplasmic or nuclear receptors. For these hormones to have an effect on immune system cells, the presence of hormone receptors in these cells is necessary. Although steroid hormones also exert effects by non-genomic mechanisms by acting on cell surface receptors and triggering signaling cascades, it is currently accepted that the main route of biological activity occurs by means of specific nuclear receptors (NR) that function as transcription factors, and coordinate, after binding to their ligand, the expression of target genes. The following NR are mediators of these effects: estrogen receptors (ER) and androgen receptor (AR); the estrogen receptors ER-α and ER-β, each coded for by an individual gene, whose predominating ligand is 17β-estradiol; progesterone receptor (PR), which has variants A and B generated from the same gene by alternative splicing, and whose main ligand is progesterone. Androgen receptors (AR), coded for by a single gene and its ligands being testosterone and dehydrotestosterone (DHT). In fact, the binding between estradiol (E_2) and its membrane ER activates group I and II of the metabotropic glutamate receptor (Boulware et al., 2005). It should here be mentioned that ER is able to bind to Src kinases through their highly conserved SH2 domains, which could considerably modify the effect of ERK 1/2 on the phosphorylation pattern of this transcription factor (Auricchio et al., 2008). Recently, three new putative membrane progesterone receptors (mPRs), mPRα, mPRβ, and mPRγ have been described and detected also on T lymphocytes (Dosiou et al., 2008). The mechanism of action of these membrane progesterone receptors is suggested to be through G_i-protein activation. Previous findings have also revealed unconventional non-genomic surface receptors for testosterone in rat T cells. These belong to the class of membrane receptors coupled to phospholipase C (PLC) via a pertussis toxin-sensitive G-protein. Binding of testosterone to these cell surface receptors causes a rapid increase in intracellular free Ca^{2+} concentration ($[Ca^{2+}]i$) and an increased formation of inositol 1,4,5-triphosphate and diacylglycerol (Benten et al., 1999). Preliminary evidence indicates that in murine T cells, testosterone also induces a rapid rise in $[Ca^{2+}]^i$, presumably due to Ca^{2+} influx triggered by binding of testosterone to receptors on the outer surface of T cells.

3. Sex steroids and immune response to helminthes parasites

Sexual dimorphism (SD) in parasitic infections it is a scarcely studied biological phenomenon of considerable significance for individual health as well as for the evolution of species. Most of the poor knowledge about this topic is related to the wrong concept of the female supremacy in infectious diseases. However, there are many notable exceptions to this rule of a favorable female bias in susceptibility to infection. Particularly in the host's sexual differences to cystercosis infection, females are more likely to become infected, to carry larger parasite loads, to be more severely affected and more reticent to develop protective immunity to variable degrees that associate with their genetic backgrounds and times of infection. The importance of the interaction between the immune and endocrine systems becomes evident in particular circumstances of the lifespan of an organism, such as pregnancy, autoimmune diseases, and some time, it is also affected by infectious diseases. In all cases, the available evidence underscores the importance of sex steroids as immunoregulators (Verthelyi, 2001).

The hormonal microenvironment and in particular the balance of male and female hormones may favor survival of certain parasites under certain circumstances. Predominance of a sex-distinctive steroid may directly induce reproduction, growth or differentiation of the parasite, and thus favor the establishment of infection. This represents a highly evolved host parasite relationship that places the parasite in an environment that, far from being hostile, endows it with growth factors that operate directly and positively on its growth and reproduction. This is independent of other elements such as the immune system. All of this amounts to the parasite exploiting endocrine mechanism developed by the host for its own advantage. It may thus be noted that the benefit of parasites to infect a host of a particular sex largely depends on the circulating steroid levels at the time of infection, and appears as the result of lengthy adaptive trials between host and parasite subjected to the same co-evolutionary process.

4. The case of Cestodes

Cestoda is the class of parasitic flatworms, commonly called tapeworms that live in the digestive tract of vertebrates as adults and often in the bodies of various animals as juveniles. There are two subclasses in class Cestoda, the Cestodaria and the Eucestoda. By far the most common and widespread are the Eucestoda, with only a few species of unusual worms in subclass Cestodaria. The cyclophyllideans are the most important to humans because they infect people and livestock. Two important tapeworms are the pork tapeworm, *Taenia solium*, and the beef tapeworms, *T. saginata* (Morales-Montor et al., 2004). Taennids, particularly *Taenia solium* (causal agent of porcine cysticercosis and human neurocysticercosis) and *Taenia crassiceps* (causal agent of murine cysticercosis) are highly evolved parasites that have developed diverse mechanisms of survival that facilitate their establishment in the hosts. Taennids can also exploit the hormonal microenvironment within the host in their favor (Escobedo et al., 2005; Locksley, 1997). Taennids have evolved structures similar to the steroid and protein hormone receptors expressed in upper vertebrates, with binding properties and terminal effects similar to the hormonal metabolites synthesized by the host (Damian, 1989; Salzet et al., 2000). In the next paragraphs, we summarize the findings on the role of sex steroids in two cestodes: *Taenia crassiceps* and *Taenia solium*.

4.1 Experimental *T. solium* Taeniosis/cysticercosis

T. solium is an ancient parasite that still threatens public health and porcine husbandry in Latin America, Africa and Asia, and is re-emerging in developed countries on account of the massive human migrations of modern times (Hoberg, 2002; DeGiorgio et al., 2005; Sorvillo et al., 2011). Cysticercosis results from the ingestion of the *T. solium* eggs by intermediate hosts (humans and pigs, principally), to then hatch in the intestines liberating motile oncospheres that penetrate the circulation and distribute in the organism. Oncospheres may establish in muscles, subcutaneous connective tissue, central nervous system, liver, and other organs of the host, where they develop into cysticerci, the larvae of *T. solium* contained within a vesicular translucent structure of about one cm in size (Sciutto et al., 2000). Once developed, many cysticerci die leaving scar tissue or nodular calcifications, while others live-on causing chronic and severe organic malfunction because of space-occupation and/or local inflammation, especially when located in the brain of the human intermediate host. Humans are also the only definitive hosts of the intestinal adult tapeworm, the stage in which the parasite is capable of sexual reproduction and of massive egg production. Pigs are nowadays the preferred intermediary host for the *T. solium*'s larval stage (i.e., cysticercus), a necessary stage in the parasite´s life cycle before its eventual transformation into an adult tapeworm upon their ingestion by humans in infected and uncooked pork meat.

Host's sexual dimorphism in *Taenia solium* infections is much less obvious than that of experimental *Taenia crassiceps* cysticercosis in laboratory mice. Nonetheless, there are various hints pointing in that direction and several speculations as to the reasons behind such low profiles of sexual differences in cysticercotic pigs and humans. Human's immunological contact with any of *T. solium*'s developmental forms is likely to induce an immune response. The high mean prevalence of seropositive individuals in the open population of Mexico (~1%) (Larralde et al., 1992), when compared with the presumed prevalence of neurocysticercosis (~0.1 to 10%) (Fleury et al., 2003; 2006), is taken to indicate that very few of the contacts result in the establishment of the cysticercus in the tissues of humans and less so in their brains. In view of the many weaknesses of such numbers and assumptions lacking the objective finding of the parasite in the suspected human cases it's somewhat adventurous to interpret them as signs of sexual dimophism in human disease, even if significant differences in serological prevalence favor women over men in Mexico (Larralde et al., 1992). The more so if no credible prevalence differences of neurocysticercosis were supported by necropsy studies (Rabiela et al., 1982). Nonetheless, there are other findings indicating to sexual dimorphism among human neurocyticercotic patients. Women develop more frequently generalized encephalitis than men and, when bearing subarchnoidal and ventricular vesicular parasites, women show higher inflammatory profiles in their cerebral spinal fluid than men (Del Brutto et al., 1988; Fleury et al., 2004). However, in those same patients there were no other immunological signs of sexual dimorphism (Chavarria et al., 2005). Also, in Peru, it was reported that subjects included a newly devised anti-helminth treatment protocol were mostly women highly suspected of carrying an adult *T. solium* in their intestines. Likewise, women were recently reported to harbor more single cysticercotic calcified lesions in their right cerebral hemisphere than in the left. Presumably, lateralization of calcified cysticerci reflects the differential immunological abilities between the cerebral hemispheres (Meador et al., 2004). Although no sexual differences in these cerebral abilities have been notified, cysticercus lateralization is not found in male neurocysticercotic patients. Gender discriminatory practices in health services also throw shadows upon morbidity and mortality differences between women and men in Mexico: men request more frequently medical attention at hospitals than women do, yet they have similar mortality rates in the many diseases not in close association with genital organs, including infections. It would then follow that Mexican women more frequently resort to informal consult and therapy of their ailments than men do, thus defaulting from morbidity data and appearing for consult in the final stages of disease. Notwithstanding the many sex and gender associated biological and social biases involved, the findings of sexual dimorphism in cysticercotic humans should not be confidently dismissed.

Sex steroids play an important role during *T. solium* infection, particularly progesterone has been proposed as a key immunomodulatory hormone involved in susceptibility to human taeniosis in woman and cysticercosis in pregnant pigs. Then, we evaluated the effect of progesterone administration upon experimental taeniosis in hamsters (*Mesocricetus auratus*). Intact female adult hamsters were randomly divided into 3 groups: progesterone-subcutaneously treated; olive oil-treated, as the vehicle group; and untreated controls. Animals were treated every other day during 4 weeks. After 2 weeks of treatment, all hamsters were orally infected with 4 viable *T. solium* cysticerci. After 2 weeks post infection, progesterone-treated hamsters showed reduction in adult worm recovery by 80%, compared

to both vehicle-treated and non-manipulated infected animals. In contrast to control and vehicle groups, progesterone diminished tapeworm length by 75% and increased proliferation rate of leukocytes from spleen and mesenteric lymph nodes of infected hamsters by 5-fold. IL-4, IL-6 and TNF-α expression at the duodenal mucosa, promoted local exacerbation of inflammatory infiltrate.
The issue of sexual dimorphism in naturally acquired porcine cysticercosis is a bit stronger than it is in human cysticercosis. Male rural pigs castrated 4 months before sacrifice show a cysticercosis prevalence double that of non-castrated male pigs, and so do pregnant sows (Morales et al., 2002; 2006). There is, however, an exposure catch obscuring the reason of such associations: castrated pigs flock around a dominant female that effectively search for foodstus in the open fields whilst sexually active boars are almost wild creatures, roaming around marginally to any flock and are thus presumed to be less well nurtured and less exposed to consuming human feces and becoming infected. Anyways, research is in progress to ascertain if any endocrinological changes in the sex steroids of rural pigs associate with cysticercosis. Moreover, frequency of *T. solium* pig cysticercosis is increased during pregnancy, when there is a significant increase in progesterone levels (Morales et al., 2002; Peña et al., 2007). It has also been demonstrated that castration in naturally infected male boars, induces an increase in the prevalence of cysticercosis, which highlights the possible role of host androgens to restrict parasite establishment and estrogens to facilitate it (Morales et al., 2002).

4.2 Sexual steroids directly act upon *Taenia solium*

The effects of progesterone and its antagonist RU486, on scolex evagination, which is the initial step in the development of the adult worm, have been demonstrated (Escobedo, et al, 2010). Interestingly, progesterone increased *T. solium* scolex evagination and worm growth, in a concentration-independent pattern. Progesterone effects could be mediated by a novel *T. solium* progesterone receptor (TsPR), since RU486 inhibits both scolex evagination and worm development induced by progesterone. By using RT-PCR and western blot, sequences related to progesterone receptor were detected in the parasite. A phylogenetic analysis reveals that TsPR is highly related to fish and amphibian progesterone receptors, whereas it has a distant relation with birds and mammals. Conclusively, progesterone directly acts upon *T. solium* cysticerci, possibly through its binding to a progesterone receptor synthesized by the parasite (Escobedo et al, 2010).

4.3 Experimental *Taenia crassiceps* murine cysticercosis

Due to the intrinsic difficulties in working with the natural hosts (pigs and humans) of *T. solium* or because of the high costs of sufficient pigs plus the slowness in data retrieval, we have used an experimental cysticercosis approach to gain knowledge of the complex host (H) parasite (P) relationship in cysticercosis. Murine intraperitoneal cysticercosis is caused by the taenid *Taenia crassiceps* and it has been useful to explore the physiological host factors associated with porcine cysticercosis, and to some degree, with human neurocysticercosis (Sciutto et al., 2011). Intraperitoneal *T. crassiceps* cysticercosis of mice lends itself well to controlled and reproducible experimentation, generating numerical data of parasite loads in individual mice in a matter of weeks after infection. Its general representation of other forms of cysticercosis has later been strengthened by similar results in other mouse and parasite strains, by the parasite's extensive sharing of antigens with other taennids and cestodes and by the DNA homology between *T. crassiceps and T. solium* (Rishi & McManus, 1988). These characteristics have made murine cysticercosis a convenient instrument to test vaccine candidates and new drugs or treatments against cysticercosis (Vargas-Villavicencio). Several features of natural cysticercotic disease have been found by extrapolation from experimental murine cysticercosis (Morales-Montor et al., 2008).

4.4 Role of sex steroids in cysticercosis

In *T. crassiceps* cysticercosis, females of all strains of mice studied sustain larger intensities of infection than males, but during chronic infection (more than 4 weeks) this difference disappears and the males of BALB/c strain show a feminization process, characterized by high serum estrogens levels (200 times the normal values) whilst those of testosterone are 90% decreased. The target organs for testosterone action, testes and seminal vesicles, have a 50% weight reduction (Larralde et al., 1995). At the same time, the cellular immune response (Th1) is markedly diminished in both sexes, and the humoral (Th2) response is enhanced (Terrazas et al., 1998). Estradiol is involved in the immunoendocrine regulation of murine *T. crassiceps* cysticercosis as a major protagonist in promoting cysticercus growth interfering with the thymus dependent cellular immune mechanisms that obstruct parasite growth (Terrazas et al., 1994). Gonadectomy alters this resistance pattern and makes intensities equal in both sexes by increasing that of males and diminishing it in females (Huerta et al., 1992), whilst the serum sex steroids level are not detectable in these animals. However, the absence of estrogens does not prevent parasite growth in both genders, demonstrating that although estradiol favours *Taenia crassiceps* development, it is not indispensable for rapid parasite growth (Larralde et al., 1995).

5. Immuno-endocrine interactions in the host

The mechanisms by which sex steroids act upon *T. crassiceps* cysticercus asexual reproduction are two: A) through the host's immune system mediation or/and B) directly through the parasites own physiological systems.

The changes in steroid production of infected male mice were found to associate with an increase in *c-fos* mRNA content in all tissues studied, whereas the *c-jun* mRNA content was increased only in the thymus. The p53 mRNA content was markedly reduced in all tissues of the parasitized animals analyzed, whereas bcl-2 gene expression was abolished only in the thymus (Morales-Montor et al., 1998).

On the other hand, thymic cell analysis performed by flow cytometry showed a diminution in the percent of $CD3^{+}CD4^{+}$, and $CD3^{+}CD8^{+}$ subpopulations in the infected mice, suggesting that the increase in estradiol levels of the host could change the expression pattern of several genes that participate in apoptosis regulation in the thymus of male mice during chronic infection with *T. crassiceps* cysticerci, and that estrogens could inhibit the specific cellular immune response to the parasite (Morales-Montor et al., 1998). Previous immunological experiments had led to suspect that estradiol positively regulates parasite reproduction in hosts of both sexes, presumably by interfering with the thymus-dependent cellular immune mechanisms that obstruct parasite growth (Th1) and favoring those that facilitate it (Th2) (Terrazas et al., 1998; Bojalil et al., 1993). A specific shift from Th1 to Th2 immune response in the course of infection was found that coincided with the initial low rate of reproduction that accelerates at later times of infection. The shift is characterized by a marked decrease of

IL-2 and IFN-γ in both sexes, while the secretion of cytokines involved in the specific humoral response (IL-6, IL-10 and IL-4) is enhanced (Terrazas et al., 1998, 1999). Thus, striking differences in susceptibility to cysticercosis between male and female mice may involve the joint action of the immune system and the gonads, both driven by a parasite that is able to change the parasite's restrictive male normal hormonal milieu during chronic infection to a more parasite's permissive female environment.

To strengthen the above notions and in an effort to identify the sex steroids involved we studied the effects of testosterone, dihydrotestosterone, and 17β-estradiol in castrated mice of both sexes infected with *Taenia crassiceps* cysticerci (Morales-Montor et al., 2002a). In this study, we found that castration and treatment with either testosterone or dihydrotestosterone before infection markedly decreased parasite loads in both gender mice, while the treatment with 17β-estradiol increased it in both genders (Morales-Montor et al., 2002a). The specific splenocyte cell proliferation and IL-2 and IFN-γ production were depressed in infected-castrated mice of both genders, while treatment with testosterone or dihydrotestosterone produced a significant cell proliferation recovery and enhanced production of IL-2 and IFN-γ (Morales-Montor et al., 2002a). An opposite effect of the same sex steroids was found on the humoral response: it was unaffected with testosterone or dihydrotestosterone restitution, while the treatment with estradiol in both genders augmented the levels of anti-cysticerci IgG, as well as IL-6 and IL-10 production. These results suggest androgens mediate immune functions, which protect mice from cysticercosis, possibly through the stimulation of the specific cellular immunity of the host (Morales-Montor et al., 2002a).

Immunoendocrine interactions during cysticercosis are the cornerstone of the feminization of male mice. When the infected male mice have an intact immune system, there is an increase in serum estradiol levels and a decrease of those of testosterone and DHT. However, when the immune system is knocked down by total irradiation or neonatal thymectomy, there is no change in the levels of serum steroids in chronically infected male mice, and the levels remain steady between infected and uninfected male mice (Morales-Montor et al., 2001).

The importance of sex-hormones driving the specific immune response during cysticercosis was assessed by administration of Fadrozole (a P450-aromatase inhibitor) in male and female mice to suppress the production of 17β-estradiol (Morales-Montor et al., 2002b). A reduction was found in parasite loads (~70%) in infected mice treated with Fadrozole. The protective effect of the P450-aromatase inhibitor was associated in male mice with a recovery of the specific cellular immune response. Furthermore, it has also been demonstrated that administration of Tamoxifen (an anti-estrogen) produced an 80% parasite load reduction in female mice, and had a weaker effect of 50% in male mice. This protective effect was associated in both sexes with an increase in the mRNA levels of IL-2 (a cytokine associated to protection against cysticerci) and IL-4 (innocuos against infection). Tamoxifen treatment modified 17β-estradiol production in females, while serum testosterone was not affected. However, the expression of the two types of estrogen receptor, ER-α and ER-β, in the spleen of infected mice of both sexes, was decreased by Tamoxifen treatment (Vargas-Villavicencio et al., 2007). The *in vitro* treatment of *T. crassiceps* with Tamoxifen, reduced reproduction and induced loss of motility in the parasite. These results indicate that Tamoxifen treatment is a new therapeutic possibility to treat cysticercosis, since it can act at both senses of the host-parasite relationship: increasing the cellular immune response protective against the parasite and acting directly upon the parasite, reducing its reproduction and increasing its mortality (Vargas-Villavicencio et al., 2007). Another steroid that was recently tested and found to be implicated in the regulation of the parasite loads during murine cysticercosis is progesterone (P_4). P_4 treatment has a dichotomic effect: if mice of both sexes are non-gonadectomized (intact), P_4 treatment increased parasite loads, possibly through manipulation of the specific cellular immune response, besides the steroid's promotion of parasite reproduction (Vargas-Villavicencio et al., 2005). However, if mice are gonadectomized, P_4 completely decreases parasite loads, an impressive and unprecedented cysticidal effect, the likes of which are absent from other preventive or therapeutic measures (Vargas-Villavicencio et al., 2006). These two experiments suggests that, in intact hosts, progesterone is metabolized to estradiol, that is permissive for parasite reproduction, while in castrated animals, there is an active metabolism of progesterone in the adrenal glands to androgens, resulting in a toxic effect in the parasite growth (Vargas-Villavicencio et al., 2005, 2006). The major steroid produced by the adrenal gland is the androgen dehydroepiandrosterone (DHEA). So, another set of experiments showed DHEA effect on male and female infected mice. DHEA treatment reduced parasite loads by 70 and 80% respectively. In contrast with the common assumption of DHEA as an immuno-stimulatory hormone, the immune responses of our mice was not affected by DHEA treatment (Vargas-Villavicencio et al., 2008). *In vitro*, treatment of *T. crassiceps* cysticerci with DHEA induced an 80% reduction in parasite reproduction, which may partially explain the reduction of parasite loads observed *in vivo* a partial effect suggesting the involvement of other unknown factors in the *in vivo* regulation of parasite loads (Vargas-Villavicencio et al., 2008).

6. Sexual steroids directly act upon *Taenia crassiceps*

Not only do sex steroids regulate parasite loads through the immune response modulation of the host, but also they directly act upon cysticerci reproduction. For instance, it has been shown that E_2 and P_4 *in vitro* treatment stimulates *T. crassiceps* reproduction, while *in vitro* treatment with T or DHT inhibit and even exert a slight toxic effect on the parasite (Escobedo et al., 2004). The possible molecular mechanisms by which sex-steroids affect *Taenia crassiceps* reproduction, imply the presence of estrogen receptors (both α and β isoforms) and androgen receptors, but no progesterone receptors. In addition, once host's E_2 has bound to its parasite estrogen receptor, the active, ligand bound complex would activate the transcription of several *Taenia crassiceps* proliferative genes, such as *c-fos, c-jun* and cyclin D1, and in that way up-regulate parasite growth and reproduction. All this hypothetical molecular mechanism could be interrupted *in vitro* by means of using tamoxifen that is well known for its anti-estrogenic effects (Vargas-Villavicencio et al., 2007), which strongly suggests a genomic action mechanism for 17-β estradiol on the parasite. On the other hand, action mechanism of the androgen is likely different from the found for estrogens and progesterone. Testosterone and DHT likely directly affect parasitic DNA integrity by activating apoptotic mechanism in the cysticercus cells. This experimental finding is not dependent of a nuclear receptor, because flutamide (a well studied and used anti-androgen) did not have effects upon parasite reproduction *in vitro* (Escobedo et al., 2004). These results demonstrate that sex steroids act directly upon parasite reproduction perhaps by binding to receptors closely resembling classic and specific sex-steroid vertebrate receptors (Escobedo et al., 2004) (64).

7. Concluding remarks

The evidence presented above illustrates the complexity and importance of neuroimmunoendocrine interactions during helminth infections, and provides clues to the many other possible mechanisms of parasite establishment, growth and reproduction in an immunocompetent host. Further, strong neuroimmunoendocrine interactions may have implications in the control of transmission and treatment of several parasitic diseases, but particularly in those produced by helminth parasites, in animals and humans. In practical importance, the complexity of the helminth-host relationship suggests that all physiological factors (i.e., sex, age) should be taken into account in the design of vaccines and new drugs. The differential response of helminthes to sex steroids may also be involved in their ability to grow faster in female or male hosts. Host and parasite sex-associated biases may be combined to favour their evolution towards a mutually acceptable relationship. Also, the strong immune-endocrine interactions observed during *Taenia crassiceps* and *Taenia solium* cysticercosis, could give ways to possible new mechanisms of parasite establishment, growth and reproduction in an immunocompetent host.

8. Acknowledgments

Financial support was provided by grant IN 214011-3 from the Programa de Apoyo a Proyectos de Innovación Tecnológica, Dirección General de Asuntos del Personal Académico, Universidad Nacional Autónoma de México to J. Morales-Montor. R. Hernández-Bello has a Posdoctoral fellowship from RED-Farmed, from CONACyT.

9. References

Angioni, S.; Petraglia, F. & Genezzani, AR. (1991). Immune-neuroendocrine correlations: a new aspect in human physiology. *Acta Eur Fertil*, Vol.22, No.3, pp. 167-170.

Auricchio, F.; Migliaccio, A. & Castoria, G. (2008). Sex-steroid hormones and EGF signalling in breast and prostate cancer cells: targeting the association of Src with steroid receptors. *Steroids*, Vol.73, No.9-10, pp.880-884.

Barrabes, A.; Duong, TH. & Combescot, C. (1979). Effect of testosterone or progesterone implants on the intensity of experimental infestation with *Schistosoma mansoni* in the female golden hamster. *C R Seances Soc Biol Fil*, Vol.173, No.1, pp. 153-156.

Bebo, B.F.; Fyfe-Johnson, A.; Adlard, K.; Beam, A. G.; Vandenbark, A.A. & Offner, H. (2001). Low-dose estrogen therapy ameliorates experimental autoimmune encephalomyelitis in two different inbred mouse strains. *J Immunol*, Vol.166, No.3, pp. 2080-2089.

Benten, W.P.; Lieberherr, M.; Giese, G.; Wrehlke, C.; Stamm, O.; Sekeris, C. E.; Mossmann, H. & Wunderlich, F. (1999). Functional testosterone receptors in plasma membranes of T cells. *FASEB J*, Vol.13, No.1, pp. 123-133.

Besedovsky, H.O. & del Rey, A. (2002). Introduction: immune-neuroendocrine network. *Front Horm Res*, Vol.29, pp. 1-14.

Bojalil, R.; Terrazas, L.I.; Govezensky, T.; Sciutto, E. & Larralde, C. (1993). Thymus-related cellular immune mechanisms in sex associated resistance to experimental murine cysticercosis (*Taenia crassiceps*). *J Parasitol*, Vol.78, pp. 471-476.

Boulware, M.I.; Weick, J.P.; Becklund, B.R.; Kuo, S.P.; Groth, R.D. & Mermelstein, P.G. (2005). Estradiol activates group I and II metabotropic glutamate receptor signaling, leading to opposing influences on cAMP response element-binding protein. *J Neurosci*, Vol.25, No.20, pp. 5066-5078.

Bouman, A.; Heineman, M.J. & Faas MM. (2005). Sex hormones and the immune response in humans. *Hum Reprod Update,* Vol.11, pp. 411-423.

Brodsky, F.M.; Lem, L.; Solache, A. & Bennett EM. (1999). Human pathogen subversion of antigen presentation. *Immunol Rev*, Vol.168, pp. 199-215.

Chavarría, A.; Fleury, A.; García, E.; Márquez, C.; Fragoso, G. & Sciutto, E. (2005). Relationship between the clinical heterogeneity of neurocysticercosis and the immune-inflammatory profiles. *Clin Immunol*, Vol.116, No.3, pp. 27127-8.

Da Silva, J.A. (1999). Sex hormones and glucocorticoids: interactions with the immune system. *Ann N Y Acad Sci*, Vol.876, pp. 102-118.

Damian, R.T. (1989). Molecular mimicry: parasite evasion and host defense. *Curr Top Microbiol Immunol*, Vol.145, pp. 101-115.

DeGiorgio, C.M.; Sorvillo, F. & Escueta, S.P. (2005). Neurocysticercosis in the United States: review of an important emerging infection. *Neurology*, Vol.64, No.8 pp. 1486

Del Brutto, O.H.; Garcia, E.; Talamas, O. & Sotelo, J. (1988). Sex-related severity of inflammation in parenchymal brain cysticercosis. *Archives of Internal Medicine*, Vol.148, pp. 544–546.

Derijk, R. & Berkenbosch, F. (1991). The immune-hypothalamo-pituitary-adrenal axis and autoimmunity. *Int J Neurosci*, Vol.59, No.1-3, pp. 91-100.

do Prado junior, J.C.; Leal Mde, P.; Anselmo-Franci, J.A.; de Andrade juniur, H.F. & Kloetzel, J.K., (1998). Influence of female gonadal hormones on the parasitemia of female *Calomys callosus* infected with the "Y" strain of *Trypanosoma cruzi. Parasitol Res*, Vol.84, No.2, pp. 100-115.

Dosiou, C.; Hamilton, A.E.; Pang, Y.; Overgaard, M.T.; Tulac, S.; Dong, J.; Thomas, P. & Giudice, L.C. (2008). Expression of membrane progesterone receptors on human T lymphocytes and Jurkat cells and activation of G-proteins by progesterone. *J Endocrinol*, Vol.196, No.1, pp. 67-77.

Escobedo, G.; Camacho-Arroyo, I.; Hernández-Hernández, O.T.; Ostoa-Saloma, P.; García-Varela, M. & Morales-Montor, J. (2010). Progesterone induces scolex evagination of the human parasite *Taenia solium*: evolutionary implications to the host-parasite relationship. *J Biomed Biotechnol.*, Vol.2010, pp. 591079.

Escobedo, G.; Roberts, C.W.; Carrero, J.C. & Morales-Montor, J. (2005) Parasite regulation by host hormones: an old mechanism of host exploitation? *Trends Parasitol* Vol.21, pp. 588-593.

Escobedo, G.; Larralde, C.; Chavarria, A.; Cerbon, M. A. & Morales-Montor, J. (2004). Molecular mechanisms involved in the differential effects of sex steroids on the reproduction and infectivity of *Taenia crassiceps*. *J Parasitol*, Vol.90, No.6, pp. 1235-1244.

Fleury, A.; Dessein, A.; Preux, P.M.; Dumas, M.; Tapia, G.; Larralde, C. & Sciutto, E. (2004). Symptomatic human neurocysticercosis--age, sex and exposure factors relating with disease heterogeneity. *J Neurol*, Vol.251, No,7, pp. 830-837.

Fleury, A.; Gomez, T.; Alvarez, I.; Meza, D.; Huerta, M.; Chavarria, A.; Carrillo Mezo, R.A.; Lloyd, C.; Dessein, A.; Preux, P.M.; Dumas, M.; Larralde, C.; Sciutto, E. & Fragoso, G. (2003). High prevalence of calcified silent neurocysticercosis in a rural village of Mexico. *Neuroepidemiology*, Vol.22, No.2, pp. 139-145.

Fleury, A.; Morales, J.; Bobes, R.J.; Dumas, M.; Yánez, O.; Piña, J.; Carrillo-Mezo, R.; Martínez, J.J.; Fragoso, G.; Dessein, A.; Larralde, C. & Sciutto, E. (2006). An epidemiological study of familial neurocysticercosis in an endemic Mexican community. *Trans R Soc Trop Med Hyg*, Vol.100, No.6, pp. 551-558.

Grossman, C.J.; Roselle, G.A. & Mendenhall, C.L. (1991). Sex steroid regulation of autoimmunity. *J Steroid Biochem Mol Biol*, Vol.40, No.4-6, pp. 649-59.

Hoberg, E.P. (2002). *Taenia* tapeworms: their biology, evolution and socioeconomic significance. *Microbes Infect*, Vol.4, No.8, pp.859-866.

Huerta, L.; Terrazas, L. I.; Sciutto, E. & Larralde, C. (1992). Immunological mediation of gonadal effects on experimental murine cysticercosis caused by *Taenia crassiceps* metacestodes. *J Parasitol*, Vol.78, pp. 471-476.

Klein, S. (2004). Hormonal and immunological mechanisms mediating sex differences in parasite infection. *Parasite Immunol*, Vol.26, pp. 247-264.

Larralde, C.; Padilla, A.; Hernández, M.; Govezensky, T.; Sciutto, E.; Gutiérrez, G.; Tapia-Conyer, R.; Salvatierra, B. & Sepúlveda, J. (1992). Seroepidemiology of cysticercosis in Mexico. *Salud Publica Mex*, Vol.34, No.2, pp. 197-210.

Larralde, C.; Morales, J.; Terrazas, I.; Govezensky, T. & Romano, M.C. (1995). Sex hormone changes induced by the parasite lead to feminization of the male host in murine *Taenia crassiceps* cysticercosis. *J Steroid Biochem Mol Biol*, Vol.52 pp. 575-581.

Libonati, R.M.; Cunha, M.G.; Souza, J.M.; Santos, M.V.; Oliveira, S.G.; Daniel-Ribeiro, C.T.; Carvalho, L.J. & do Nascimento, J.L. (2006). Estradiol, but not dehydroepiandrosterone, decreases parasitemia and increases the incidence of cerebral malaria and the mortality in *Plasmodium berghei* ANKA-infected CBA mice. *Neuroimmunomodulation*, Vol.13, No.1, pp. 28-35.

Liesenfeld, O.; Nguyen, T.A.; Pharke, C. & Suzuki, Y. (2001). Importance of gender and sex hormones in regulation of susceptibility of the small intestine to peroral infection with *Toxoplasma gondii* tissue cysts. *J Parasitol*, Vol.87, No.6, pp. 1491-1493

Locksley, R.M. (1997). Exploitation of immune and other defence mechanisms by parasites: an overview. *Parasitology*, Vol.115, Suppl.S5-7.

Meador, K.J.; Loring, D.W.; Ray, P.G.; Helman, S.W.; Vazquez, B.R. & Neveu, P.J. 2004. Role of cerebral lateralization in control of immune processes in humans. *Ann Neurol*, Vol.55, No.6, pp. 840-844.

Morales, J.; Martínez, J.J.; Garcia-Castella, J.; Peña, N.; Maza, V.; Villalobos, N.; Aluja, A.S.; Fleury, A.; Fragoso, G.; Larralde, C. & Sciutto, E. (2006). *Taenia solium*: the complex interactions, of biological, social, geographical and commercial factors, involved in the transmission dynamics of pig cysticercosis in highly endemic areas. *Ann Trop Med Parasitol*, Vol.100, No.2, pp. 123-135.

Morales, J.; Velasco, T.; Tovar, V.; Fragoso, G.; Fleury, A.: Beltrán, C.; Villalobos, N.; Aluja, A.; Rodarte, L.F.; Sciutto, E. & Larralde, C. (2002). Castration and pregnancy of rural pigs significantly increase the prevalence of naturally acquired *Taenia solium* cysticercosis. *Vet Parasitol*, Vol.108, No.1, pp. 41-48.

Morales-Montor, J.; Escobedo, G.; Vargas-Villavicencio, J.A. & Larralde, C. (2008). The neuroimmunoendocrine network in the complex host-parasite relationship during murine cysticercosis. *Curr Top Med Chem*, Vol.8, No.5, pp. 400-407.

Morales-Montor, J.; Baig, S.; Hallal-Calleros, C. & Damian, R.T. (2002a). *Taenia crassiceps*: androgen reconstitution of the host leads to protection during cysticercosis. *Exp. Parasitol*, Vol.100, pp. 209-216.

Morales-Montor, J.; Baig, S.; Mitchell, R.; Deway, K.; Hallal-Calleros, C. & Damian, R.T. (2001). Immunoendocrine interactions during chronic cysticercosis determine male mouse feminization: role of IL-6. *J Immunol*, Vol.167, pp. 4527-4533.

Morales-Montor, J.; Chavarria, A.; De Leon, M. A.; Del Castillo, L. I.; Escobedo, E. G.; Sanchez, E. N.; Vargas, J. A.; Hernandez-Flores, M.; Romo-Gonzalez, T. & Larralde, C. (2004). Host gender in parasitic infections of mammals: an evaluation of the female host supremacy paradigm. *J Parasitol*, Vol.90, No.3, pp. 531-546.

Morales-Montor, J.; Hallal-Calleros, C.; Romano, M. & Damian, R.T. (2002b). Inhibition of P-450 aromatase prevents feminization and induces protection during cysticercosis. *Int J Parasitol*, Vol. 32, pp. 1379-1387.

Morales-Montor, J.; Rodriguez-Dorantes, M.; Mendoza-Rodriguez, C.A.; Camacho-Arroyo, I. & Cerbon, M.A. (1998). Differential expression of the estrogen-regulated proto-oncogenes *c-fos*, *c-jun*, *bcl-2* and of the tumor-suppressor *p53* gene in the male mouse chronically infected with *Taenia crassiceps* cysticerci. *Parasitol Res*, Vol.84, pp. 616-622.

Munoz-Cruz, S.; Togno-Pierce, C. & Morales-Montor, J. (2011). Non-Reproductive Effects of Sex Steroids: Their Immunoregulatory Role. Curr Top Med Chem, Vol.11, No.13, pp. 1714-1727.

Peña, N.; Morales, J.; Morales-Montor, J.; Vargas-Villavicencio, A.; Fleury, A.; Zarco, L.; de Aluja, A.S., Larralde, C.; Fragoso, G. & Sciutto, E.. (2007) Impact of naturally acquired *Taenia solium* cysticercosis on the hormonal levels of free ranging boars. *Vet Parasitol*, Vol.21, pp. 134-137.

Rabiela, M.T.; Rivas, A.; Rodriguez, J.; Castillo, S. & Cancino, F.M. (1982). Anatomopathological aspects of human brain cysticercosis. In: *Cysticercosis: present state of knowledge and perspectives*, Flisser A, Willms K, Laclette JP, Larralde C, Ridaura C, Beltran F, (Ed.), pp. 179–200, Academic Press, ISBN 978-0122607400, New York.

Remoué, F.; Mani, J.C.; Pugnière, M.; Schacht, A.M., Capron, A. & Riveau, G. (2002). Functional specific binding of testosterone to *Schistosoma haematobium* 28-kilodalton glutathione S-transferase. *Infect Immun*, Vol.70, No.2, pp. 601-605.

Remoué, F.; To Van, D.; Schacht, A. M.; Picquet, M.; Garraud, O.; Vercruysse, J.; Ly, A.; Capron, A. & Riveau, G. (2001). Gender-dependent specific immune response during chronic human *Schistosomiasis haematobia*. *Clin Exp Immunol*, Vol.124, No.1, pp. 62-68.

Rishi, A.K. & McManus, D.P. (1988). Molecular cloning of *Taenia solium* genomic DNA and characterization of taeniid cestodes by DNA analysis. *Parasitology*, Vol.97, (Pt 1), pp. 161-76.

Roberts, C.W.; Walker, W. & Alexander, J. (2001) Sex-associated hormones and immunity to protozoan parasites. *Clin Microbiol Rev*, Vol.14, pp. 476-88.

Salzet, M.; Capron, A. & Stefano, G. B. (2000). Molecular crosstalk in host-parasite relationships: schistosome- and leech-host interactions. *Parasitol Today*, Vol.16, No.12, pp. 536-540.

Satoskar, A. & Alexander, J. (1995). Sex-determined susceptibility and differential IFN-gamma and TNF-alpha mRNA expression in DBA/2 mice infected with *Leishmania mexicana*. *Immunology*, Vol.84, No.1, pp. 1-4.

Sciutto, E.; Fragoso, G.; Fleury, A.; Laclette, J.P.; Sotelo, J.; Aluja, A.; Vargas, L. & Larralde, C. (2000). *Taenia solium* disease in humans and pigs: an ancient parasitosis disease rooted in developing countries and emerging as a major health problem of global dimensions. *Microbes Infect*, Vol.2, No.15, pp. 1875-1890.

Sciutto, E.; Fragoso, G. & Larralde, C. (2011). *Taenia crassiceps* as a model for *Taenia solium* and the S3Pvac vaccine. *Parasite Immunol*, Vol.33, No.1 pp. 79-80.

Sorvillo, F.; Wilkins, P.; Shafir, S. & Eberhard, M. (2011). Public health implications of cysticercosis acquired in the United States. *Emerg Infect Dis*, Vol.17, No.1, pp. 1-6.

Tait, A.S.; Butts, C.L. & Sternberg, E.M. (2008). The role of glucocorticoids and progestins in inflammatory, autoimmune, and infectious disease. *J Leukoc Biol*, Vol.84, pp. 924-931.

Terrazas, L.I., Bojalil, R., Govezensky, T., & Larralde, C. (1998). Shift from an early protective Th1 immune response to a late permissive Th2-type response in murine cysticercosis (*Taenia crassiceps*). *Journal of Parasitology*, Vol.84, pp. 74-81.

Terrazas, L.I.; Bojalil, R.; Govezensky, T. & Larralde, C. (1994). A role for 17b-estradiol in immunoendocrine regulation of cysticercosis (*Taenia crassiceps*). *J Parasitol*, Vol.80, pp. 563-568.

Terrazas, L.I.; Cruz, M.; Rodríguez-Sosa, M.; Bojalil, R.; García-Tamayo, F. & Larralde, C. (1999). Th1-type cytokines improve resistance to murine cysticercosis caused by *Taenia crassiceps*. *Parasitol Res*, Vol.85, pp. 135.

Vargas-Villavicencio, J.A.; Larralde, C.; De León-Nava, M.A.; Escobedo, G.; Morales-Montor, J. (2007). Tamoxifen treatment induces protection in murine cysticercosis. *J Parasitol*, Vol. 93, No.6, pp. 1512-1517.

Vargas-Villavicencio, J.A.; Larralde, C. & Morales-Montor, J. (2008). Treatment with dehydroepiandrosterone *in vivo* and *in vitro* inhibits reproduction, growth and viability of *Taenia crassiceps* metacestodes. *Int J Parasitol*, Vol.38, No.7, pp. 775-781.

Vargas-Villavicencio, J.A.; Larralde, C.; De Leon-Nava, M. A. & Morales-Montor, J. (2005). Regulation of the immune response to cestode infection by progesterone is due to its metabolism to estradiol. *Microbes Infect*, Vol.7, pp. 485-493.

Vargas-Villavicencio, J.A.; Larralde, C. & Morales-Montor, J. (2006). Gonadectomy and progesterone treatment induce protection in murine cysticercosis. *Parasite Immunol*, Vol.28, No.12, pp. 667-674.

Verthelyi, D. (2001). Sex hormones as immunomodulators in health and disease. *Int Immunopharmacol*, Vol.1, No.6, pp. 983-993.

Zahner, H.; Sani, B.P.; Shealy, Y.F. & Nitschmann, A. (1989) Antifilarial activities of synthetic and natural retinoids *in vitro*. *Trop Med Parasitol*, Vol.40, No.3, pp. 322-326.

Zuk, M. & McKean, K.A. (1996). Sex differences in parasite infections: patterns and processes. *Int J Parasitol*, Vol.26, No.10, pp. 1009-1023.

Part 4

Therapy

14

Adipose Tissue Metabolism and Effect of Postmenopausal Hormone Therapy on Change of Body Composition

Kyong Wook Yi[1] and Seung Yup Ku[2]
[1]*Department of Obstetrics and Gynecology, College of Medicine, Korea University,*
[2]*Department of Obstetrics and Gynecology, College of Medicine, Seoul National University, Seoul, Korea*

1. Introduction

Obesity is a process by which excess energy accumulates and results in increasing fat deposition in various parts of the body. Obesity is associated with economic, social, and lifestyle factors, and is commonly induced by imbalanced energy intake and consumption of high calorie foods or low physical activity. Obesity is a worldwide issue in public health that significantly increases the risk for type 2 diabetes, metabolic syndrome, atherosclerosis, and cardiovascular disease.

Body weight increases with aging in both genders, irrespective of the baseline weight in normal and obese individuals [1]. This increase in body weight is attributed to a reduction in energy expenditure with decreased physical activity. The global prevalence of obesity has been reported to be higher in females than males [2]. A US population survey estimated that approximately two thirds of women 40 - 60 years of age are overweight or obese [3].

In addition to aging, the menopause is considered an important factor for contributing to altered adiposity in women. Menopause is defined as a decline in endogenous estrogen production from the ovaries, and clinically represents cessation of menstruation and loss of fertility. Estrogen loss is the most significant event impacting a variety of physiologic and psychological changes in women. In the peri- or postmenopausal period, a change in adiposity has been well described. Weight gain during the menopausal transition has been scrutinized as a critical factor to midlife body weight in women [1]. Several observational studies have shown increased weight gain during the menopausal transition [4, 5]. A number of clinical trials have demonstrated a significant association between menopausal status with changes in anthropometry, blood pressure, lipid profile, and glucose/insulin metabolism [6-11], which can be linked to increased cardiovascular morbidity and mortality during the postmenopausal period [12].

Given the collective evidence on the change in adiposity across the menopausal transition, the roles of sex hormones, especially estrogen, are of increased interest in understanding the regulation of adiposity. This review discusses the association between estrogen and adiposity, and the interaction of estrogen with other biological metabolites and substances involved in obesity. In addition we summarize evidence for the effect of postmenopausal hormone therapy (HT) on changes in body composition.

2. Adipose tissue

Adipose tissue has a vital role in the lives of mammals. The primary function of adipose tissue is to store excess energy within the body in the form of free fatty acids (FFAs) and heat production. However, adipocytes are currently regarded as an independent endocrine organ since the metabolic and endocrine actions have been revealed.

In mammals, two types of adipose tissue exist (white adipose tissue [WAT] and brown adipose tissue [BAT]) [13]. WAT represents the major component of adipose tissue and provides most of the total body fat [13]. Moreover, WAT is the main source of FFAs that are available as energy substrates for generation through oxidative phosphorylation of adenosine triphosphate (ATP) high-energy bonds [13, 14]. Excess WAT in the upper parts of the body (android type obesity) represents a strong risk factor for some inflammatory pathologies [15]. In contrast, accumulation of WAT in lower body parts (gynecoid type obesity) is not associated with metabolic complications [13, 15].

In contrast to WAT, BAT participates in energy expenditure from non-oxidative phosphorylation in the form of heat for cold adaption [16]. The uncoupling of phosphorylation in BAT is attributed to the activity of uncoupling protein-1, which is expressed on the mitochondrial membrane, by creating a proton leak that depletes the electrochemical gradient needed for oxidative phosphorylation [14, 16]. BAT represents a smaller number of fat cells that have a rich vascular supply, which can respond more rapidly to sympathetic nervous system stimulation, and elicits heat production, rather than ATP production from nonshivering cold adaptive thermogenesis [14, 16]. In humans, BAT helps to maintain body temperature in newborns, but BAT regresses with increasing age and is completely lost in adulthood [17, 18]. Recently, Virtanen et al. studied BAT deposition in healthy adults using the glucose analogue, ^{18}F-flurodeoxyglucose, uptake by PET and computed tomography [18]. Metabolically-active BAT depots in paracervical and supraclavicular adipose tissue, which can be induced in response to cold and sympathetic nervous system activation, has been reported [14, 16, 18]. The presence of BAT in human adults is of potential interest in understanding the mechanism of obesity, and may provide a rationale for pharmacologic and gene expression manipulation to combat human obesity [14, 18, 19].

3. Deposition and distribution of adipose tissue

Deposition of the fat mass has a different pattern between the genders. Young males have little subcutaneous fat and do not show a central-peripheral difference [20], whereas women of reproductive age have more subcutaneous fat than men at all measured subcutaneous regions [21]. In addition, with an increasing severity of obesity, adipose tissue thickness is higher in the central regions in men, but women exhibit a peripheral deposition [20]. This pattern of fat deposition is altered in women across the menopausal transition; specifically, the total amount of body fat increases, and the peripheral fat shifts around the abdomen. Furthermore, the change in visceral adipose tissue has been ascribed to both chronologic aging and menopause [22, 23]. The results from a clinical study with 156 healthy women during 4 years of follow-up showed an increase in visceral adipose tissue and total body fat, and a 32% reduction in fat oxidation during the menopausal transition [4]. In the study, the subcutaneous adipose tissue increased in accordance with age independent of menopausal status, while the findings of increased visceral adipose tissue and total body fat were noted only in postmenopausal women. This distinctive physiologic change in amount and distribution of fat in women is noteworthy because the central fat deposition has a more deleterious effect on the development of cardiovascular and metabolic disease [24, 25].

Although the exact mechanism regarding fat redistribution after menopause remains unclear, the phenomenon with declining estrogen level may be due to alterations in adipose tissue metabolism [4]. Several studies have shown that estrogen directly promotes subcutaneous fat accumulation [26], and the loss of estrogen by menopause is associated with an increase in central fat. Several longitudinal studies lend support in suggesting that estrogen plays an important role in regulating body fat distribution. Postmenopausal women who receive estrogen replacement have significantly lower waist-to-hip ratios and less visceral adipose tissue than women who have never received estrogen replacement therapy [27, 28].

In experimental studies, 17β-estradiol (E2) has been shown to regulate adipose tissue by increasing the number of adipocytes through effects on proliferation and differentiation [29, 30]. The number and size of adipocytes is a determining factor for adiposity, and the adipocyte size is balanced by lipogenesis and the lipolysis pathway. Palin et al. have found a direct regulatory effect of E2 on the expression of lipoprotein lipase (LPL) and hormone-sensitive lipase (HSL) in human subcutaneous abdominal adipose tissue [31]. LPL is a major modulator of lipid deposition as triglycerides into adipocytes, and HSL is the rating-limiting enzyme involved in the process of lipolysis. Therefore, the direct effect of estrogen on these enzymes might lead to fat redistribution in postmenopausal women.

As other mechanisms suggest, the role of the estrogen receptor (ER) is focused on estrogen-related action on the regulation of adiposity. Adipocytes express two main subtypes of ERs (alpha [ERα] and beta [ERβ]). ERα was discovered first, and the biological effects of ERα on adiposity have been thoroughly described. ERα is considered to be essential for genomic actions of E2 on the regulation of body fat [32]. Because the hypothalamic nuclei that regulate energy homeostasis express ERα, E2 action could affect adiposity [33-35]. An animal study conducted by Heine et al. demonstrated that glucose intolerance, hypertrophy, and hyperplasia of adipocytes are induced in ERα knockout mice [36], thus supporting a critical role of ERα in determining adiposity.

In contrast, the biological implications of the more recently discovered ERβ have been less revealing than ERα. The binding affinity of estrogen to ERα and ERβ is known to be similar, but the two subtypes of ER only have 56% identity in the ligand binding domain [26, 37, 38]. Therefore, different or competitive roles between both ERs have been repeatedly suggested. Naaz et al. studied the role of ERβ in adipose tissue [39] in mice with ERαKO. When compared to the results generated in ERαKO mice, it was shown that removing E2/ERβ signaling induced a decrease in body weight, the amount of fat, and adipocyte size. Therefore, the authors suggested a potential role for ERβ in regulating adiposity, as well as ERα, but with opposing actions. Thus, the roles for ERs in adipocytes might be an interesting target to further elucidate the estrogen effects on regulating adiposity.

4. Proinflammatory cytokines production

Obesity is a low grade systemic inflammatory state; several studies have addressed adipocyte-related mechanisms involved in regulating proinflammatory [15, 40] and adipocyte-specific cytokines. Systemic chronic inflammation is due to an inflammatory response in adipose tissues that are under quick expansion, and in which macrophages and adipocytes are activated and stimulate the production of proinflammatory cytokines and adipokines [41]. Visceral WAT is considered a main source of inflammation related to obesity. Obese subjects with higher visceral fat exhibit monocyte-chemotactic protein (MCP)-1 expression and infiltration of macrophages in visceral fat compared to subcutaneous fat [42]. Also, several *in vivo* studies have shown higher levels of plasminogen activator inhibitor (PAI)-1, IL-6, and TNF-α in visceral obesity [43, 44].

Recent studies have shown the inhibitory role of estrogen to the inflammatory response in adipose tissue, and cardiovascular and nervous systems [35]. ERα is located in cytokine-producing cells, such as macrophages and microglia, and several *in vitro* studies have reported that E2/ ERα decreases the number of pro-inflammatory cytokines [35, 45, 46]. Another *in vivo* study has demonstrated that both ERα and ERβ regulate proinflammatory cytokine and chemokine production through E2-dependent and independent mechanisms [47].

Because energy expenditure is related to inflammation, a role for nuclear receptor kappa B (NF-κB) has been suggested. NF-κB is a protein complex that controls transcription factor, and is known to have a crucial role in regulating immune responses to infection or stress. NF-κB induces the transcription of inflammatory cytokines, such as TNF-α, IL-1, IL-6, and MCP-1 [41]. In the classical pathway, NF-κB is mediated through IKKβ-induced phosphorylation and proteasome-mediated degradation of IkBα [48]. The other pathway is the activation by hypoxia in the absence of IkBα degradation, a pathway in adipocytes and macrophages which contributes to chronic inflammation in the adipose tissues of obese subjects [41, 49]. Limited evidence has proposed an inhibitory effect of E2 via ERα on NF-κB [50, 51], which partially explains the anti-inflammatory properties of estrogen.

5. Adipokine expression/secretion

Adipokines are a family of cytokines which include leptin, resistin, adiponectin, and TNF-α and are primarily secreted from adipocytes. These adipokines are released from different tissues and organs, and are not exclusively produced by WAT [14, 52].

Leptin, the product of the *ob* gene, has been shown to be a key metabolic hormone in regulating appetite body weight and energy homeostasis [53, 54]. In humans, circulating leptin levels have a parallel correlation with the amount of body fat. In addition, serum levels of leptin have been shown to be higher in women than men [55]. This finding has been hypothesized to be due to a different pattern in fat deposition between the genders and/or the effects of a different hormonal milieu [56]. With respect to the change in leptin levels according to menopausal status, data are inconsistent; some data have shown no change in leptin levels between the pre- and post-menopause [57], while other studies have demonstrated a decrease in leptin levels during the menopausal transition [58, 59]. Some investigators have suggested that the low amount of visceral fat compared with subcutaneous fat in the genders [60, 61] makes it unlikely that the leptin secretion rates from these two depots differ, and may therefore be the cause for the sexual dimorphism in leptin concentrations, suggesting an important role for sex steroid hormones [53]. According to recent data derived from healthy pre- and post-menopausal women, postmenopausal women had increased levels of tissue plasminogen activator antigen (tPA), MCP-1, and adiponectin [24]. Furthermore, an increase in intraabdominal fat was correlated with C-reactive protein, tPA, and leptin, and negatively with adiponectin levels. The results imply that during the menopausal transition, women have adverse changes in inflammatory markers and adipokines which correlate with increased visceral obesity.

Several animal studies have indicated a stimulatory effect of estrogen on leptin expression and secretion in rat adipose tissues [59, 62]. Machinal et al. reported that there are regional differences in leptin expression between subcutaneous and deep fat tissues in rats, and that leptin secretion increased in the deep fat tissue tissues [63]. Based on one study involving human adipocytes, estrogen is likely to stimulate leptin expression [53]. In a previous study, the association between ER and adipokine expression in 3T3-L1 adipocytes was investigated [64]. The results showed that ERα has a stimulatory effect on leptin expression, while the expression of ERβ is inversely correlated with leptin expression. Therefore, discordant findings regarding the estrogen effect on leptin expression/secretion from other studies can be explained by the different expression of the two ER subtypes, which have opposite actions on the expression of leptin. In addition, if there are regulating factors (genetic or environmental) for ERα or ERβ expression in adipocytes, this may explain how the different expression of ER in adipose tissue can affect the diverse obesity phenotypes.

Adiponectin is a 30 kDa protein secreted abundantly from adipocytes [65, 66], and functions to exert anti-diabetic and anti-atherogenic properties. The serum adiponectin levels are decreased in obese individuals, metabolic syndrome, and type 2 DM [67, 68]. Similar to leptin, circulating adiponectin levels show a sexual dimorphism with higher levels in women than men [69]. Although the estrogen effects for adiponectin expression are limited, some *in vitro* studies have reported no direct regulatory effect in humans and mouse adipocytes [64, 70].

Resistin is a cysteine-rich protein that was originally described as an adipose-derived protein in rodents that links obesity to insulin resistance [71]. However, in human data, the relationship of resistin with obesity and insulin metabolism is still debated. A widely reported biological role of resistin is the regulatory effect involved in inflammatory processes. In addition to adipocytes, resistin is induced by lipopolysaccharides and TNF-α in macrophages [72]. The other data showed that resistin induces or is induced by IL-6 and TNF-α via NF-κB in human monocytes [73, 74]. Data on estrogen effects for resistin expression are limited. In a mouse adipocyte model, the regulatory effect of 17β-E2 on resistin expression is discordant [64, 75].

Recently described novel adipokines, such as visfatin, retinol binding protein-4, and omentin, have been shown to exert some metabolic properties, but their biological actions linked to obesity and interactions with estrogen need to be elucidated.

6. Postmenopausal hormone therapy and change in body composition

Hormone therapy (HT) is widely used for the treatment of menopausal symptoms and preventing bone loss in postmenopausal women. Estrogen replacement, when combined with various progestogens for endometrial protection, has been established as a conventional formulation. The benefit of HT is known to reduce vasomotor symptoms, prevent osteoporotic fractures, and improve well-being and quality of life during the menopausal period. In contrast, the risks for breast cancer and thromboembolic disease may increase, and cardiovascular effects remain controversial.

As previously mentioned, aging and menopause in women are related to an increase in body fat and redistribution of fat mass to the central portion of the body. These changes are linked to an increase in metabolic and cardiovascular disease after the menopause. Therefore, it has been continuously questioned and theorized that HT may have a favorable effect on change in body composition and anthropometries in postmenopausal women. With respect to this issue, data are still debated. In a meta-analysis of 24 RCTs, no effect of ET or HT on body weight was described [76]. However, subsequent studies suggested some beneficial effects of HT on body composition. A sub-study of the estrogen plus progestin trial of the Women's Health Initiative (WHI) investigated whether or not postmenopausal HT affects age-related changes in body composition [77]. The WHI study was originally designed to evaluate the risks and benefits of HT (EPT/ET) with an enrollment of 16,608 postmenopausal women between 1993 and 1998 [78]. The sub-analysis included 835 women who had whole-body dual-energy X-ray absorptiometry scans for measurement of body composition at baseline and year 3. Based on the results of the study, women who received EPT lost less lean soft tissue mass (-0.04 kg) than women who received placebo (-0.44 kg) 3 year after intervention. Furthermore, less upper-body fat distribution was noted in the EPT group than the placebo group (ratio of trunk to leg fat mass, -0.025 for the EPT group and 0.004 for the placebo group, P = 0.003). The investigators concluded that EPT has a favorable effect by reducing central fat deposition, but the real health benefits of this effect remains to be confirmed due to the small size of the effect. In a randomized, single-blind study, the effects of HT on body fat composition were studied in 59 postmenopausal women (mean age 49.9 ± 3.8 years) [79]. The participants were assigned into the following three groups according to the type of HT: transdermal estradiol (E2)/norethisterone acetate (NETA); transdermal continuous E2/ oral medroxyprogesterone acetate (MPA); and oral continuous E2/NETA. The results showed that all types of HT caused a significant decrease in WC, subcutaneous fat, and WHR. Thus, HT reduced fat deposition in the central part of the body, and such an effect was more marked in women with a WC ≥ 88 cm and subcutaneous fat ≥ 33 cm. Another placebo-controlled study investigated the effects of oral continuous E2/NETA on anthropometric changes and serum leptin levels in postmenopausal women [80]. In agreement with a previous study, WC and HC decreased significantly in the E2/NETA group, while the body weight (BW) increased in the placebo group. With this reduction in central fat deposition, the serum leptin levels were positively related to the changes in subcutaneous fat tissue. The authors advocated that HT may have a protective effect on CVD via a slimming effect on the central region in postmenopausal women.

Although the effect of postmenopausal HT on the change of body composition is not clearly understood, the limited data have suggest that HT has a small, but significant effect on preventing an android fat shift (central fat depot) regardless of the body weight.

Tibolone is a synthetic steroid hormone that exerts estrogenic, androgenic, and progestogenic properties. The biological actions of tibolone are mediated through the metabolites of tibolone (3α-OH-tibolone, 3β-OH-tibolone, and Δ^4-isomer) by binding estrogen or progesterone receptors in multiple target tissues and organs (brain, bone, breast, and endometrium). Based on several randomized trials, tibolone has shown comparable effects with traditional estrogen therapy (ET)/HT on relieving vasomotor symptoms/ genital atrophy, improving the quality of life, and preventing bone loss in postmenopausal women [81-84]. Currently 4 studies have shown the effects of tibolone on BW or body composition in postmenopausal women. In a 2-year follow up study comparing three regimens of HRT, tibolone had a stable effect on body fat and lean mass [85]. However, the fat mass increased (+3.6%) and the lean body mass decreased (-1.7%) in the control group. Another study demonstrated that tibolone significantly increased fat-free mass by 0.85 kg and total body water by 0.78 liter during a 1-year observation period [86]. The authors reported an effect of tibolone on preventing a decline in lean body mass, but mentioned the need for a long-term observational study.

Arabi et al. compared the effects of tibolone with EPT (E2/NETA) on changes in body composition and bone densitometry in postmenopausal women [87]. Both EPT and tibolone increased lean body mass, whereas the android fat and android obesity index decreased.

Tibolone might provide further benefits in increasing lean body mass and decreasing the fat component. Steroid hormones exert their action by binding to an intra-nuclear receptor [88]. Therefore, like estrogen, tibolone might have a direct effect on skeletal muscle by binding to ERα or ERβ expressed within human skeletal muscle [88-90]. In addition, tibolone increases the serum IGF-1 levels [91], which promotes muscle protein synthesis, and increases the number of myogenic satellite cells and the proliferation of myogenic satellite cells. The anabolic effect of tibolone on muscle has been suggested to be mediated in part by local IGF-1, independent of the serum IGF-1 level [92].

7. Summary

Adipose tissue is the largest endocrine organ in the human body. The amount and distribution of adipose tissue reflects energy balance. Adipose tissue also releases a variety of biologically active molecules or cytokines. Adipocyte metabolism and physiology have been extensively studied over recent years, but the exact mechanism and effect of sex steroid hormones involved in regulating adiposity remain to be defined.

Current data give evidence that estrogen appears to have direct effects on cell proliferation or differentiation for adipocytes, and in regulating key enzymes involved in fat deposition. Another possible mechanism involves the hormonal or paracrine effects by secretion of various adipokines and cytokines, in which interactions with estrogen are promising and need additional studies.

At present, it is not known whether or not HT provides a significant effect on modulating fat mass or preventing fat redistribution. Furthermore, in recent years the HT formulations have been changed to include lower doses of estrogen (< 50 μg) in combination with new progestins. The effects of the currently used HT regimens on changes in body fat composition are limited and require more data. Tibolone includes estrogenic, androgenic, and progestogenic properties which may affect the body composition (adipose tissue or lean mass) differently than conventional HT.

The respective roles of sex steroid hormones and their receptors (ER subtypes and PR) on body fat distribution could be an interesting target for understanding the estrogen effect on adiposity, and may provide selective therapeutic approaches, such as hormonal manipulation for adiposity related to estrogen change throughout the menopausal period.

8. References

[1] H. N. Polotsky, and A. J. Polotsky, "Metabolic implications of menopause," *Semin Reprod Med*, vol. 28, no. 5, pp. 426-434.

[2] "Obesity: preventing and managing the global epidemic. Report of a WHO consultation," *World Health Organization Technical Report Series*, vol. 894, pp. i-xii, 1-253, 2000.

[3] C. L. Ogden, M. D. Carroll, L. R. Curtin et al., "Prevalence of overweight and obesity in the United States, 1999-2004," *JAMA*, vol. 295, no. 13, pp. 1549-1555, 2006.

[4] J. C. Lovejoy, C. M. Champagne, L. de Jonge et al., "Increased visceral fat and decreased energy expenditure during the menopausal transition," *Int J Obes (Lond)*, vol. 32, no. 6, pp. 949-958, 2008.

[5] R. R. Wing, K. A. Matthews, L. H. Kuller et al., "Weight gain at the time of menopause," *Archives of Internal Medicine*, vol. 151, no. 1, pp. 97-102, 1991.

[6] J. F. Owens, C. M. Stoney, and K. A. Matthews, "Menopausal status influences ambulatory blood pressure levels and blood pressure changes during mental stress," *Circulation*, vol. 88, no. 6, pp. 2794-2802, 1993.

[7] J. H. Shin, J. Y. Hur, H. S. Seo et al., "The ratio of estrogen receptor alpha to estrogen receptor beta in adipose tissue is associated with leptin production and obesity," *Steroids*, vol. 72, no. 6-7, pp. 592-599, 2007.

[8] M. P. Brincat, Y. M. Baron, and R. Galea, "Estrogens and the skin," *Climacteric*, vol. 8, no. 2, pp. 110-123, 2005.

[9] F. A. Tremollieres, J. M. Pouilles, C. Cauneille, and C. Ribot, "Coronary heart disease risk factors and menopause: a study in 1684 French women," *Atherosclerosis*, vol. 142, no. 2, pp. 415-423, 1999.

[10] K. Fukami, K. Koike, K. Hirota et al., "Perimenopausal changes in serum lipids and lipoproteins: a 7-year longitudinal study," *Maturitas*, vol. 22, no. 3, pp. 193-197, 1995.

[11] M. E. Piche, S. J. Weisnagel, L. Corneau et al., "Contribution of abdominal visceral obesity and insulin resistance to the cardiovascular risk profile of postmenopausal women," *Diabetes*, vol. 54, no. 3, pp. 770-777, 2005.

[12] K. A. Matthews, E. Meilahn, L. H. Kuller et al., "Menopause and risk factors for coronary heart disease," *New England Journal of Medicine*, vol. 321, no. 10, pp. 641-646, 1989.

[13] S. Gesta, Y. H. Tseng, and C. R. Kahn, "Developmental origin of fat: tracking obesity to its source," *Cell*, vol. 131, no. 2, pp. 242-256, 2007.

[14] C. R. Balistreri, C. Caruso, and G. Candore, "The role of adipose tissue and adipokines in obesity-related inflammatory diseases," *Mediators of Inflammation*, vol. 2010, p. 802078.

[15] R. Cancello, and K. Clement, "Is obesity an inflammatory illness? Role of low-grade inflammation and macrophage infiltration in human white adipose tissue," *BJOG*, vol. 113, no. 10, pp. 1141-1147, 2006.

[16] R. N. Redinger, "Fat storage and the biology of energy expenditure," *Transl Res*, vol. 154, no. 2, pp. 52-60, 2009.

[17] M. E. Lean, "Brown adipose tissue in humans," *Proceedings of the Nutrition Society*, vol. 48, no. 2, pp. 243-256, 1989.

[18] K. A. Virtanen, M. E. Lidell, J. Orava et al., "Functional brown adipose tissue in healthy adults," *New England Journal of Medicine*, vol. 360, no. 15, pp. 1518-1525, 2009.

[19] G. Fruhbeck, S. Becerril, N. Sainz et al., "BAT: a new target for human obesity?," *Trends in Pharmacological Sciences*, vol. 30, no. 8, pp. 387-396, 2009.
[20] P. Bjorntorp, "Adipose tissue distribution and function," *International Journal of Obesity*, vol. 15 Suppl 2, pp. 67-81, 1991.
[21] L. Sjostrom, U. Smith, M. Krotkiewski, and P. Bjorntorp, "Cellularity in different regions of adipose tissue in young men and women," *Metabolism: Clinical and Experimental*, vol. 21, no. 12, pp. 1143-1153, 1972.
[22] C. J. Ley, B. Lees, and J. C. Stevenson, "Sex- and menopause-associated changes in body-fat distribution," *American Journal of Clinical Nutrition*, vol. 55, no. 5, pp. 950-954, 1992.
[23] H. Shimokata, R. Andres, P. J. Coon et al., "Studies in the distribution of body fat. II. Longitudinal effects of change in weight," *International Journal of Obesity*, vol. 13, no. 4, pp. 455-464, 1989.
[24] C. G. Lee, M. C. Carr, S. J. Murdoch et al., "Adipokines, inflammation, and visceral adiposity across the menopausal transition: a prospective study," *Journal of Clinical Endocrinology and Metabolism*, vol. 94, no. 4, pp. 1104-1110, 2009.
[25] W. B. Kannel, L. A. Cupples, R. Ramaswami et al., "Regional obesity and risk of cardiovascular disease; the Framingham Study," *Journal of Clinical Epidemiology*, vol. 44, no. 2, pp. 183-190, 1991.
[26] M. Krotkiewski, P. Bjorntorp, L. Sjostrom, and U. Smith, "Impact of obesity on metabolism in men and women. Importance of regional adipose tissue distribution," *Journal of Clinical Investigation*, vol. 72, no. 3, pp. 1150-1162, 1983.
[27] J. Munoz, A. Derstine, and B. A. Gower, "Fat distribution and insulin sensitivity in postmenopausal women: influence of hormone replacement," *Obesity Research*, vol. 10, no. 6, pp. 424-431, 2002.
[28] M. A. Espeland, M. L. Stefanick, D. Kritz-Silverstein et al., "Effect of postmenopausal hormone therapy on body weight and waist and hip girths. Postmenopausal Estrogen-Progestin Interventions Study Investigators," *Journal of Clinical Endocrinology and Metabolism*, vol. 82, no. 5, pp. 1549-1556, 1997.
[29] M. N. Dieudonne, R. Pecquery, M. C. Leneveu, and Y. Giudicelli, "Opposite effects of androgens and estrogens on adipogenesis in rat preadipocytes: evidence for sex and site-related specificities and possible involvement of insulin-like growth factor 1 receptor and peroxisome proliferator-activated receptor gamma2," *Endocrinology*, vol. 141, no. 2, pp. 649-656, 2000.
[30] D. A. Roncari, and R. L. Van, "Promotion of human adipocyte precursor replication by 17beta-estradiol in culture," *Journal of Clinical Investigation*, vol. 62, no. 3, pp. 503-508, 1978.
[31] S. L. Palin, P. G. McTernan, L. A. Anderson et al., "17Beta-estradiol and anti-estrogen ICI:compound 182,780 regulate expression of lipoprotein lipase and hormone-sensitive lipase in isolated subcutaneous abdominal adipocytes," *Metabolism: Clinical and Experimental*, vol. 52, no. 4, pp. 383-388, 2003.
[32] S. Musatov, W. Chen, D. W. Pfaff et al., "Silencing of estrogen receptor alpha in the ventromedial nucleus of hypothalamus leads to metabolic syndrome," *Proceedings of the National Academy of Sciences of the United States of America*, vol. 104, no. 7, pp. 2501-2506, 2007.

[33] I. Merchenthaler, M. V. Lane, S. Numan, and T. L. Dellovade, "Distribution of estrogen receptor alpha and beta in the mouse central nervous system: in vivo autoradiographic and immunocytochemical analyses," *Journal of Comparative Neurology*, vol. 473, no. 2, pp. 270-291, 2004.

[34] D. L. Voisin, S. X. Simonian, and A. E. Herbison, "Identification of estrogen receptor-containing neurons projecting to the rat supraoptic nucleus," *Neuroscience*, vol. 78, no. 1, pp. 215-228, 1997.

[35] L. M. Brown, and D. J. Clegg, "Central effects of estradiol in the regulation of food intake, body weight, and adiposity," *Journal of Steroid Biochemistry and Molecular Biology*, vol. 122, no. 1-3, pp. 65-73.

[36] P. A. Heine, J. A. Taylor, G. A. Iwamoto et al., "Increased adipose tissue in male and female estrogen receptor-alpha knockout mice," *Proceedings of the National Academy of Sciences of the United States of America*, vol. 97, no. 23, pp. 12729-12734, 2000.

[37] S. Mosselman, J. Polman, and R. Dijkema, "ER beta: identification and characterization of a novel human estrogen receptor," *FEBS Letters*, vol. 392, no. 1, pp. 49-53, 1996.

[38] G. G. Kuiper, E. Enmark, M. Pelto-Huikko et al., "Cloning of a novel receptor expressed in rat prostate and ovary," *Proceedings of the National Academy of Sciences of the United States of America*, vol. 93, no. 12, pp. 5925-5930, 1996.

[39] A. Naaz, M. Zakroczymski, P. Heine et al., "Effect of ovariectomy on adipose tissue of mice in the absence of estrogen receptor alpha (ERalpha): a potential role for estrogen receptor beta (ERbeta)," *Hormone and Metabolic Research*, vol. 34, no. 11-12, pp. 758-763, 2002.

[40] C. E. Juge-Aubry, E. Henrichot, and C. A. Meier, "Adipose tissue: a regulator of inflammation," *Best Pract Res Clin Endocrinol Metab*, vol. 19, no. 4, pp. 547-566, 2005.

[41] J. Ye, and J. N. Keller, "Regulation of energy metabolism by inflammation: a feedback response in obesity and calorie restriction," *Aging (Albany NY)*, vol. 2, no. 6, pp. 361-368.

[42] I. Harman-Boehm, M. Bluher, H. Redel et al., "Macrophage infiltration into omental versus subcutaneous fat across different populations: effect of regional adiposity and the comorbidities of obesity," *Journal of Clinical Endocrinology and Metabolism*, vol. 92, no. 6, pp. 2240-2247, 2007.

[43] G. Winkler, S. Kiss, L. Keszthelyi et al., "Expression of tumor necrosis factor (TNF)-alpha protein in the subcutaneous and visceral adipose tissue in correlation with adipocyte cell volume, serum TNF-alpha, soluble serum TNF-receptor-2 concentrations and C-peptide level," *European Journal of Endocrinology / European Federation of Endocrine Societies*, vol. 149, no. 2, pp. 129-135, 2003.

[44] G. He, S. B. Pedersen, J. M. Bruun et al., "Differences in plasminogen activator inhibitor 1 in subcutaneous versus omental adipose tissue in non-obese and obese subjects," *Hormone and Metabolic Research*, vol. 35, no. 3, pp. 178-182, 2003.

[45] E. Vegeto, S. Belcredito, S. Etteri et al., "Estrogen receptor-alpha mediates the brain antiinflammatory activity of estradiol," *Proceedings of the National Academy of Sciences of the United States of America*, vol. 100, no. 16, pp. 9614-9619, 2003.

[46] E. Vegeto, C. Bonincontro, G. Pollio et al., "Estrogen prevents the lipopolysaccharide-induced inflammatory response in microglia," *Journal of Neuroscience*, vol. 21, no. 6, pp. 1809-1818, 2001.
[47] C. M. Brown, T. A. Mulcahey, N. C. Filipek, and P. M. Wise, "Production of proinflammatory cytokines and chemokines during neuroinflammation: novel roles for estrogen receptors alpha and beta," *Endocrinology*, vol. 151, no. 10, pp. 4916-4925.
[48] M. Karin, and Y. Ben-Neriah, "Phosphorylation meets ubiquitination: the control of NF-[kappa]B activity," *Annual Review of Immunology*, vol. 18, pp. 621-663, 2000.
[49] J. Ye, Z. Gao, J. Yin, and Q. He, "Hypoxia is a potential risk factor for chronic inflammation and adiponectin reduction in adipose tissue of ob/ob and dietary obese mice," *Am J Physiol Endocrinol Metab*, vol. 293, no. 4, pp. E1118-1128, 2007.
[50] S. Ghisletti, C. Meda, A. Maggi, and E. Vegeto, "17beta-estradiol inhibits inflammatory gene expression by controlling NF-kappaB intracellular localization," *Molecular and Cellular Biology*, vol. 25, no. 8, pp. 2957-2968, 2005.
[51] B. Stein, and M. X. Yang, "Repression of the interleukin-6 promoter by estrogen receptor is mediated by NF-kappa B and C/EBP beta," *Molecular and Cellular Biology*, vol. 15, no. 9, pp. 4971-4979, 1995.
[52] F. Lago, R. Gomez, J. J. Gomez-Reino et al., "Adipokines as novel modulators of lipid metabolism," *Trends in Biochemical Sciences*, vol. 34, no. 10, pp. 500-510, 2009.
[53] C. Di Carlo, G. A. Tommaselli, and C. Nappi, "Effects of sex steroid hormones and menopause on serum leptin concentrations," *Gynecological Endocrinology*, vol. 16, no. 6, pp. 479-491, 2002.
[54] Y. Zhang, R. Proenca, M. Maffei et al., "Positional cloning of the mouse obese gene and its human homologue," *Nature*, vol. 372, no. 6505, pp. 425-432, 1994.
[55] M. Maffei, J. Halaas, E. Ravussin et al., "Leptin levels in human and rodent: measurement of plasma leptin and ob RNA in obese and weight-reduced subjects," *Nature Medicine*, vol. 1, no. 11, pp. 1155-1161, 1995.
[56] C. Di Carlo, G. A. Tommaselli, A. Sammartino et al., "Serum leptin levels and body composition in postmenopausal women: effects of hormone therapy," *Menopause*, vol. 11, no. 4, pp. 466-473, 2004.
[57] P. J. Havel, S. Kasim-Karakas, G. R. Dubuc et al., "Gender differences in plasma leptin concentrations," *Nature Medicine*, vol. 2, no. 9, pp. 949-950, 1996.
[58] M. Rosenbaum, M. Nicolson, J. Hirsch et al., "Effects of gender, body composition, and menopause on plasma concentrations of leptin," *Journal of Clinical Endocrinology and Metabolism*, vol. 81, no. 9, pp. 3424-3427, 1996.
[59] H. Shimizu, Y. Shimomura, Y. Nakanishi et al., "Estrogen increases in vivo leptin production in rats and human subjects," *Journal of Endocrinology*, vol. 154, no. 2, pp. 285-292, 1997.
[60] K. Kotani, K. Tokunaga, S. Fujioka et al., "Sexual dimorphism of age-related changes in whole-body fat distribution in the obese," *International Journal of Obesity and Related Metabolic Disorders*, vol. 18, no. 4, pp. 207-202, 1994.
[61] R. Leenen, K. van der Kooy, P. Deurenberg et al., "Visceral fat accumulation in obese subjects: relation to energy expenditure and response to weight loss," *American Journal of Physiology*, vol. 263, no. 5 Pt 1, pp. E913-919, 1992.

[62] T. Murakami, M. Iida, and K. Shima, "Dexamethasone regulates obese expression in isolated rat adipocytes," *Biochemical and Biophysical Research Communications*, vol. 214, no. 3, pp. 1260-1267, 1995.

[63] F. Machinal, M. N. Dieudonne, M. C. Leneveu et al., "In vivo and in vitro ob gene expression and leptin secretion in rat adipocytes: evidence for a regional specific regulation by sex steroid hormones," *Endocrinology*, vol. 140, no. 4, pp. 1567-1574, 1999.

[64] K. W. Yi, J. H. Shin, H. S. Seo et al., "Role of estrogen receptor-alpha and -beta in regulating leptin expression in 3T3-L1 adipocytes," *Obesity (Silver Spring)*, vol. 16, no. 11, pp. 2393-2399, 2008.

[65] E. Hu, P. Liang, and B. M. Spiegelman, "AdipoQ is a novel adipose-specific gene dysregulated in obesity," *Journal of Biological Chemistry*, vol. 271, no. 18, pp. 10697-10703, 1996.

[66] P. E. Scherer, S. Williams, M. Fogliano et al., "A novel serum protein similar to C1q, produced exclusively in adipocytes," *Journal of Biological Chemistry*, vol. 270, no. 45, pp. 26746-26749, 1995.

[67] K. Hotta, T. Funahashi, Y. Arita et al., "Plasma concentrations of a novel, adipose-specific protein, adiponectin, in type 2 diabetic patients," *Arteriosclerosis, Thrombosis, and Vascular Biology*, vol. 20, no. 6, pp. 1595-1599, 2000.

[68] Y. Arita, S. Kihara, N. Ouchi et al., "Paradoxical decrease of an adipose-specific protein, adiponectin, in obesity," *Biochemical and Biophysical Research Communications*, vol. 257, no. 1, pp. 79-83, 1999.

[69] H. Nishizawa, I. Shimomura, K. Kishida et al., "Androgens decrease plasma adiponectin, an insulin-sensitizing adipocyte-derived protein," *Diabetes*, vol. 51, no. 9, pp. 2734-2741, 2002.

[70] S. Horenburg, P. Fischer-Posovszky, K. M. Debatin, and M. Wabitsch, "Influence of sex hormones on adiponectin expression in human adipocytes," *Hormone and Metabolic Research*, vol. 40, no. 11, pp. 779-786, 2008.

[71] C. M. Steppan, S. T. Bailey, S. Bhat et al., "The hormone resistin links obesity to diabetes," *Nature*, vol. 409, no. 6818, pp. 307-312, 2001.

[72] P. D. Anderson, N. N. Mehta, M. L. Wolfe et al., "Innate immunity modulates adipokines in humans," *Journal of Clinical Endocrinology and Metabolism*, vol. 92, no. 6, pp. 2272-2279, 2007.

[73] S. S. Pang, and Y. Y. Le, "Role of resistin in inflammation and inflammation-related diseases," *Cell Mol Immunol*, vol. 3, no. 1, pp. 29-34, 2006.

[74] M. Bokarewa, I. Nagaev, L. Dahlberg et al., "Resistin, an adipokine with potent proinflammatory properties," *Journal of Immunology*, vol. 174, no. 9, pp. 5789-5795, 2005.

[75] Y. H. Chen, M. J. Lee, H. H. Chang et al., "17 beta-estradiol stimulates resistin gene expression in 3T3-L1 adipocytes via the estrogen receptor, extracellularly regulated kinase, and CCAAT/enhancer binding protein-alpha pathways," *Endocrinology*, vol. 147, no. 9, pp. 4496-4504, 2006.

[76] R. J. Norman, I. H. Flight, and M. C. Rees, "Oestrogen and progestogen hormone replacement therapy for peri-menopausal and post-menopausal women: weight and body fat distribution," *Cochrane Database Syst Rev*, no. 2, p. CD001018, 2000.

[77] Z. Chen, T. Bassford, S. B. Green et al., "Postmenopausal hormone therapy and body composition--a substudy of the estrogen plus progestin trial of the Women's Health Initiative," *American Journal of Clinical Nutrition*, vol. 82, no. 3, pp. 651-656, 2005.

[78] J. E. Rossouw, G. L. Anderson, R. L. Prentice et al., "Risks and benefits of estrogen plus progestin in healthy postmenopausal women: principal results From the Women's Health Initiative randomized controlled trial," *JAMA*, vol. 288, no. 3, pp. 321-333, 2002.

[79] H. Yuksel, A. R. Odabasi, S. Demircan et al., "Effects of postmenopausal hormone replacement therapy on body fat composition," *Gynecological Endocrinology*, vol. 23, no. 2, pp. 99-104, 2007.

[80] H. Yuksel, A. R. Odabasi, S. Demircan et al., "Effects of oral continuous 17beta-estradiol plus norethisterone acetate replacement therapy on abdominal subcutaneous fat, serum leptin levels and body composition," *Gynecological Endocrinology*, vol. 22, no. 7, pp. 381-387, 2006.

[81] S. R. Cummings, B. Ettinger, P. D. Delmas et al., "The effects of tibolone in older postmenopausal women," *New England Journal of Medicine*, vol. 359, no. 7, pp. 697-708, 2008.

[82] E. A. Nijland, W. C. Weijmar Schultz, and S. R. Davis, "Effects of tibolone and raloxifene on health-related quality of life and sexual function," *Maturitas*, vol. 58, no. 2, pp. 164-173, 2007.

[83] M. L. Hammar, P. van de Weijer, H. R. Franke et al., "Tibolone and low-dose continuous combined hormone treatment: vaginal bleeding pattern, efficacy and tolerability," *BJOG*, vol. 114, no. 12, pp. 1522-1529, 2007.

[84] M. L. Bots, G. W. Evans, W. Riley et al., "The effect of tibolone and continuous combined conjugated equine oestrogens plus medroxyprogesterone acetate on progression of carotid intima-media thickness: the Osteoporosis Prevention and Arterial effects of tiboLone (OPAL) study," *European Heart Journal*, vol. 27, no. 6, pp. 746-755, 2006.

[85] W. Hanggi, K. Lippuner, P. Jaeger et al., "Differential impact of conventional oral or transdermal hormone replacement therapy or tibolone on body composition in postmenopausal women," *Clinical Endocrinology*, vol. 48, no. 6, pp. 691-699, 1998.

[86] I. B. Meeuwsen, M. M. Samson, S. A. Duursma, and H. J. Verhaar, "The effect of tibolone on fat mass, fat-free mass, and total body water in postmenopausal women," *Endocrinology*, vol. 142, no. 11, pp. 4813-4817, 2001.

[87] A. Arabi, P. Garnero, R. Porcher et al., "Changes in body composition during post-menopausal hormone therapy: a 2 year prospective study," *Human Reproduction*, vol. 18, no. 8, pp. 1747-1752, 2003.

[88] D. E. Jacobsen, M. M. Samson, S. Kezic, and H. J. Verhaar, "Postmenopausal HRT and tibolone in relation to muscle strength and body composition," *Maturitas*, vol. 58, no. 1, pp. 7-18, 2007.

[89] A. Wiik, M. Ekman, G. Morgan et al., "Oestrogen receptor beta is present in both muscle fibres and endothelial cells within human skeletal muscle tissue," *Histochemistry and Cell Biology*, vol. 124, no. 2, pp. 161-165, 2005.

[90] S. Lemoine, P. Granier, C. Tiffoche et al., "Estrogen receptor alpha mRNA in human skeletal muscles," *Medicine and Science in Sports and Exercise*, vol. 35, no. 3, pp. 439-443, 2003.

[91] A. Porcile, E. Gallardo, P. Duarte, and S. Aedo, "[Differential effects on serum IGF-1 of tibolone (5 mg/day) vs combined continuous estrogen/progestagen in post menopausal women]," *Revista Medica de Chile*, vol. 131, no. 10, pp. 1151-1156, 2003.

[92] M. I. Lewis, G. D. Horvitz, D. R. Clemmons, and M. Fournier, "Role of IGF-I and IGF-binding proteins within diaphragm muscle in modulating the effects of nandrolone," *Am J Physiol Endocrinol Metab*, vol. 282, no. 2, pp. E483-490, 2002.

15

Standard Gonadotropin-Suppressive Therapy in Japanese Girls with Idiopathic Central Precocious or Early Puberty Does Not Adversely Affect Body Composition

Toshihide Kubo
National Hospital Organization, Okayama Medical Center
Japan

1. Introduction

Estrogen deprivation, for instance after ovariectomy or natural menopause, is associated with significant bone loss in adult women. (Lindsay, 1995) Gonadotropin-releasing hormone agonist (GnRHa) inhibits hypothalamo-pituitary-gonadal hormone secretion and gradually reduces the estrogen level. (Wacharawsindhu et al., 2006) Consequently, decreases in bone mineral density, which are also observed after ovariectomy and natural menopause, have been observed during GnRHa therapy in women with endometriosis and men with benign prostatic hyperplasia. (Goldray et al., 1993) Moreover, women who were treated with this analog showed body composition changes, including a decrease in lean mass and an increase in fat mass, which resemble the body changes that occur during the menopause. (Revila et al., 1998)

Meanwhile, GnRHa has also been the treatment of choice for central precocious puberty (CPP) since the mid-1980s. (Crowley et al., 1981) Many of the previous studies on the auxological effects of GnRHa treatment on CPP have focused on assessing the patient's final height, whereas much less attention has been paid to changes in their weight and body composition. (Arrigo et al., 2004)

However, concern has been expressed that CPP might be associated with increases in body mass index (BMI) both at the initial presentation and during GnRHa treatment (Boot et al., 1998) and that individuals with the condition are prone to developing obesity. This concern is supported by adult cases that were treated with GnRHa, as described above.

On the other hand, it is well known that BMI and percentage body fat increase during puberty. Consequently, gonadotropin-suppressive therapy can theoretically halt the progression to obesity by inhibiting pubertal development.

Recently, there have been many reports about the changes in body composition that occur in children with CPP who are treated with GnRHa (Wacharsindhu et al., 2006, Arrigo et al., 2004, Boot et al., 1998, Feuillan et al.,1999, Palmert et al., 1999, Chiumello et al., 2000, van der Sluis et al., 2002, Paterson et al., 2004, Oosdijk et al., 1996, Traggiai et al., 2005, Herger et al., 1999, Pasuquino et al., 2008). Some reports have shown that obesity occurs at a high frequency among children with CPP (Arrigo et al., 2004, Feuillan et al., 1999, Palmert et al.,

1999, Chiumello et al., 2000, van der Sluis et al., 2002, Paterson et al., 2004). However, most of these reports studied populations in Western countries, and almost none investigated Asian children (Wacharsindhu et al., 2006). Furthermore, in these studies, GnRHa was administered at higher doses (Boot et al., 1998, Chiumello et al., 2000, van der Sluis et al., 2002) than are used in the standard gonadotropin-suppressive therapy protocol that is currently in operation in Japan. With some exceptions, all these reports showed that obesity is aggravated during GnRHa therapy (Wacharsindhu et al., 2006, Boot et al., 1998, Chiumello et al., 2000, van der Sluis et al., 2002, Paterson et al., 2004, Oosdijk et al., 1996, http://www.iotf.org/documents/iotfsocplan251006.pdf). Therefore, we assessed the effects of the standard gonadotropin-suppressive therapy protocol that is currently used in Japan on body composition in order to review the optimal dose of GnRHa.

The aims of the present study were to prospectively evaluate whether obesity occurs at a high frequency among Japanese children with CPP and to longitudinally evaluate the body composition of Japanese children with CPP before and during GnRHa therapy.

2. Subjects and methods

2.1 Patients

Eighteen patients participated in the study. At diagnosis, all of the patients had a history of increased growth velocity, breast development of Tanner stage 2 or more, and a bone age that was more than 1 yr above their chronological age. Ten girls had idiopathic central precocious puberty (ICPP), and 8 girls had idiopathic central early puberty (ICEP). The diagnosis of ICPP was made based upon the onset of breast development before the age of 7 yr and 6 mo, the generation of pubic hair before the age of 9 yr, or the onset of menses before the age of 10 yr and 6 mo, according to the diagnostic criteria currently used in Japan. ICEP was defined as the appearance of pubertal signs between 8 -10 yr of age. Furthermore, neither set of patients showed any evidence of hypothalamo-pituitary lesions on magnetic resonance imaging or additional conditions that might have affected their body mass index (BMI).

The median age at the start of treatment was 8.3 yr (range: 6 to 11). All patients received leuprolide acetate (LUPRON DEPOT, Takeda, Osaka, Japan) at an initial dose of 30 μg/kg, which was administered subcutaneously every 4 weeks according to the standard gonadotropin-suppressive therapy currently used in Japan.

2.2 Methods

Standard anthropometric measurements were taken at the baseline and during the 2-year GnRHa treatment period. BMI was calculated as weight (kg)/height (m^2), compared with age- and sex-matched reference values, and expressed as a standard deviation score (SDS) according to the method of Inokuchi (Inokuchi, 2009). The percentage of overweight (POW) was calculated as 100 x (the measured weight – normal weight)/normal weight (%). Normal weight data were derived from the 1990 Ministry of Health and Welfare data (Yamazaki et al., 1994). A POW of ≥ 20% was considered to indicate obesity (Asayama et al., 2003). Pubertal development was determined according to the method of Tanner (Tanner & Whitehouse, 1976).

Pituitary-gonadal axis function was considered to be adequately suppressed during treatment if the concentrations of LH and E2 were maintained within the prepubertal normal ranges of our laboratory; i.e., if a) the basal serum LH level was below 0.5 mIU/ml and b) the basal serum E2 level was below 10 pg/ml. In the patients that demonstrated incomplete suppression, the dose of leuprolide acetate was increased to 150 μg/kg. Bone age (BA) was assessed by one investigator using an x-ray of the left hand, according to the method of Greulich and Pyle (Greulich & Pyle, 1959).

2.3 Statistical analysis

For statistical purposes, the Wilcoxon test was used when appropriate in order to estimate the significance of differences between groups. The correlations between individual values were examined using Pearson's test. All values are given as the mean ± S.E. The significance threshold was set at $p < 0.05$.

3. Results

3.1 Prevalence of obesity

In our recent study of 18 girls with CPP or early puberty, five girls (27.8%) were diagnosed with obesity because their BMI values were higher than the 95th centile (Inokuchi, 2009) at the initiation of therapy. Moreover, the BMI standard deviation score (SDS) for chronological age (CA) was higher than zero in 14 (77.8%) patients, and the mean BMI SDS for CA was 1.07±0.32 at the baseline. Even when it was corrected for bone age (BA), the BMI SDS was still higher than zero in 9 (50.0%) patients, and the mean BMI SDS was 0.33±0.25 at the baseline. On the other hand, the POW was higher than 20% (indicating obesity) in 5 patients (27.8%) at the baseline.

3.2 BMI and POW during follow-up

The mean BMI was significantly increased after 1 year and increased further afterwards (Fig.1). BMI was higher than the 95th centile in 5 patients (27.8%) at the initiation of therapy, which was also true after 2 years treatment.

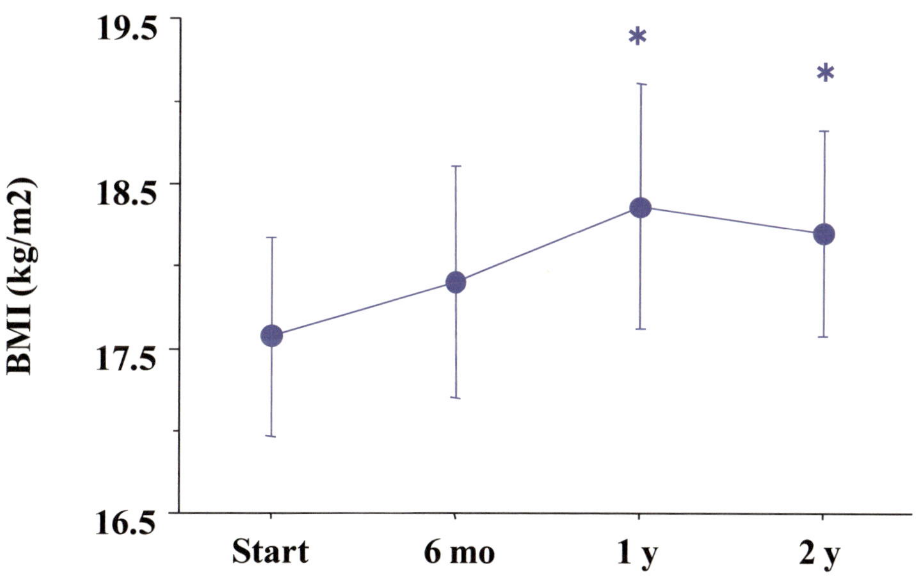

Fig. 1. Changes in BMI during GnRHa therapy

The BMI SDS for CA was higher than zero in 14 patients (77.8%) at the initiation of therapy, which was also the case for 13 individuals (72.2%) after 2 years treatment. Furthermore, 5 patients had BMI SDS of higher than 2 SD at the baseline, and 4 patients had BMI SDS of higher than 2 SD after 2 years treatment. The mean BMI SDS for CA was 1.07 ± 0.32 at the baseline and changed little during the therapy (Fig. 2).

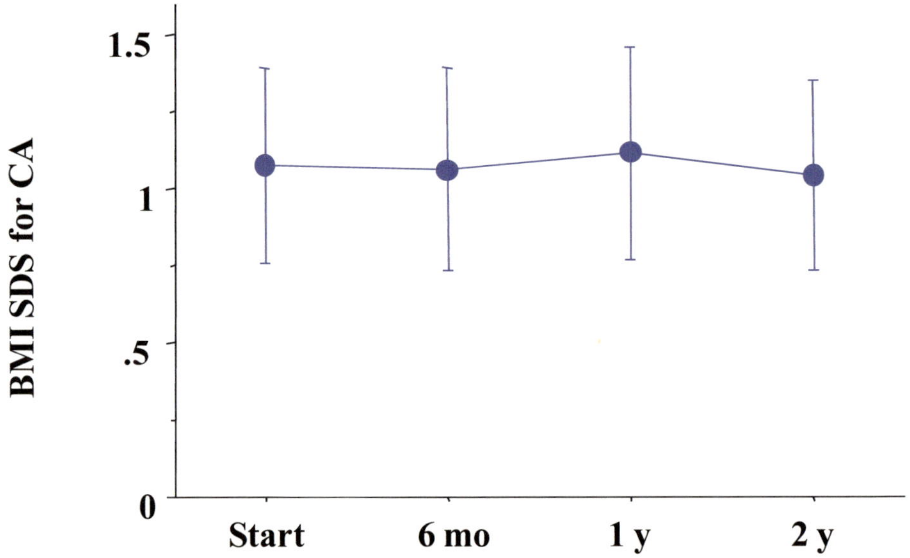

Fig. 2. Changes in the BMI SDS for CA during GnRHa therapy

On the other hand, the mean BMI SDS for BA was 0.33 ± 0.25 at the baseline and slightly but not significantly increased during the GnRHa therapy (Fig.3).

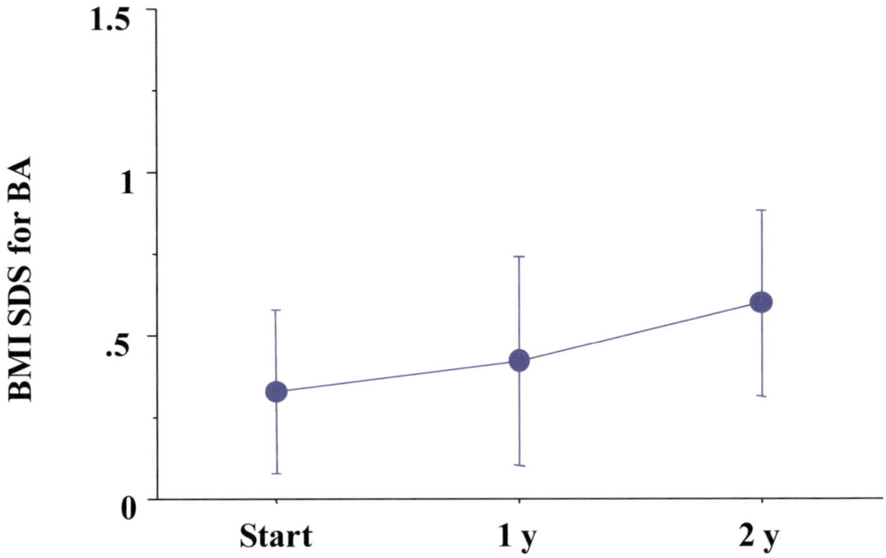

Fig. 3. Changes in the BMI SDS for BA during GnRHa therapy

In addition, the POW was higher than 20% (indicating obesity) in 5 patients (27.8%) at the baseline, which was also true after 2 yrs treatment. The mean POW was 8.2 ± 4.0% at the baseline and changed little during the GnRHa therapy (Fig. 4).

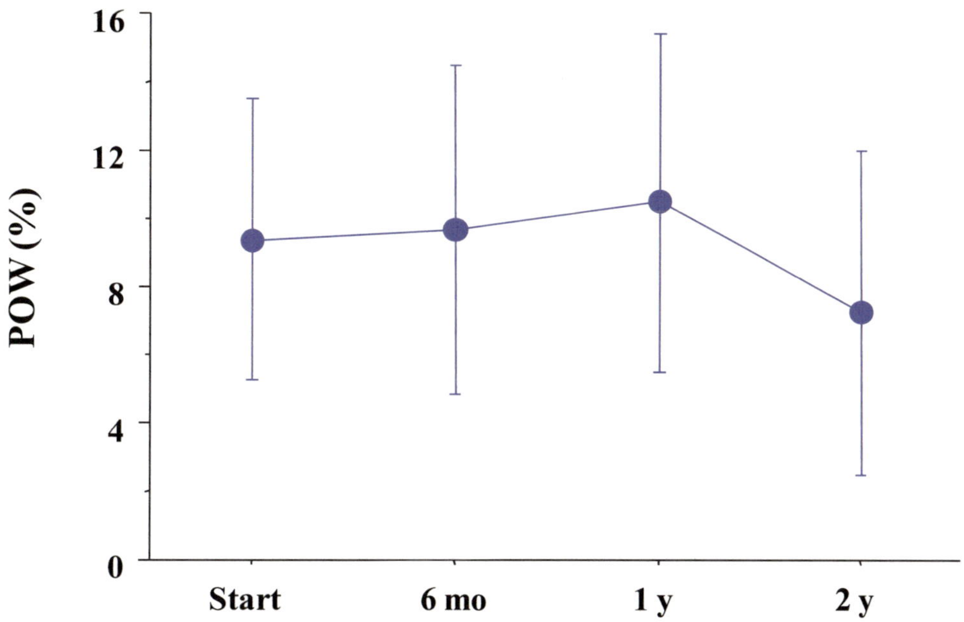

Fig. 4. Changes in POW during GnRHa therapy

3.3 Correlation between the BMI SDS at the start of treatment and that during treatment for CA and BA

Regression analysis showed that the BMI SDS for CA and BA at the start of treatment were positively correlated with those during treatment (Table 1, 2).

	r
After 6 months of therapy	0.963
After 1 year of therapy	0.971
After 2 years of therapy	0.975

Table 1. Relationship among BMI SDS for CA during therapy

	r
After 1 year or therapy	0.947
After 2 years of therapy	0.926

Table 2. Relationship among BMI SDS for BA during therapy

4. Discussion

Many reports have shown that obesity occurs at a high frequency among children with CPP. (Arrigo et al., 2004, Boot et al., 1998, Feuillan et al., 1999, Palmert et al., 1999, Chiumello et al., 2000, van der Sluis et al., 2002, Paterson et al., 2004) Feuillan et al. reported that the mean BMI of 18 girls with precocious puberty due to hypothalamic hamartoma (HH) and 32 with ICPP was higher than normal before GnRHa treatment (Feuillan et al., 1999), and Arrigo et al. reported that 23.6% of the 101 girls with ICPP that they studied were obese before the start of therapy. (Arrigo et al., 2004) Our results confirm that obesity is a common problem in children with CPP in Japan. Indeed, in this study, a quarter of our patients were found to be obese according to both BMI and POW before the start of therapy. Moreover, the BMI SDS for CA and BA were higher than zero in more than half of the patients at the baseline. Since the prevalence of obesity in girls in later childhood is 14.3% in Japan (http://www.iotf.org/documents/iotfsocplan251006.pdf), the above figure indicates that the prevalence of obesity in children with CPP is unusually high.

Although several reports have stated that obesity is a common problem in girls with CPP, as mentioned above, the reason why so many girls with CPP have an increased BMI is unclear. A decrease in lean body mass and an increase in fat mass leads to obesity. Chiumello et al. suggested that girls with CPP undergo a shortened period of prepubertal lean mass development and so possess an insufficient lean body mass, leading to obesity. (Chiumello et al., 2000) Recently, Arrigo et al. hypothesized that the pre-treatment increase in BMI is caused pubertal hormonal changes and secondary changes in body fat rather than CPP itself, as in their series they found that the suppression of pituitary-gonadal axis function was accompanied by a significant decrease in excess weight (Arrigo et al., 2004). However, our results showed that the suppression of the pituitary-gonadal axis did not bring about a significant change in excess weight, as described below. Furthermore, as for the number of patients whose BMI SDS for CA was higher than zero, it decreased from 14 (77.8%) to 9 (50%) after correcting for BA, and the mean BMI SDS for CA (1.07±0.32) also decreased to 0.33±0.25 after correcting for BA at the start of treatment. Moreover, Oostdijk et al. reported that the BMI SDS for CA of CPP patients was higher than that of the reference population, whereas their BMI SDS for bone age (BA) was normal at the start of treatment. (Oosdijk et al., 1996) Taken together, the BMI of children with CPP might be appropriate for the onset of adolescence, even though they are indicated to be overweight by BMI calculations. Therefore, it is reasonable to suggest that the pre-treatment overweightness observed in CPP girls is due to pubertal hormonal changes and secondary changes in body fat, rather than being a cause of their CPP.

As for the progression of baseline overweightness in CPP patients, the available data in the literature are very inconsistent; however, many reports have suggested that obesity progresses in this group (Wacharsindhu et al., 2006, Boot et al., 1998, Chiumello et al., 2000, van der Sluis et al., 2002, Paterson et al., 2004, Oosdijk et al., 1996, Traggiai et al., 2005). Oostdijk et al. treated 31 girls with CPP with triptorelin for a mean period of 3.4 years. (Oosdijk et al., 1996) The mean BMI SDS for CA at the start of treatment was higher than that of the reference population, and it did not change significantly during treatment. However, the mean BMI SDS for BA at the start of treatment was normal and increased during treatment. Boot et al. treated 32 girls and 2 boys with CPP or early puberty with leuprolide-acetate for 2 years. (Boot et al., 1998) Their lean tissue mass SDS decreased significantly during treatment, whereas their fat mass SDS and percentage body fat SDS increased. In addition, their mean BMI SDS was higher than zero at the baseline and increased during treatment. Chiumello et al. treated 14 girls and 2 boys with CPP with leuprolide and triptorelin for at least 1 year. (Chiumello et al., 2000) They concluded that fat mass is increased by GnRHa therapy and that this could lead to obesity; therefore, they suggested that CPP patients undergo a shortened period of pubertal lean mass development and that while the progression of puberty in these patients is associated with increases in fat and lean mass, only the latter is blocked by the "menopausal effect" or the GnRHa therapy itself. van der Sluis et al., who belong to the same group as Boot, reported 47 patients (36 girls and 11 boys) with CPP or early puberty who received leuprolide-acetate for a mean period of 2.7 years. (van der Sluis et al., 2002) In this cohort, BMI SDS increased significantly during treatment, whereas lean body mass decreased significantly during treatment, and percentage body fat increased. Paterson et al. reported 46 girls with CPP or early puberty who received goserelin for a mean period of 1.6 years. (Paterson et al., 2004) In this group, there was a marked increase in BMI following treatment. On average, the girls were fatter than the general population before treatment (BMI SDS: 0.93) and were significantly fatter (BMI SDS: 1.2) than the general population after the completion of therapy. Before treatment, 19 (41%) girls were overweight (BMI > 85th centile), 13 (28%) of whom were obese (BMI > 95th centile), which rose to 27 (59%) overweight patients, of whom 18 (39%) were obese, after the completion of therapy. Wacharasindhu et al. treated 10 Thai girls with CPP for a period of 1 year and reported that their percentage fat values increased significantly. (Wacharsindhu et al., 2006) So far, this is the only report in an Oriental population.

In contrast, some authors have reported no change throughout the observation period. (Palmert et al., 1999, Herger et al., 1999, Pasuquino et al., 2008) For example, Heger et al. treated 50 girls with CPP with depot triptorelin for a mean period of 4.4 years and reported that their BMI SDS values at pretreatment, at the end of treatment, and at final height were not significantly different. (Herger et al., 1999) Palmert et al. treated 96 girls and 14 boys with CPP with deslorelin or histrelin for 36 months. (Palmert et al., 1999) Among the girls, multiple regression analysis indicated that the BMI SDS for CA at the pretherapy visit was the greatest predictor of the BMI SDS for CA at the end of treatment. They concluded that the administration of GnRHa did not influence the progression of adolescent CPP patients toward obesity. Pasquino et al. reported 87 girls with CPP who received depot triptorelin for a mean period of 4.2 years. (Pasuquino et al., 2008) Their BMI increased markedly during treatment, but their BMI SDS for CA did not change significantly. In addition, 14.3% of the girls were overweight and 9.1 % were obese at the start of therapy, and both categories contained 11.7% of patients at the discontinuation of treatment. Although the patients' overall BMI increased, they remained in the same BMI centile and had the same BMI SDS throughout the treatment period. Regression analysis showed that the BMI SDS for CA at the end of treatment was positively correlated with the BMI SDS for CA at the start of treatment. As a result, they concluded that GnRHa treatment did not result in a significant BMI increase.

On the other hand, Arrigo et al. reported 101 girls with CPP who received decapeptyl depot for over 2 years. (Arrigo et al., 2004) As described above, a quarter of the girls were classified as obese at the start of therapy, and only 4% of them were still obese at the end of therapy. BMI SDS did not increase in any of the patients during the therapy period. In fact, both the mean BMI SDS and obesity prevalence significantly decreased during the treatment period. This is the only report to state that BMI and the prevalence of obesity decreased during GnRHa therapy.

In our study, although on the whole BMI increased, the SDS for both CA and BA remained the same throughout the treatment period. Moreover, POW also changed little during the therapeutic period, as reported by Chiumello (who described it as relative body weight) (Chiumello et al., 2000). It should be noted that we used a small amount of GnRHa in relation to body weight in accordance with the standard treatment protocol used in Japan, as described above (we used 2.5mg or less) and were able to control CPP. In the reports from Western countries in which the same leuprolide acetate drug was used, a dose of 3.75mg was used from the first stage onwards, and all showed a significant increase in BMI during treatment (Boot et al., 1998, Chiumello et al., 2000, van der Sluis et al., 2002). The doses used in other reports were also larger than the dose that is usually administered in Japan.
In this study, regression analysis showed that the BMI SDS for both CA and BA during treatment were positively correlated with those observed at the start of treatment, as reported by Pasquino et al. (Pasuquino et al., 2008) and Palmert (Palmert et al., 1999). Therefore, we consider that the initial BMI SDS is a predictor of BMI SDS at subsequent visits.
Taken together, the administration of GnRHa according to the standard Japanese protocol does not seem to influence the progression of children with CPP towards obesity. One possible reason for this is the suitability of the standard gonadotropin-suppressive therapy administered to girls with CPP in Japan, although racial differences might also be relevant.

5. Conclusion

In conclusion, the standard gonadotropin-suppressive therapy protocol used to treat girls with ICCP or ICEP in Japan does not adversely affect body composition, at least when administered for up to 2 years.

6. References

Arrigo T., De Luca F., Antoniazzi F., Galluzzi F., Segni M., Rosano M., Messnia MF., & Lombardo F. (2004). Reduction of baseline body mass index under gonadotropin-suppressive therapy in girls with idiopathic precocious puberty. European Journal of Endocrinology Vol.150, pp. 533-537

Asayama K., Ozeki T., Sugihara S., et al. (2003). Criteria for medical intervention in obese children: a new definition of 'obesity disease' in Japanese children. Pediatr Int. Vol.45, pp. 642-646

Boot AM., de Muinck Keizer-Schrama SMPF., Pols HAP., Krenning EP., & Drop SLS. (1998). Bone mineral density and body composition before and during treatment with gonadotropin-releaseing hormone agonist in children with central precocious and early puberty. J Clin Endocrinol Metab Vol.83, No.2, pp. 370-373

Chiumello G., Brambilla P., Guarneri M.P, Russo G., Manzoni P., & Sgaramella P. (2000). Precious puberty and body composition: Effects of GnRH analog treatment. J Ped Endocrinol Metab V13: 791-794

Crowley WF., Comite F., Vale W, Rivier J., Loriauz DL., & Cutler GB. (1981). Therapeutic use of pituitary desensitization with a long-acting LHRH agonist: a potential new treatment for idiopathic precocious puberty. J Clin Endocrinol MetabVol.52, pp. 370-372

Feuillan PP., Jones JV., Barnes K., Oerter-Klein K., & Cutler Jr GB. (1999). Reproductive axis after discontinuation of gonadotropin-releasing hormone analog treatment of girls with precocious puberty: Long term follow-up comparing girls with hypothalamic hamartoma to those with idiopathic precocious puberty. J Clin Endocrinol Metab Vol.84, No.1, pp. 44-49

Goldray D., Weisman Y., Laccard N., Merdler C., Chen J., & Matzkin H. (1993). Decreased bone density in elderly men treated with the gonadotropin-relseasing hormone agonist decapeptyl(D-Trp6-GnRH). J Clin Endocrinol Metab Vol.76, pp. 288-90

Greulich WW., & Pyle SI. (1959). Radiographic atlas of skeletal development of the hand and wrist. 2nd ed. Stanford; USA

Heger S., Partsch C-J., & Sippell WG. (1999). Long-term outcome after gonadotropin-releasing hormone agonist treatment of central precocious puberty: Final height, body proportions, body composition, bone mineral density, and reproductive function. J Clin Endocrinol Metab Vol.84, No.12, pp. 4583-4590

http://www.iotf.org/documents/iotfsocplan251006.pdf

Inokuchi M. (2009).Obesity in Japanese children The Keio Journal of the Keio Medical Society Vol.85, No.2, pp. T53-T85 (in Japanese)

Lindsay, R. (1995). Estrogen deficiency. In: Osteoporosis, etiology, diagnosis, and management, 2nd ed. Riggs BL, Melton LJ, (Ed.), 133-160, Philadelphia, USA

Oostdijk W., Rikken B., Schrerude S., Otten B., Odink R., Rouwe C., et al. (1996). Final height in central precocious puberty after long term treatment with a slow release GnRH agonist. Arch Dis Child Vol.75, pp. 292-297

Palmert MR, Mansfield MJ., Crowley Jr WF., Crigler Jr JF., Crawford JD., & Boepple PA. (1999). Is obesity an outcome of gonadotropin-releasing hormone agonist administration? Analysis of growth and body composition in 110 patients with central precocious puberty. J Clin Endocrinol Metab Vol.84, No.12, pp. 480-4488

Pasquino AM., Pucarelli I., Accardo F., Demiraj V., Segni M., & di Nardo R. (2008). Long-term observation of 87 girls with idiopathic central precocious puberty treated with gonadotropin-releasing hormone analogs: Impact on adult height, body mass index, bone mineral content, and reproductive function. J Clin Endocrinol Metab Vol.93, No.1, pp. 190-195

Paterson WF., McNeill E, Young D., & Donaldson MDC. (2004). Auxological outcome and time menarche following long-acting goserelin therapy in girls with central precocious or early puberty. Clinical Endocrinology Vol.61, pp. 626-634

Revila R., Revilla M., Villa LF., Cortes ., Arribas J., & Rico H. (1998). Changes in body composition in women treated with gonadotropin-releasing hormone agonist. Maturitas pp. 3163-68

Tanner JM., & Whitehouse R. (1976). Longitudinal standards for height, weight-height, weight-height, weight-velocity and stages of puberty. Arch Dis Child. Vol.51, pp. 170-179

Traggiai C., Perucchin PP., Zerbini K., Gastaldi R., De Biasio P., & Lorini R. (2005). Outcome after depot gonadotropin-releasing hormone agonist treatment for central precocious puberty: effects on body mass index and final height. European Journal of Endocrinology Vol.153, pp. 463-464

Wacharasindhu, S., Petwijit, T., Aroonparkmongkol S., Srivuthana S,. & Kingpetch K. (2006). Bone mineral density and body composition in Thai precocious puberty girls treated with GnRH agonist. J Med Assoc Thai Vol.89, No.8, pp.1194-1198 van der Sluis IM., Boot AM., Krenning EP., Drop SLS., & de Muinck Keizer-Schrama SMPF. (2002). Longitudinal follow-up of bone density and body composition in children with precocious or early puberty before, during and after cessation of GnRH agonist therapy. J Clin Endocrinol Metab 2Vol.87, No.2, pp. 506-512

Yamazaki K., Matsuoka H., Kawanobe S., Hujita Y., & Murata M. (1994). Evaluation of standard body weight by sex, age, and height. On the basis of 1990 school year data. J Jpn. Pediatr. Soc. Vol.98, pp. 96-102(in Japanese)

16

Hormone Therapy for the Treatment of Patients with Malignant Salivary Gland Tumor (MSGT)

Tomoki Sumida and Akiko Ishikawa
Department of Oral & Maxillofacial Surgery, Ehime University School of Medicine
Japan

1. Introduction

Malignant salivary gland tumors (MSGTs) account for 2-6% of all head and neck cancers (Glisson et al., 2004; Milano et al., 2007). Despite their rarity, MSGTs have been of great interest because of their wide variety of pathological features and high rates of metastasis, which result in poor prognoses. Surgical resection followed by radiation therapy is the primary therapy for this malignancy. Adjuvant therapy is reserved for the management of local recurrence no longer amenable to additional local therapy and for metastasis. Based on studies of other types of tumors, particularly breast cancer, the expression and function of sex steroid hormone receptors in cancer have been extensively studied and the findings applied to diagnosis and treatment (Clarke & Sutherland, 1990; Kester et al., 1997). Although a number of studies have been published, the rationale for hormone therapy of MSGTs remains controversial because of disparate results and an insufficient number of cases. However, some recent studies have shown that certain salivary gland neoplasms are similar to breast cancer, not only in terms of their pathological features, but also at the molecular level (Pia-Foschini, 2003; Wick et al., 1998; Yoshimura et al., 2007). Here, we shed light on the biological similarity between MSGTs and certain types of breast cancer, and describe the potential use of hormone and additional therapies for MSGTs.

2. The role of sex steroid hormone receptors in cancer therapy

The function of sex steroid hormone receptors in breast cancer has been extensively studied and the findings applied to diagnosis and treatment (Clarke & Sutherland, 1990; Kester et al., 1997) Estrogen stimulates cell proliferation of breast epithelial cells, and the close relationship between the expression of estrogen receptor (ER) and the prognosis of breast cancer has been well characterized (Ma et al., 2009). Progesterone levels fluctuate during the menstrual cycle and regulate cell proliferation and differentiation; however, less is known regarding its role in breast cancer (Jeng et al., 1992; Sutherland et al., 1988; van der Burg et al., 1992) We have previously reported that introducing progesterone receptor (PR) into hormone-independent breast cancer cells significantly suppresses their proliferative and invasive activities upon progesterone treatment (Sumida et al., 2004). Several drugs, such as

Tamoxifen, an estrogen receptor antagonist, and a synthetic progestin similar to progesterone, are considered to be effective at inhibiting tumor cell proliferation. These drugs are given as adjuvant therapies to breast cancer patients when immunohistochemical staining of their tumor tissue indicates that >10% of the breast cancer cells express ER or PR (Horwitz, 1993; Williams et al., 2007). Molecular-targeted drug therapy is generally less toxic than traditional chemotherapy; however, some studies have reported severe side effects, and carefully designed and regulated clinical trials are necessary to confirm their safety. Moreover, these types of therapies are not viable when a tumor expresses a low level of a molecular target such as a receptor (Ismail-Khanet al., 2010). This problem is exemplified by breast cancers that do not express ER, PR, or HER2 receptors, that is, in triple negative cases. It is a challenge for clinicians to provide efficacious treatments for this patient population.

Sex steroid hormone therapy in prostate cancers is based on their high sensitivity to androgen inhibition. The most common hormone therapy is initiated by reducing the concentration of circulating androgens through surgical or medical castration and/or by administering anti-androgens such as flutamide or bicalutamide (Klotz et al., 2005; Miyake et al., 2005). However, in almost all patients, the efficacy of the treatment decreases over time as the tumor becomes "androgen-refractory" (Yuan et al., 2009). As a result, these patients develop distant metastases, such as in the bone, which eventually proves fatal to the patient. Therefore, the molecular events that control the transition from androgen-sensitive prostate cancer to androgen-refractory prostate cancer need to be elucidated.

Accumulating evidence suggests that the androgen receptor (AR) plays a critical role in regulating the growth of both androgen-sensitive and androgen-refractory prostate cancer (Chen et al., 2004; Debes et al., 2004; Grossmann et al., 2001; Hara et al., 2003; Scher et al., 2005; Taplin et al., 2004). In addition, recent studies have shown that the AR can regulate invasion and metastasis (Hara et al., 2008). In AR-negative cell lines such as PC3 and DU145, it has been shown that forced AR expression decreases their invasive properties and treatment with androgen further reduces invasion by these cells (Bonaccorsi et al., 2000; Cinar et al., 2001). Moreover, it has been reported that hormone-refractory prostate cancers have a variety of AR alterations that are either not found in hormone-naive tumors or are found at a lower frequency (Taplin et al., 2004). A more recent investigation demonstrated that forced expression of AR in a subline of a metastatic androgen-dependent prostate cancer cell line led to increased invasion (Hara et al., 2008). It is clear that a more detailed understanding of the AR alterations in the evolution of androgen-refractory prostate cancer is needed to help drive the development of potential new therapies.

Few studies of ovarian and colon cancer have addressed the potential application of hormone therapies (Burkman, 2002). In ovarian cancer, the use of estrogen as a menopausal therapy has frequently been associated with an increased risk of ovarian cancer, and there is still conflicting evidence regarding the impact of hormone therapy in terms of decreasing the risk of cancer (Greiser et al., 2010). A recent study, however, suggested that this problem can be circumvented by co-administering progestin and estrogen (Pearce et al., 2009). Further, experiments in culture showed that progesterone reduced the proliferation of both benign and malignant ovarian tumor cells (Zhou et al., 2002). Therefore, progestin might be a key factor for preventing and suppressing ovarian cancer cell growth. In contrast to ovarian cancer, estrogen appears to have protective effects against colon cancer (Kennelly et al., 2008). However, the role of hormone replacement therapy with estrogen for the treatment of colon cancer is poorly understood, and further analyses are needed.

3. Pathological and biological similarities between MSGTs and breast cancer

Mammary and salivary glands are tubulo-acinar exocrine glands that share similar morphological characteristics. Similar histological features are observed when the tumors arising from these 2 sites are compared (Camelo-Piragua et al., 2009; Hellquist et al., 1994; Marchio et al., 2010; Pia-Foschini et al., 2003). Although the cancers differ in terms of their incidence and clinical behavior, certain biological features have been described in both entities and potential common therapeutic approaches have been considered. The WHO classification of MSGTs lists more than 20 different histological subtypes (Laurie et al., 2006; Milano et al., 2007). The majority of these are divided into 2 groups—those of secretory duct origin (including mucoepidermoid carcinoma [MEC] and salivary duct carcinoma [SDC]) and those of intercalated origin (including adenoid cystic carcinoma [ACC]) (Batsakis et al., 1989; Dardick et al., 1987). Most of these tumors occur in the parotid gland (70%), and less than 25% are malignant (Glisson et al., 2004). Although the incidence of tumors at other sites such as the submandibular, sublingual, and minor salivary glands is less common, malignancy at these sites is higher, approximating 50% (Glisson et al., 2004). Most aggressive breast cancers are composed of invasive ductal carcinomas, and other histologic features such as MEC and ACC are relatively rare. Below, we briefly describe some of the types of MSGTs that display features (at the morphological and molecular level) that they have in common with breast cancers, and could therefore provide potential common therapeutic strategies.

3.1 Mucoepidermoid carcinoma (MEC)

MEC is the most common salivary gland neoplasm, accounting for 29–34% of all malignancies of the major and minor salivary glands (Milano et al., 2007). These tumors grow slowly and present as painless masses in most cases. They are primarily composed of intermediate, mucous, and epidermoid cells. The cell types are classified histologically as low-, intermediate-, and high-grade; 5-year overall survival (OS) varies from 92% to 100% for low-grade tumors, 62% to 92% for intermediate-grade tumors, and 0% to 43% for high-grade tumors (Pires et al., 2004). High-grade MEC is an aggressive malignancy, characterized by high rates of local recurrence and distant metastasis. On the contrary, low-grade MECs generally do not metastasize. MEC of the breast is a rare entity with an estimated incidence of 0.2% and is composed of a mixture of basaloid, intermediate, epidermoid, and mucinous cells (Camelo-Piragua et al., 2009; Fisher et al., 1983). Since Patchefsky et al. first described breast MEC in 1979, only 28 cases have been reported (Berry et al., 1998; Chang et al., 1998; Di Tommaso et al., 2004; Fisher et al., 1983; Gomez-Aracil et al., 2006; Hanna et al., 1985; Hastrup et al., 1985; Hornychova et al., 2007; Kovi et al., 1981; Leong et al., 1985; Luchtrath et al., 1989; Markopoulos et al., 1998; Patchefsky et al., 1979; Pettinato et al., 1989; Ratanarapee et al., 1983; Tjalma et al., 2002). Because of its rarity, the prognosis remains controversial debatable matter. However, MECs from the breasts and salivary glands have been shown to share similar biological features and morphologies (Camelo-Piragua et al., 2009). Researchers have classified breast MECs into 3 grades by using the same grading system as for salivary gland tumors and have demonstrated that high-grade tumors are associated with high mortality as a result of lymph node and distant metastases. These results suggest that MECs from both mammary and salivary glands have similar morphological features, and thus could have similar treatment strategies. Further, a common cytogenetic alteration of breast and salivary MECs has been reported. A reciprocal translocation t(11;19)(q21;p13) (MAML2: MECT) was identified in breast MEC; this is the most frequent genetic alteration in the salivary glands (Tonon et al., 2003). The translocation creates a fusion product (MAML2: MECT1) that activates transcription of cAMP/CREB target genes (Tonon et al., 2003; Tonon et al., 2004). Another report noted that patients in whom the protein fusion gene is expressed have a significantly lower risk of death compared to patients without the fusion protein MAML2:MECT1 (Behboudi et al., 2006). It has also been shown that other subtypes of breast cancer are negative for this gene, suggesting that this fusion gene is specific to MEC. This translocation is likely to be a promising marker of MECs from both the mammary and salivary glands (Nordkvist et al., 1994).

3.2 Adenoid cystic carcinoma (ACC)

ACCs account for 22% of MSGTs (Hotte et al., 2005). There are 3 histological subtypes: tubular; cribriform; and solid (Da Silva et al., 2009; Pia-Foschini et al., 2003). In contrast to the squamous cell carcinomas that account for the vast majority of head and neck malignancies, ACC often spreads systemically, especially to the lung and bone, and the metastatic proportion of this type of neoplasm is 24–55% (Dodd et al., 2006). Because of the high metastatic rate, prognosis is poor. The 10-year OS is 39–55% and the 20-year OS is 21–25% (Dodd et al., 2006).

On the other hand, breast ACC is a rare malignancy, accounting for 0.1–1% of all breast cancers (Marchio et al., 2010). In addition, these neoplasms show different clinical behaviors than their salivary gland counterparts. The 10-year OS is >90%, and lymph node and distant metastases are generally rare (Marchio et al., 2010). However, the histological features of breast ACCs are very similar to ACCs originating from the salivary glands (as shown in Fig. 1). Ro et al. applied the same grading system to ACCs from both types of tissues, and both breast and salivary gland tumors are characterized by expression of c-KIT and share a common chromosomal translocation t(6;9) leading to the fusion gene MYB-NFIB (Marchio et al., 2010; Persson et al., 2009; Ro et al., 1987). c-KIT has been shown to be expressed in 80–100% of ACCs of the salivary glands and in almost all ACCs from the breast (Azoulay et al., 2005; Crisi et al., 2005; Edwards et al., 2003; Holst et al., 1999; Jeng et al., 2000; Mastropasqua et al., 2005; Vila et al., 2009; Weigelt et al., 2008). The genetic alteration t(6;9)(q22-23;p23-24) was first identified as a characteristic of salivary gland ACCs (Nordkvist et al., 1994). Since then, the same translocation has been detected in breast tumors (Persson et al., 2009). The fusion gene is highly expressed in proliferating cells and is downregulated as the cells become more differentiated. Therefore, this gene may provide new therapeutic approaches for the management of ACCs.

3.3 Salivary duct carcinoma (SDC)

SDC is a rare and highly aggressive neoplasm with histologic features very similar to that of invasive ductal carcinoma of the breast (IDC) (Barneset al., 1994; Hellquist et al., 1994; Kleinsasser et al., 1968). SDC is generally more aggressive and has lower survival rates than other MSGTs. The epithelium tends to form cribriform, papillary, and solid growth patterns along with duct-like structures (Hellquist et al., 1994). The morphology of SDC is characterized by cuboidal and polygonal cells forming distended ducts and solid nests (often with central necrosis) that are very similar to comedocarcinoma (Hellquist et al., 1994). In addition to the histopathological resemblance, both entities have similar clinical behaviors, that is, they have highly metastatic features leading to a poor prognosis. A wide variety of molecular studies have led to the identification of certain biological markers of SDCs. Among these is HER-2, which is amplified in 20–25% of breast cancers (Moy et al., 2006; Press et al., 1997). Various studies of HER-2 in SDC have shown variable results, with amplification occurring in 25–100% of tumors (Jaspers et al., 2011). Nonetheless, the proportion is much higher than that observed in the other histological subtypes, such as the ACCs and MECs described above (Etges et al., 2003; Giannoni et al., 1995; Gibbons et al., 2001; Glisson et al., 2004; Hellquist et al., 1994; Jaehne et al., 2005; Locati et al., 2009; Milanoet al., 2007; Nguyen et al., 2003; Press et al., 1994; Skalova et al., 2001; Williams et al., 2007). HER-2 expression is considered to correlate with histological grade in both salivary gland neoplasms as well as breast cancer, and represents a potential attractive therapeutic approach for SDCs. Since HER-2 can also enhance AR function, anti-androgen therapy may be effective against MSGTs when HER-2 is overexpressed.

Previous studies have shown that high EGFR expression in SDCs may contribute to tumor growth (Fan et al., 2001; Locati et al., 2009). EGFR has also been shown to enhance tumorigenesis in several human carcinomas by blocking apoptosis and promoting angiogenesis (Kari et al., 2003). An interaction between both EGFR and HER-2 and hormonal pathways has also been described. In breast and uterine cancers, treatment with anti-EGF antibodies reduces tumor proliferation induced by treatment with estradiol. Likewise, the antiestrogen ICI 164,384 reduces the effects of EGF-induced tumor proliferation (Shupnik, 2004).

Hoang et al. performed molecular studies with microsatellite markers and DNA flow cytometry to compare the biological characteristics of SDC and IDC. They found that there were similar allelic alterations on chromosomal arms 6q, 16q, 17p, and 17q, and DNA aneuploidy in both malignancies; these alterations may contribute to the aggressive behavior (Hoang et al., 2001). Recently, polysomy of chromosome 7 was detected in 25% of SDCs, and this alteration correlated with poor OS (Williams et al., 2010). This correlation was also reported in IDCs, and supports the notion that EGFR gene mutations may guide therapy (Shien et al., 2005). Taken together, gene alterations of both EGFR and HER-2 may define the molecular features of these 2 types of malignancies, and these receptors may be candidates for targeted therapy.

4. Hormone therapy for the treatment of patients with MSGTs

As described above, several types of MSGTs are morphologically and biologically similar to malignant breast cancers (Pia-Foschini et al., 2003; Wick et al., 1998) (Fig. 1). Further, the clinical significance of sex hormone receptors has been debated since White and Garcelon first described therapy with estrogen against salivary gland neoplasms in 1955 (White & Garcelon, 1955). Previous reports obtained using a low number of biopsy samples have shown conflicting results regarding the expression of sex hormone receptors, making it difficult to determine the potential benefits of hormone therapy (Barnes et al., 1994; Barrera et al., 2008; Dimery et al., 1987; Dori et al., 2000; Jeannon et al., 1999; Lamey et al., 1987; Lewis et al., 1996; Miller et al., 1994; Nasser et al., 2003; Pires et al., 2004; Shick et al., 1995). Therefore, additional studies are required in order to clarify the role of hormone receptors in MSGTs. Although several studies have examined ER and PR expression in MSGTs, there is substantial disparity in the results: the expression of ER and PR varies from 0 to 86% and 0 to 50%, respectively (Barnes et al., 1994; Barrera et al., 2008; Dimery et al., 1987; Dori et al., 2000; Jeannon et al., 1999; Lamey et al., 1987; Lewis et al., 1996; Miller et al., 1994; Nasser et al., 2003; Pires et al., 2004; Shick et al., 1995). These disparities may be explained by differences in the antibodies used, the experimental methods of detection (e.g., Western blotting vs. immunohistochemistry), and the criteria used for ruling out false positives and negatives. It is therefore particularly critical to standardize protocols in a way similar to that described for the analysis of breast cancer tissues. Some of the differences might also result from an insufficient number of samples.

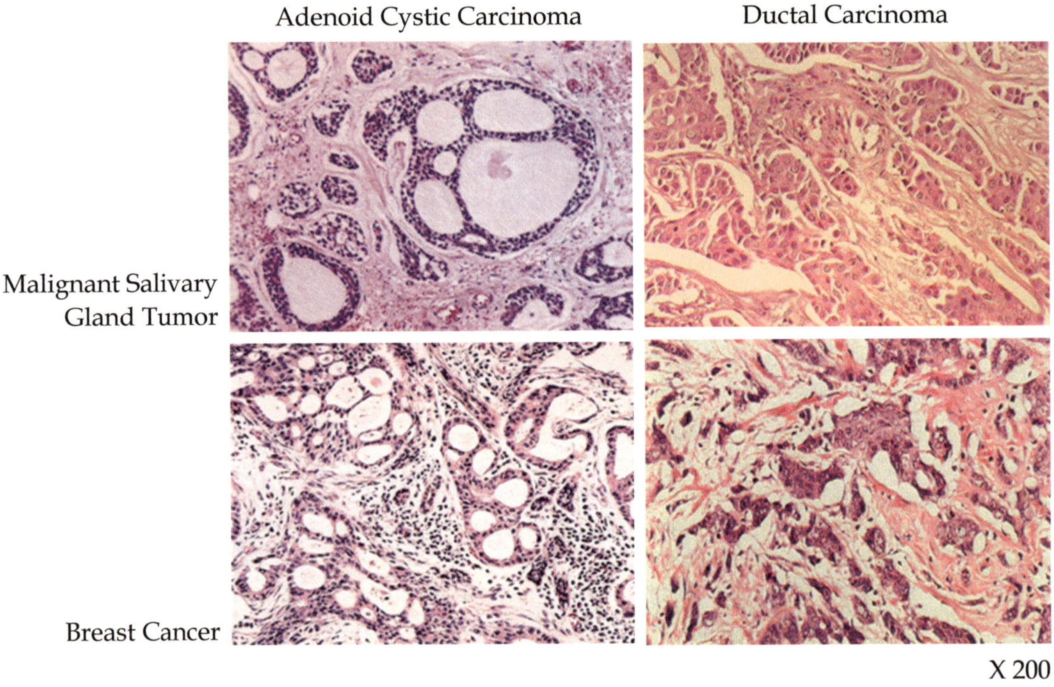

Salivary glands and mammary glands are both tubulo-acinar exocrine tissues sharing similar morphological features. It is therefore expected that the tumors originating from these two different glands would show similarities in their response to hormonal treatment.

Fig. 1. Histological comparison of malignant salivary and mammary gland tumors.

Even though ER expression is unlikely to represent a useful marker for detecting MSGTs, a subset of MSGTs clearly expresses hormone receptors, and these receptors could control disease progression. Thus, current therapeutic strategies in breast cancer patients may also be effective for the treatment of MSGTs. Moreover, the feasibility of hormone therapy seems to be supported by accumulating reports of AR expression in SDCs. Although the expression of AR is generally rare in salivary gland neoplasms, SDCs commonly express AR in 92–100% of cases (Fan et al., 2001; Kapadia et al., 1998; Moriki et al., 2001). Recently, Jaspers et al. reported that androgen deprivation therapy (ADT) in patients with recurrent or disseminated disease showed a clinical benefit in 5 out of 10 cases, and 2 of these had partial responses (Jaspers et al., 2011). This approach is therefore more effective than the results obtained with chemotherapy. Given the fact that ADT generally has less adverse effects than chemotherapy, anti-androgen therapy may lead to better clinical outcomes and could become a standard treatment for SDCs.

Williams et al. reported that most tumors derived from breast and salivary glands expressed estrogen receptor-beta (ER-β) and that the patients whose tumors lacked ER-β were at higher risk for local recurrence (Williams et al., 2007). In addition, previous studies have linked the loss of ER expression to aggressive features in adenocarcinomas of the breast, prostate, and colon (Foley et al., 2000; Fuqua et al., 2003; Leygue et al., 1999; Maggiolini et al., 2004; Strom et al., 2004; Wong et al., 2005). In breast and prostate carcinoma, ER-β has been shown to inhibit cell proliferation via the cyclin D1 pathway, and to induce apoptosis by downregulating bcl-2 and/or by inducing Bax expression (Bardin et al., 2004; Pettersson et al., 2000). Targeting ER-β may therefore become a useful approach for the management of salivary duct carcinoma.

In our previous studies, we determined that MSGT cell lines in culture lacked estrogen and progesterone receptors. However, the lack of hormone receptors may be a consequence of malignant transformation and may represent a requirement for the establishment of immortal cell lines. Other clinical studies have reported the efficacy of Tamoxifen against MSGTs (Elkin & Jacobs, 2008; Shadaba et al., 1997), and one resulted in long-term survival even though in these patients, no ER was detected by immunohistochemistry. This result appears to be supported by another case report where Tamoxifen could reactivate ER expression (Sharma et al., 2006). Our previous studies showed that progesterone could suppress MGST cell aggressiveness in a manner similar to that observed in breast cancer cells (Fig. 2). Specifically, we demonstrated that after transduction of PR, progesterone could significantly suppress the proliferation (and invasion) of MSGT cells (Yoshimura et al., 2007). This suppression did not lead to cell death, but instead to cell cycle arrest. These data suggest that if MSGTs express significant levels of PR, then progesterone treatment may slow the growth of the primary tumor and potentially shift it to a dormant state. Since most MSGTs occur in elderly patients, triggering tumor dormancy could improve the quality of

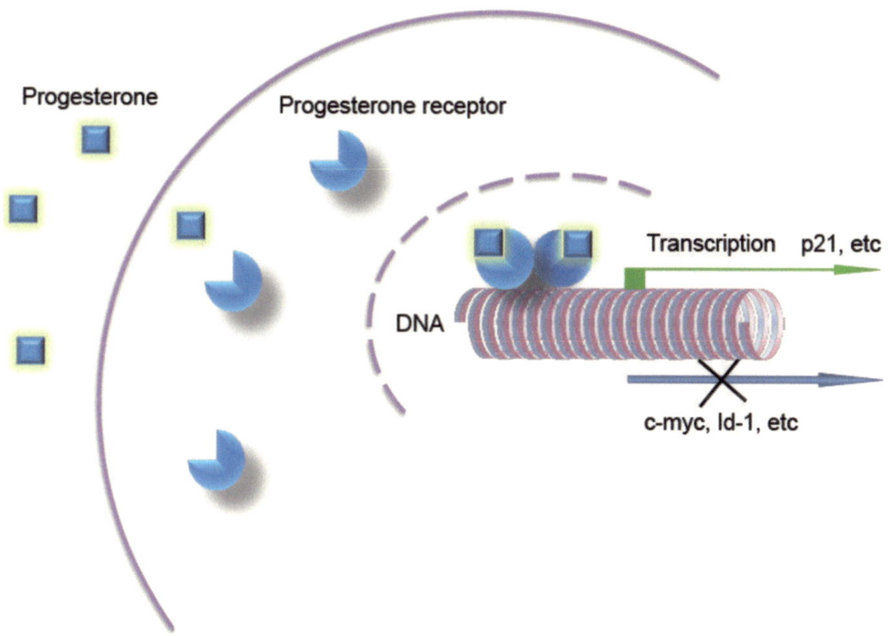

Fig. 2. Pg suppresses proliferation and invasion of both salivary gland and breast cancer cells.

life, and may be a successful way to allow the patient to live a normal lifespan. Although the 5-year OS in patients with MSGTs represents the average, extended survival rates are extremely low (Lones et al., 1997; Lopes et al., 1998; Spiro, 1997). MSGTs show low sensitivity to chemotherapy and surgery because of anatomical limitations (Marabdas et al., 1990; Takagi et al., 2001). Since radiation is also less effective, novel therapeutic approaches are eagerly anticipated. Triggering tumor dormancy as a consequence of hormone therapy could represent a novel strategy for the treatment of patients with MSGTs.

In our recent studies, the inhibitory effect of Pg on the proliferative and invasive activities of the salivary gland and breast tumor cells was demonstrated, suggesting some common mechanisms. In both types of cancers, expression of Id-1 and c-myc was down-regulated after Pg treatment, whereas p21 expression level was up-regulated.

5. Conclusions

Besides surgical resection and radiation of MSGTs, there are no other effective therapies. Adjuvant therapy is generally reserved for palliative treatment; however, there is no clear evidence that such treatment can bring clinical benefits. Since adverse effects caused by chemotherapy often threaten the life of a patient, and since some patients with specific MSGTs, especially ACCs, show long survival even with multiple metastases, the adoption of adjuvant therapy should be carefully considered. To achieve new therapeutic methods, it is now necessary to clarify several unanswered questions regarding the expression and/or function of sex steroid hormone receptors in MSGTs. As indicated by AR expression in SDCs, there is now evidence linking hormone receptors and growth factor receptors to the disease. Expression of these receptors could render tumors sensitive to hormone therapy. However, to improve clinical outcomes of patients with rather rare malignancies, more accurate data obtained from multiple and larger studies are required. MSGTs tend to occur in elderly patients, and triggering tumor dormancy could be a successful means of slowing disease progression, therefore providing an improvement in their quality of life. Our studies on PR-negative cells also suggest that induction of hormone receptor gene expression might be an option for delaying disease progression. Based on multiple lines of evidence from a range of cancers, sex steroid hormone receptors may prove to be appropriate targets for the establishment of novel treatments for patients with MSGTs.

6. References

Azoulay S, Laé M, Fréneaux P, Merle S, Al Ghuzlan A, Chnecker C, Rosty C, Klijanienko J, Sigal-Zafrani B, Salmon R, Fourquet A, Sastre-Garau X, Vincent-Salomon A. (2005) KIT is highly expressed in adenoid cystic carcinoma of the breast, a basal-like carcinoma associated with a favorable outcome. *Mod Pathol*, 18, 12, pp1623-31.

Bardin A, Boulle N, Lazennec G, Vignon F, Pujol P. (2004) Loss of ERbeta expression as a common step in estrogen-dependent tumor progression. *Endocr Relat Cancer*, 11, 3, pp537-51.

Barnes L, Rao U, Contis L, Krause J, Schwartz A, Scalamogna P. (1994) Salivary duct carcinoma. Part II. Immunohistochemical evaluation of 13 cases for estrogen and progesterone receptors, cathepsin D, and c-erbB-2 protein. *Oral Surg Oral Med Oral Pathol,* 78, 1, pp74-80.

Barnes L, Rao U, Krause J, Contis L, Schwartz A, Scalamogna P. (1994) Salivary duct carcinoma. Part I. A clinicopathologic evaluation and DNA image analysis of 13 cases with review of the literature. *Oral Surg Oral Med Oral Pathol*, 78, 1, pp64-73.

Barrera JE, Shroyer KR, Said S, Hoernig G, Melrose R, Freedman PD, Wright TA, Greer RO. (2008) Estrogen and progesterone receptor and p53 gene expression in adenoid cystic cancer. *Head Neck Pathol*, 2, 1, pp13-8.

Batsakis JG, Regezi JA, Luna MA, el-Naggar A. (1989) Histogenesis of salivary gland neoplasms: a postulate with prognostic implications. *J Laryngol Otol*, 103, 10, pp 939-44.

Behboudi A, Enlund F, Winnes M, Andrén Y, Nordkvist A, Leivo I, Flaberg E, Szekely L, Mäkitie A, Grenman R, Mark J, Stenman G. (2006) Molecular classification of mucoepidermoid carcinomasprognostic significance of the MECT1-MAML2 fusion oncogene. *Genes Chromosomes Cancer*, 45, 5, pp470-81.

Berry MG, C Caldwell, R Carpenter. (1998) Mucoepidermoid carcinoma of the breast: a case report and review of the literature. *Eur J Surg Oncol*, 24, 1, pp78-80.

Bonaccorsi L, Carloni V, Muratori M, Salvadori A, Giannini A, Carini M, Serio M, Forti G, Baldi E. (2000) Androgen receptor expression in prostate carcinoma cells suppresses alpha6beta4 integrin-mediated invasive phenotype. *Endocrinology*, 141, 9, pp3172-82.

Burkman RT. (2002) Reproductive hormones and cancer: ovarian and colon cancer. *Obstet Gynecol Clin North Am*, 29, 3, pp527-40.

Camelo-Piragua SI, Habib C, Kanumuri P, Lago CE, Mason HS, Otis CN. (2009) Mucoepidermoid carcinoma of the breast shares cytogenetic abnormality with mucoepidermoid carcinoma of the salivary gland: a case report with molecular analysis and review of the literature. *Hum Pathol*, 40, 6, pp887-92.

Chang LC, Lee N, Lee CT, Huang JS. (1998) High-grade mucoepidermoid carcinoma of the breast: case report. *Changgeng Yi Xue Za Zhi*, 21, 3, pp352-7.

Chen CD, Welsbie DS, Tran C, Baek SH, Chen R, Vessella R, Rosenfeld MG, Sawyers CL. (2004) Molecular determinants of resistance to antiandrogen therapy. *Nat Med*, 10, 1, pp 33-9.

Cinar B, Koeneman KS, Edlund M, Prins GS, Zhau HE, Chung LW. (2001) Androgen receptor mediates the reduced tumor growth, enhanced androgen responsiveness, and selected target gene transactivation in a human prostate cancer cell line. *Cancer Res*, 61, 19, pp7310-7.

Clarke CL and RL Sutherland, (1990) Progestin regulation of cellular proliferation. *Endocr Rev*, 11, 2, pp266-301.

Crisi GM, Marconi SA, Makari-Judson G, Goulart RA. (2005) Expression of c-kit in adenoid cystic carcinoma of the breast. *Am JClin Pathol*, 124, 5, pp733-9.

Da Silva L、 Buck L, Simpson PT, Reid L, McCallum N, Madigan BJ, Lakhani SR. (2009) Molecular and morphological analysis of adenoid cystic carcinoma of the breast with synchronous tubular adenosis. *Virchows Arch*, 454, 1, pp107-14.

Dardick I, AW van Nostrand. (1987) Morphogenesis of salivary gland tumors. A prerequisite to improving classification. *Pathol Annu*, 22, Pt 1, pp1-53.

Debes JD, DJ Tindall. (2004) Mechanisms of androgen-refractory prostate cancer. *N Engl J Med*, 351, 15, pp1488-90.

Di Tommaso L, Foschini MP, Ragazzini T, Magrini E, Fornelli A, Ellis IO, Eusebi V. (2004) Mucoepidermoid carcinoma of the breast. *Virchows Arch*, 444, 1, pp13-9.

Dimery IW, Jones LA, Verjan RP, Raymond AK, Goepfert H, Hong WK. (1987) Estrogen receptors in normal salivary gland and salivary gland carcinoma. *Arch Otolaryngol Head Neck Surg*, 113, 10, pp1082-5.

Dodd RL, NJ Slevin. (2006) Salivary gland adenoid cystic carcinoma: a review of chemotherapy and molecular therapies. *Oral Oncol*, 42, 8, pp759-69.

Dori S, Trougouboff P, David R, Buchner A. (2000) Immunohistochemical evaluation of estrogen and progesterone receptors in adenoid cystic carcinoma of salivary gland origin. *Oral Oncol*, 36, 5, pp450-3.

Edwards PC, T Bhuiya, RD Kelsch. (2003) C-kit expression in the salivary gland neoplasms adenoid cystic carcinoma, polymorphous low-grade adenocarcinoma, and monomorphic adenoma. *Oral Surg Oral Med Oral Pathol Oral Radiol Endod*, 95, 5, pp586-93.

Elkin AD, CD Jacobs. (2008) Tamoxifen for salivary gland adenoid cystic carcinoma: report of two cases. *J Cancer Res Clin Oncol*, 134, 10, pp1151-3.

Etges A, Pinto DS Jr, Kowalski LP, Soares FA, Araújo VC. (2003) Salivary duct carcinoma: immunohistochemical profile of an aggressive salivary gland tumour. *J Clin Pathol*, 56, 12, pp914-8.

Fan CY, Melhem MF, Hosal AS, Grandis JR, Barnes EL. (2001) Expression of androgen receptor, epidermal growth factor receptor, and transforming growth factor alpha in salivary duct carcinoma. *Arch Otolaryngol Head Neck Surg*, 127, 9, pp1075-9.

Fisher ER, Palekar AS, Gregorio RM, Paulson JD. (1983) Mucoepidermoid and squamous cell carcinomas of breast with reference to squamous metaplasia and giant cell tumors. *Am J Surg Pathol*, 7, 1, pp15-27.

Foley EF, Jazaeri AA, Shupnik MA, Jazaeri O, Rice LW. (2000) Selective loss of estrogen receptor beta in malignant human colon. *Cancer Res*, 60, 2, pp245-8.

Fuqua SA, Schiff R, Parra I, Moore JT, Mohsin SK, Osborne CK, Clark GM, Allred DC. (2003) Estrogen receptor beta protein in human breast cancer: correlation with clinical tumor parameters. *Cancer Res*, 63, 10, pp2434-9.

Giannoni C, el-Naggar AK, Ordoñez NG, Tu ZN, Austin J, Luna MA, Batsakis JG. (1995) c-erbB-2/neu oncogene and Ki-67 analysis in the assessment of palatal salivary gland neoplasms. *Otolaryngol Head Neck Surg*, 112, 3, pp391-8.

Gibbons MD, Manne U, Carroll WR, Peters GE, Weiss HL, Grizzle WE. (2001) Molecular differences in mucoepidermoid carcinoma and adenoid cystic carcinoma of the major salivary glands. *Laryngoscope*, 111, 8, pp1373-8.

Glisson B, Colevas AD, Haddad R, Krane J, El-Naggar A, Kies M, Costello R, Summey C, Arquette M, Langer C, Amrein PC, Posner M. (2004) HER2 expression in salivary gland carcinomas: dependence on histological subtype. *Clin Cancer Res*, 10, 3, pp944-6.

Gomez-Aracil V, Mayayo Artal E, Azua-Romeo J, Mayayo Alvira R, Azúa-Blanco J, Arraiza Goicoechea A. (2006) Fine needle aspiration cytology of high grade mucoepidermoid carcinoma of the breast: a case report. *Acta Cytol*, 50, 3, pp344-8.

Greiser CM, EM Greiser, M Doren. (2010) Menopausal hormone therapy and risk of lung cancer-Systematic review and meta-analysis. *Maturitas*, 65, 3, pp198-204.

Grossmann ME, H Huang, DJ Tindall. (2001) Androgen receptor signaling in androgen-refractory prostate cancer. *J Natl Cancer Inst*, 93, 22, pp1687-97.

Hanna W, HJ Kahn. (1985) Ultrastructural and immunohistochemical characteristics of mucoepidermoid carcinoma of the breast. *Hum Pathol*, 16, 9, pp941-6.

Hara T, Miyazaki H, Lee A, Tran CP, Reiter RE. (2008) Androgen receptor and invasion in prostate cancer. *Cancer Res*, 68, 4, pp1128-35.

Hara T, Nakamura K, Araki H, Kusaka M, Yamaoka M. (2003) Enhanced androgen receptor signaling correlates with the androgenrefractory growth in a newly established MDA PCa 2b-hr human prostate cancer cell subline. *Cancer Res*, 63, 17, pp5622-8.

Hastrup N, M Sehested. (1985) High-grade mucoepidermoid carcinoma of the breast. *Histopathology*, 9, 8, pp887-92.

Hellquist HB, MG Karlsson, C Nilsson. (1994) Salivary duct carcinoma--a highly aggressive salivary gland tumour with overexpression of c-erbB-2. *J Pathol*, 172, 1, pp35-44.

Hoang MP, Callender DL, Sola Gallego JJ, Huang Z, Sneige N, Luna MA, Batsakis JG, El-Naggar AK. (2001) Molecular and biomarker analyses of salivary duct carcinomas: comparison with mammary duct carcinoma. *Int J Oncol*, 19, 4, pp865-71.

Holst VA, Marshall CE, Moskaluk CA, Frierson HF Jr. (1999) KIT protein expression and analysis of c-kit gene mutation in adenoid cystic carcinoma. *Mod Pathol*, 12, 10, pp956-60.

Hornychova H, Ryska A, Betlach J, Bohác R, Cízek T, Tomsová M, Obermannová R. (2007) Mucoepidermoid carcinoma of the breast. *Neoplasma*, 54, 2, pp168-72.

Horwitz KB. Mechanisms of hormone resistance in breast cancer. (1993) *Breast Cancer Res Treat*, 26, 2, pp119-30.

Hotte SJ, Winquist EW, Lamont E, MacKenzie M, Vokes E, Chen EX, Brown S, Pond GR, Murgo A, Siu LL. (2005) Imatinib mesylate in patients with adenoid cystic cancers of the salivary glands expressing c-kit: a Princess Margaret Hospital phase II consortium study. *J Clin Oncol*, 23, 3, pp585-90.

Ismail-Khan R, MM Bui. (2010) A review of triple-negative breast cancer. *Cancer Control*, 17, 3, pp173-6.

Jaehne M, Roeser K, Jaekel T, Schepers JD, Albert N, Löning T. (2005) Clinical and immunohistologic typing of salivary duct carcinoma: a report of 50 cases. Cancer, 103, 12, pp2526-33.

Jaspers HC, Verbist BM, Schoffelen R, Mattijssen V, Slootweg PJ, van der Graaf WT, van Herpen CM. (2011) Androgen receptor-positive salivary duct carcinoma: a disease entity with promising new treatment options. *J Clin Oncol*, 29, 16, ppe473-6.

Jeannon JP, Soames JV, Bell H, Wilson JA. (1999) Immunohistochemical detection of oestrogen and progesterone receptors in salivary tumours. *Clin Otolaryngol Allied Sci*, 24, 1, pp52-4.

Jeng, MH, CJ Parker, VC Jordan. (1992) Estrogenic potential of progestins in oral contraceptives to stimulate human breast cancer cell proliferation. *Cancer Res*, 52, 23, pp6539-46.

Jeng YM, CY Lin, HC Hsu. (2000) Expression of the c-kit protein is associated with certain subtypes of salivary gland carcinoma. *Cancer Lett*, 154, 1, pp107-11.

Jones AS, Hamilton JW, Rowley H, Husband D, Helliwell TR. (1997) Adenoid cystic carcinoma of the head and neck. *Clin Otolaryngol Allied Sci*, 22, 5, pp434-43.

Kapadia SB, L Barnes. (1998) Expression of androgen receptor, gross cystic disease fluid protein, and CD44 in salivary duct carcinoma. *Mod Pathol*, 11, 11, pp1033-8.

Kari C, Chan TO, Rocha de Quadros M, Rodeck U. (2003) Targeting the epidermal growth factor receptor in cancer: apoptosis takes center stage. *Cancer Res*, 63, 1, pp1-5.

Kennelly R, Kavanagh DO, Hogan AM, Winter DC. (2008) Oestrogen and the colon: potential mechanisms for cancer prevention. *Lancet Oncol*, 9, 4, pp385-91.

Kester HA, van der Leede BM, van der Saag PT, van der Burg B. (1997) Novel progesterone target genes identified by an improved differential display technique suggest that progestin-induced growth inhibition of breast cancer cells coincides with enhancement of differentiation. *J Biol Chem*, 272, 26, pp16637-43.

Kleinsasser O, HJ Klein, G Hubner. (1968) Salivary duct carcinoma. A group of salivary gland tumors analogous to mammary duct carcinoma. *Arch Klin ExpOhren Nasen Kehlkopfheilkd*, 192, 1, pp100-5.

Klotz L, P Schellhammer. (2005) Combined androgen blockade: the case for bicalutamide. *Clin Prostate Cancer*, 3, 4, pp215-9.

Kovi J, HD Duong, LS Leffall Jr. (1981) High-grade mucoepidermoid carcinoma of the breast. *Arch Pathol Lab Med*, 105, 11, pp612-4.

Lamey PJ, Leake RE, Cowan SK, Soutar DS, McGregor IA, McGregor FM. (1987) Steroid hormone receptors in human salivary gland tumours. *J Clin Pathol*, 40, 5, pp532-4.

Laurie SA, L Licitra. (2006) Systemic therapy in the palliative management of advanced salivary gland cancers. *J Clin Oncol*, 24, 17, pp2673-8.

Leong AS, JA Williams. (1985) Mucoepidermoid carcinoma of the breast: high grade variant. *Pathology*, 17, 3, pp516-21.

Lewis JE, McKinney BC, Weiland LH, Ferreiro JA, Olsen KD. (1996) Salivary duct carcinoma. Clinicopathologic and immunohistochemical review of 26 cases. *Cancer*, 77, 2, pp223-30.

Leygue E, Dotzlaw H, Watson PH, Murphy LC. (1999) Expression of estrogen receptor beta1, beta2, and beta5 messenger RNAs in human breast tissue. *Cancer Res*, 1999. 59, 6, pp1175-9.

Locati LD, Perrone F, Losa M, Mela M, Casieri P, Orsenigo M, Cortelazzi B, Negri T, Tamborini E, Quattrone P, Bossi P, Rinaldi G, Bergamini C, Calderone RG, Liberatoscioli C, Licitra L. (2009) Treatment relevant target immunophenotyping of 139 salivary gland carcinomas (SGCs). *Oral Oncol*, 45, 11, pp986-90.

Lopes MA, GC Santos, LP Kowalski. (1998) Multivariate survival analysis of 128 cases of oral cavity minor salivary gland carcinomas. *Head Neck*, 20, 8, pp699-706.

Luchtrath H, R Moll. (1989) Mucoepidermoid mammary carcinoma. Immunohistochemical and biochemical analyses of intermediate filaments. *Virchows Arch A Pathol Anat Histopathol*, 416, 2 pp105-13.

Ma CX, CG Sanchez, MJ Ellis. (2009) Predicting endocrine therapy responsiveness in breast cancer. *Oncology (Williston Park)*, 23, 2, pp133-42.

Maggiolini M, Recchia AG, Carpino A, Vivacqua A, Fasanella G, Rago V, Pezzi V, Briand PA, Picard D, Andò S. (2004) Oestrogen receptor beta is required for androgen-stimulated proliferation of LNCaP prostate cancer cells. *J Mol Endocrinol*, 32, 3, pp777-91.

Marandas P, Dharkar D, Davis A, Leridant AM, Pacheco Ojeda L, Micheau C, Wibault P, Schwaab G. (1990) Malignant tumours of the parotid: a study of 76 patients. *Clin Otolaryngol Allied Sci*, 15, 2, pp103-9.

Marchio C, B Weigelt, JS Reis-Filho. (2010) Adenoid cystic carcinomas of the breast and salivary glands (or 'The strange case of Dr Jekyll and Mr Hyde' of exocrine gland carcinomas). *J Clin Pathol*, 63, 3, pp220-8.

Markopoulos C, Gogas H, Livaditou A, Floros D. (1998) Mucoepidermoid carcinoma of the breast. *Eur J Gynaecol Oncol*, 19, 3, pp291-3.

Mastropasqua MG, Maiorano E, Pruneri G, Orvieto E, Mazzarol G, Vento AR, Viale G. (2005) Immunoreactivity for c-kit and p63 as an adjunct in the diagnosis of adenoid cystic carcinoma of the breast. *Mod Pathol*, 18, 10, pp1277-82.

Milano A, Longo F, Basile M, Iaffaioli RV, Caponigro F. (2007) Recent advances in the treatment of salivary gland cancers: emphasis on molecular targeted therapy. *Oral Oncol*, 43, 8, pp729-34.

Miller AS, Hartman GG, Chen SY, Edmonds PR, Brightman SA, Harwick RD. (1994) Estrogen receptor assay in polymorphous low-grade adenocarcinoma and adenoid cystic carcinoma of salivary gland origin. An immunohistochemical study. *Oral Surg Oral Med Oral Pathol*, 77, 1, pp36-40.

Miyake H, I Hara, H Eto. (2005) Clinical outcome of maximum androgen blockade using flutamide as second-line hormonal therapy for hormone-refractory prostate cancer. *BJU Int*, 96, 6, pp791-5.

Moriki T, Ueta S, Takahashi T, Mitani M, Ichien M. (2001) Salivary duct carcinoma: cytologic characteristics and application of androgen receptor immunostaining for diagnosis. *Cancer*, 93, 5, pp344-50.

Moy B, PE Goss. (2006) Lapatinib: current status and future directions in breast cancer. *Oncologist*, 11, 10, pp1047-57.

Nasser SM, WC Faquin, Y Dayal. (2003) Expression of androgen, estrogen, and progesterone receptors in salivary gland tumors. Frequent expression of androgen receptor in a subset of malignant salivary gland tumors. *Am J Clin Pathol*, 119, 6, pp801-6.

Nguyen LH, Black MJ, Hier M, Chauvin P, Rochon L. (2003) HER2/neu and Ki-67 as prognostic indicators in mucoepidermoid carcinoma of salivary glands. *J Otolaryngol*, 32, 5, pp328-31.

Nordkvist A, Gustafsson H, Juberg-Ode M, Stenman G. (1994) Recurrent rearrangements of 11q14-22 in mucoepidermoid carcinoma. *Cancer Genet Cytogenet*, 74, 2, pp77-83.

Nordkvist A, Mark J, Gustafsson H, Bang G, Stenman G. (1994) Non-random chromosome rearrangements in adenoid cystic carcinoma of the salivary glands. *Genes Chromosomes Cancer*, 10, 2, pp115-21.

Patchefsky AS, Frauenhoffer CM, Krall RA, Cooper HS. (1979) Low-grade mucoepidermoid carcinoma of the breast. *Arch Pathol Lab Med*, 103, 4, pp196-8.

Pearce CL, Chung K, Pike MC, Wu AH. (2009) Increased ovarian cancer risk associated with menopausal estrogen therapy is reduced by adding a progestin. *Cancer*, 115, 3, pp531-9.

Persson M, Andrén Y, Mark J, Horlings HM, Persson F, Stenman G. (2009) Recurrent fusion of MYB and NFIB transcription factor genes in carcinomas of the breast and head and neck. *Proc Natl Acad Sci U S A*, 106, 44, pp18740-4.

Pettersson K, F Delaunay, JA Gustafsson. (2000) Estrogen receptor beta acts as a dominant regulator of estrogen signaling. *Oncogene*, 19, 43, pp4970-8.

Pettinato G, Insabato L, De Chiara A, Manco A, Petrella G. (1989) High-grade mucoepidermoid carcinoma of the breast. Fine needle aspiration cytology and clinicopathologic study of a case. *Acta Cytol*, 33, 2, pp195-200.

Pia-Foschini M, Reis-Filho JS, Eusebi V, Lakhani SR. (2003) Salivary gland-like tumours of the breast: surgical and molecular pathology. *J Clin Pathol*, 56, 7, pp497-506.

Pires FR, de Almeida OP, de Araújo VC, Kowalski LP. (2004) Prognostic factors in head and neck mucoepidermoid carcinoma. *Arch Otolaryngol Head Neck Surg*, 130, 2, pp174-80.

Pires FR, da Cruz Perez DE, de Almeida OP, Kowalski LP. (2004) Estrogen receptor expression in salivary gland mucoepidermoid carcinoma and adenoid cystic carcinoma. *Pathol Oncol Res*, 10, 3, pp166-8.

Press MF, Bernstein L, Thomas PA, Meisner LF, Zhou JY, Ma Y, Hung G, Robinson RA, Harris C, El-Naggar A, Slamon DJ, Phillips RN, Ross JS, Wolman SR, Flom KJ. (1997) HER-2/neu gene amplification characterized by fluorescence in situ hybridization: poor prognosis in node-negative breast carcinomas. *J Clin Oncol*, 15, 8, pp2894-904.

Press MF, Pike MC, Hung G, Zhou JY, Ma Y, George J, Dietz-Band J, James W, Slamon DJ, Batsakis JG, AK El-Naggar. (1994) Amplification and overexpression of HER-2/neu in carcinomas of the salivary gland: correlation with poor prognosis. *Cancer Res*, 54, 21, pp5675-82.

Ratanarapee S, Prinyar-Nussorn N, Chantarakul N, Pacharee P. (1983) High-grade mucoepidermoid carcinoma of the breast. A case report. *J Med Assoc Thai*, 66, 10, pp642-8.

Ro JY, EG Silva, HS Gallager. (1987) Adenoid cystic carcinoma of the breast. *Hum Pathol*, 18, 12, pp1276-81.

Scher HI, CL Sawyers. (2005) Biology of progressive, castration-resistant prostate cancer: directed therapies targeting the androgen-receptor signaling axis. *J Clin Oncol*, 23, 32, pp8253-61.

Skalova A, Stárek, Kucerová V, Szépe P, Plank L. (2001) Salivary duct carcinoma--a highly aggressive salivary gland tumor with HER-2/neu oncoprotein overexpression. *Pathol Res Pract*, 197, 9, pp621-6.

Shadaba A, MN Gaze, HR Grant. (1997) The response of adenoid cystic carcinoma to tamoxifen. *J Laryngol Otol*, 111, 12, pp1186-9.

Sharma D, Saxena NK, Davidson NE, Vertino PM. (2006) Restoration of tamoxifen sensitivity in estrogen receptor-negative breast cancer cells: tamoxifen-bound reactivated ER recruits distinctive corepressor complexes. *Cancer Res*, 66, 12, pp6370-8.

Shick PC, GP Riordan, RD Foss. (1995) Estrogen and progesterone receptors in salivary gland adenoid cystic carcinoma. *Oral Surg Oral Med Oral Pathol Oral Radiol Endod*, 80, 4, pp440-4.

Shien T, Tashiro T, Omatsu M, Masuda T, Furuta K, Sato N, Akashi-Tanaka S, Uehara M, Iwamoto E, Kinoshita T, Fukutomi T, Tsuda H, Hasegawa T. (2005) Frequent overexpression of epidermal growth factor receptor (EGFR) in mammary high grade ductal carcinomas with myoepithelial differentiation. *J Clin Pathol*, 58, 12, pp1299-304.

Shupnik MA. (2004) Crosstalk between steroid receptors and the c-Src-receptor tyrosine kinase pathways: implications for cell proliferation. *Oncogene*, 23, 48, pp7979-89.

Spiro RH. (1997) Distant metastasis in adenoid cystic carcinoma of salivary origin. *Am J Surg*, 174, 5, pp495-8.

Strom A, Hartman J, Foster JS, Kietz S, Wimalasena J, Gustafsson JA. (2004) Estrogen receptor beta inhibits 17beta-estradiol-stimulated proliferation of the breast cancer cell line T47D. *Proc Natl Acad Sci U S A*, 101, 6, pp1566-71.

Sumida, T. Itahana Y, Hamakawa H, Desprez PY. (2004) Reduction of human metastatic breast cancer cell aggressiveness on introduction of either form A or B of the progesterone receptor and then treatment with progestins. *Cancer Res*, 64, 21, pp7886-92.

Sutherland RL, Hall RE, Pang GY, Musgrove EA, Clarke CL. (1988) Effect of medroxyprogesterone acetate on proliferation and cell cycle kinetics of human mammary carcinoma cells. *Cancer Res*, 48, 18, pp5084-91.

Takagi D, Fukuda S, Furuta Y, Yagi K, Homma A, Nagahashi T, Inuyama Y. (2001) Clinical study of adenoid cystic carcinoma of the head and neck. *Auris Nasus Larynx*, 28, Suppl, ppS99-102.

Taplin ME, SP Balk. (2004) Androgen receptor: a key molecule in the progression of prostate cancer to hormone independence. *J Cell Biochem*, 91, 3, pp483-90.

Tjalma WA, Verslegers IO, De Loecker PA, Van Marck EA. (2002) Low and high grade mucoepidermoid carcinomas of the breast. *Eur J Gynaecol Oncol*, 23, 5, pp423-5.

Tonon G, Gehlhaus KS, Yonescu R, Kaye FJ, Kirsch IR. (2004) Multiple reciprocal translocations in salivary gland mucoepidermoid carcinomas. *Cancer Genet Cytogenet*, 152, 1, pp15-22.

Tonon G, Modi S, Wu L, Kubo A, Coxon AB, Komiya T, O'Neil K, Stover K, El-Naggar A, Griffin JD, Kirsch IR, Kaye FJ. (2003) t(11;19)(q21;p13) translocation in mucoepidermoid carcinoma creates a novel fusion product that disrupts a Notch signaling pathway. *Nat Genet*, 33, 2, pp208-13.

van der Burg, B, Kalkhoven E, Isbrücker L, de Laat SW. (1992) Effects of progestins on the proliferation of estrogendependent human breast cancer cells under growth factor-defined conditions. *J Steroid Biochem Mol Biol*, 42, 5, pp457-65.

Vila L, Liu H, Al-Quran SZ, Coco DP, Dong HJ, Liu C. (2009) Identification of c-kit gene mutations in primary adenoid cystic carcinoma of the salivary gland. *Mod Pathol*, 22, 10, pp1296-302.

Weigelt B. Horlings HM, Kreike B, Hayes MM, Hauptmann M, Wessels LF, de Jong D, Van de Vijver MJ, Van't Veer LJ, Peterse JL. (2008) Refinement of breast cancer classification by molecular characterization of histological special types. *J Pathol*, 216, 2, pp141-50.

White G, GG Garcelon. (1955) Estrogen and combined estrogen and x-ray therapy; their effects on advanced malignant salivary-gland tumors. *N Engl J Med*, 253, 10, pp410-2.

Wick MR, Ockner DM, Mills SE, Ritter JH, Swanson PE. (1998) Homologous carcinomas of the breasts, skin, and salivary glands. A histologic and immunohistochemical comparison of ductal mammary carcinoma, ductal sweat gland carcinoma, and salivary duct carcinoma. *Am J Clin Pathol*, 109, 1, pp75-84.

Williams, MD, Roberts D, Blumenschein GR Jr, Temam S, Kies MS, Rosenthal DI, Weber RS, El-Naggar AK. (2007) Differential expression of hormonal and growth factor receptors in salivary duct carcinomas: biologic significance and potential role in therapeutic stratification of patients. *Am J Surg Pathol*, 31, 11, pp1645-52.

Williams MD, Roberts DB, Kies MS, Mao L, Weber RS, El-Naggar AK. (2010) Genetic and expression analysis of HER-2 and EGFR genes in salivary duct carcinoma: empirical and therapeutic significance. *Clin Cancer Res*, 16, 8, pp2266-74.

Wong NA, Malcomson RD, Jodrell DI, Groome NP, Harrison DJ, Saunders PT. (2005) ERbeta isoform expression in colorectal carcinoma: an in vivo and in vitro study of clinicopathological and molecular correlates. *J Pathol*, 207, 1, pp53-60.

Yoshimura T, Sumida T, Liu S, Onishi A, Shintani S, Desprez PY, Hamakawa H. (2007) Growth inhibition of human salivary gland tumor cells by introduction of progesterone (Pg) receptor and Pg treatment. *Endocr Relat Cancer*, 14, 4, pp1107-16.

Yuan X, SP Balk. (2009) Mechanisms mediating androgen receptor reactivation after castration. *Urol Oncol*, 27, 1, pp36-41.

Zhou H, Luo MP, Schönthal AH, Pike MC, Stallcup MR, Blumenthal M, Zheng W, Dubeau L. (2002) Effect of reproductive hormones on ovarian epithelial tumors: I. Effect on cell cycle activity. *Cancer Biol Ther*, 1, 3, pp300-6.